AF342671

Urogenital Imaging

Urogenital Imaging

A Problem-Oriented Approach

Editors

Sameh K. Morcos

Northern General Hospital, Sheffield, UK

and

Henrik S. Thomsen

Copenhagen University Hospital at Herlev, Denmark

WILEY-BLACKWELL

A John Wiley & Sons, Ltd., Publication

This edition first published 2009 © 2009, John Wiley & Sons Ltd

Wiley-Blackwell is an imprint of John Wiley & Sons, formed by the merger of Wiley's global Scientific, Technical and Medical business with Blackwell Publishing.

Registered office: John Wiley & Sons Ltd, The Atrium, Southern Gate, Chichester, West Sussex, PO19 8SQ, UK

Other Editorial Offices:
9600 Garsington Road, Oxford, OX4 2DQ, UK
111 River Street, Hoboken, NJ 07030-5774, USA

For details of our global editorial offices, for customer services and for information about how to apply for permission to reuse the copyright material in this book please see our website at www.wiley.com/wiley-blackwell

The right of the author to be identified as the author of this work has been asserted in accordance with the Copyright, Designs and Patents Act 1988.

All rights reserved. No part of this publication may be reproduced, stored in a retrieval system, or transmitted, in any form or by any means, electronic, mechanical, photocopying, recording or otherwise, except as permitted by the UK Copyright, Designs and Patents Act 1988, without the prior permission of the publisher.

Wiley also publishes its books in a variety of electronic formats. Some content that appears in print may not be available in electronic books.

Designations used by companies to distinguish their products are often claimed as trademarks. All brand names and product names used in this book are trade names, service marks, trademarks or registered trademarks of their respective owners. The publisher is not associated with any product or vendor mentioned in this book. This publication is designed to provide accurate and authoritative information in regard to the subject matter covered. It is sold on the understanding that the publisher is not engaged in rendering professional services. If professional advice or other expert assistance is required, the services of a competent professional should be sought.

The contents of this work are intended to further general scientific research, understanding, and discussion only and are not intended and should not be relied upon as recommending or promoting a specific method, diagnosis, or treatment by physicians for any particular patient. The publisher and the author make no representations or warranties with respect to the accuracy or completeness of the contents of this work and specifically disclaim all warranties, including without limitation any implied warranties of fitness for a particular purpose. In view of ongoing research, equipment modifications, changes in governmental regulations, and the constant flow of information relating to the use of medicines, equipment, and devices, the reader is urged to review and evaluate the information provided in the package insert or instructions for each medicine, equipment, or device for, among other things, any changes in the instructions or indication of usage and for added warnings and precautions. Readers should consult with a specialist where appropriate. The fact that an organization or Website is referred to in this work as a citation and/or a potential source of further information does not mean that the author or the publisher endorses the information the organization or Website may provide or recommendations it may make. Further, readers should be aware that Internet Websites listed in this work may have changed or disappeared between when this work was written and when it is read. No warranty may be created or extended by any promotional statements for this work. Neither the publisher nor the author shall be liable for any damages arising herefrom.

Library of Congress Cataloging-in-Publication Data

Urogenital imaging : a problem-oriented approach/edited by Sameh Morcos and Henrik Thomsen.
    p. ; cm.
  Includes bibliographical references and index.
  ISBN 978-0-470-51089-6 (cloth)
  1. Genitourinary organs – Imaging. 2. Genitourinary organs – Diseases – Diagnosis. I. Morcos, Sameh K. II. Thomsen, Henrik Klem.
  [DNLM: 1. Female Urogenital Diseases – diagnosis. 2. Male Urogenital Diseases – diagnosis. 3. Diagnostic Imaging – methods. WJ 141 U773 2009]
  RC874.U72 2009
  616.6′0754 – dc22

                                                                2008047080

ISBN 978-0-470-51089-6 (H/B)

A catalogue record for this book is available from the British Library.

Set in 10/12 Times New Roman by Laserwords Private Ltd, Chennai, India.
Printed and bound in Great Britain by CPI Antony Rowe, Chippenham, Wiltshire

First Impression   2009

To the memory of my late parents Kamel and Monira who gave me so much unconditionally.

To my beloved wife and daughters Sandra, Sarah, Hannah and Rebecca whose tremendous love and support I will always cherish.

Sameh K. Morcos, Sheffield, UK

Contents

Foreword   xiii

Preface   xv

Contributors   xvii

1 Adrenal Imaging   1
Khaled M. Elsayes, Isaac R. Francis, Melvyn Korobkin and Gerard M. Doherty   1

  1.1   Introduction   1
  1.2   Cushing's syndrome   2
  1.3   Primary hyperaldosteronism   5
  1.4   Pheochromocytoma   8
  1.5   Adrenal cortical carcinoma   12
  1.6   Adrenal incidentaloma   15

2 Retroperitoneal Masses   21
Pietro Pavlica, Massimo Valentino and Libero Barozzi   21

  2.1   Introduction   21
  2.2   Retroperitoneal anatomy   21
  2.3   Pathological conditions   22
  2.4   Primary solid retroperitoneal tumors   22
  2.5   Retroperitoneal lymphoma   27
  2.6   Cystic retroperitoneal masses   30
  2.7   Retroperitoneal metastases   32
  2.8   Retroperitoneal fibrosis (Ormond's disease)   33
  2.9   Retroperitoneal fluid collections (traumatic and non-traumatic)   35
  References   41

3 Imaging of Renal Artery Stenosis   43
Robert Hartman   43

  3.1   Introduction   43
  3.2   Clinical features   43
  3.3   Pathology   45

　　3.4　Imaging of suspected renal artery stenosis　　45
　　References　　51

4　Renal Masses　　**53**
Philip J. Kenney　　53
　　4.1　Introduction　　53
　　4.2　Symptomatic renal carcinoma　　53
　　4.3　Incidental renal masses　　55
　　4.4　Patients with a known cancer (other than RCC)　　62
　　4.5　Renal mass in patients with symptoms　　63
　　4.6　Vascular lesions presenting as a renal mass　　68
　　4.7　Renal mass in patients with cystic disease　　72
　　4.8　Treatment　　73
　　References　　73

5　Non-neoplastic Renal Cystic Lesions　　**75**
Sameh K. Morcos　　75
　　5.1　Introduction　　75
　　5.2　Classification　　75
　　5.3　Cystic lesions affecting renal cortex　　76
　　5.4　Cystic lesions of renal medulla　　80
　　5.5　Cystic diseases affecting both the cortex and medulla　　86
　　References　　97

6　Urological and Vascular Complications Post-renal Transplantation　　**99**
Tarek El-Diasty and Yasser Osman　　99
　　6.1　Introduction　　99
　　6.2　Vascular complications　　99
　　6.3　Urological complications　　107
　　6.4　Ureteric strictures　　110
　　6.5　Post-transplant lymphocele　　113
　　6.6　Delayed graft function (DGF)　　116
　　6.7　Post-transplant bladder malignancy　　119
　　References　　120

7　Urinary Tract Injuries　　**121**
Elliott R. Friedman, Stanford M. Goldman and Tung Shu　　121
　　7.1　Introduction　　121
　　7.2　Renal trauma　　121
　　7.3　Adrenal trauma　　130
　　7.4　Ureteral trauma　　131
　　7.5　Bladder trauma　　133
　　7.6　Urethral trauma　　136
　　7.7　Penile and scrotal trauma　　142
　　References　　147

8 Urinary Tract Infections — 149
Mikael Hellström, Ulf Jodal, Rune Sixt and Eira Stokland — 149

8.1	Symptomatic urinary tract infection in children	149
8.2	Symptomatic upper urinary tract infection in adults	167
8.3	Emphysematous pyelonephritis	173
8.4	Xanthogranulomatous pyelonephritis	174
8.5	Urinary tract infection in the immunocompromised patient	177
8.6	Tuberculosis	179
8.7	Schistosomiasis	183
8.8	Hydatid disease (echinococcosis)	188
8.9	Urethritis	191
	References	193

9 Imaging of the Genitourinary System – Urolithiasis — 195
Sami A Moussa and Paramananthan Mariappan — 195

9.1	Introduction	195
9.2	Pathology	195
9.3	Clinical features	197
9.4	Evaluation of patients with suspected urinary stones	198
9.5	Treatment	198
9.6	Imaging	199
	References	218

10 Hematuria — 219
Thomas Bretlau, Kirstine L. Hermann, Jørgen Nordling and Henrik S. Thomsen — 219

10.1	Definition	219
10.2	Clinical considerations	219
10.3	Diagnosis of hematuria	220
10.4	Epidemiology	220
10.5	Distribution of malignancy in patients with hematuria	223
10.6	Imaging	223
10.7	Summary	230
	References	234

11 Bladder Cancer — 235
G. Heinz-Peer and C. Kratzik — 235

11.1	Introduction	235
11.2	Clinical features	237
11.3	Pathology	239
11.4	Imaging findings	243
11.5	Treatment planning	253
11.6	Post-treatment Imaging	254

11.7   Summary   254
References   255

12 Imaging of Urinary Diversion   257
Sameh Hanna and Hesham Badawy   257
12.1   Introduction   257
12.2   Indications for urinary diversion   257
12.3   Types of urinary diversion   257
12.4   Non-continent cutaneous form of diversion   258
12.5   Continent cutaneous urinary diversion (*Continent Catheterizing Pouches*)   258
12.6   Non-orthotopic continent diversion, relying on the anal sphincter for
continence   260
12.7   Orthotopic form of diversion to the native, intact urethra (neobladder)   261
12.8   Contraindications to urinary diversion   264
12.9   Complications of urinary diversions   264
12.10   The role of radiologist in urinary diversion includes   267
12.11   Imaging studies   268
12.12   Imaging of complications   269
12.13   Summary   271
References   271

13 Imaging of the Prostate Gland   273
François Cornud   273
13.1   Introduction   273
13.2   Zonal anatomy and benign prostatic hypertrophy   273
13.3   Diagnosis of prostate cancer: TRUS features   276
13.4   Diagnostic of prostate cancer: MRI   284
13.5   Contrast-enhanced (dynamic) MRI   285
13.6   Magnetic Resonance Spectroscopic Imaging (MRSI)   290
13.7   Diffusion-weighted imaging   292
13.8   Indications of functional MRI   295
13.9   Extension of prostate cancer   297
13.10   Local extension by TRUS and TRUS-guided biopsy   297
13.11   MRI and staging of prostate cancer   298
13.12   Local staging   299
13.13   Lymph node metastases: lympho-MRI   304
13.14   Bone metastases: whole marrow MRI   304
13.15   Benign disorders of the prostate (BPH excluded)   305
References   321

14 Haemospermia   323
Drew A. Torigian, Keith N. Van Arsdalen and Parvati Ramchandani   323
14.1   Introduction   323
14.2   Clinical features   323

14.3 Pathology 325
14.4 Imaging findings 325
14.5 Summary 337
References 337

15 Scrotal Masses
Lorenzo E. Derchi and Alchiede Simonato　　339

339

15.1 Introduction 339
15.2 Clinical features 339
15.3 Pathology 340
15.4 Imaging 340
15.5 Important principles in assessment of scrotal masses 341
15.6 Important problems in differentiating benign from malignant lesions 345
References 350

16 Gynaecological Adnexal Masses
John A. Spencer and Michael J. Weston　　351

351

16.1 Introduction 351
16.2 Clinical features 351
16.3 Pathology 352
16.4 Imaging 354
16.5 Standard radiographic techniques 355
16.6 Ultrasound (US) 355
16.7 MR Imaging (MRI) 366
16.8 Computed Tomography 373
References 379

17 Imaging of Abnormal Uterine Bleeding
Patricia Noël, Evis Sala and Caroline Reinhold　　381

381

17.1 Abnormal uterine bleeding 381
17.2 Adenomyosis 382
17.3 Leiomyomas 385
17.4 Endometrial polyp 389
17.5 Endometrial hyperplasia 391
17.6 Endometrial carcinoma 394
17.7 Summary 396
References 397

18 Female Pelvic Floor Dysfunction
Rania Farouk El Sayed　　399

399

18.1 Introduction 399
18.2 Anatomical considerations 399
18.3 Pathophysiology of pelvic floor dysfunction 401

18.4 Clinical features 401

18.5 Imaging of pelvic floor dysfunction 404

18.6 Magnetic resonance imaging (MRI) 407

References 413

19 Imaging of female infertility 415

Ahmed-Emad Mahfouz and Hanan Sherif 415

19.1 Introduction 415

19.2 Polycystic ovary syndrome 415

19.3 Abnormalities of the fallopian tubes (Hydrosalpinx/Hematosalpinx, tubal block) 418

19.4 Fibroids 421

19.5 Adenomyosis 423

19.6 Developmental anomalies of the uterus 424

19.7 Endometriosis 429

19.8 Imaging 430

Index 431

Index 431

Foreword

This book has the unique aim to provide the greatest utility to the modern radiologist practicing diagnostic imaging of the genitourinary system. In this time of great pressure within the medical environment, where time is always of the essence, one can even question the usefulness of any book. Many practitioners quickly go the internet for a "google search". Unfortunately, although the internet can provide extremely valuable information quickly, it also can provide an enormous amount of misinformation quickly. Unless one knows and trusts the source, the internet although readily available may lead to uncertainty. In addition, the internet often provides "factoids" bereft of context.

This book is designed for the busy modern world, by providing key information representing a consensus of current practice in a very accessible fashion. The nineteen chapters cover, in moderate depth, all the most important topics relating to the male and female genital and urinary tracts. The forty three authors are truly an international group of experts in the field. Each chapter provides information on usual presentation of disorders, clinical, laboratory and pathologic features and the best current information on imaging features critical for diagnosis. A brief presentation on current therapy is also included.

A critical decision was made in the preparation of this book as to the style of presentation of the information. Elegant phraseology has been bypassed in favor of a "bullet point" approach, along with heavy use of tables and extensive illustration of typical features of common lesions. This results in an "information dense" text. Despite the relative brevity of the chapters, each is packed with useful information. That information can be accessed by the reader extremely quickly – whether searching for a single key point, such as how to calculate relative washout of an adrenal mass and the best diagnostic cutoffs, or whether desirous of a quick overview of a topic. This book in fact would be an excellent choice for someone reviewing for a radiology exam such as ABR MOC. The authors have concentrated in each chapter on accepted key diagnostic features; the character of the authors makes this truly an international consensus.

What one will not find in the book is extensive discussion of the history of imaging of any area. It does not include the initial description of some sign, or the early attempts for criteria that failed. There is not an extensive list of references, nor a discussion of controversial areas. Rare entities or extremely unusual presentations of common lesions are not included in general. Rather the focus is on well accepted key points on clinical aspects of the more common diseases and the accepted findings that allow one to make an imaging diagnosis. Some presentation, although limited, is given of imaging techniques. This is not meant to teach in detail how to perform exams correctly. The heavy emphasis in most chapters is on Computed Tomography (CT) and Magnetic Resonance Imaging (MRI), as those methods currently are most useful for final diagnosis in most areas. However, in appropriate areas, such as kidney transplant, prostate disease, female pelvis and male scrotum, ultrasound is well covered. As it has been largely superseded, little attention is paid to intravenous urography or to most radiologic methods. This is not a text that extensively reviews nuclear medicine techniques.

I am proud to have been a contributor to this text. I expect many radiologists will find it a most useful guide to the best of current practice of imaging diagnosis of the genitourinary tract. The size of the book is designed such that it can be kept close at hand for easy and frequent use.

Professor Philip J. Kenney

Preface

This book is designed to offer both radiologists and clinicians focused information about different important aspects of the urogenital system. Each chapter provides concise information about clinical features, pathology and imaging findings of the aspect under consideration.

The book does not follow the traditional style of scientific textbooks. The text is presented mainly in bullet format which the reader will find easy to follow and remember. Many images demonstrating important diagnostic features of different diseases are provided in each chapter. A list of key references is provided at the end of each chapter. A diagnostic algorithm is also provided whenever appropriate.

The book is aimed mainly at urologists, nephrologists, gynecologists, general radiologists and trainee radiologists. Specialized urogenital radiologists will also find the book a quick reminder of important features of different conditions in their field of interest.

We are most grateful to all the authors who covered their topics expertly and clearly. We are fortunate to have so many eminent colleagues contributing to this book.

We hope you will find the book informative and a good reference to refresh your knowledge in the field of urogenital imaging.

SK Morcos
Sheffield, UK

HS Thomsen
Copenhagen, Denmark

Contributors

Hesham Badawy
Urology Department,
Kasr El Aini Hospital – Faculty of Medicine,
Cairo University,
Egypt

Libero Barozzi,
Radiology Unit,
S. Orsola-Malpighi University Hospital,
Via Massarenti, 9,
40138 Bologna
Italy

Thomas Bretlau,
Departments of Diagnostic Radiology and Urology,
Copenhagen University Hospital at Herlev,
Herlev Ringvej 75,
DK-2730 Herlev
Denmark

François Cornud,
Service de Radiologie B (Pr Chevrot),
Hôpital Cochin,
27 rue du Faubourg St Jacques,
75014 Paris,
France

Lorenzo E. Derchi,
DICMI-Radiologia,
Universitá di Genova,
I-16132 Genova,
Italy

Gerard M. Doherty
Department of Surgery,
University of Michigan,
Ann Arbor,
Michigan, 48109
USA

Tarek El-Diasty
Radiology Department,
Urology & Nephrology Center,
Mansoura University,
Mansoura,
Egypt.

Rania Farouk El Sayed
Radiology Department,
Cairo University Hospitals,
Cairo,
Egypt

Khaled M. Elsayes
Dept. of Radiology,
University of Michigan,
Ann Arbor,
Michigan 48109
USA

Isaac R. Francis
Department of Radiology,
University of Michigan,
Ann Arbor,
Michigan 48109
USA

Elliott R. Friedman
Diagnostic and Interventional Imaging,
University of Texas Health Science Center at
Houston,
Texas,
USA

Stanford M. Goldman
Diagnostic and Interventional Imaging and
Urology,
University of Texas Health Science Center at
Houston,
Texas,
USA

Sameh A.Z. Hanna
Radiology Department,
Kasr El Aini Hospital – Faculty of Medicine,
Cairo University,
Egypt

Robert Hartman,
Department of Diagnostic Radiology,
Mayo Clinic,
Rochester MN,
USA

Gertraud Heinz-Peer
Department of Radiology,
Medical University of Vienna,
Währinger Gürtel 18-20,
1090 Vienna,
Austria

Mikael Hellström,
Department of Radiology,
The Sahlgrenska University Hospital,
Göteborg,
Sweden

Kirstine L. Hermann,
Departments of Diagnostic Radiology and
Urology,
Copenhagen University Hospital at
Herlev,
Herlev Ringvej 75,
DK-2730 Herlev
Denmark

Ulf Jodal,
Department of Pediatric Nephrology,
The Queen Silvia Children's Hospital,
Göteborg,
Sweden

Philip J. Kenney
University of Arkansas for Medical
Science,
4301 W. Markham St.,
Little Rock, AR 72205
USA

Melvyn Korobkin
Department of Radiology,
University of Michigan,
Ann Arbor,
Michigan 48109
USA

C.Kratzik
Department of Urology,
Medical University of Vienna,
Währinger Gürtel 18-20,
1090 Vienna,
Austria

Ahmed-Emad Mahfouz
Radiology Departments,
Hamad Medical Corporation,
POB 3050, Doha
Qatar and
Cairo University, Cairo
Egypt

Mr Paramananthan Mariappan,
Department of Urology,
Western General Hospital,
Crewe Road South,
Edinburgh, EH4 2XU,
UK

Sameh K. Morcos
Sheffield Teaching Hospitals NHS Foundation
Trust,
Department of Diagnostic Imaging,
Northern General Hospital,
Herries Rd, Sheffield S5 7AU UK

Sami A. Moussa,
Department of Radiology,
Western General Hospital,
Crewe Road South,
Edinburgh, EH4 2XU,
UK

Patricia Noël
Department of Radiology
CHUQ Hôtel-Dieu de Québec
11, Côte du Palais Québec,
Québec, G1R 2J6
Canada

Jørgen Nordling
Departments of Diagnostic Radiology and Urology,
Copenhagen University Hospital at Herlev,
Herlev Ringvej 75,
DK-2730 Herlev
Denmark

Yasser Osman
Urology and Nephrology Center,
Mansoura University,
Mansoura
Egypt

Pietro Pavlica,
Radiology Unit,
S. Orsola-Malpighi University Hospital,
Via Massarenti, 9
40138 Bologna
Italy

Parvati Ramchandani
University of Pennsylvania School of Medicine,
Philadelphia, PA 19104,
USA

Caroline Reinhold
Department of Radiology,
McGill University Health Center,
1650 Cedar Ave.,
Montreal, Quebec, H3G 1A4
Canada

Evis Sala
University Department of Radiology,
5, Addenbrooke's Hospital,
Hills Road,
Cambridge CB2 0QQ,
UK

Hanan Sherif
Radiology Departments,
Hamad Medical Corporation,
POB 3050, Doha
Qatar and
Cairo University, Cairo
Egypt

Tung Shu
University of Texas Health Sciences Center at Houston,
Houston,
Texas,
USA

Alchiede Simonato,
Clinica Urologica, Universitá di Genova,
Ospedale San Martino,
Largo R. Benzi, 10
I-16132 Genova
Italy

Rune Sixt,
Department of Clinical Physiology,
The Queen Silvia Children's Hospital,
Göteborg,
Sweden

Eira Stokland
Department of Radiology,
The Queen Silvia Children's Hospital,
Göteborg,
Sweden

John A. Spencer,
Department of Clinical Radiology,
St James's University Hospital,
Leeds LS9 7TF,
UK

Henrik S. Thomsen,
University of Copenhagen,
Department of Diagnostic Radiology,
Copenhagen University Hospital at Herlev,
Herlev Ringvej 75, DK-2730 Herlev,
Denmark

Drew A. Torigian
Department of Radiology,
Hospital of the University of Pennsylvania,
3400 Spruce Street,
Philadelphia, PA 19104,
USA

Massimo Valentino,
Radiology Unit,
S. Orsola-Malpighi University Hospital,
Via Massarenti, 9
I-40138 Bologna
Italy

Keith N. Van Arsdalen
University of Pennsylvania School of
Medicine,
Philadelphia, PA 19104,
USA

Michael J Weston
Department of Clinical Radiology
St James's University Hospital,
Leeds LS9 7TF,
UK

1
Adrenal Imaging

Khaled M. Elsayes[1], Isaac R. Francis[1], Melvyn Korobkin[1] and Gerard M. Doherty[2]

[1]*Department of Radiology, University of Michigan*
[2]*Department of Radiology and Surgery, University of Michigan*

1.1 Introduction

Most adrenal adenomas are initially detected incidentally by computed tomography (CT), in patients who undergo the examination for other indications. But CT and magnetic resonance imaging (MRI) are also used in the investigation of adrenal hyperfunction.

Adrenal adenoma is the most common adrenal mass that is seen on cross-sectional imaging, usually CT and MRI. The majority of these lesions contain abundant lipid and can be seen on unenhanced CT as low density masses measuring less than 10 Hounsfield units [HU], and exhibit loss of signal intensity on out-of-phase (opposed phase) gradient-echo MR images. Adenomas also exhibit rapid intravenous iodinated contrast enhancement washout and therefore can be distinguished from malignant lesions which do not exhibit this feature.

CT and MRI can be used to stage adrenal cortical carcinomas and detect pheochromocytomas. FDG PET scans can help differentiate adrenal metastases from adenomas by their strong avidity for FDG, but some adenomas show mild tracer uptake.

There are several masses such as uncomplicated adrenal cysts, adrenal myelolipomas and acute adrenal hemorrhage which can be readily characterized on CT and MRI.

Utility of various imaging modalities in diagnosis of adrenal gland masses:

- Ultrasound: Ultrasound is sensitive but not specific for diagnosis adrenal masses
- Computed Tomography (CT):
  - Most commonly used modality for detection and characterization of adrenal masses
  - Measuring the unenhanced attenuation value of adrenal mass is important for diagnosing lipid rich adenoma

Urogenital Imaging: A Problem-oriented Approach   Edited by Sameh K. Morcos and Henrik S. Thomsen
© 2009 John Wiley & Sons, Ltd

- o Use of contrast enhancement washout values are also useful in distinguishing between adenomas and malignant lesions
- o The absolute per cent enhancement washout can be calculated by measuring the enhanced attenuation, the delayed enhanced, the unenhanced values and using the following formula:

$$\text{Absolute enhancement Washout} = \frac{\text{Enhanced attenuation value} - \text{Delayed attenuation value}}{\text{Enhanced attenuation value} - \text{Unenhanced attenuation value}}$$

- o When non-contrast scans have not been obtained, and only contrast enhanced scans have been obtained, delayed images of the adrenal mass can be performed at 15 min following initial injection of intravenous contrast, and relative enhancement washout calculated as follows:

$$\text{Relative enhancement Washout} = \frac{\text{Enhanced attenuation value} - \text{Delayed attenuation value}}{\text{Enhanced attenuation value}}$$

- o Threshold values of greater 60% for absolute and 40% for relative enhancement washout have been found to be over 90% specific for adenoma diagnosis.

- Magnetic Resonance Imaging (MRI):

  - o Qualitative analysis: The most important sequence of the adrenal MR imaging protocol is chemical shift imaging sequence. Chemical shift imaging is performed with in-phase and out-of-phase sequences. Loss of signal intensity of the adrenal mass using the spleen as reference organ, on out-of-phase, compared with in-phase pulse sequence is diagnostic for the presence of intracellular lipid

  - o Quantitative Analysis:

$$\text{Percentage loss of signal} = \frac{{}^{*}\text{SI on in-phase} - \text{SI on opposed-phase}}{\text{SI on in-phase}} \times 100$$

$$^{*}\text{SI: Signal Intensity}$$

$>$16.5% loss of SI on out-of-phase images as compared with in-phase images has $>$90% specificity for adenoma diagnosis.

1.2 Cushing's syndrome

The most common cause of adrenocortical steroid hormone excess is Cushing's disease due to pituitary hypersecretion of ACTH. However, primary adrenal causes are an important part of the differential diagnosis, and diagnostic plan.

Clinical features

- Facial plethora, dorsocervical fat pad, supraclavicular fat pad, truncal obesity, easy bruisabililty, purple striae, hirsutism, impotence or amenorrhea, muscle weakness, and psychosis.

- Hypertension.

- Hyperglycemia.

- Includes Cushing's disease (excess adrenocorticotropic hormone [ACTH] produced by pituitary adenomas) and Cushing's syndrome (ectopic ACTH syndrome or primary adrenal disease resulting in glucocorticoid secretion independent of ACTH stimulation).

- Symptoms and Signs

  o Truncal obesity, hirsutism, moon facies, acne, buffalo hump, purple striae

  o Hypertension

  o Hyperglycemia

  o Weakness

  o Depression

  o Growth retardation or arrest in children.

- Laboratory Findings

  o Overnight, low-dose dexamethasone suppression test and measurement of urinary free cortisol establishes diagnosis

    - No suppression and elevated urinary cortisol suggest Cushing's syndrome.

  o Detection of elevated midnight cortisol level suggests Cushing's syndrome (midnight plasma level or late-night salivary cortisol sampling).

  o Once Cushing's syndrome established, measure plasma ACTH level

    - A normal or elevated ACTH level suggests pituitary adenoma or ectopic ACTH secretion.

    - Suppressed ACTH is diagnostic of hyperadrenocorticism due to primary adrenal disease.

  o If ACTH-dependent Cushing's disease and no clear pituitary lesion on MRI, may proceed to petrosal sinus sampling with corticotropin-releasing hormone (CRH) stimulation: a central to peripheral ACTH gradient suggests Cushing's disease, while no gradient suggests ectopic ACTH secretion.

Pathophysiology

- Rare forms of ACTH-independent Cushing's syndrome include macronodular hyperplasia.

- Pigmented micronodular hyperplasia is associated with the syndrome of Carney complex (also includes cardiac myxomas and lentigines).

- Rarely, ectopic adrenal tissue can be the source for excess cortisol secretion; most common location is along the abdominal aorta.

- Ectopic ACTH syndrome usually caused by small-cell lung cancers or carcinoids but can result from tumors of the pancreas, thyroid, thymus, prostate, esophagus, colon, ovaries, pheochromocytoma, and malignant melanoma.

Treatment

- Resection is best treatment for cortisol-producing adrenal tumors or ACTH-producing tumors.

- Pituitary irradiation may be necessary if pituitary surgery fails.

- Medical treatment may be indicated to control hypercortisolism, or when patients not cured by resection or when complete resection is impossible.

Imaging findings

Adrenal hyperplasia

- Often seen in patients with Cushing's syndrome and less commonly in Conn's syndrome.

- May be diffuse or nodular and is typically bilateral (Figs 1.1 and 1.2).

Adrenal adenoma

- Most are less than 3 cm in size.

- Can be of varying density on CT and MRI.

- Lipid-rich adenoma. Attenuation value of 10 HU or less at unenhanced CT (Fig. 1.3).

- Adenomas usually have absolute enhancement washout of >60% (Fig. 1.4) and relative enhancement washout of >40%.

- Greater than 16.5% loss of signal intensity on out-of-phase, compared with in-phase MRI pulse sequences (Fig. 1.5).

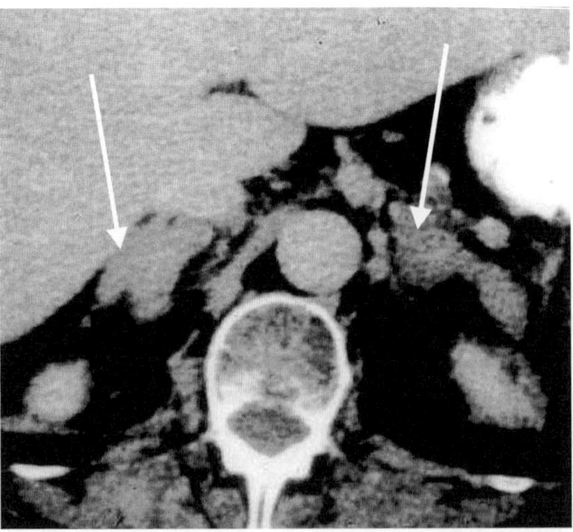

Figure 1.1 Bilateral adrenal cortical hyperplasia. Axial contrast-enhanced CT image shows nodular thickening of adrenal glands bilaterally in patient with Cushing's syndrome.

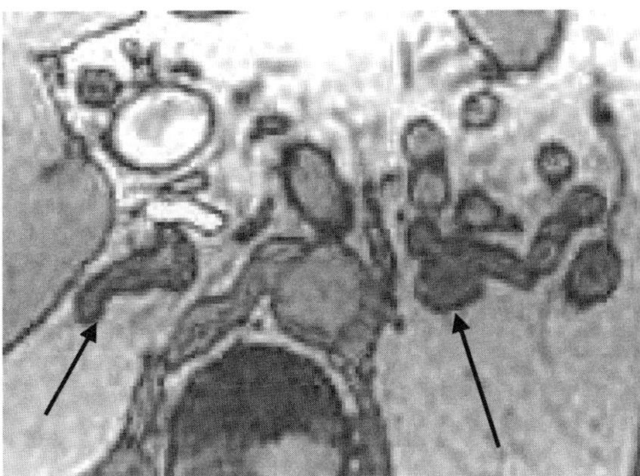

Figure 1.2 Bilateral adrenal cortical hyperplasia. Axial out-of-phase MR image shows nodular thickening of adrenal glands bilaterally in patient with Cushing's syndrome.

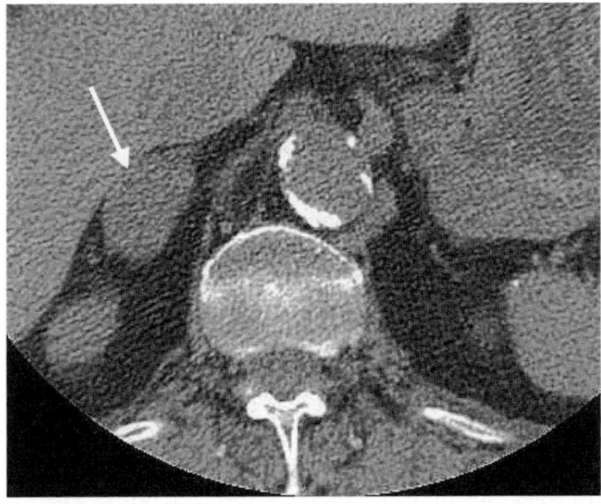

Figure 1.3 Lipid-rich adenoma. Axial unenhanced CT shows a right adrenal mass measuring 8 HU.

- Functioning and non-functioning adenomas, appear similar based on imaging as do Cushing's and Conn's adenomas.

Adrenal cortical carcinomas can also cause Cushing's syndrome (see below for imaging appearances of adrenal cortical carcinoma).

1.3 Primary hyperaldosteronism

Introduction

Primary hyperaldostronism is a relatively common and underdiagnosed condition that contributes to hypertension in about 1% of hypertensive people. The condition is very effectively treated, and so screening programs have become routine in some places.

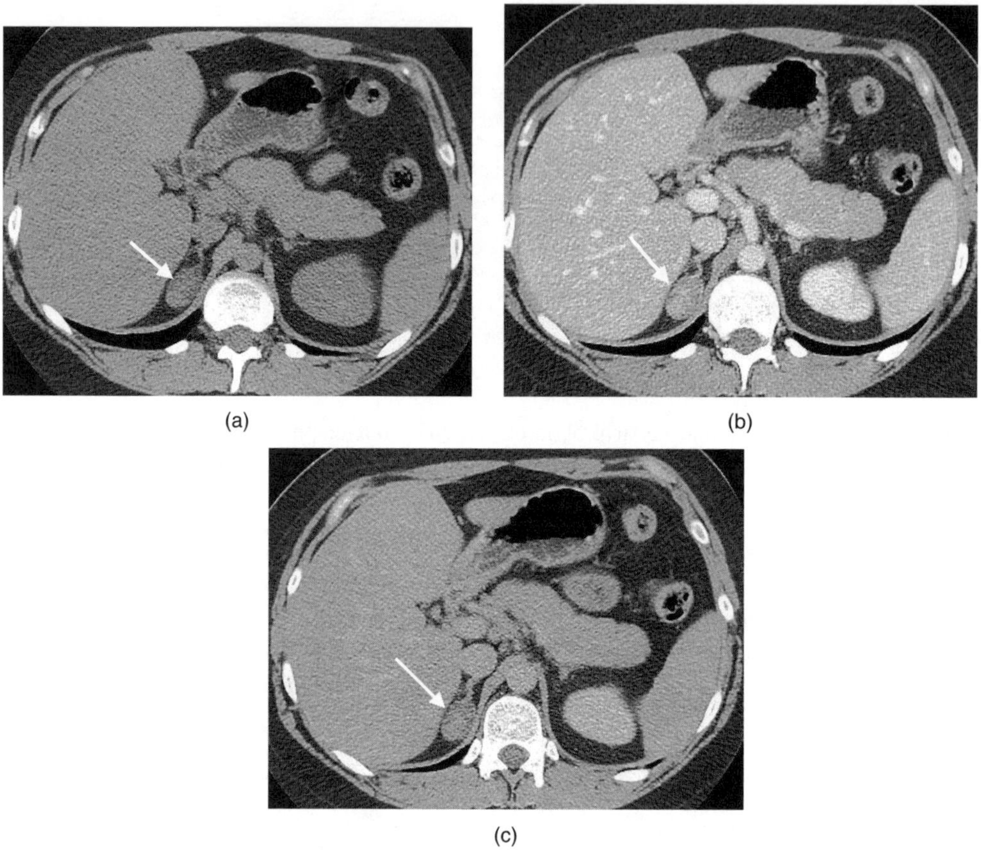

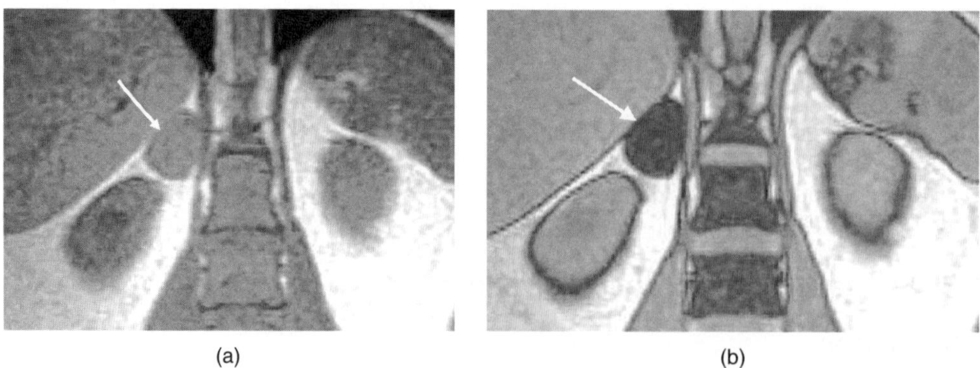

Figure 1.4 Lipid-poor adenoma. Axial unenhanced CT shows a right adrenal mass measuring 27 HU (arrow) (a). Following intravenous contrast enhancement the mass measures 96 HU (arrow) (b) and 50 HU (arrow) on delayed images (c), respectively. This mass had an absolute enhancement washout of 67%. Absolute Washout = 96 − 50/96 − 27 × 100 = 67%.

Figure 1.5 Adrenal adenoma. Coronal in-phase (a) and out-of-phase (b) MR images show an adrenal mass (arrow) which exhibits a typical decrease in signal intensity on the out-of-phase image.

Clinical features

- Hypertension with or without hypokalemia.

- Elevated aldosterone secretion and suppressed plasma renin activity.

- Metabolic alkalosis, relative hypernatremia.

- Weakness, polyuria, paresthesias, tetany, cramps due to hypokalemia.

- Common subtypes of primary hyperaldosteronism: aldosteronoma (75%) and bilateral adrenal hyperplasia (25%).

- Rare subtypes of primary hyperaldosteronism: unilateral primary adrenal hyperplasia, aldosterone-producing adrenocortical carcinoma, glucocorticoid-remediable hyperaldosteronism (familial hyperaldosteronism type 1).

- Symptoms and signs

  - Hypertension
  - Headaches
  - Malaise
  - Muscle weakness
  - Polyuria
  - Polydipsia
  - Cramps
  - Paresthesias
  - Hypokalemic paralysis (rare).

- Laboratory findings

  - Hypokalemia
  - Hypernatremia
  - Metabolic alkalosis
  - Elevated plasma aldosterone to renin ratio ($\gg$ 20)
  - Elevated plasma aldosterone concentration ($\gg$ 15 ng/dL)
  - Elevated urine/serum aldosterone level with PO or IV sodium challenge.

Treatment

- Surgical therapy for patients with aldosteronoma and unilateral primary adrenal hyperplasia.

- Medical therapy for bilateral adrenal hyperplasia, or poor surgical candidates.

- Surgery

  - Nearly always laparoscopic approach.
  - Unilaterality best defined by adrenal vein sampling for aldosterone and cortisol

- ■ Indications
    - Unilateral aldosteronoma
    - Unilateral primary adrenal hyperplasia.
  - ■ Contraindications
    - Bilateral adrenal hyperplasia.
  - ○ Removal of aldosteronoma normalizes potassium, but hypertension is not always cured.
  - ○ 33% of patients have persistent, mild hypertension (easier to control than before operation).
- Medications
  - ○ Spironolactone: competitive aldosterone antagonist.
  - ○ Amiloride: potassium-sparing diuretic.
  - ○ Other antihypertensive agents such as ACE inhibitors and calcium channel blockers.

Imaging findings

Adrenal hyperplasia

- May be diffuse or nodular and is typically bilateral (Figs 1.1 and 1.2).

Adrenal adenoma

- Most are small and less than 2 cm in size.
- Usually much smaller than Cushing's adenoma.
- Can have varying appearances of CT and MRI.
- Lipid-rich adenoma- Attenuation value of 10 HU or less at unenhanced CT (Fig. 1.3).
- Absolute enhancement washout >60% (Fig. 1.4) and relative enhancement washout >40%.
- Greater than 16.5% loss of signal intensity on out-of-phase, compared with in-phase MRI pulse sequences (Fig. 1.5).
- Functioning and non-functioning adenomas, appear similar based on imaging as do Cushing's and Conn's adenomas.

Adrenal cortical carcinomas rarely cause Conn's syndrome.

1.4 Pheochromocytoma

Introduction

Pheochromocytomas are tumors that develop from the adrenal medulla. The hormonal function typically includes production of catecholamines, and the characteristic syndrome that follows. These tumors can be benign or malignant.

Clinical features

- Episodic headache, excessive sweating, palpitations, and visual blurring.

- Hypertension, frequently sustained, with or without paroxysms.

- Postural tachycardia and hypotension.

- Elevated urinary catecholamines or their metabolites, hypermetabolism, hyperglycemia.

- Early recognition during pregnancy is key because if left untreated, half of fetuses and nearly half of the mothers will die.

- Epidemiology.
  - Found in <0.1% of patients with hypertension.
  - 5% of tumors discovered incidentally on CT scan.
  - Most occur sporadically.
  - Associated with familial syndromes, such as:
    - Multiple endocrine neoplasia type 2A (MEN 2A)
    - MEN 2B
    - Recklinghausen disease
    - von Hippel-Lindau disease.
  - Pheochromocytomas are present in 40% of patients with MEN 2
  - 90% of patients with pheochromocytoma are hypertensive.
  - Rule of 10s:
    - 10% malignant
    - 10% familial
    - 10% bilateral
    - 10% multiple tumors
    - 10% extra-adrenal.
  - Hypertension less common in children.
  - In children, 50% of patients have multiple or extra-adrenal tumors.

- Symptoms and signs
  - Episodic or sustained hypertension.
  - Triad of palpitation, headache, and diaphoresis.
  - Anxiety, tremors.
  - Weight loss.
  - Dizziness, nausea, and vomiting.
  - Abdominal discomfort, constipation, diarrhea.
  - Visual blurring.
  - Tachycardia, postural hypotension.
  - Hypertensive retinopathy.

- Laboratory findings
  - Hyperglycemia.
  - Elevated plasma metanephrines.
  - Elevated 24-h urine metanephrines and free catecholamines.
  - Elevated urinary vanillylmandelic acid (VMA).
  - Elevated plasma catecholamines.
- Avoid arteriography or fine-needle aspiration as they can precipitate a hypertensive crisis.

Treatment

α-Adrenergic blocking agents should be started as soon as the biochemical diagnosis is established to restore blood volume, to prevent a severe crisis, and to allow recovery from the cardiomyopathy.

- β-blockade should generally be established after α-blockade, and prior to operation
- surgery
  - Indications
    - All resectable pheochromocytomas should be excised.
  - Contraindications
    - Unresectable systemic disease.
    - Inadequate medical preparation (α-blockade).
- Medications
  - α-Adrenergic blocking agents, such as phenoxybenzamine.
  - Other agents include metyrosine, prazosin, and calcium channel blockers.
  - β-Adrenergic blocking agents can be used only after full α-blockade has been achieved.
  - Avoid opioids as they stimulate histamine release.
- Prognosis
  - Operative mortality is 1–2%.
  - Mild to moderate essential hypertension may persist after surgery.
  - Treatment with ^{131}I-MIBG may help patients with metastatic or recurrent malignant pheochromocytomas.

Imaging findings

- May be homogeneous or heterogeneous, solid or cystic complex masses.
- May show calcification.
- Smaller tumors tend to have a more uniform attenuation.

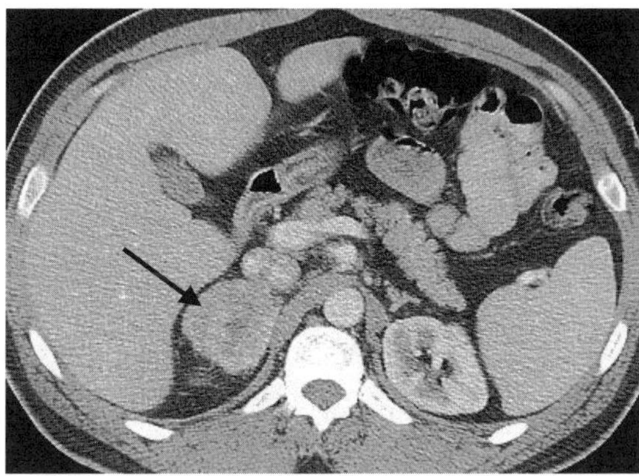

Figure 1.6 Adrenal pheochromocytoma. Axial contrast enhanced CT shows a heterogeneously enhancing right adrenal mass (arrow).

- Typically enhance avidly with intravenous contrast administration but can be heterogeneous (Fig. 1.6).

- Most have an absolute enhancement washout of less than 60%, and a relative enhancement of less than 40%, but washout features are variable.

- Show less than 16.5% loss of signal intensity on out-of-phase, compared with in-phase MRI pulse sequences.

- The classic 'light bulb bright' signal on T2-weighted images is infrequently seen.

- Pheochromocytomas occur in association with various syndromes such as; multiple endocrine neoplasias (MEN2), Von Recklinghausen neurofibromatosis (NF1), and Von Hippel-Lindau disease (VHL) (Fig. 1.7).

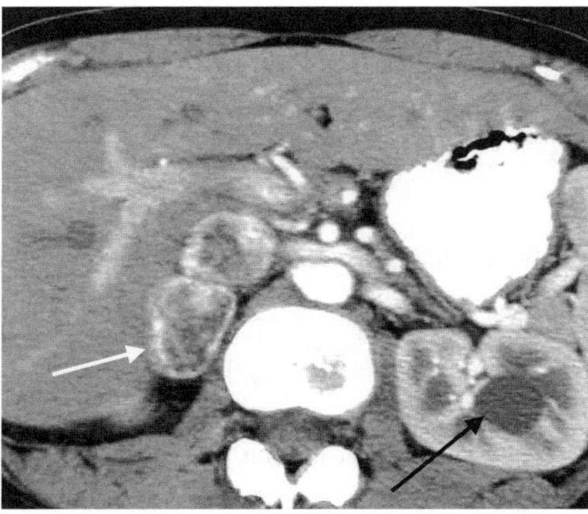

Figure 1.7 Adrenal pheochromocytoma. Axial contrast enhanced CT shows a heterogeneously enhancing right adrenal mass (arrow). Also note visualization of a left renal cyst (arrow) in this patient with Von Hippel Lindau disease.

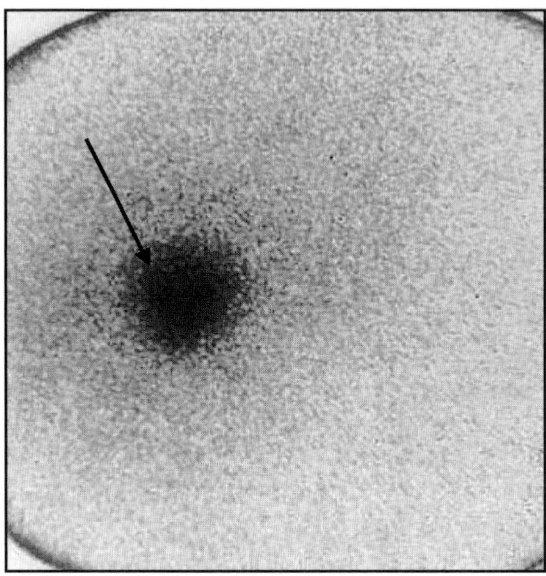

Figure 1.8 Adrenal pheochromocytoma. Radionuclide MIBG scan shows increased tracer uptake in the region of a right adrenal mass.

- Pheochromocytomas usually exhibit high uptake on MIBG scintigraphic examination (Fig. 1.8).

1.5 Adrenal cortical carcinoma

Introduction

Adrenocortical carcinoma is typically an aggressive malignancy with a poor prognosis, though less aggressive forms do occur. The tumors can present either due to hormone production, or due to mass effect from the primary or metastatic lesions.

Clinical features

- Variety of clinical symptoms through excess production of adrenal hormones.

- Complete surgical removal of the primary lesion and symptomatic metastatic sites, if possible, has been the mainstay of treatment.

- Epidemiology

  o These tumors are rare; 1–2 cases per million persons in the USA.

  o Less than 0.05% of newly diagnosed cancers per year.

  o Bimodal occurrence, with tumors developing in children less than 5 years of age and in adults in their fifth through seventh decade of life.

  o Male:female ratio is 2:1, with functional tumors being more common in women.

- o Left adrenal involved slightly more often than the right (53% vs. 47%); bilateral tumors are rare (2%).
- o 50–60% of patients have symptoms related to hypersecretion of hormones (most commonly Cushing's syndrome and virilization).
- o Feminizing and purely aldosterone-secreting carcinomas are more rare.
- o 50% of patients have metastases at the time of diagnosis.
- Symptoms and signs
  - o Symptoms of specific hormone excess (cortisol excess, virilization, feminization).
  - o Palpable abdominal mass.
  - o Abdominal pain.
  - o Fatigue, weight loss, fever, hematuria.
- Laboratory findings
  - o All laboratory abnormalities depend on hormonal status of tumor.
  - o Elevated urinary free cortisol or steroid precursors.
  - o Loss of normal circadian rhythm for serum cortisol.
  - o Low serum adrenocorticotropic hormone (ACTH).
  - o Abnormal dexamethasone suppression test.
  - o Elevated serum testosterone, estradiol, or aldosterone levels.

Treatment

- Surgery is the only treatment that can cure or prolong survival.
- Laparoscopic surgery not recommended because of spread of tumor, fragility of tumor, and the possible need to resect adjacent involved organs.
- For local recurrent disease, reoperation is the only effective therapy and may prolong life.
- Surgery
  - o Indications
    - Disease localized to the adrenal, or local spread.
  - o Contraindications
    - Widely metastatic disease.
- Medications
  - o Mitotane (an adrenolytic agent) can be used as adjuvant therapy; controls endocrine symptoms in 50% of patients but does not generally affect survival.
- Prognosis
  - o Tumor stage at the initial operation predicts survival.
  - o Median survival is 25 months.
  - o 5-year actuarial survival is 25%.
  - o 5-year survival with grossly complete surgical resection is 50%.

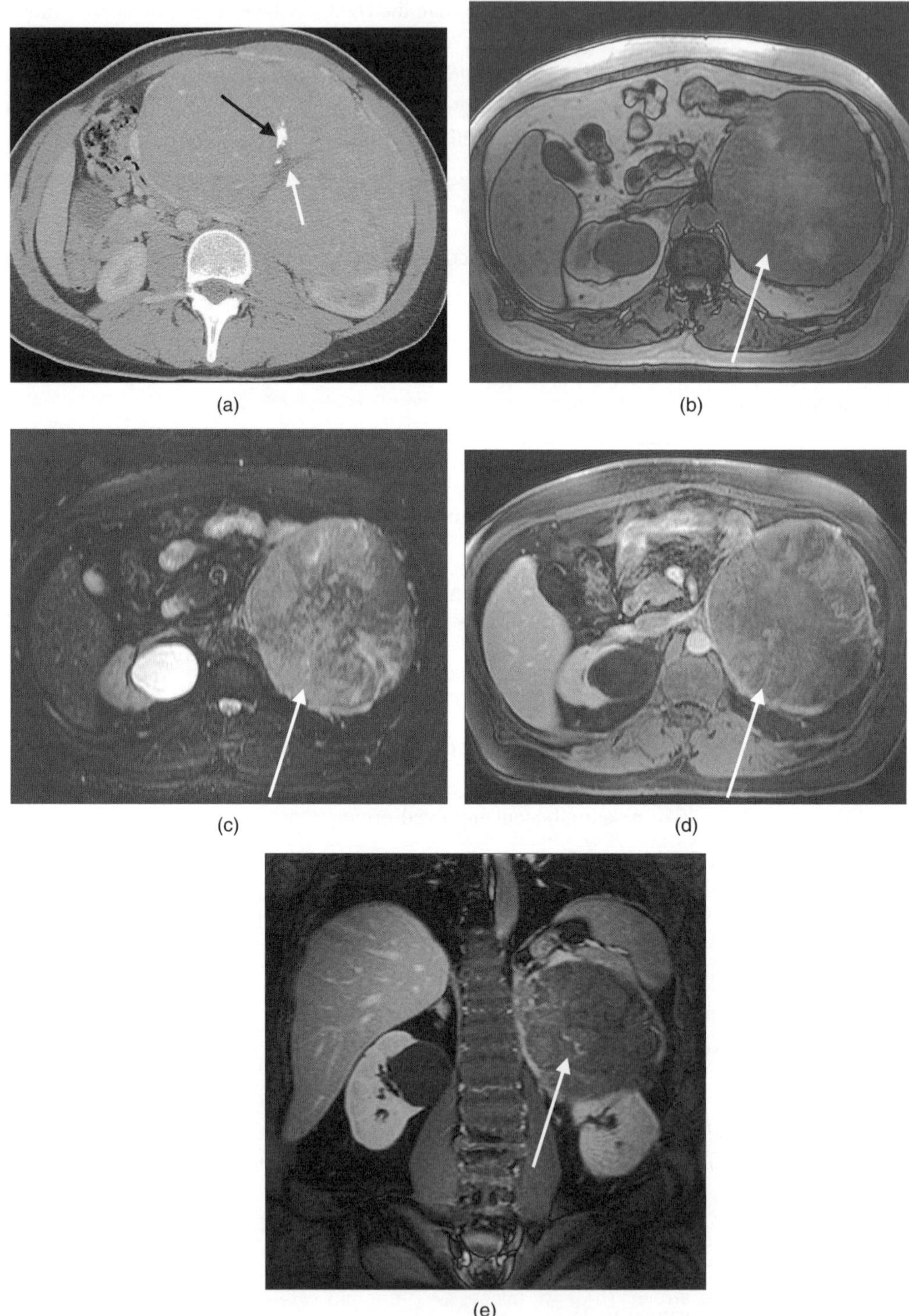

Imaging findings

- Usually large tumors at diagnosis, most larger than 6 cm.

- Heterogeneous on CT and MRI, owing to the presence of internal hemorrhage, calcification and necrosis (Fig. 1.9).

- Large tumors tend to invade the adrenal vein and inferior vena cava.

1.6 Adrenal incidentaloma

Introduction

Incidentally identified adrenal tumors found on studies performed for other indications than symptomatic adrenal disease are common. Evaluation of patients who have these tumors can depend on the age of the patient and the size of the tumor. Although adrenal cortical adenomas are the most common lesions that present as incidentalomas, a wide variety of benign and malignant masses as well as non-hyperfunctioning and subclinical hormonally active masses can present in this manner.

Clinical features

- Incidence of diagnosis has increased with use of ultrasonography, CT, and MRI for various, non-related conditions of the abdomen.

- Diagnosis includes such conditions as non-functioning adrenocortical adenoma, functioning adenoma, pheochromocytomas with subclinical secretion of hormones, and adrenocortical carcinomas.

- Major issues are to determine whether the tumor is hormonally active, or a carcinoma, or neither.

- Most simple adrenal cysts, myelolipomas, and adrenal hemorrhages can be identified by the imaging characteristics alone.

- Adrenal cysts can be very large.

- Since most tumors are non-functioning adenomas, the work-up should avoid unnecessary procedures and expense.

- Non-functioning adrenal tumors that are greater than 5 cm have a higher risk of cancer.

- An adrenal mass {≫} 3 cm in a patient with a previously treated malignancy is very likely a metastasis.

Figure 1.9 Adrenal cortical carcinoma. (a) Axial contrast enhanced CT shows a large heterogeneously enhancing left adrenal mass containing calcification (black arrow) and low attenuation area of necrosis (white arrow). (b-e) MR images in a different case of adrenal carcinoma shows heterogeneous regions (arrows) prior to and following intravenous gadolinium administration due to degeneration and necrosis.

- Primary tumors that metastasize to the adrenal gland include: lung, breast, colon, renal cell carcinoma, malignant melanoma, uterine, and prostate.

- Epidemiology

  o Found in 1–4% of CT scans.

  o Found in 6% of random autopsies.

  o Incidence increases with age.

  o Over 80% are non-functioning cortical adenomas.

  o 5% each are preclinical Cushing's syndrome, pheochromocytoma, and adrenocortical carcinoma.

  o 2% are metastatic carcinoma.

  o 1% are aldosteronoma.

  o 25% of pheochromocytomas are found incidentally.

Workup and treatment

- Complete history and physical exam, with specific reference to previous malignancies, symptoms of Cushing's syndrome, hypertension, virilization, or feminization.

- All patients, even those without hypertension, should have plasma metanephrines and 24-h urinary fractionated catecholamines determined to evaluate for pheochromocytoma.

- All patients should have a serum cortisol, 24-h urine collection for cortisol, and an overnight dexamethasone suppression test.

- Patients who are hypertensive should have serum potassium, and plasma aldosterone and renin activity measured.

- Consider obtaining a dehydroepiandrosterone (DHEA) level (potential marker for adreno-cortical carcinoma).

- If above studies show the tumor to be non-functional, the size of the tumor and the patient's overall medical condition determine management.

- If metastasis is suspected and pheochromocytoma is ruled out, then CT-guided biopsy is useful.

Imaging findings

Most commonly these are 'non-functioning' adrenal cortical adenomas, but functioning tumors such as adrenal cortical carcinoma and pheochromocytoma may also present as 'incidental' adrenal masses.

Adrenal adenoma

- Most are less than 3 cm in size.

- Can have varying appearances on CT.

- Lipid-rich adenoma. Attenuation value of 10 HU or less on unenhanced CT.

- Absolute enhancement washout >60% and relative enhancement washout >40%.

- Greater than 16.5% loss of signal intensity on out-of-phase, compared with in-phase MRI pulse sequences.

Other masses include the following:

Adrenal cyst

- Can have features of simple cyst such as attenuation of less than 20 HU on unenhanced image and no enhancement following intravenous contrast administration (Fig. 1.10).

- Hypointense on T1-weighted images and hyperintense on T2-weighted images, with no soft-tissue component and no internal enhancement (Fig. 1.11).

- Pseudocysts typically arise after an episode of adrenal hemorrhage or trauma.

- Adrenal pseudocysts may have a complicated appearance on CT and MR images, with septations, blood products, soft-tissue component secondary to hemorrhage or hyalinized thrombus, and curvilinear calcification (Fig. 1.12). Pseudocysts can be indistinguishable from malignant tumors.

Adrenal myelolipoma

- Benign tumor composed of marrow elements such as mature adipose tissue (fat), hematopoietic tissue and calcification/ossification.

- Fat can be diagnosed by the presence of areas of negative attenuation value by CT (Fig. 1.13) and on MR, by suppression of signal intensity on fat suppressed images, when compared with non-fat suppressed images.

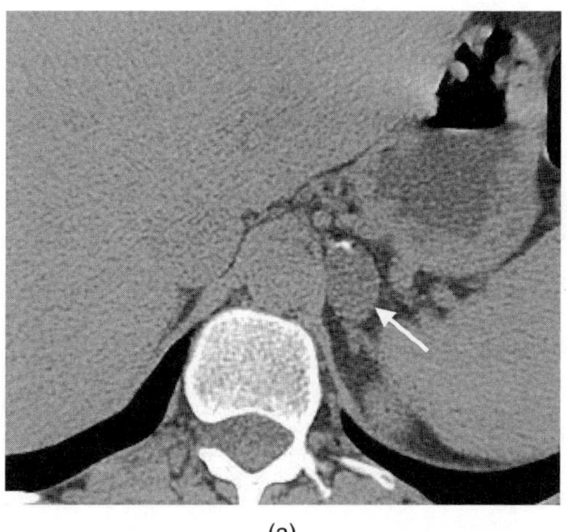
(a)

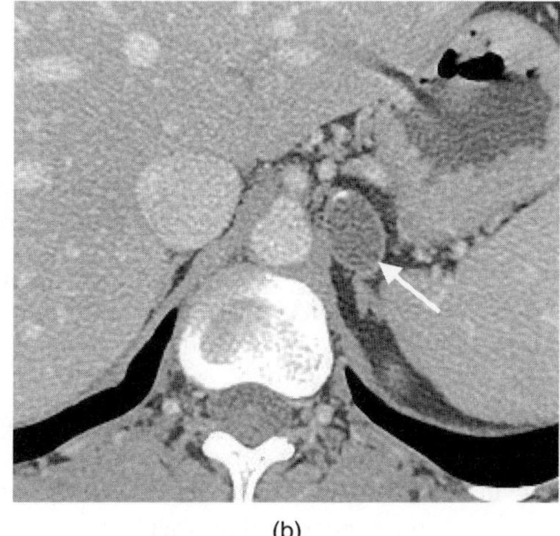
(b)

Figure 1.10 Adrenal cyst. Axial unenhanced CT shows a left adrenal mass measuring 18 HU (arrow) (a). Following intravenous contrast enhancement the mass did not show significant enhancement (arrow) (b).

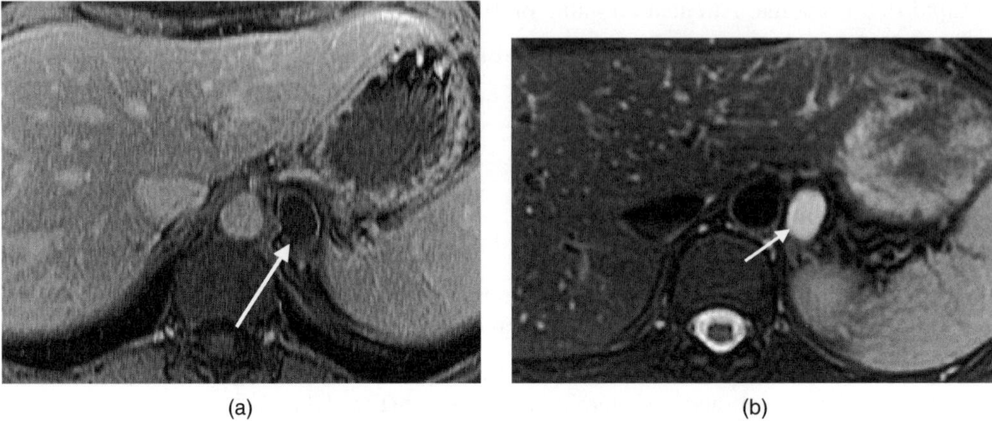

(a)   (b)

Figure 1.11   Adrenal cyst. Axial contrast enhanced T1 weighted (a), and axial fat suppressed T2 weighted (b) MR show a left adrenal mass exhibiting a hypointense signal on T1-weighted images (arrow) and hyperintense signal on T2-weighted images (arrow) with no soft-tissue component and no internal enhancement.

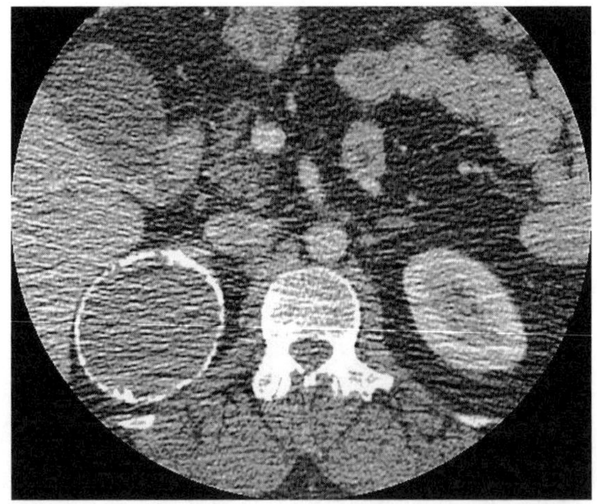

Figure 1.12   Adrenal pseudocyst. Axial contrast enhanced CT shows a right calcified adrenal mass measuring 19 HU.

Adrenal hemorrhage

- Usually bilateral.

- Can be seen in post-operative states, trauma, sepsis and in patients with blood dyscrasias or receiving anticoagulant therapy.

- If unilateral usually due to trauma or following liver transplantation (right sided)

- High density on unenhanced images (Fig. 1.14).

- Appearance overlaps that of other lesions following contrast enhancement.

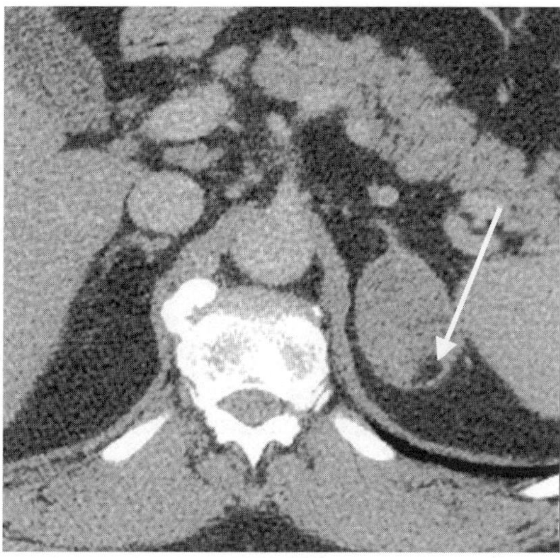

Figure 1.13   Adrenal myelolipoma. Axial contrast enhanced CT shows a left adrenal mass with an intralesional area of fat indicated by a negative attenuation value of −28 HU (arrow). Note that qualitatively this area is of similar attenuation to the adjacent intra-abdominal fat.

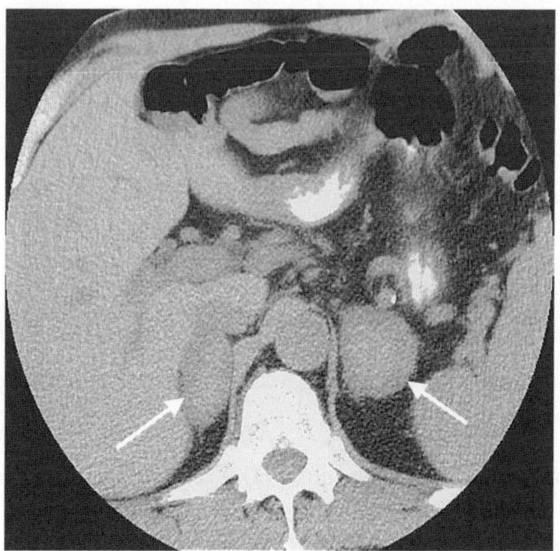

Figure 1.14   Bilateral adrenal hemorrhage. Unenhanced CT shows bilateral adrenal masses (arrows) with high attenuation.

Metastases (Fig. 1.15)

- Common primary tumors include the lung, breast, GI tract and pancreas.

- Can be of varying size.

- Attenuation higher than 10 HU on unenhanced CT, as they do not typically contain intracellular lipid.

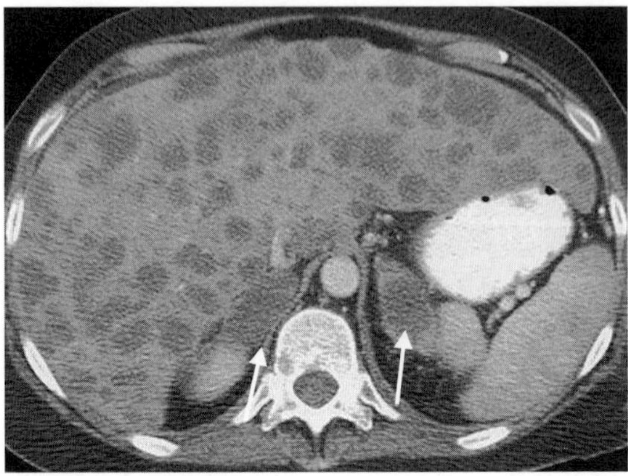

Figure 1.15 Adrenal metastases. Contrast-enhanced CT shows diffuse hepatic and bilateral adrenal metastases (arrows) in patient with advanced melanoma.

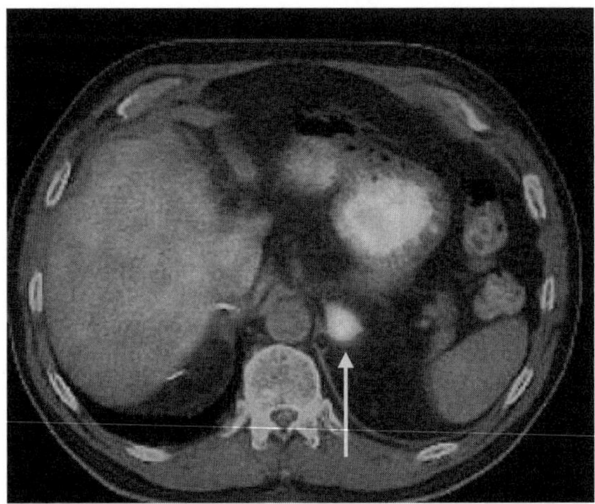

Figure 1.16 Adrenal metastasis. Fused PET/CT scan shows marked tracer uptake in a small left adrenal mass (arrow).

- Absolute enhancement washout of less than 60%, and a relative enhancement of less than 40%.

- Usually heterogeneous.

- Less than 16.5% loss of signal intensity on out-of-phase, compared with in-phase MRI pulse sequences, except in metastatic clear cell renal carcinoma which may contain foci of lipid.

- High tracer activity on FDG PET scans usually differentiates malignancy (metastasis or adrenal cortical carcinoma) from adenoma. Comparison to liver uptake is often useful for this assessment (Fig. 1.16).

2
Retroperitoneal Masses

Pietro Pavlica[1], Massimo Valentino[1] and Libero Barozzi[1]

[1] *Radiology Unit*

2.1 Introduction

The retroperitoneum is the portion of the abdomen located posterior to the peritoneal cavity. It extends from the diaphragm to the pelvic inlet and includes portions of the colon, duodenum, pancreas, kidneys, adrenals, abdominal aorta, inferior vena cava, lymph nodes, fat, and much of the abdominal wall musculature.

It is clearly displayed by computed tomography (CT) and magnetic resonance (MR). Both have the advantages over ultrasonography (US) of being panoramic, not limited by the artefacts of the overlying structures and able to explore skeleton and muscle at the same time.

This chapter outlines the normal retroperitoneal anatomy, and describes different pathological diseases involving the retroperitoneal spaces.

2.2 Retroperitoneal anatomy

The retroperitoneum is traditionally divided into three distinct compartments (Fig. 2.1) by the renal fascia (Gerota's fascia):

1. posterior pararenal space containing only fat and muscles;

2. perirenal spaces containing kidneys with proximal ureters, adrenal glands, and perirenal fat; and

3. anterior pararenal space containing the pancreas, ascending and descending colon, 2nd and 3rd portion of duodenum, and the mesenteric root.

Urogenital Imaging: A Problem-oriented Approach   Edited by Sameh K. Morcos and Henrik S. Thomsen
© 2009 John Wiley & Sons, Ltd

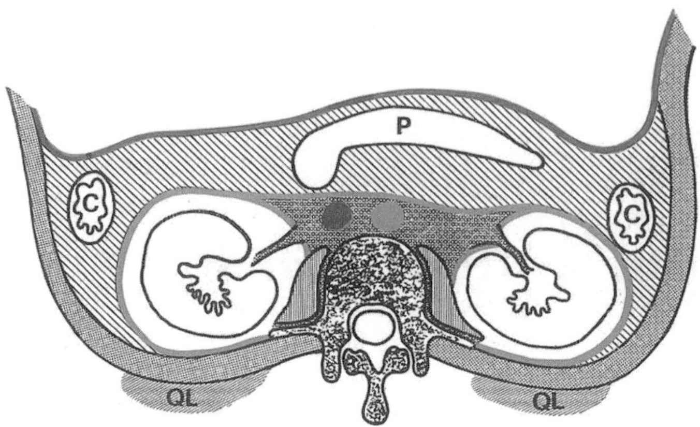

Figure 2.1 Graphic shows the main division of the retroperitoneal space. The parietal peritoneum (blue line) separates the peritoneal cavity from the retroperitoneum. The anterior renal fascia of Gerota (yellow line) separates the perirenal space from the anterior retroperitoneum. The posterior renal fascia separates the perirenal space from the posterior retroperitoneum.

The retroperitoneum is bounded anteriorly by the parietal peritoneum and posteriorly by the transversalis fascia. It extends from the diaphragm down to the level of the pelvic fossa. These spaces are separated but they are opened inferiorly at the level of the pelvis where the retroperitoneum space communicates with the extraperitoneal space of the pelvis, and the two compartments become continuous.

These anatomic features explain why effusion or other retroperitoneal diseases can spread a long distance from the origin.

2.3 Pathological conditions

- Identification of the retroperitoneal spaces on diagnostic imaging is useful in elucidating the etiologies of various solid or cystic masses.

- Neoplastic and inflammatory processes can initially cause thickening of the retroperitoneal fasciae.

- Fluid collections from pancreatic or gastro-intestinal tract diseases, hematomas, or urinomas can develop in the retroperitoneal spaces.

- Localization of retroperitoneal origin is sometimes difficult for large masses.

2.4 Primary solid retroperitoneal tumors

Clinical problem – key concepts

- The complex embryological structure of the retroperitoneal space explains the wide pathological variety of different tumors.

- Pathologists are not always able to clarify the origin and nature of the growing mass and imaging can sometimes be useful to define this problem.

- Diagnosis of retroperitoneal tumors is generally delayed due to the lack of clinical signs and they are detected when already large.

- Abdominal pain of non-defined origin and localization is the most common presenting symptom and in about 30% of cases an abdominal mass is the first presenting sign. Vague gastrointestinal symptoms can be caused by the displacement or compression of the bowel, while urological or neurological signs are uncommon. There are some exceptions in hormonally active tumors or in lesions observed in risk group patients (Von Hippel Lindau disease, MEN syndrome, tuberous sclerosis, neurofibromatosis).

- The majority (80–85%) of primary retroperitoneal tumors are malignant, but they represent only 0.4% of all malignancies. The benign lesions are less frequent and generally detected serendipitously.

- Retroperitoneal primary tumors can be schematically divided into two groups on the basis of their frequency in clinical practice: common retroperitoneal tumors and rare primary retroperitoneal masses (Tables 1.1 and 1.2).

Role of diagnostic imaging

- Conventional radiology (barium small bowel, barium enema and urography) does not have any diagnostic role today because only the indirect signs of the mass can be detected (Fig. 2.2).

- Computed Tomography (CT) is the first line procedure to detect, stage and follow-up retroperitoneal masses. It is the most diffuse and reliable method and sometimes allows a tissue-specific diagnosis. Multiplanar reconstructions allow a precise definition of the vascular supply and vascular infiltration before a therapeutic planning.

- Magnetic Resonance Imaging (MRI) is currently a second line diagnostic procedure and allows a better differentiation between benign and malignant lesions.

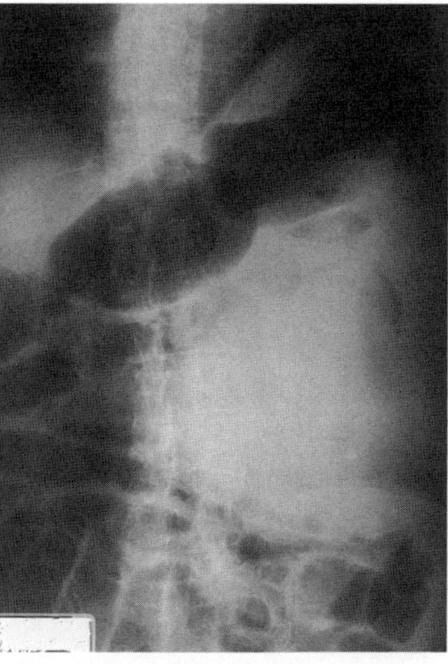

Figure 2.2 Retroperitoneal sarcoma. Large left retroperitoneal mass displacing the stomach and the bowel loops to the right. Small calcification is visible. Plain film of the abdomen.

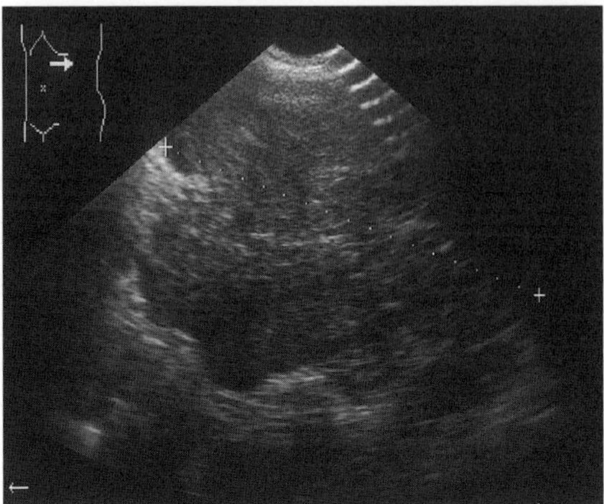

Figure 2.3 Retroperitoneal fibrosarcoma. Sonography of the abdomen in longitudinal scan showing a large retroperitoneal abdomen solid mass with not well defined profiles and infiltrating the different abdominal structures.

- Angiography which was formerly used to define the vascular anatomy before surgical planning, has now been replaced by angio-CT and angio-MR imaging with 3D reconstructions.

- Sonography has a limited role in the detection and staging of the retroperitoneal masses (Fig. 2.3).

General imaging criteria

- Large soft tissue mass displacing neighboring organs

- Large vessel dislocation and/or wall infiltration

- Psoas muscle infiltration

- Central areas of necrosis or hemorrhage (Fig. 2.4)

- Calcifications

- Lymph node enlargement

- CT density values before and after contrast medium administration

- Signal intensity values at MR before and after contrast media

- Other organ metastases.

There are no specific signs of malignancy but the main criteria to consider are:

- Infiltration of psoas muscle and other organs

- Fascial overlapping

- Vascular wall infiltration

- Neoangiogenesis.

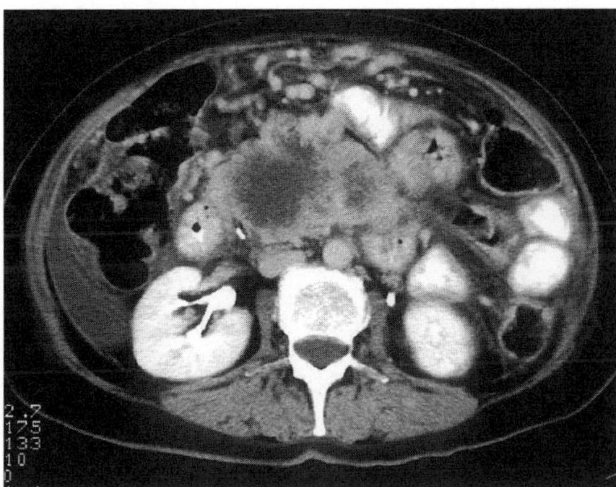

Figure 2.4 Primary fibrosarcoma of the retroperitoneum. CT in transversal scan at the level of the kidney, after contrast injection. Large necrotic mass, with fuzzy margins and peripheral contrast enhancement.

Specific imaging criteria

- **Lipoma.** Benign tumor originating from the fat tissue of the retroperitoneal space. It can be very large with no signs of infiltrations, no solid mass and no vascularization. The main diagnostic sign is the detection of fat-tissue density at CT (about – 100HU) and high intensity signal in MR images or dark images with fat saturation sequences.

- **Leiomyoma.** This originates from the blood vessels, vas deferens or embryonal remnants. Usually it shows a rapid growth and necrotic or cystic central degeneration is observed. Contrast medium reveals a moderate enhancement mainly at the periphery with internal septa.

- **Benign teratoma.** A specific diagnosis can be made in 70–90% of cases because of typical CT or MR aspects owing to the contemporaneous presence of fat tissue, bone, teeth and fluid. Malignant components can not be ruled out with certainty on the basis of imaging.

- **Rare mesenchymal, neurogenic and dysgenetic benign tumors.** (Table 2.1). No specific diagnostic features are detectable and the final definition is made by biopsy or surgery.

- **Liposarcoma.** The most common malignant mesenchymal tumor and more frequent in women. It does not arise from a benign lipoma and the CT density is correlated to the degree of histological differentiation. Lipoma-like liposarcomas with low grade malignancy are present, formed mainly of fat and show negative density values at CT or high signals in MR images.

- **Leiomyosarcoma.** Can arise from retroperitoneal smooth muscle (Fig. 2.5) or vascular wall (cava or aorta). Necrotic or hemorrhagic areas inside the mass can frequently be seen and they show peripheral contrast enhancement. The differential diagnosis from the benign leiomyoma is made on the base of a more aggressive and infiltrating aspect. The thrombotic obstruction of the inferior vena cava is common in primary leiomyosarcoma and the lesion can manifest itself with edema of the legs, nephritic syndrome or Budd-Chiari syndrome.

Table 2.1 Primary retroperitoneal tumors

Benign	**Malignant**
Mesenchymal (40–80%)	
Lipoma	Liposarcoma
Leiomyoma	Leiomyosarcoma
Fibroma	Fibrosarcoma
Rhabdomioma	Rhabdomyosarcoma
Hemangioma	Hemangiosarcoma
Angiomyolipoma	Hemangiopericytoma
Lymphangioma	Lymphangiosarcoma
Xantogranuloma	Malignant fibrous histiocytoma
Neurogenic(10–50%)	
Neurinoma	
Neurofibroma	Neurofibrosarcoma
Benign neuroblastoma	Malignant neuroblastoma
Benign ganglioneuroma	Malignant ganglioneuroma
Benign sympathicoblastoma	Malignat sympathicoblastoma
Paraganglioma	Malignant paraganglioma
Dysgenetic and epithelial (5–19%)	
Benign teratoma	Malignant teratoma
Chordoma	
Urogenital remnant tumors	

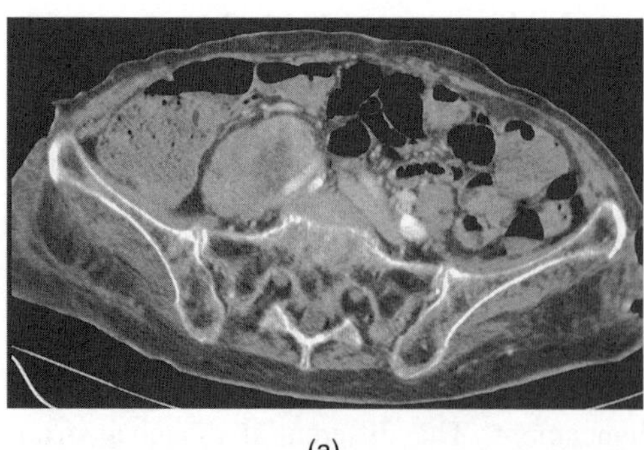

(a)

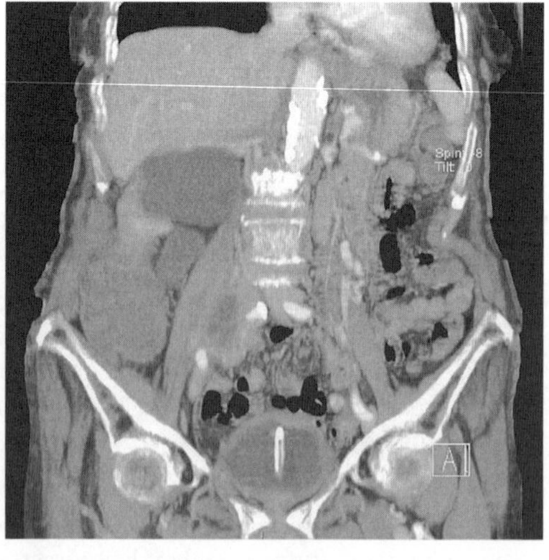

(b)

Figure 2.5 Leiomyosarcoma of the retroperitoneum originating from the right psoas muscle. CT in transversal scan (a) and coronal reconstruction (b) after contrast medium administration. The mass develops in front of the sacrum, displacing the bowel loops and compressing the iliac vessels.

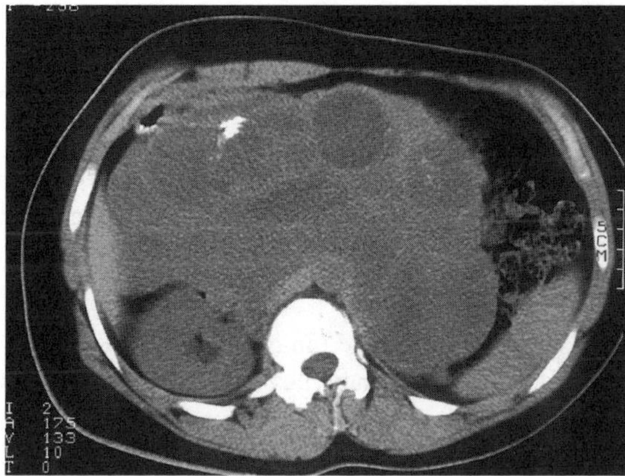

Figure 2.6 Primary malignant histiocytoma. Large retroperitoneal mass that develops into the abdominal cavity. CT without contrast administration. The mass has a dishomogeneous density with areas of low density and an area of calcification.

- **Malignant fibrous histiocytoma.** More common in men than in women. The mass does not contain fat or involve the vena cava. It has muscle density values at CT and larger masses show central necrotic areas. Calcifications are observed in 25% of cases (Fig. 2.6).

- **Neurofibrosarcoma.** Occurs in young patients and the malignant form is not distinguishable with imaging from the benign form. They may be multiple especially when associated with neurofibromatosis.

- **Rare mesenchymal, neurogenic and dysgenetic malignat tumors of the retroperitoneum.** (Table 2.2). These tumors are impossible to differentiate from other masses and require biopsy. Malignancy can be suspected on the basis of the infiltrating nature and the detection of metastasis.

- **Very rare primary retroperitoneal tumors.** They consist of a heterogeneous group of lesions, rarely observed and with no specific criteria at imaging.

2.5 Retroperitoneal lymphoma

Clinical problem – key concepts

- Lymphomas are frequent in clinical settings and represent about 5% of newly-diagnosed cancers.

- Fever, night sweating, weight loss and superficial nodal enlargement are the most common presenting signs.

- Hodgkin's and non-Hodgkin's lymphoma are frequently localized in retroperitoneal lymph nodes.

- Incidence has increased in patients with AIDS or organ transplantation.

- Imaging is the first diagnostic procedure to detect and stage retroperitoneal nodes in patients with systemic lymphatic disease.

Table 2.2 Rare primary retroperitoneal tumors

Tumor	Clinic/Pathology	Imaging
Hemangiopericytoma	20% originate in the retroperitoneum	Lobulated lesion with calcifications, cystic structure and contrast enhancement at CT and MR
Castelman tumor	Benign lymphatic tumor with 2 histological subtypes: vascular-hyaline (90%; benign) and plasmacellular (symptomatic with fever, anemia, hyper-gammaglobulin)	Richly vascularized mass with evident enhancement, associated cystic changes, necrosis. May be very large and involve the blood vessel
Neurogenic tumors	Common in risk patients (VHL syndrome, neurofibromatosis, tuberous sclerosis) Malignant transformation is observed in 10% of patients	Septated mass with hypervascularized capsule. Multiple simultaneous lesions
Cystic lymphangioma	Origin from embryonal lymphatic tissue. Rare.	Unilocular or multilocular cystic mass with water density and mild contrast enhancement of the wall. Septa can be thick and contain calcifications
Lymphangiomatosis	Very rare tumor, almost exclusive in women.	Inhomogeneous mass
Xanthogranulomatosis	Multicentric or systemic tumor of the histiocytes. The disease is frequently related with retroperitoneal fibrosis. Generally benign.	Soft tissue dense mass. Infiltrations of retroperitoneal structures
Extra-adrenal pheochromocytoma	Develops from the sympathetic chain	No specific signs
Extra-adrenal neuroblastoma	Located in the sympathetic chain outside the adrenals	Large mass with frequent calcifications (80%). Central necrosis
Extra-osseous chondrogenic neoplasms	Atypical retroperitoneal location	Large mass, occasionally with calcifications. Cystic or necrotic areas are common

- Lymphangiography is now rarely performed and the increase in sensitivity and specificity compared with CT is low.

Role of diagnostic imaging

- Detects enlarged retroperitoneal nodes in para-aortic, aortocaval, retrocaval and iliac nodal groups.

- Sonography can not be proposed as a standard of care. Nodes are enlarged and hypoechoic without sound transmission.

- MR imaging is not superior to CT

- The best diagnostic procedure is PET-TC with FDG because the false-positive and false-negative rates are lower since PET allows a functional imaging which is expression of the activity of the disease even in normal sized nodes

- PET has a sensitivity of 90–95% compared with 80–85% of CT. Detects more lesions and is responsible for stage change in 30% of patients

- PET is particularly helpful to differentiate residual active lymphoma from post-therapeutic fibrosis

Imaging criteria

- Nodal enlargement with increase in number and size of normal nodes (Fig. 2.7).

- The majority of normal para-aortic and paracaval nodes measure less than 1 cm, while nodes larger than 1.5 cm are always considered pathologic.

- Node identification caudal to the bifurcation and in the pelvis is more difficult because of the multiple small arteries and veins that can mimic small lymph nodes.

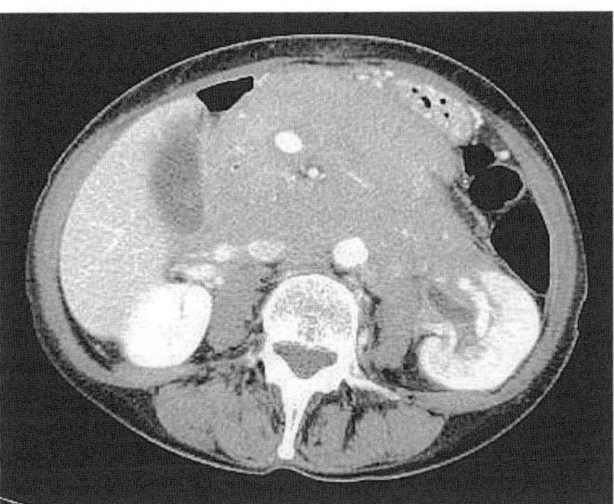

Figure 2.7 Primary non-Hodgkin's lymphoma of the retroperitoneum. CT of the abdomen after contrast administration. Enlarged nodes involving the retroperitoneal nodal chains with displacement of vessels.

- Enlarged nodes can form a conglomerate masses or a large homogeneous mass in which individual nodes are no longer recognized.

- The nodal masses show a soft tissue density as the other solid viscera and sometimes areas of reduced density due to tissue degeneration.

2.6 Cystic retroperitoneal masses

Clinical problem – key concepts

- Retroperitoneal cystic masses are uncommon. They can be classified as either neoplastic or non-neoplastic.

- Neoplastic lesions include cystic lymphangioma, mucinous cystadenoma, cystic teratoma, müllerian cyst, epidermoid cyst, and cystic change in solid neoplasms. Non-neoplastic lesions include pancreatic pseudocyst, non-pancreatic pseudocyst, lymphocele, urinoma, and hematoma.

- The most important clinical parameters include patient gender, age, symptoms, and clinical history.

Role of diagnostic imaging

- The widespread use of axial imaging modalities has increased the detection rate of retroperitoneal cystic lesions.

- Some features may suggest a specific diagnosis. Imaging may provide important information regarding lesion location, size, and shape; the presence and thickness of a wall; the presence of septa, calcifications, or fat; and involvement of adjacent structures.

- Conventional radiology does not offer any utility in detection and characterization of cystic masses.

- Sonography can detect easily urinomas and hemorrhage as fluid collections but it is not always able to differentiate between them.

- CT and MR are the preferred diagnostic modalities to investigate retroperitoneal cystic masses.

General imaging criteria

- low-attenuation mass sometimes containing tiny calcifications

- localization characteristics for some pathologies (e.g. presacral, or in the obturator space)

- absence of infiltration

- no lymph nodes enlargement

- small variations in density values at CT after contrast administration

- solid signal intensity at MR T2-weighted sequences

Specific imaging criteria

- **Cystic lymphangioma.** Uncommon, congenital benign tumors and occur due to failure of the developing lymphatic tissue. Cystic lymphangiomas can develop anywhere in the perirenal, pararenal, or pelvic extraperitoneal spaces. They may cross more than one compartment of the retroperitoneum.

- **Mucinous cystadenoma.** Rare retroperitoneal cystic lesions that occur in women with normal ovaries. Early diagnosis of primary mucinous cystadenoma is important because of its malignant potential. They usually appear as a homogeneous, unilocular cystic mass at CT. Differentiating this mass from cystic mesothelioma, cystic lymphangioma, and non-pancreatic pseudocyst is difficult.

- **Cystic teratoma.** Retroperitoneal cystic teratomas are composed of well-differentiated derivations from at least two of the three germ layers (ectoderm, mesoderm, endoderm). A cystic teratoma is likely to be benign, whereas a solid teratoma is likely to be malignant. At CT, a mature teratoma of the retroperitoneum consist of a complex mass containing a well-circumscribed fluid component, adipose tissue, and calcification (Fig. 2.8).

- **Müllerian cyst.** Müllerian cyst of the retroperitoneum is an extremely rare disease that is thought to be a subtype of urogenital cyst. At CT, müllerian cyst appear as a unilocular or multilocular thin-walled cyst containing clear fluid.

- **Epidermoid cyst.** Epidermoid cysts are rare congenital lesions of ectodermal origin and can occur anywhere from the head to the foot. At CT, epidermoid cysts generally appear as thin-walled, unilocular cystic masses with fluid attenuation.

- **Cystic change in solid neoplasm.** Occasionally, paraganglioma and neurogenic tumor can be cystic. They can be associated to clinical symptoms because of the catecholamines they produce. At CT, retroperitoneal paragangliomas usually have homogeneous soft-tissue attenuation or central areas of low attenuation.

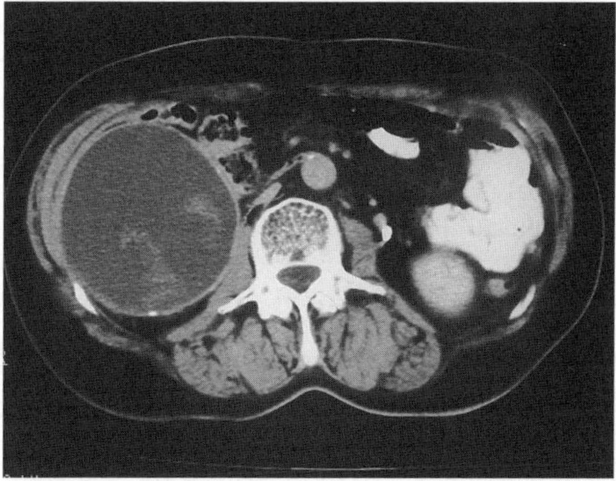

Figure 2.8 Retroperitoneal cystic teratoma. CT scan after contrast medium administration. A large well defined mass with fluid content and solid internal areas, involving the right retroperitoneal space and displacing the adjacent structures. A regular enhanced capsula and a small calcification is present.

- **Lymphocele.** Lymphoceles are fluid-filled cysts without an epithelial lining that occur after pelvic or retroperitoneal lymphadenectomy or renal transplant surgery. They occur in 12–24% of patients who undergo radical lymphadenectomy. At CT, a lymphocele appear as a low-attenuation mass. Negative attenuation values due to fat within the fluid are rare but are highly suggestive of a lymphocele.

2.7 Retroperitoneal metastases

Clinical problem – key concepts

- Retroperitoneal and pelvic lymph nodes can be the site of spread of malignant cell secondary to testicular tumors, melanoma, prostate cancer, bladder TCC, ovarian carcinoma, or lung and breast tumors.

- Enlarged lymph nodes can be observed in patients without malignancies and accounts for 6% of nodes disease. Sarcoidosis, tuberculosis, rheumatoid arthritis, amyloidosis, Whipple and Crohn's disease, cirrhosis and chronic hepatitis have to be considered in the differential diagnosis.

- Lymph node enlargement is frequent in AIDS patients as part of systemic lymphatic disease. A non-Hodgkin's lymphoma is the most frequent type of AIDS-related lymphoma. Kaposi's sarcoma can manifest as bulky retroperitoneal adenopathy and tumor infiltrating the retroperitoneum. Opportunistic infections are common in AIDS patients, most often caused by tuberculosis or fungal infection.

Imaging criteria

- In testicular tumors the lymphatic drainage follows the gonadal vessels and the metastases are generally located at the level of the renal hilum and in the adjacent para-aortic and paracaval space. Rapidly growing discrete or confluent low density nodes are characteristic of seminomas. MR imaging can be used because the young age of patients with testicular tumors. Retroperitoneal nodes show a low or intermediate signal intensity in T1-weighted images and high intensity signal in T2. Nodes may enhance after contrast administration like the primary tumor.

- Tumors that origin from pelvic organs as prostate, bladder, uterus and ovary usually show initial met to the obturator and iliac nodes and to the retroperitoneal nodes in advanced stage (Fig. 2.9). They are usually smaller in size compared to node enlargement observed in lymphomas or testicular cancer.

- Melanoma node metastases generally have high intensity signal in T1-weighted images.

- The CT or MR diagnosis of pathological lymph nodes is based on the enlargement of normally oval-shaped and smooth nodes. The upper limit of normality varies according to the site: 6–7 mm for retrocrural, 12–15 for para-aortic and paracaval, and 18–20 mm for iliac and obturatory nodes.

- Enlargement is not pathognomonic for malignancy because inflammatory or reactive changes are a very common cause of increased size.

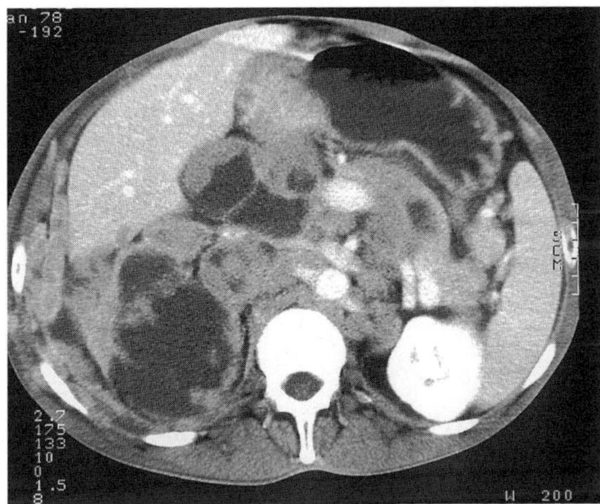

Figure 2.9 Retroperitoneal metastases secondary to colonic carcinoma. CT of the abdomen in transversal scan at the level of the kidney, with contrast medium. Multiple confluent nodules of different size displacing the main vessels and the bowel. Some nodules show extensive necrotic areas, while others are still homogeneous.

- The detection of multiple nodes of 10 mm or the presence of a bulky mass is indicative of malignancy.

- The loss of the normally present peri-aortic and pericaval fat layer is considered a sign of infiltration.

- Central hypodense areas in enlarged nodes is generally indicative of necrosis, fat deposition and is nor specific for malignancy.

- Hydronephrosis due to ureteral compression or infiltration is often observed in retroperitoneal metastastasis and is indicative of malignancy.

- Bone destruction or muscular infiltration with nerve infiltration is very common in secondary lymph node involvement.

2.8 Retroperitoneal fibrosis (Ormond's disease)

Clinical problem – key concepts

- Chronic inflammatory fibrosing disease localized in the connective tissue of the lumbar retroperitoneum which may compromise ureters and blood vessels.

- Primary idiopathic form is observed in 70% of patients, while the other 30% is secondary to drug abuse, aortic aneurysm, tumors and other rare causes.

- The clinical symptoms are non-specific and the most commonly observed are abdominal pain extended from the back to the genital area (80–90%), weight loss (40–50%), gastrointestinal discomfort (25–50%), anorexia (13%), anuria (10–16%), progressive renal failure (40%).

- The majority of patients come to observation because of renal insufficiency, lower-extremity or scrotal edema, venous insufficiency.

- Pathology shows a firm grayish fibrosis, beginning at the level of the lower lumbar vertebral bodies and extending cranially to the renal hilum and caudally into the pelvis.

- Caudally the process can extend in the parailiacal and periureteral direction and involve the gonadal vessels, uterus, bladder, sigmoid colon and seminal vesicles.

Imaging criteria

Conventional radiology

- Excretory urography, retrograde pyelography and barium enema are still used procedures and the main diagnostic signs are bilateral hydronephrosis with gradual tapering of both ureters in the lumbar area. The medial displacement of the ureters is observed in 75–90% of the cases in the middle third.

- Retrograde pyelography shows pyeloureteral ectasia extending to the level of L4 and L5, medial deviation of ureters and normal appearing pelvic ureters.

- Barium enema is indicated in cases with extension to the pelvis and can detect extrinsic compression or displacement of the rectum and sigmoid.

CT imaging

- CT is superior to conventional radiology and sonography and is actually the first line procedure.

- A soft tissue density plaque or mass is observed in para-aortic and paracaval region, surrounding aorta, inferior vena cava and ureters (Fig. 2.10).

- The vascular structures are poorly delineated on non-contrast images, while compression on the vena cava is observed in post-contrast scanning. Aortic wall infiltration is very rare.

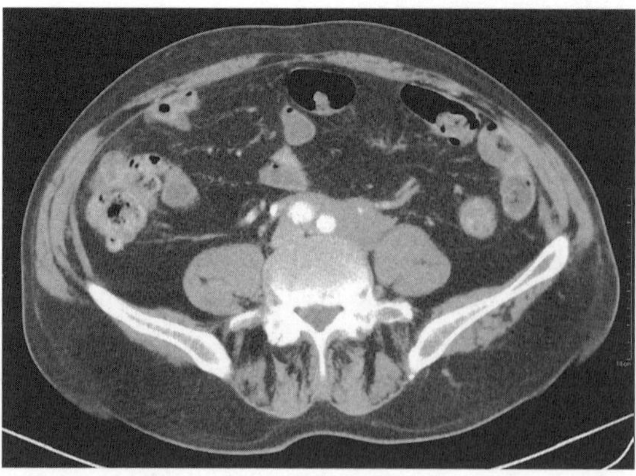

Figure 2.10 Retroperitoneal fibrosis. CT transversal scan after contrast medium. A soft tissue density mass surrounding the retroperitoneal vessels, without enhancement due to well organized fibrous tissue.

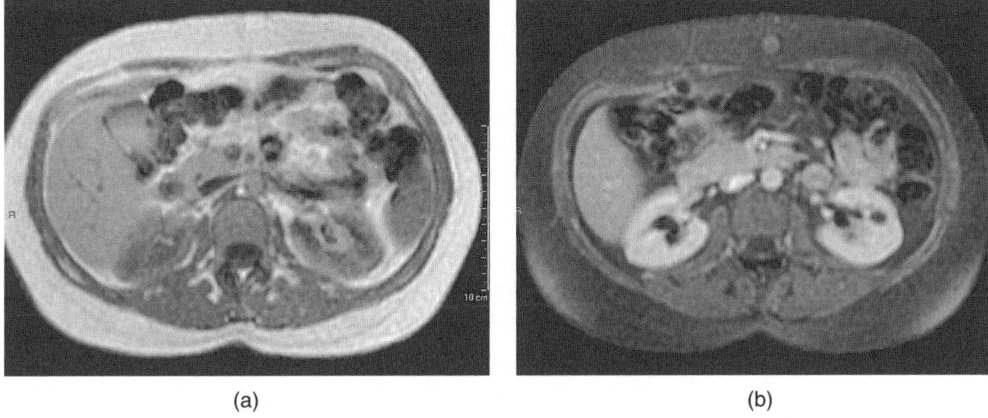

(a)   (b)

Figure 2.11   Retroperitoneal fibrosis. MR axial scans in T1WI (a) and T1WI after contrast medium (b). Low-moderate signal intensity mass located in front of inferior vena cava showing a contrast enhancement due to active inflammatory process.

- The main lesion is usually observed at the level of the lower lumbar bodies.

- After contrast injection the fibrotic mass can show mainly marginal enhancement due to the active inflammatory peripheral components of the fibrotic process. When the fibrous tissue is organized and dense there is no contrast enhancement.

Magnetic resonance imaging

- It can be applied as problem-solving method in particular cases.

- In T1-weighted images the retroperitoneal fibrosis appears as a mass or plaque of low-medium homogeneous signal intensity.

- In T2 images it has low-moderate heterogeneous signal intensity, less than fat but more than muscle.

- After contrast medium injection a dishomogeneous enhancement can be observed in relation to the activity of the fibrotic process (Fig. 2.11).

2.9 Retroperitoneal fluid collections (traumatic and non-traumatic)

Retroperitoneal traumatic hematomas

Clinical problem – key concepts

- Retroperitoneal injuries are quite unusual and tipically are caused by adjacent fractures or are associated with retroperitoneal organ injuries (i.e. kidney, pancreas or duodenum). They can be associated with vascular pedicle avulsion. Incidence of retroperitoneal hematomas has been reported in 2.5–12% of blunt abdominal trauma.

- Clinical examination is often unreliable, due to the lack of signs or complaints. When present, the most common signs are pain, tenderness with guarding, hypovolemic shock with decreased sensorium.

- Mechanisms of injuries can be 1) an increased intra-abdominal pressure, which can cause a rupture of a hollow viscus (e.g. seat-belt injury); 2) crushing effect caused by compression of viscera between the offending force and the body structures; 3) sudden shearing forces of viscera at fixed points of attachment.

- Detection and quantification of retroperitoneal hematomas following blunt or penetrating abdominal trauma are crucial in detecting the sites of possible significant but often clinically occult blood loss in planning the necessary management.

- To facilitate clinical management of hematomas resulting from blunt trauma the retroperitoneum can be anatomically divided into three zones. **Zone I** is the upper central area, extending caudally from the aortic hiatus of the diaphragm to the sacral promontory. A zone I retroperitoneal hematoma require surgical intervention in 75% of the cases. **Zone II** refers to the flank or lateral retroperitoneum and includes the kidneys. Retroperitoneal hematomas in this zone can typically be managed without surgery if shown to be stable at CT. **Zone III** includes pelvic space and is the most common affected location. In blunt trauma, pelvic hematomas should not be investigated surgically because of the risk for detamponade of bleeding and lack of control of hemorrhage with occlusion of both internal iliac arteries.

- The kidney is the most commonly injured organ seen in association with retroperitoneal hematomas, followed by pancreas and duodenum.

Role of diagnostic imaging

- Clinically unstable patients are investigated immediately by surgery, although interventional angiography may be utilized to control the hemorrhage.

- The clinically stable patients are usually evaluated by focused abdominal sonography for trauma (FAST) or, more in the past, diagnostic peritoneal lavage (DPL) to exclude the presence of free fluid within the peritoneal cavity. Both the modality are not reliable in retroperitoneal hematomas and a large bleed limited to this space can go undetected. CT is the imaging modality of choice to evaluate stable patients with blunt or penetrating trauma.

- CT is accurate in defining retroperitoneal effusion and vascular injuries; it is very sensitive for kidney and pancreatic lesions, and mild sensitive for hollow viscous injuries. It is fully capable of simultaneous evaluation of the intraperitoneal and retroperitoneal compartments as well as spine and pelvis skeleton in one rapid pass (Fig. 2.12).

- Diagnostic angiography is replaced at present by CT, whether interventional angiography can provide endovascular treatment or bleeding control. Pelvic arterial hemorrhage is best managed by embolization. Endovascular treatment is more effective than surgical intervention.

- Plain radiography and pelvic radiographs can provide information suggesting the presence of retroperitoneal hematoma, as an area of increased density or by a 'mass' displacing or cancelling anatomical structures.

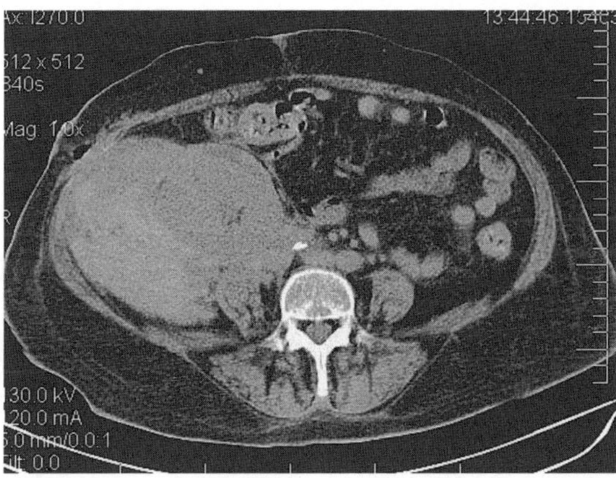

Figure 2.12 Traumatic retroperitoneal hematoma. CT transversal scan without contrast medium shows a non-homogeneous collection with high density values du to recent bleeding.

General diagnostic criteria

- CT with contrast injection identifies the site of active bleeding, indicating the likely vascular origins and providing a map for surgical or angiographic investigation.

- Serial CT can be used to document stability or expansion of retroperitoneal hematoma.

- The detection of a focal retroperitoneal hematoma may act as a 'sentinel clot' for a particular organ. The presence of thickening or hemorrhage along the anterior Gerota's fascia or lateral conal fascia has been an indirect sign for injury to colon or pancreas. In these cases a careful clinical and repeat CT is recommended.

- Administration of oral contrast material can be helpful in identifying bowel injuries.

Retroperitoneal non-traumatic hematomas

Clinical problem – key concepts

- Hemorrhage is an often serious complication of anticoagulant therapy, reported in up to 4% of treated patients.

- CT is the imaging modality used in assessing patients with anticoagulant therapy complaining acute abdominal or back pain.

- Clinical symptoms can be related to acute anemia or palpable abdominal mass.

- After catheterization, hematomas may appear in four different location: retroperitoneal, intraperitoneal, groin and thigh muscle, abdominal wall.

Role of diagnostic imaging

- Hematomas undergo evolutionary changes that are reflected by their appearance on CT. Hyperdensity is a CT feature of a recent bleed. In the acute phase, within 3 days of bleeding, hematomas appear as a hyperdense mass, measuring between 60 and 80 HU. The mass

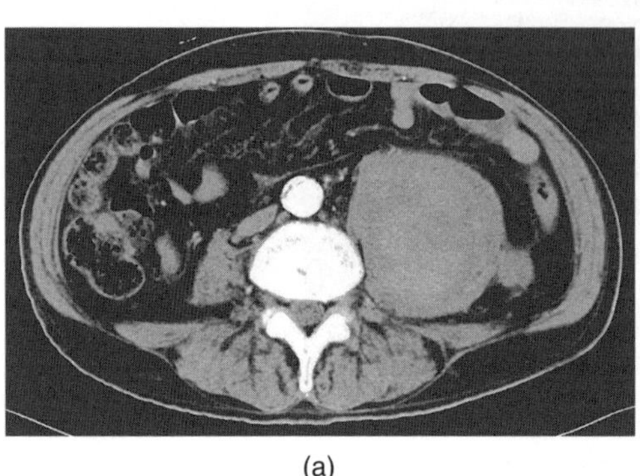
(a)

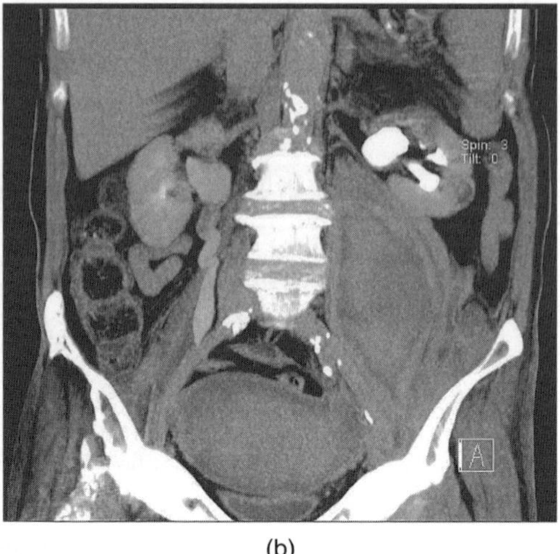
(b)

Figure 2.13 Spontaneous hematoma of the left psoas muscle. CT transversal scan (a) and coronal reconstruction (b) after contrast injection. Large fluid collection extending from the left retroperitoneum to the pelvis with swelling of the psoas and iliac muscle. High attenuation value due to recent bleeding.

is often non-homogeneous and typically contains hyperdense foci and fluid-level. Over time, hematomas decrease in size along with diminution of their attenuation. Resolving hematomas may show peripheral rim enhancement (Fig. 2.13).

- Ultrasonography may identify retroperitoneal hematomas as non-homogeneous mass but is less effective than CT at establishing the extent of the lesion.

- Plain radiography can provide the same information described in the post-traumatic retroperitoneal hematomas.

- Angiography can provide endovascular treatment or bleeding control. Surgical or endovascular treatment are related to the Zones I–III of location and to the expansion of hematoma.

Retroperitoneal urinoma

Clinical problem – key concepts

- A urinoma is an encapsulated collection of extravasated urine. Both obstructive causes and non-obstructive causes (including abdominal trauma and injury to the collecting system during surgery or diagnostic instrumentation) can lead to urinary extravasation.

- Most commonly, it results from renal trauma. It may also be the result of transmitted back pressure caused by obstruction of the genitourinary system due to a ureteral stone or pelvic mass, pregnancy, retroperitoneal fibrosis, posterior urethral valves, or bladder outlet obstruction. Iatrogenic injury during surgical or percutaneous procedures is another possible cause of renal injury.

- Retroperitoneal urinoma may also result from ureter or bladder injury. Ureteral urine leaks most commonly occur as a result of iatrogenic injury following genitourinary, retroperitoneal, pelvic, or gynecologic surgery Ureteral anastomotic dehiscence may occur following renal transplantation or ureteral diversion procedures.

- Urinomas may initially be clinically occult and may manifest with delayed complications such as hydronephrosis, paralytic ileus, electrolyte imbalances, and abscess formation.

- They have a variety of appearances and may be misdiagnosed as ordinary ascites, abdominal or pelvic abscesses or hematomas, cystic masses, or pancreatic pseudocysts.

Diagnostic criteria

- CT is the study of choice. CT protocol in patients with such suspect require a delayed phase obtained 5–20 min after contrast material injection.

- At unenhanced CT, urinoma usually manifests as a fluid collection with water attenuation.

- After contrast media administration, the attenuation increase over time after intravenous administration of contrast material because contrast-enhanced urine enters the urinoma (Fig. 2.14).

- Absence of distal ureteral opacification is a sentinel CT finding of ureteral disruption, but a ureter distal to the injury can contain opacified urine when the ureter is only lacerated.

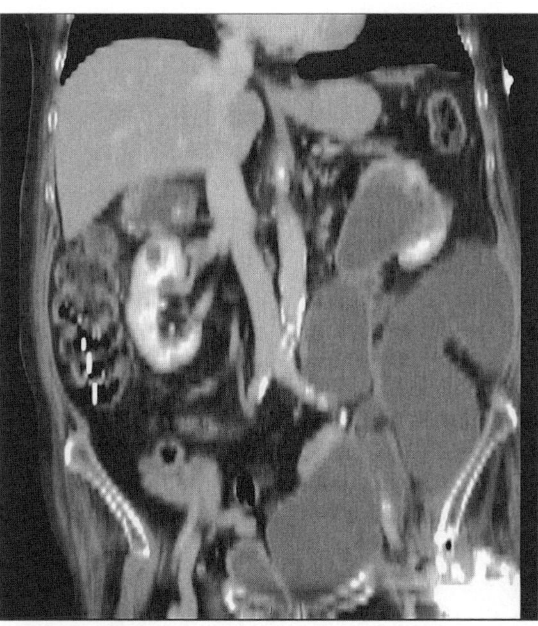

Figure 2.14   Retroperitoneal urinoma. CT with contrast medium coronal reconstruction. Large multiloculated collection extending from the left kidney to the pelvis with low density values due to a long-standing urinoma.

- Bone scintigraphy or renal scintigraphy may also allow a diagnosis of urinoma. They are useful particularly in patients who cannot receive a CT with intravenous contrast material due to elevated creatinine levels, or are allergic to the iodinated contrast medium, or have received a renal transplant.

- Percutaneous aspiration and drainage may allow confirmation of the diagnosis and treatment.

Retroperitoneal abscesses

Iliopsoas abscesses

- A iliopsoas abscess is a rarely encountered form of retroperitoneal infection. In the majority of cases, it results from adjacent infection of the kidneys, aortic bed, spine, pancreas, or bowel. Pyogenic infections are most frequent. Iliopsoas abscess from tuberculous spondylitis is possible.

Diagnostic criteria

- Asymmetry in the size and/or density of the muscles is the most consistent radiological finding.

- On CT iliopsoas inflammatory disease displays a variety of appearances, ranging from diffuse enlargement of the muscle to a mass containing areas of low attenuation.

- Gas bubble may be seen in approximately 50% of abscesses, more rarely in tumors.

- Presence of gas suggests infection, while bone destruction other than spondylitis is a sign of tumor. Nevertheless, in the most of patients the history and appearance are not specific and necessitate needle aspiration biopsy.

- Scanning with ^{67}Ga has been reported to be helpful in cause of fever of unknown origin, to identify the location of pathological process. [67]Ga scanning is superior to CT in demonstrating concomitant infectious foci at other sites, which are common in these patients.

Psoas abscess from tuberculosis

- Psoas abscesses are a well-known accompaniment of tuberculous spondylitis, due to destruction of the cortical bone and formation of a paraspinal abscess.

- Lymph nodes are sites of disease and they may be the cause of recurrence.

Diagnostic criteria

- Radiologic patterns for psoas abscess include loss of the psoas shadow, abnormal soft-tissue shadows, gas inclusions, bony destruction of the spine, and abscess calcification.

- CT scan demonstrates psoas abscess (see above) with gas inclusions, extending from the spine.

- Enlarged retroperitoneal lymphoadenopathies are usually detected. Adenopathies have low attenuation centers consistent with necrosis.

- Treatment includes percutaneous drainage and antibiotic therapy. Surgical intervention is performed in the delayed phase.

References

Federle MP, Jeffrey RB, Desser TS *et al.* (2004) *Diagnostic Imaging. Abdomen.* Amirsys Inc, Salt Lake City, Utah.

Nishino M, Hayakawa K, Minami M *et al.* (2003) Primary retroperitoneal neoplasms CT and MR imaging findings with anatomic and pathologic diagnostic clues. *Radiographics* **23**: 45–57.

Yang DM, Fung DH, Kim H *et al.* (2004) Retroperitoneal cystic masses: CT, clinical and pathological findings and literature review. *Radiographics* **24**: 1353–1365

Vivas I, Nicolàs AI, Velazquez P *et al.* (2000) Retroperitoneal fibrosis: typical and atypical manifestations. *Br. J. Radiol.* **73**: 214–222.

Falcone RA, Luchette FA, Choe KA *et al.* (1999) Zone I retroperitoneal hematoma identified by computed tomography scan as an indicator of significant abdominal injury. *Surgery* **126**: 608–614.

Roberts J. (1996) CT of abdominal and pelvic trauma. *Semin. Ultrasound CT MR.* **17**: 142–169.

3
Imaging of Renal Artery Stenosis

Robert Hartman

Department of Diagnostic Radiology, Mayo clinic, Rochester MN

3.1 Introduction

Currently it is estimated that approximately 50 million or more Americans suffer from hypertension. The worldwide figures may include as many as 1 billion individuals with over 7 million deaths per year attributable to the disease. The vast majority of these individuals have essential hypertension but a significant subset have a secondary cause for the hypertension. Within this group of patients the largest single cause of secondary hypertension is renal mediated hypertension, of which renal artery stenosis is the leading pathology. It is estimated that as many as 5% of all cases of hypertension in the entire population is caused by renal artery stenosis equating to as many as 3 million cases in the USA of this potentially treatable form of hypertension. The detection of renal artery stenosis is of particular importance to ensure this group of patients with a potentially curable form of hypertension is identified and treated properly. Treatment of renal artery stenosis by angioplasty, with or without stenting, may cure or improve hypertension in many cases.

3.2 Clinical features

The initial evaluation of a patient with hypertension should include a comprehensive history and physical. Information from the examination should be focused on answering questions regarding:

- Lifestyle assessment and identification of other cardiovascular risk factors that may affect prognosis and help to guide treatment.
- Detection of identifiable causes of hypertension.

Urogenital Imaging: A Problem-oriented Approach   Edited by Sameh K. Morcos and Henrik S. Thomsen
© 2009 John Wiley & Sons, Ltd

- Assessment for the presence or absence of end-organ damage and cardiovascular disease.

Potential causes of secondary hypertension include:

- Renal artery stenosis
- Chronic kidney disease
- Primary hyperaldosteronism
- Coarctation of the aorta
- Cushing's syndrome
- Pheochromocytoma
- Thyroid/parathyroid disorders

In certain cases a secondary cause of hypertension can be suspected. These situations include:

- Patients whose age, history, physical examination, severity of hypertension, or initial laboratory findings suggests such causes.
- Patients whose BP responds poorly to multidrug therapy.
- Patients whose BP begins to increase for uncertain reason after being well controlled.
- Patients with sudden onset of hypertension.

In particular, findings that suggest renal artery stenosis as the cause of secondary hypertension include:

- Rapid onset of hypertension or uncontrollable hypertension in a middle age female.
- Rapid onset of hypertension in patient over the age of 55.
- Abdominal bruit.
- Azotemia occurring on angiotensin converting enzyme (ACE) inhibitor or angiotensin receptor blocker (ARB).
- Previously well controlled hypertension becoming more resistant to drug therapy.
- Flash pulmonary edema.
- Renal failure of unknown cause.
- Hypokalemia.

In cases where there is a high clinical suspicion of renal artery stenosis and secondary hypertension radiological evaluation can often be helpful.

3.3 Pathology

Renal vascular hypertension, particularly hypertension secondary to renal artery stenosis, is due to activation of the renin-angiotensin cascade. The affected kidney experiences decreased blood flow and activates the renin-angiotensin cascade in order to establish a normotensive state. The cascade consists of:

- Renin released form the juxtaglomerular cell of the kidney.

- Circulating renin in the blood leads to conversion of angiotensinogen to angiotensin I.

- Angiotensin converting enzymes (ACE) in the lung convert angiotensin I to angiotensin II.

- Angiotensin II has effects on the adrenal glands stimulating release of aldosterone. It also has direct effect on the blood vessels causing vasoconstriction.

- Aldosterone affects the kidney resulting in Na^+ and H_2O retention leading to overall vascular volume increase.

- The combined effects of vasoconstriction and increased intravascular volume result in systemic hypertension.

3.4 Imaging of suspected renal artery stenosis

A number of exams utilizing a variety of modalities are available for the evaluation of suspected renal artery stenosis (RAS). These include:

- Grayscale and Doppler US

- ACE inhibitor Nuclear Medicine Renogram

- Computed tomography (CT) angiography

- Magnetic resonance (MR) angiography

- Digital subtraction arteriography

The choice of initial examination requires consideration of a number of factors including the availability of a particular exam, the invasiveness of a particular examination, the level of comfort of radiology personnel performing and interpreting individual examinations, as well as the suspected etiology of the RAS. The initial examination of choice will therefore vary from practice to practice in many instances.

In general catheter directed digital subtraction arteriography (DSA) is only used as the initial exam in cases where the clinical suspicion of RAS is very high and intervention is anticipated. Although DSA is the gold standard for the evaluation of RAS, allowing the performing Radiologist the ability to identify anatomic areas of stenosis as well as determine the presence or absence of a pressure gradient across the stenosis, the invasiveness of the exam has delegated it to use primarily in the treatment of stenoses identified via less invasive modalities (Fig. 3.1).

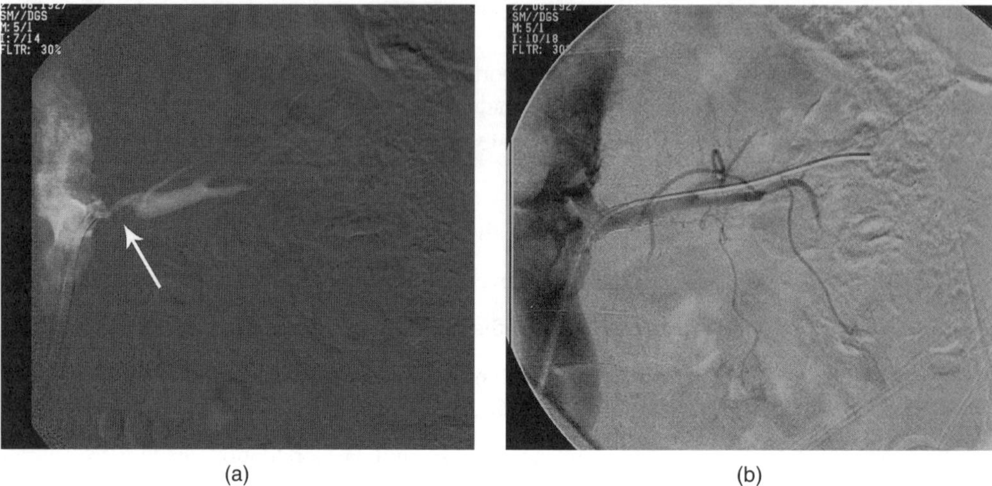

(a)   (b)

Figure 3.1 Conventional catheter directed angiogram (a) demonstrating an eccentric high grade stenosis near the origin of the left renal artery (arrow) secondary to atherosclerotic disease. Angiogram following angioplasty and stent placement demonstrating complete reduction of the stenotic segment (b).

The following sections describe the remaining modalities used for the evaluation of suspected RAS and particular typical findings.

Ultrasound

Ultrasound evaluation for suspected RAS requires both grayscale images of the kidney as well as Doppler examination of the renal vessels. These images are used to evaluate not only the vessels for demonstration of stenotic segments but also for parenchymal changes secondary to the RAS.

Grayscale images are used for:

- Evaluation of renal parenchymal thickness.

- Determination of parenchymal echogenicity.

Doppler examination is used to:

- Determine the location and number of renal arteries to each kidney.

- Examine the entire length of all renal arteries to identify areas of stenosis based on elevated velocities of blood flow.

- Evaluate segmental renal arteries to identify abnormal arterial waveforms typical of main renal artery stenoses.

Ultrasound findings in RAS

In RAS grayscale images may show changes in the affected kidney consisting of:

- Global parenchymal thinning relative to the unaffected kidney secondary to decreased blood-flow and ischemia.

- Increased echogenicity of renal parenchyma.

Doppler evaluation is capable of imaging changes in flow velocity and waveform. (Fig. 3.2) The main renal artery is examined to detect the specific site of the stenosis. In this region findings consist of:

- Abnormal waveform with spectral widening secondary to turbulent flow.

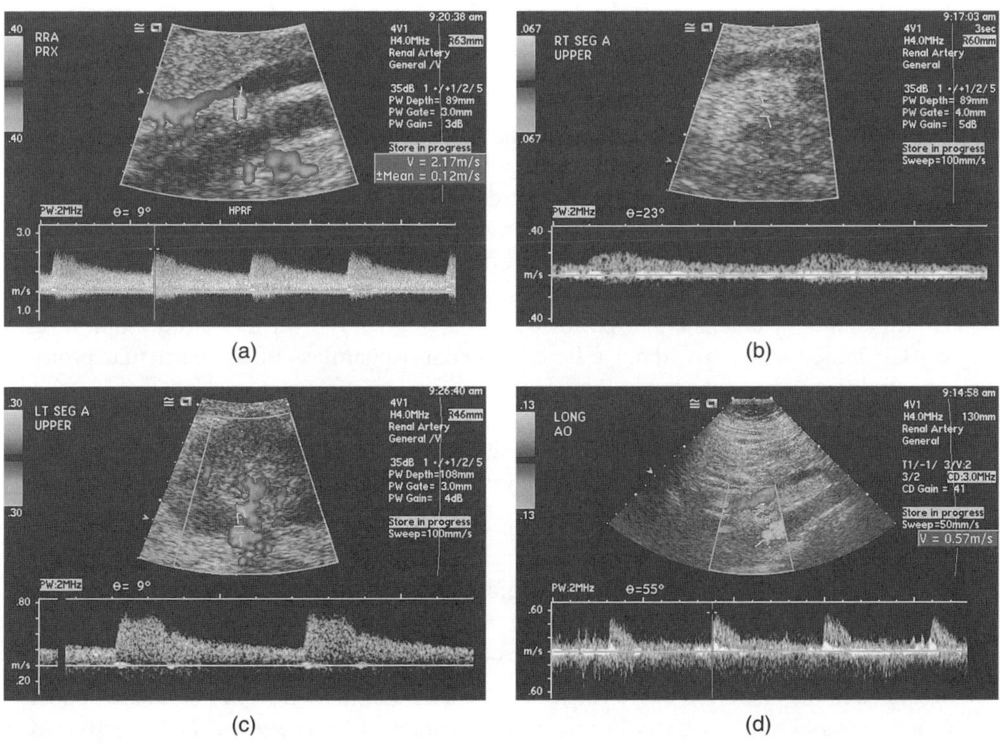

Figure 3.2 Doppler ultrasound evaluation of a stenotic right renal artery. Elevated peak systolic velocity of 2.17 m/s (normal <2.0 m/s) within the main renal artery is identified (a). The waveform of the segmental renal artery on the affected side is dampened (b) relative to the normal waveform from the contralateral kidney (c). The ratio of the peak systolic velocity in the stenotic segment relative to the systolic velocity in the aorta (d) is abnormally high, greater than 3.5 (2.17 m/s/0.57 m/s = 3.8).

- Color Doppler aliasing.

- Increased peak systolic velocity greater than 2.0 m/s.

- Increased renal artery velocity/aorta velocity ratio exceeding 3.5.

Examination of the segmental renal arteries primarily shows changes in the arterial waveform typical of flow downstream from a stenosis. This produces a Tardus (late)-parvus (small) waveform in which the usual rapid systolic upstroke and early peak is dampened and delayed. Specific quantitative measures of this abnormal waveform have been determined. These include:

- Acceleration time (time from start of systole to peak systole). Normally this is less than 0.07 s.

- Acceleration index (slope of the systolic upstroke). Normally this at least 300 cm/s.

Nuclear Medicine Angiotensin Converting Enzyme (ACE) Inhibition Renogram

Nuclear medicine renograms for the detection of RAS make use of ACE-inhibitors to eliminate elevated circulating levels of angiotensin II. Angiotensin II has effects on the efferent arteriole of the renal glomerulus causing vasoconstriction. This effect maintains glomerular filtration rate (GFR) in a kidney downstream from RAS and can mask abnormalities expected on a renogram. By blocking the conversion of angiotensin I to angiotensin II the efferent arteriole does not constrict and the effects of decreased GFR in the affected kidney become evident. Different institutions use a variety of protocols consisting of baseline versus ACE inhibitor exams either performed on a single day over a two day exam or as a single ACE inhibitor exam without a baseline exam. Regardless of the particular protocol the abnormalities used to diagnose RAS include: (Fig. 3.3)

- Changes on renogram images from 1 to 20 min consisting of delayed cortical uptake (delayed nephrogram) and/or delayed excretion from the affected kidney.

- Alterations of the cortical uptake curve (measure of tracer activity in the renal parenchyma) consisting of delayed tracer activity in the affected kidney relative to the unaffected kidney due to alterations in blood-flow to the kidney. This is often most evident if Tc-99m DTPA is the radiopharmaceutical used. This may not be as apparent when MAG3 is the radiopharmaceutical used.

- Alterations in the excretion curve (measure of tracer elimination from the kidney) consisting of prolonged tracer activity in the affected kidney. This is evident in Tc-99m MAG3 exams as there is decreased urine flow to wash out the secreted tracer.

- Quantitative measurement of the excretion curve will demonstrate prolongation of the $t^{1/2}$ (time required to eliminated $1/2$ of the tracer activity from the kidney).

CT Angiography

Useful in the anatomic depiction of the renal artery allowing for differentiation of some causes of RAS particularly fibromuscular dysplasia and atherosclerotic disease. (Fig. 3.4)

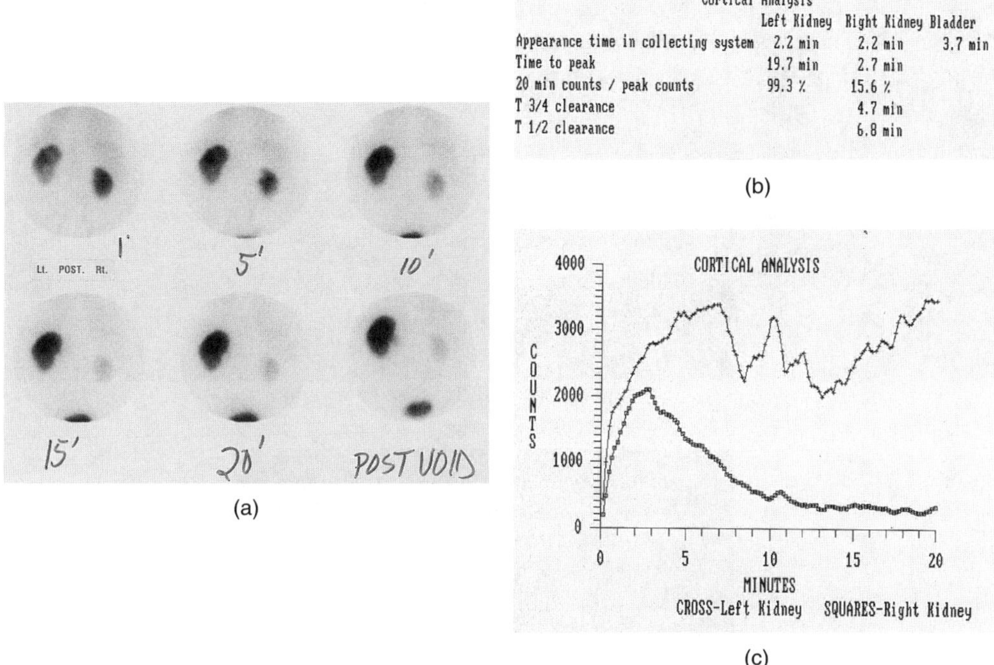

Figure 3.3 Nuclear medicine Tc99m-MAG 3 ACE-inhibitor renogram. Images of the kidneys from 1–20 min (a) demonstrate prolonged cortical retention in the left kidney relative to the right. This is the result of decreased urine flow in the left kidney from renal artery stenosis. The cortical analysis (b, c) confirm the visual evidence by demonstrating quantitative marked retention of tracer activity in the left kidney.

In patients with atherosclerosis the use of iodinated contrast is a relative contraindication as this group often has renal impairment increasing their risk of contrast induced nephropathy. Abnormalities identified include:

- Region of stenosis depicted as a site of focal narrowing of the arterial caliber.

- Associated post-stenotic dilatation in the artery distal to the stenosis from turbulent high velocity flow.

- An eccentric area of narrowing near the renal artery origin, often containing calcification, indicative of atherosclerotic RAS.

- Multiple web-like areas of narrowing interspersed with focal areas of dilatation (beaded appearance) in the mid to distal main renal artery indicative of the most common form of fibromuscular dysplasia.

MR Angiography

Like CT angiography MRA is useful in the depiction of the anatomic appearance of RAS. MRA has an advantage over CTA as it is performed without iodinated contrast which has

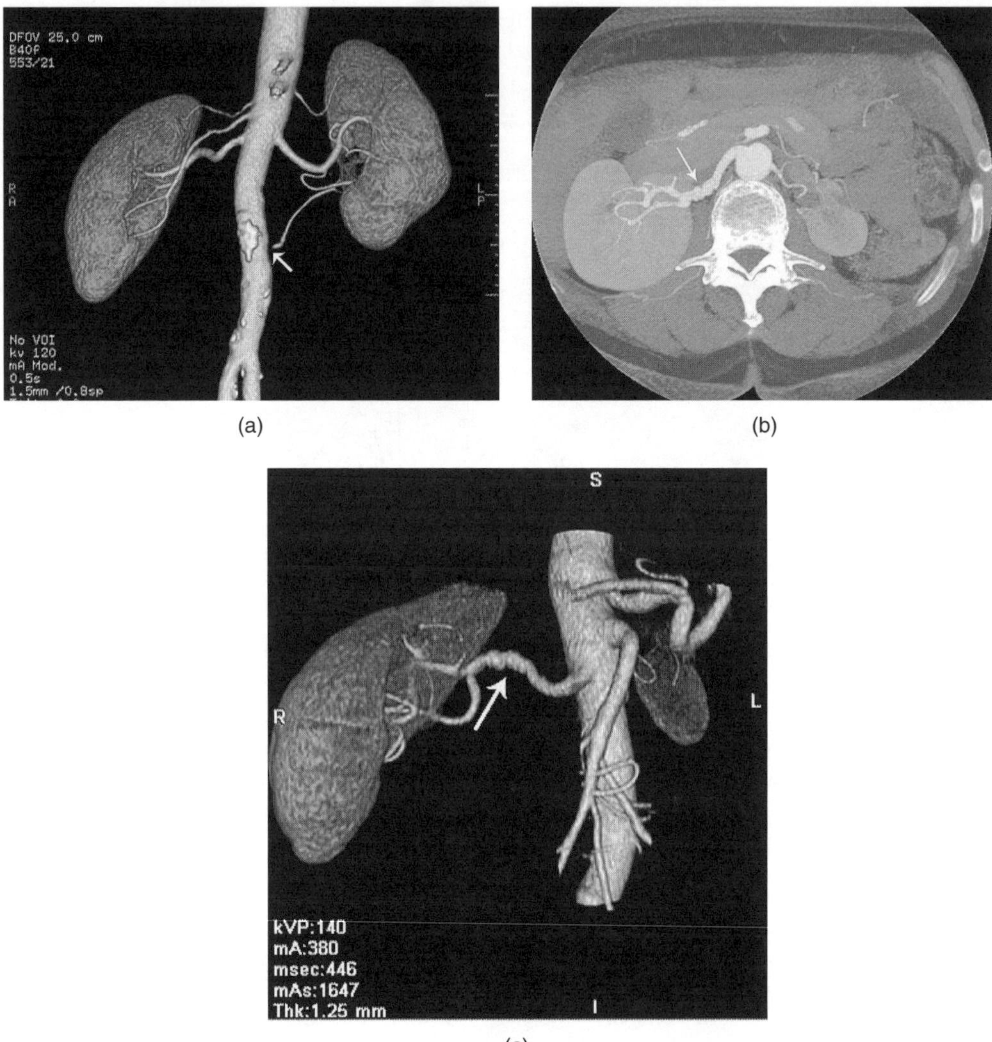

Figure 3.4 3D volume rendering from CT angiogram demonstrates multiple bilateral renal arteries. (a) The most inferior left renal artery has a high-grade stenosis at the origin typical of atherosclerosis (arrow). Axial maximum intensity projection (b) demonstrates multiple stenoses in the mid right renal artery resulting in a 'beaded' appearance (arrow) typical of fibromuscular dysplasia. 3D volume rendering from the same patient (c) showing the same findings (arrow).

a risk of contrast induced nephropathy, and does not use ionizing radiation. Abnormalities identified are similar to CTA and include (Fig. 3.5):

- Region of stenosis depicted as a site of focal narrowing of the arterial caliber.

- Associated post-stenotic dilatation in the artery distal to the stenosis from turbulent high velocity flow.

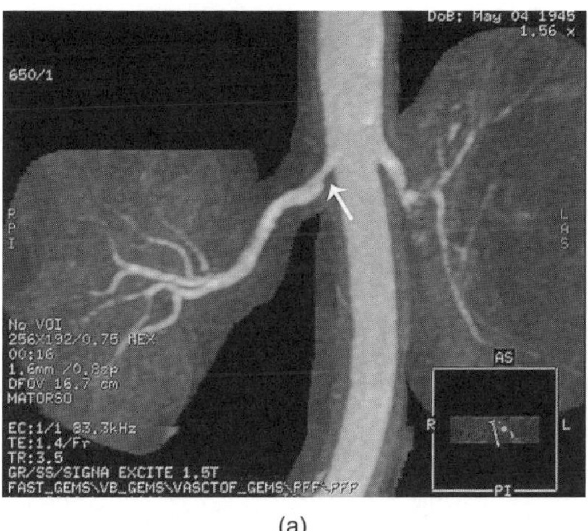 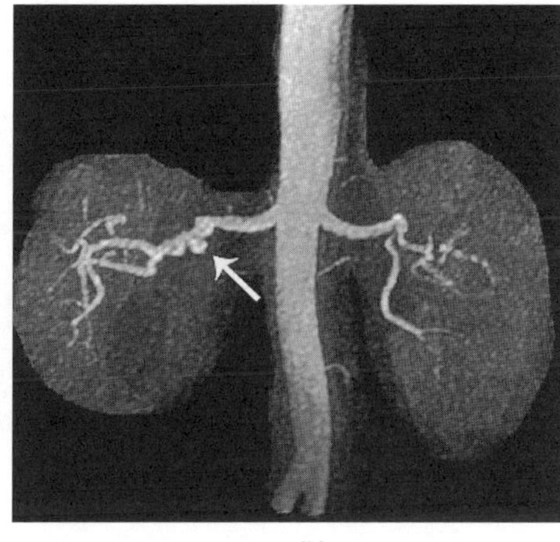

(a)   (b)

Figure 3.5 Oblique coronal maximum intensity projection (MIP) images from a 3D MR angiograms. An eccentric narrowing at the origin of the right renal artery (arrow) typical of a stenosis secondary to atherosclerosis (a) is contrasted with the multiple stenoses in the mid right renal artery (arrow) of a patient with fibromuscular dysplasia (b).

- An eccentric area of narrowing near the renal artery origin indicative of atherosclerotic RAS. Calcification of the eccentric plaque is not as well depicted with MRA as with CTA.

- Multiple web-like areas of narrowing interspersed with focal areas of dilatation (beaded appearance) in the mid to distal main renal artery indicative of the most common form of fibromuscular dysplasia.

References

Chobanian AV, Bakris GL, Black HR *et al.* (2003) Seventh report of the Joint National Committee on Prevention, Detection, Evaluation, and Treatment of High Blood Pressure. *Hypertension* **42**(6): 1206–1252.

Glockner JF, Vrtiska TJ. (2007) Renal MR and CT angiography: current concepts. *Abdom. Imaging* **32**(3): 407–420.

Pellerito JS, Zwiebel WJ. (2005) Ultrasound assessment of native renal vessels and renal allografts. In: Zwiebel WJ, Pellerito JS (eds) *Introduction to Vascular Ultrasonography*, 5th edn. Elsevier Saunders, Philadelphia, pp. 611–636.

Ziessman HA, O'Malley JP, Thrall JH. (2006) Genitourinary system. In: Thrall JH (Ed.), *Nuclear Medicine: The Requisites in Radiology*, 3rd edn. Elsevier Mosby, Philadelphia, pp. 215–262.

4
Renal Masses

Philip J. Kenney

Professor and Chair of Radiology, University of Arkansas for Medical Science

4.1 Introduction

Renal masses are detected in several different clinical scenarios. This chapter will present cases illustrative of the most common such settings, demonstrating methods of diagnosis. In general, there are three main goals of imaging:

- *detection* – is there in fact a pathologic mass;
- *diagnosis* – what is the specific etiology of the mass;
- *if the mass is malignant* – what is the stage, which will have critical impact on treatment.

4.2 Symptomatic renal carcinoma

Clinical features

- The classic triad:
  - palpable mass
  - flank pain
  - hematuria.

Urogenital Imaging: A Problem-oriented Approach   Edited by Sameh K. Morcos and Henrik S. Thomsen
© 2009 John Wiley & Sons, Ltd

Imaging approach

- Sonography often will detect the presence of a renal mass.

  - Computed Tomography (CT) is the best choice for initial evaluation, as it has high sensitivity and specificity as well as staging accuracy (Fig. 4.1).

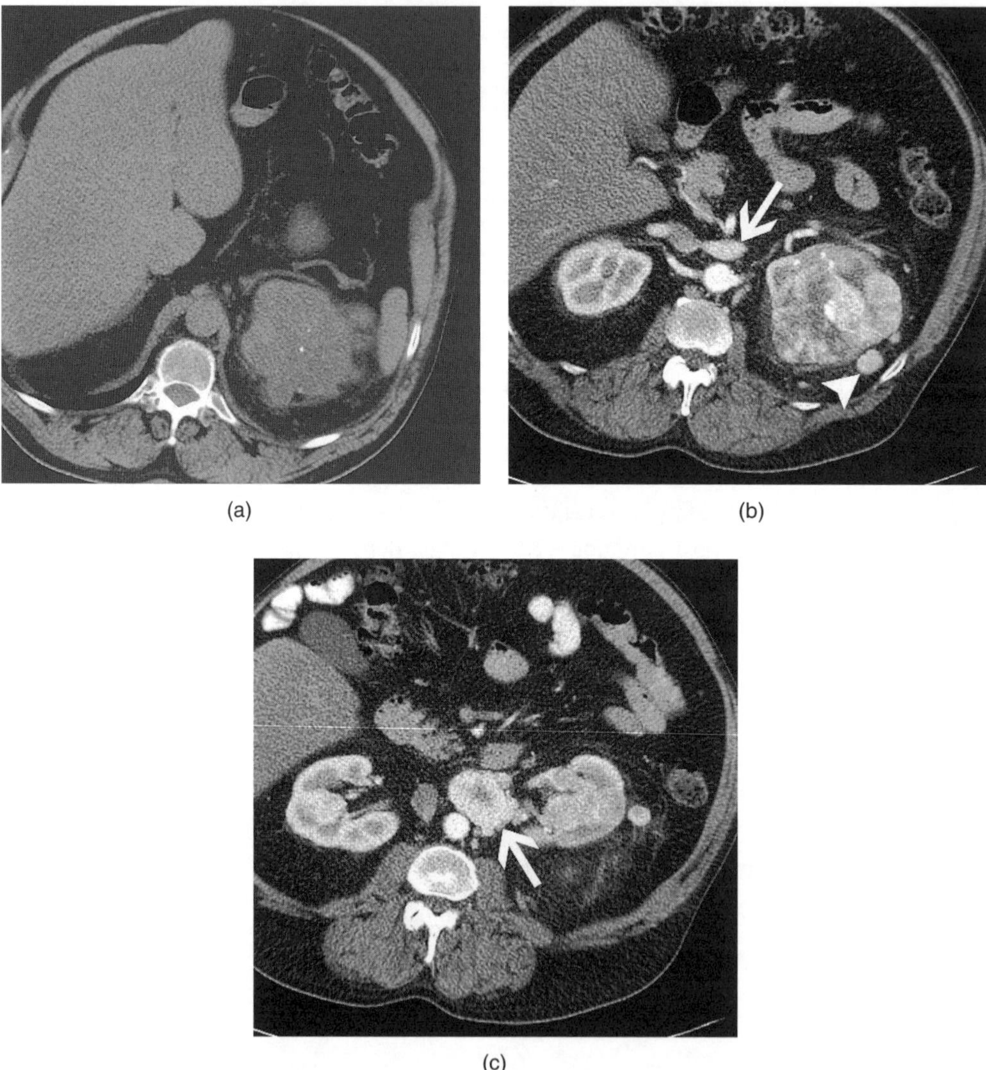

(a)

(b)

(c)

Figure 4.1 A 70-year-old male, left flank pain, and hematuria, palpable mass in left abdomen. (a) Unenhanced CT shows lobular soft tissue mass of upper pole left kidney. (b) Contrast enhanced CT shows heterogeneous enhancement. Note nodule in perirenal space (arrowhead) indicating extension beyond renal capsule (Stage 2); left renal vein is uninvolved (arrow). (c) More caudal image shows more perirenal extension but also enlarged node (4 cm) (Arrow). At open nephrectomy a 10.7 × 6.7 cm clear cell carcinoma with positive nodes was resected; patient later developed recurrence.

Table 4.1 Features of classic renal carcinoma

Solid, may be higher or lower attenuation than normal parenchyma precontrast
Clear enhancement, often very vascular and heterogeneous
Calcification common (20%)
Tendency for renal vein and caval invasion
Nodal disease
Liver, bone lung metastases
MRI: medium signal intensity T1, may be hemorrhagic high signal areas; heterogeneous high signal T2, heterogeneous enhancement following intravenous gadolinium compounds

- ○ Technique
  - CT scanning should be done with images both before and after intravenous contrast.
  - Because hypervascular liver metastases may occur, imaging in arterial as well as portal venous phases is preferred.
  - Such masses are easily detected, and have typical imaging features (Table 4.1).

- If a patient cannot tolerate intravenous iodinated contrast for any reason, MRI without and with intravenous gadolinium contrast including T1- and T2-weighted images is an excellent alternative, with diagnostic accuracy similar to CT and perhaps better staging accuracy.

- MRI is particularly effective at detecting or excluding venous invasion and graphically displaying the exact extent (Fig. 4.2). Most masses in this category are readily recognizable as malignant, typical renal carcinomas (RCC).

4.3 Incidental renal masses

- Very commonly, as non-invasive imaging is used for an ever wider variety of indications, a renal mass may be detected when unsuspected.

- An increasing proportion of RCC are discovered incidentally, and such tumors tend to be smaller, lower stage and more curable than those presenting symptomatically.

- There are many non-malignant etiologies of incidental renal masses.

- A solid mass or complex renal cyst seen at sonography may need further evaluation with CT (or MRI) done with images before and after contrast.

- Doppler evidence of flow within the mass, including flow within septations in a cystic mass, usually indicates the mass is malignant (Fig. 4.3), although benign renal lesions (including angiomyolipoma and oncocytoma) may show internal flow.

- The incidental renal masses should fall into one of several categories after diagnostic CT (or MRI): Clearly malignant (usually RCC), clearly benign (including typical simple cyst), or indeterminate.

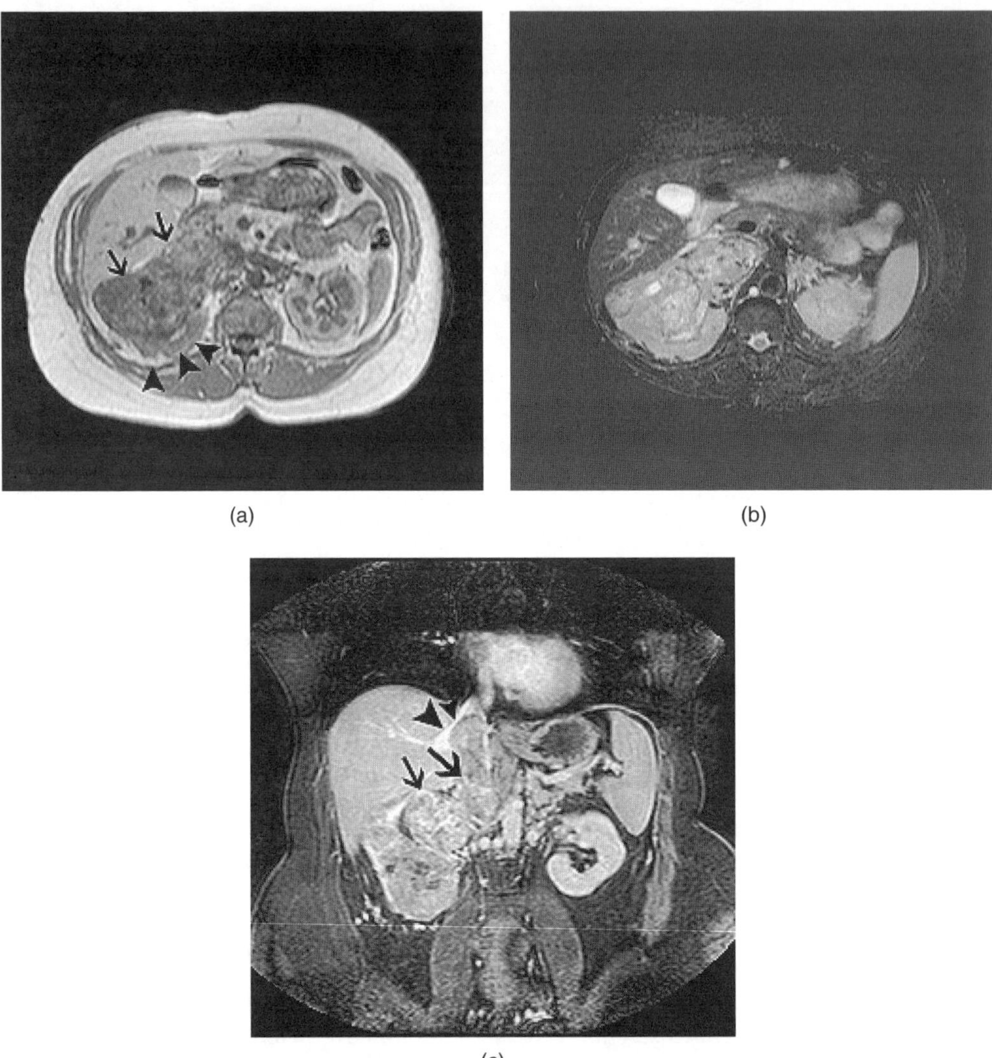

(a)

(b)

(c)

Figure 4.2　A 61-year-old female with right abdominal mass on exam, gross hematuria and flank pain. A right renal mass with probable caval extension of uncertain degree was seen on CT. (a) An axial T1 MRI shows a heterogeneous medium signal intensity mass (arrows) arising from the right kidney (arrowheads remaining normal parenchyma). The mass bulges medially into the location of the inferior vena cava. (b) On fat suppressed T2-weighted image the tumor is of overall high signal and very heterogeneous typical of RCC. No liver metastases or adenopathy were evident. (c) Coronal gadolinium enhanced T1-weighted image shows the mass enhances, and clearly extends into the inferior vena cava, with enhancement of the tumor thrombus (arrows). The upper extent of the tumor thrombus is clearly shown at the diaphragm (arrowheads) but not extending into right atrium. This large stage 3B clear cell carcinoma was successfully resected and the patient shows no recurrence 2 years later.

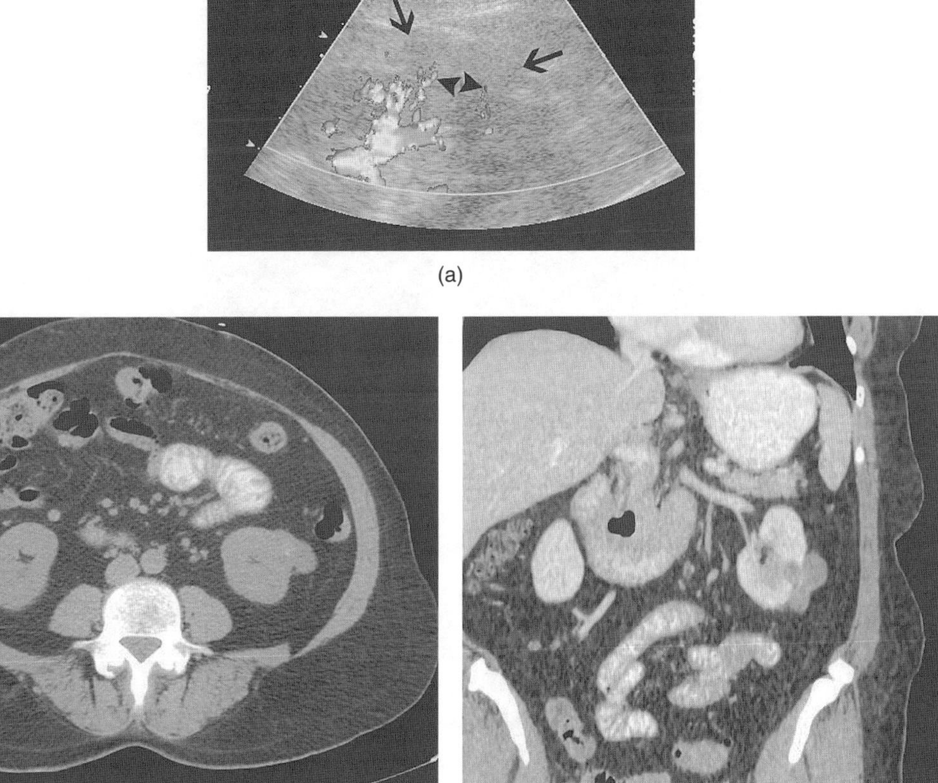

Figure 4.3 This 54-year-old female had sonography done because of abdominal pain later discovered to be diverticulitis. (a) There is a left lower pole hypoechoic mass(arrows) with flow in septations on color Doppler(arrowheads). (b) Unenhanced CT image shows the lobular mass with fleck of calcification; attenuation 41 Hounsfield units (HU). (c) Coronal reformatted image of post-contrast CT shows the exophytic mass with septal enhancement (attenuation 66 HU). This typical cystic RCC should be classified Bosniak Type 4 by imaging.

- Often, it is readily recognizable that the mass is most likely a primary renal carcinoma, with typical features as described in Table 4.1 (Fig. 4.4).
- It is often possible to determine that a mass is a recognizable benign entity:
  - Benign cysts are very common and can usually be recognized as such.
  - The classification developed by Bosniak may be useful to place cysts in appropriate category according to risk of malignancy (Table 4.2) (Figs 4.3 and 4.4).
  - A renal mass containing true fat is almost always a benign angiomyolipoma (Fig. 4.5).

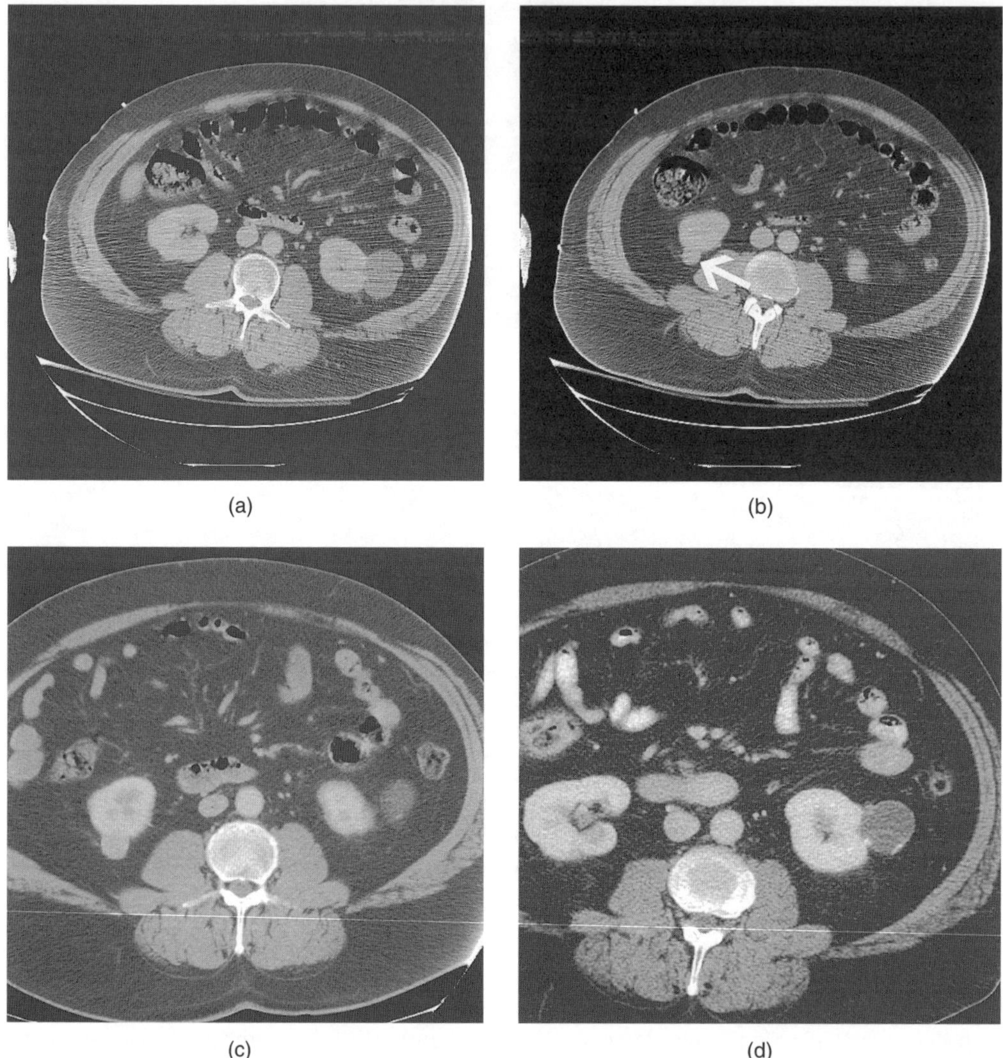

(a)

(b)

(c)

(d)

Figure 4.4   This 55-year-old male had routine contrast enhanced CT after motor vehicle collision. (a) A probably simple cyst is seen at lower pole of left kidney. (b) A smaller lesion (arrow) at lower pole of right kidney appears similar in attenuation to renal parenchyma worrisome for neoplasm. (c) Follow-up CT after contrast showed enhancement in the right lower pole mass (was 36 HU before and 78 HU after contrast). The left sided lesion showed no contrast enhancement (13 HU before and after contrast). A 1.8 cm clear cell carcinoma was removed with partial nephrectomy from the lower pole of the right kidney. The left renal lesion was followed up. (d) Follow-up CT 3 years later shows the cyst is stable although has developed peripheral calcification.

Table 4.2 Bosniak Classification

Category 1: meets all criteria of simple cyst, 100% should be benign

Category 2: minimally complicated cyst-lack of through transmission, internal echoes, high attenuation on CT, thin septae, few small calcifications on septae or wall, but no enhancing solid component: 90–95% benign

Category 3: Moderately complex cyst-more internal echoes, thick or irregular septations, thick or nodular wall, extensive calcifications, questionable enhancement (8–15 HU change): 50% malignant

Category 4: Cystic malignancy: complex largely cystic mass but with definite solid component with flow on US, or definite enhancement on CT or MRI

- Sometimes incidental renal masses do not fall into either clearly malignant or clearly benign lesions:
  - Complex cysts (Fig. 4.3) including hemorrhagic cysts or lesions with questionable enhancement.
  - Multilocular cystic nephroma produces a multiseptated solitary mass in a single kidney-although benign such lesions are difficult to distinguish from cystic RCC.
  - A multicystic dysplastic kidney in the adult is usually seen as a small collection of cysts in the renal fossa without function and usually no enhancement-these are usually incidental and can be followed (Fig. 4.6).
  - Enhancement after contrast is the most critical feature of a malignant lesion.
    - An increase of over 15–20 Hounsfield units (HU) after contrast is virtually certain enhancement; a change of less than 10 is not considered significant.
    - Small increase in attenuation (10–15 HU) can result artifactually from volume averaging with small lesion, or pseudoenhancement.
    - The majority of renal masses of soft tissue attenuation with clear enhancement are malignant, however, benign renal masses uncommonly occur with those characteristics, including oncocytoma, lipid poor angiomyolipomas and leiomyomas.
    - PET is of limited use, as only about half of the malignant renal masses show abnormal uptake (Fig. 4.7).
    - *Oncocytomas*
      - Small oncocytoma demonstrate features and enhancement similar to small RCC
      - Large oncocytoma often have central scar that simulates central necrosis, so that these are often treated as if RCC.
      - Diagnosis may be possible with biopsy especially if immunostains are done, but it is controversial whether all solid renal masses should be biopsied.
    - Lesions that remain indeterminate after optimal quality CT or MRI often are followed.
      - Over time lesions may evolve, making diagnosis of RCC possible, and if small when presenting rarely metastasize until well over 3 cm.

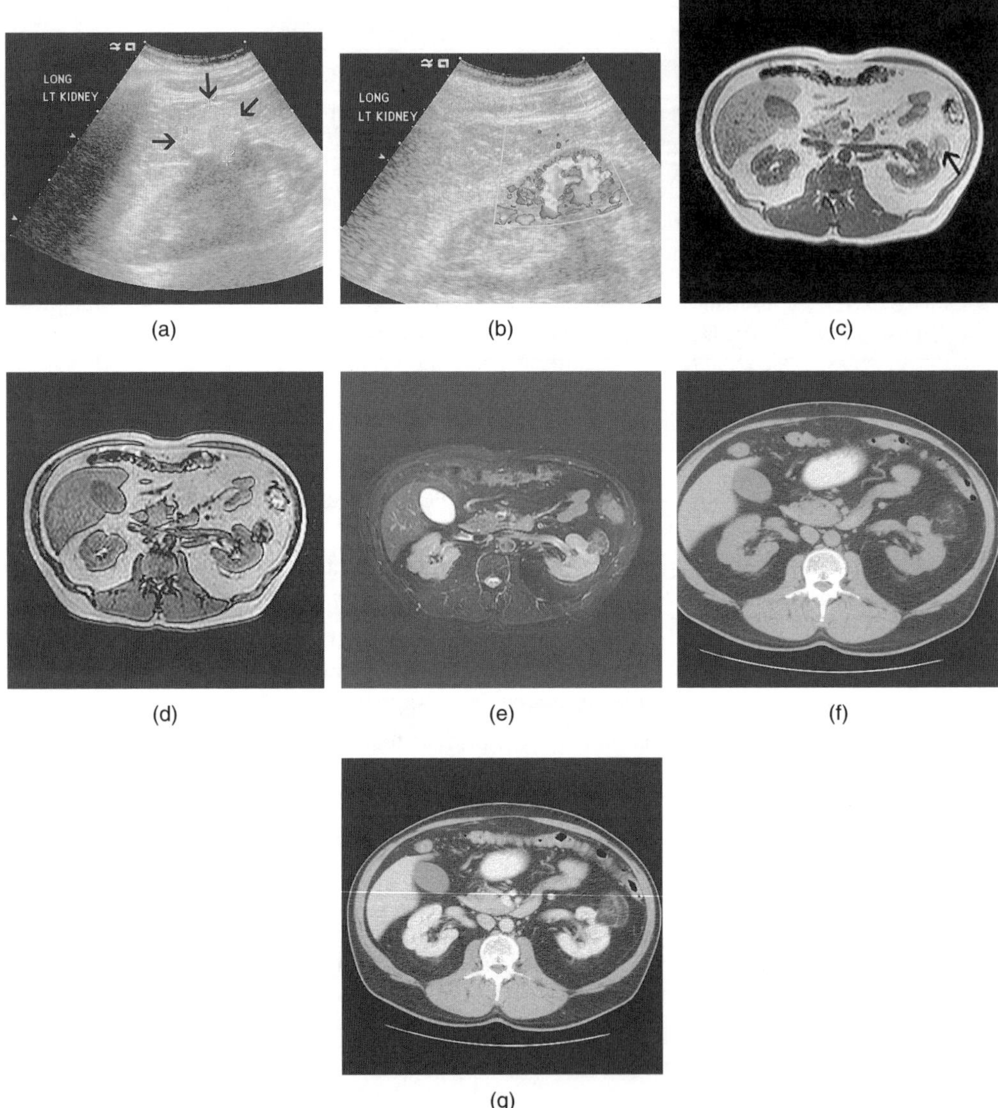

Figure 4.5 Sonography was requested due to abnormal liver enzymes. (a) An exophytic hyperechoic (3.4 × 3.7 cm) mass protrudes from the left kidney (arrows). (b) Internal flow is shown on color Doppler. (c) MRI T1 axial image shows hyperintensity within the mass (arrow). (d) Opposed phase image shows areas of signal drop within the mass, indicating fat. (e) The mass is low attenuation on fat suppressed T2 image, excluding RCC. (f) One year follow-up was done with CT due to pain; unenhanced image shows the lesion is of fat attenuation. (g) Some enhancement is noted following contrast; note the markedly exophytic growth pattern with small footprint on the kidney, typical of many AML's. Although this is clearly a benign AML, due to increasing size (4.8 × 5.2 cm) it was embolized.

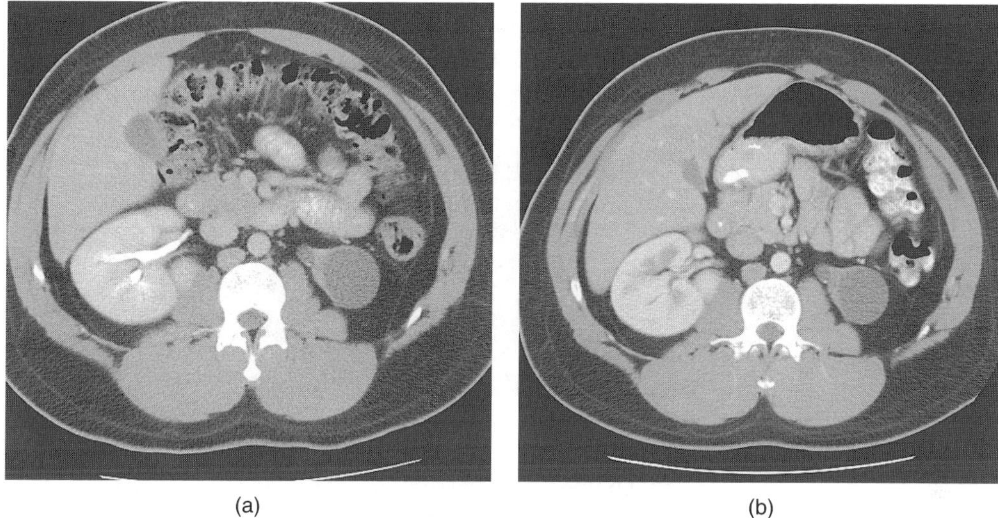

(a)   (b)

Figure 4.6 Due to back pain, CT was done in this 30-year-old male. (a) A non-functioning atrophic left kidney with numerous cysts is noted. (b) Follow-up 3 years later shows the lesion is stable, with no enhancement on post-contrast images. This is typical appearance of multicystic dysplastic kidney presenting in adulthood.

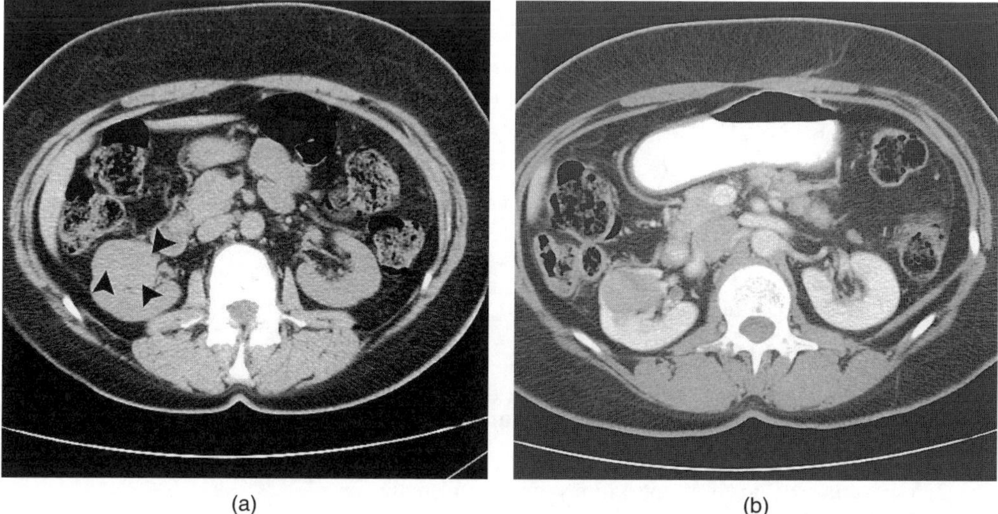

(a)   (b)

Figure 4.7 This 48-year-old female developed right flank pain. (a) Unenhanced CT was done searching for kidney stones. No stone or evidence of obstruction was seen, but a suspicious area of fullness in mid right kidney (arrowheads) which measured 32 HU was noted. (b) Further evaluation with enhanced CT shows the lesion is homogeneously enhancing, 104 HU, with no evidence of metastases. (c) Since CT showed a pulmonary nodule, a PET/CT was carried out. The mass showed no FDG uptake. Nephrectomy was done revealing Stage 1 granular cell RCC.

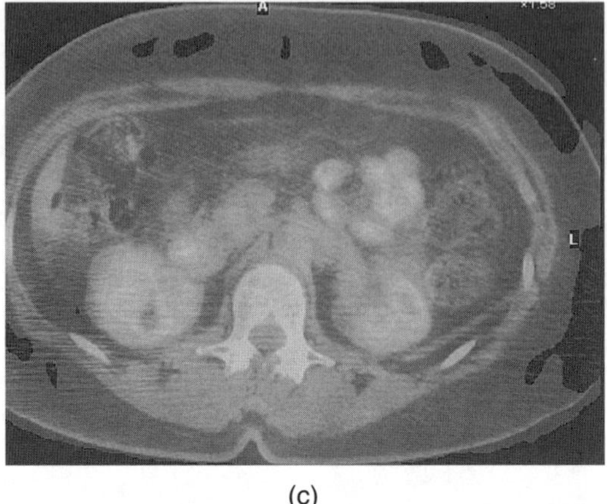

(c)

Figure 4.7   *(Continued)*

    ○ How long a renal mass must be followed remains controversial; since some low grade RCC is slow growing. At least 2 years and possibly 5 years follow-up may be advised.

4.4 Patients with a known cancer (other than RCC)

- A renal mass with features typical of RCC (single medium to large, enhancing mass, with exophytic growth pattern – ball rather than bean) should be considered RCC until proven otherwise by biopsy (Fig. 4.10).

- A patient with two primary cancers may be cured of both if each is treated optimally.

- Metastases to the kidney commonly have a distinctive pattern:

  ○ They are often found in association with metastases in other organs.

  ○ They are usually small, bilateral and/or multiple.

  ○ They usually do not have an exophytic growth pattern, and even when large tend to expand the kidney but do not alter the surface contour (bean not ball effect (Figs. 4.11 and 4.12).

  ○ Lymphoma may involve the kidney in several patterns:

    ■ direct extension from retroperitioneal disease (Fig. 4.13)

    ■ multifocal small hypovascular renal masses

    ■ perirenal disease or

    ■ diffuse enlargement of the kidney.

  ○ Biopsy may be useful in confirming the nature of renal metastases, which may respond well to systemic therapy (Fig. 4.13) while RCC is best treated surgically.

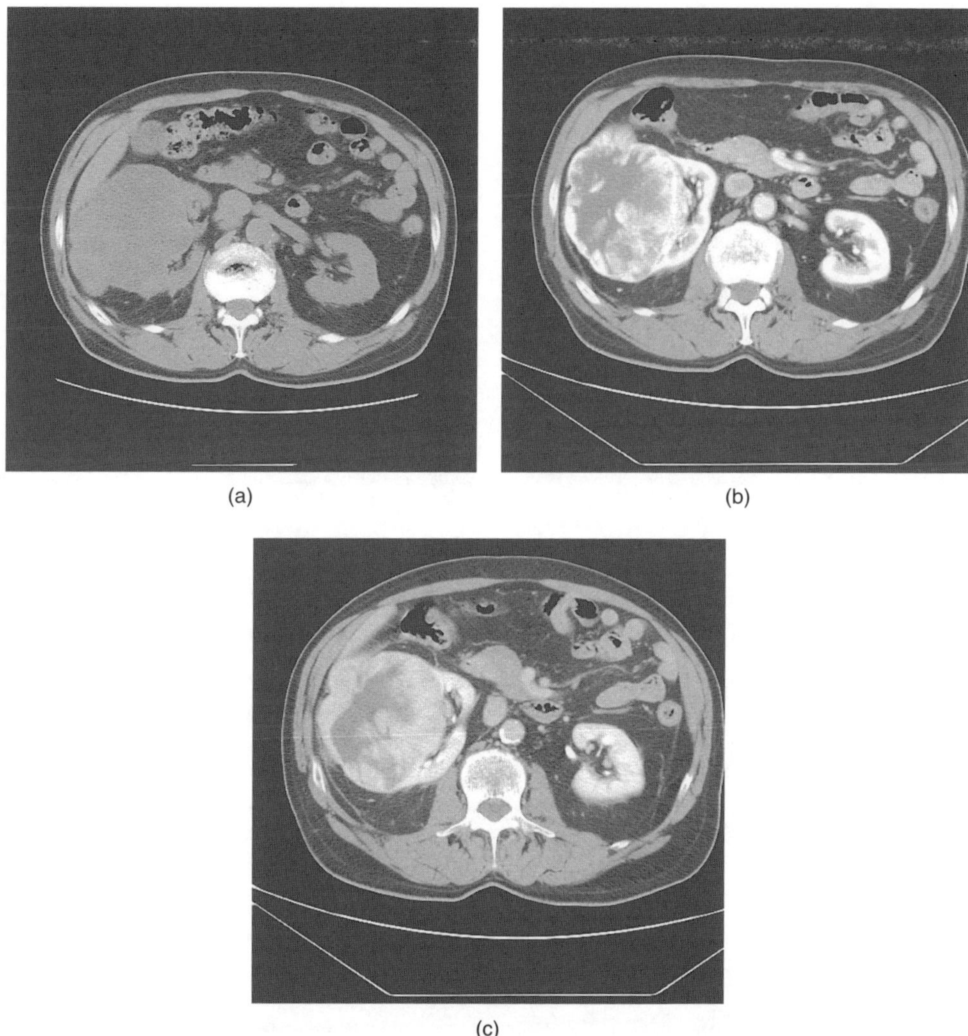

Figure 4.8 A nuclear bone scan done for research on bone aging showed a defect in the right kidney in this asymptomatic 75-year-old male. (a) Unenhanced CT reveals a very large low attenuation mass involving the right kidney. (b) Arterial phase CT shows exuberant peripheral enhancement. (c) Delayed image shows considerable enhancement but central low attenuation. Nephrectomy was done after indeterminate biopsy and revealed a large oncocytoma Large lesions such as this commonly have central scar which is not clearly distinguishable from central necrosid thus there is overlap of imaging features between large RCC and large oncocytoma.

4.5 Renal mass in patients with symptoms

- A renal mass may be detected in a patient with signs or symptoms which may be non-specific but possibly associated with a renal source.

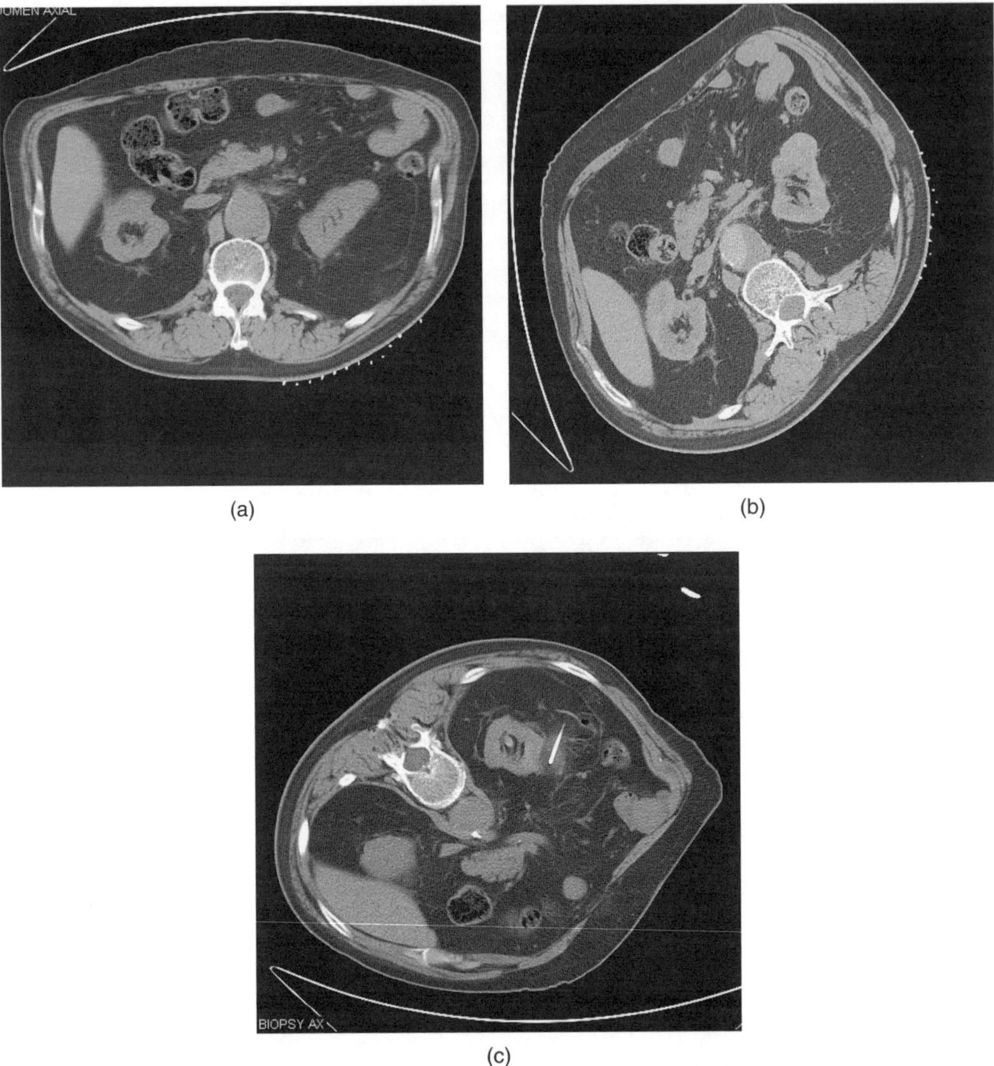

(a)   (b)

(c)

Figure 4.9   A solid mass lesion in the left kidney treated with ablative therapy. (a) Unenhanced image shows bulge from upper pole of left (attenuation 22 HU). (b) After contrast for better definition of mass, attenuation was increased to 79 HU. (c) Percutaneous biopsy was performed followed by ablation with cryotherapy. The pathology result of the biopsy was oncocytoma.

- *Flank pain, back pain, renal colic with or without hematuria* commonly is investigated with unenhanced CT.

  - If an exophytic renal mass is seen, particularly if the attenuation is higher than water (>20 HU), a contrast enhanced study should be done (Fig. 4.7).

  - Small non-contour deforming renal masses can be missed with unenhanced CT. Thus, persistent hematuria without an explanation such as urolithiasis, should also stimulate contrast enhanced examination.

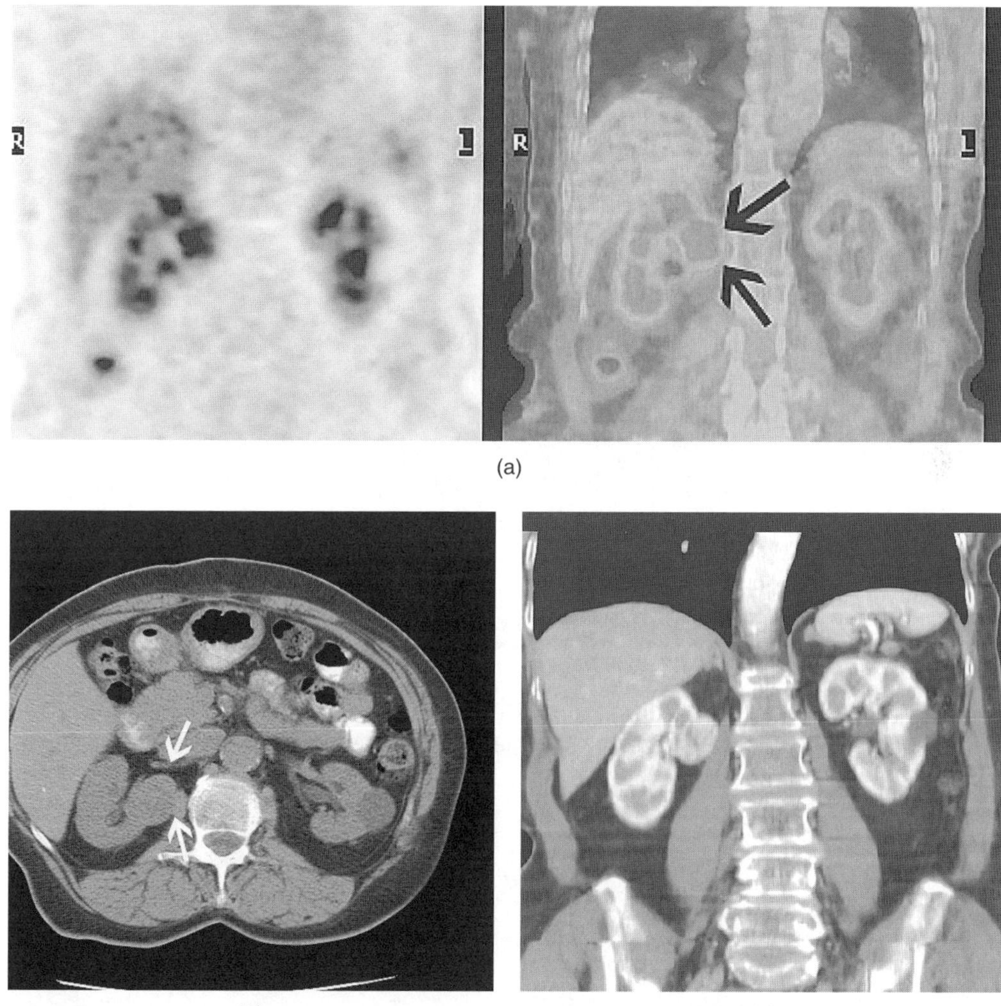

Figure 4.10 Evaluation for breast cancer in the 54-year-old female included PET/CT. (a) A coronal PET and Fused image of the kidneys reveals a hypermetabolic bulging region in the upper pole of the right kidney (arrows). (b) Unenhanced CT shows a right sided mass (arrows) with attenuation 31 HU and left sided mass 10 HU. (c) Coronal reformatted enhanced CT image shows the mass (148 HU) bulging medially from the right kidney whose shape is otherwise preserved. This is the typical exophytic growth pattern of RCC. Note the left sided Bosniak 1 simple cyst with no enhancement post contrast.

- Investigation of hematuria is covered else where in the book. RCC is a not uncommon cause of hematuria (Figs. 4.1 and 4.2).

- Urothelial tumors also can cause hematuria, although upper tract transitional carcinoma (TCC) is considerably less common than RCC.

  - TCC can usually be detected with pre- and post-contrast axial CT (Fig. 4.14).

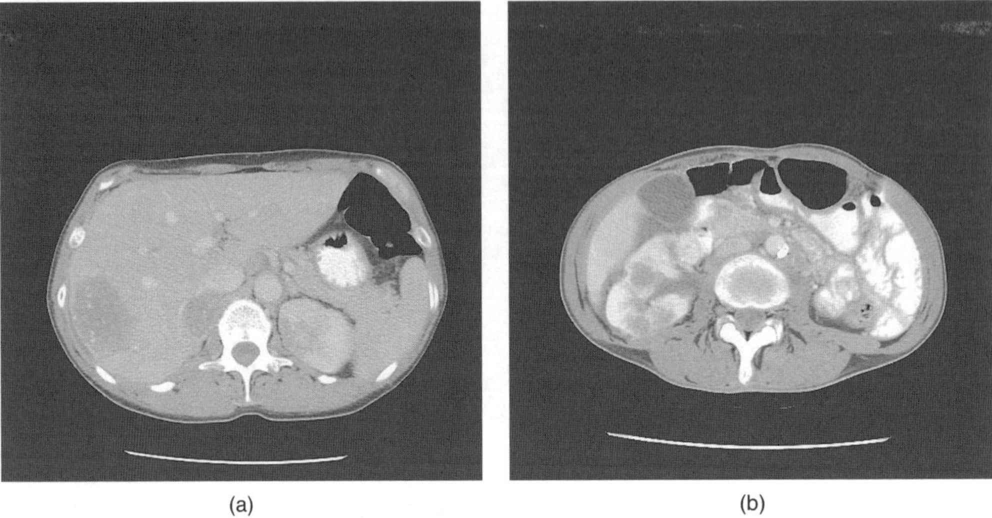

(a)   (b)

Figure 4.11 A 50-year-old female have lung secondaries from cancer of the colon. (a) Staging CT demonstrates metastases in liver, right adrenal and upper pole of left kidney. (b) A more caudal image shows right renal lesions typical of metastases to the kidney (small, multiple with endophytic growth pattern, no bulging of the renal contour). This patient was treated with chemotherapy.

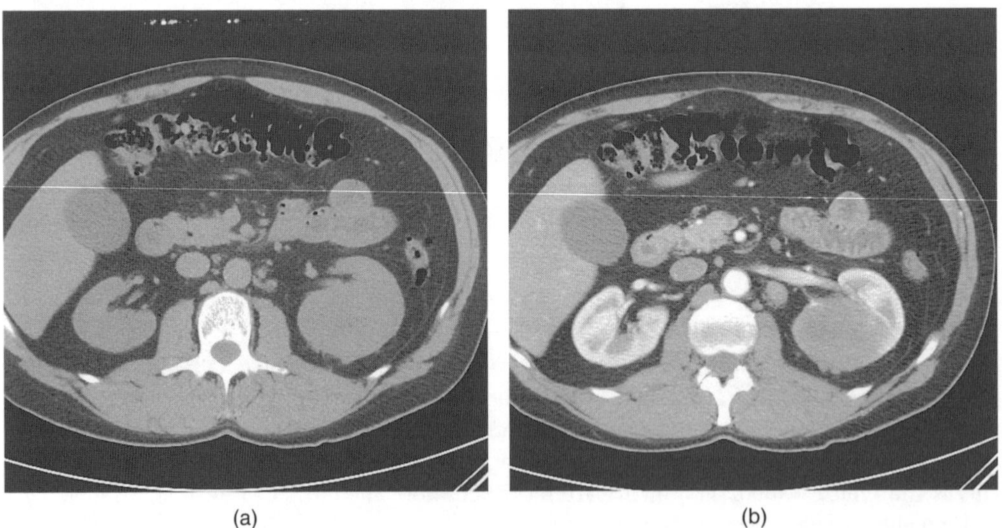

(a)   (b)

Figure 4.12 A 51-year-old male suffering from lung cancer. (a) Staging CT shows soft tissue fullness in upper pole of the left kidney. (b) Contrast enhanced CT shows a large mildly enhancing lesion in left kidney, not causing bulging of the renal contour. (c) Coronal reformatted image nicely demonstrates the 'bean' growth pattern of this mass, although the kidney is slightly expanded there is no alteration of contour. Since this was somewhat atypical of metastasis (single large renal mass without other abdominal metastases) a biopsy was done which revealed metastatatic bronchogenic carcinoma.

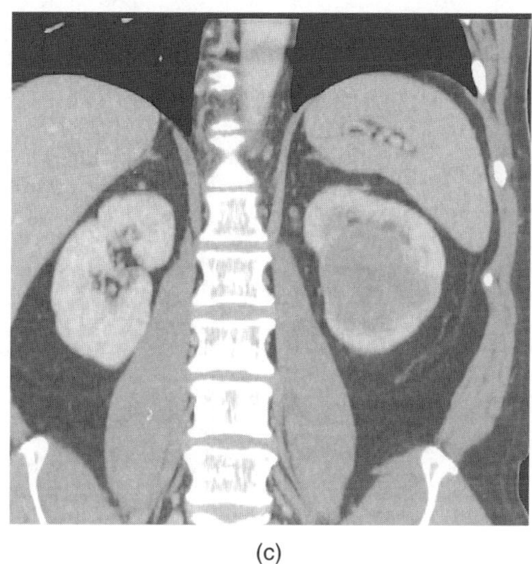

(c)

Figure 4.12 *(Continued)*

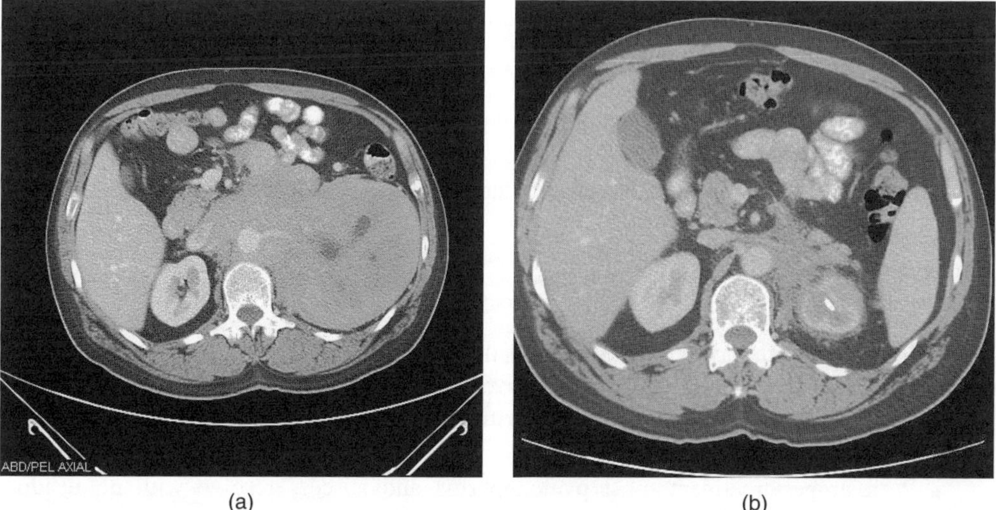

(a) (b)

Figure 4.13 A 56-year-old male presented with hematuria. (a) A CT of the abdomen reveals very extensive retroperitoneal lymphadenopathy extending directly into and expanding the left kidney. This is a typical growth pattern of renal lymphoma, with multifocal renal masses, perirenal disease, or diffuse enlargement also occurring. Percutaneous biopsy of the retroperitoneal mass was done revealing B cell lymphoma. (b) Follow-up after chemotherapy 4 months later shows marked improvement with the kidney returning to near normal.

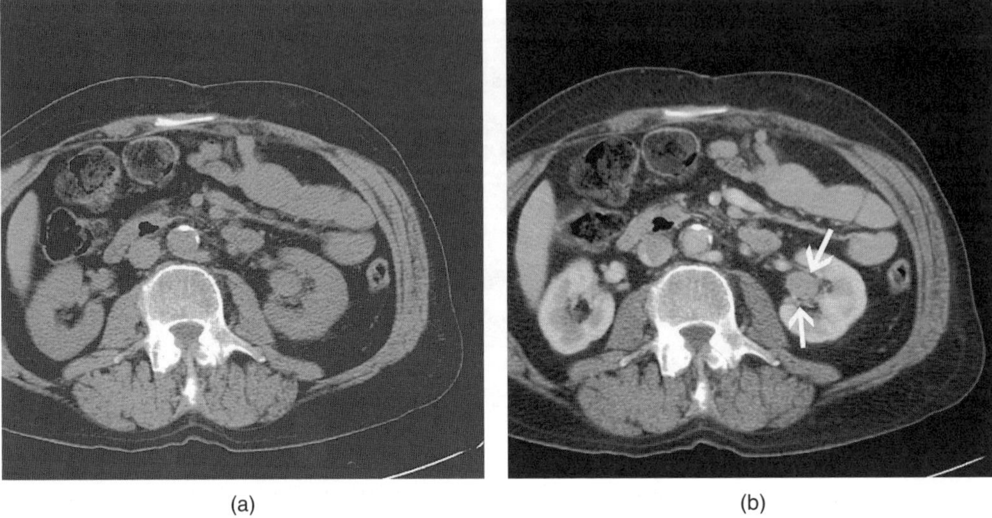

(a)　　(b)

Figure 4.14 A 76-year-old male with long smoking history developed hematuria. (a) Unenhanced CT image shows expansion of renal pelvis, measuring 28 HU thus of soft tissue attenuation, not hydronephrosis. (b) After contrast the region (arrows) measures 65 HU, thus is enhancing excluding blood clot. Even without opacification of collecting system, or reformatted images, this is diagnostic of renal pelvic TCC. High grade TCC confined to collecting system was confirmed at nephroureterectomy.

- Most renal TCC occurs in the renal pelvis, but may produce a central infiltrative mass with endophytic (bean not ball) growth pattern which is more typical of TCC rather than RCC, although there can be overlap, and RCC can invade the pelvis (Fig. 4.15).

- *A renal mass may be discovered in a patient with signs and symptoms of urinary tract infection*

  - A renal abscess produces a focal mass
    - Imaging appearance of an abscess whether on US, CT, or MRI can overlap with that of tumor with central necrosis. However, in the clinical setting, of infection correct diagnosis can be suggested with confirmation by percutaneous aspiration, culture and drainage (Fig. 4.16).
    - With proper treatment most pyelonephritis and abscess resolve with no residua, except for possible focal scar.
    - Chronic, indolent, or previously treated pyogenic infections including uncommon infections such as tuberculosis and echinococcus can result in a complex, often calcified mass (Fig. 4.17). In such cases, prior imaging studies may be useful, as the appearance can simulate a renal tumor.

4.6 Vascular lesions presenting as a renal mass

- Renal artery aneurysms and arteriovenous malformations can produce a mass-like lesion.

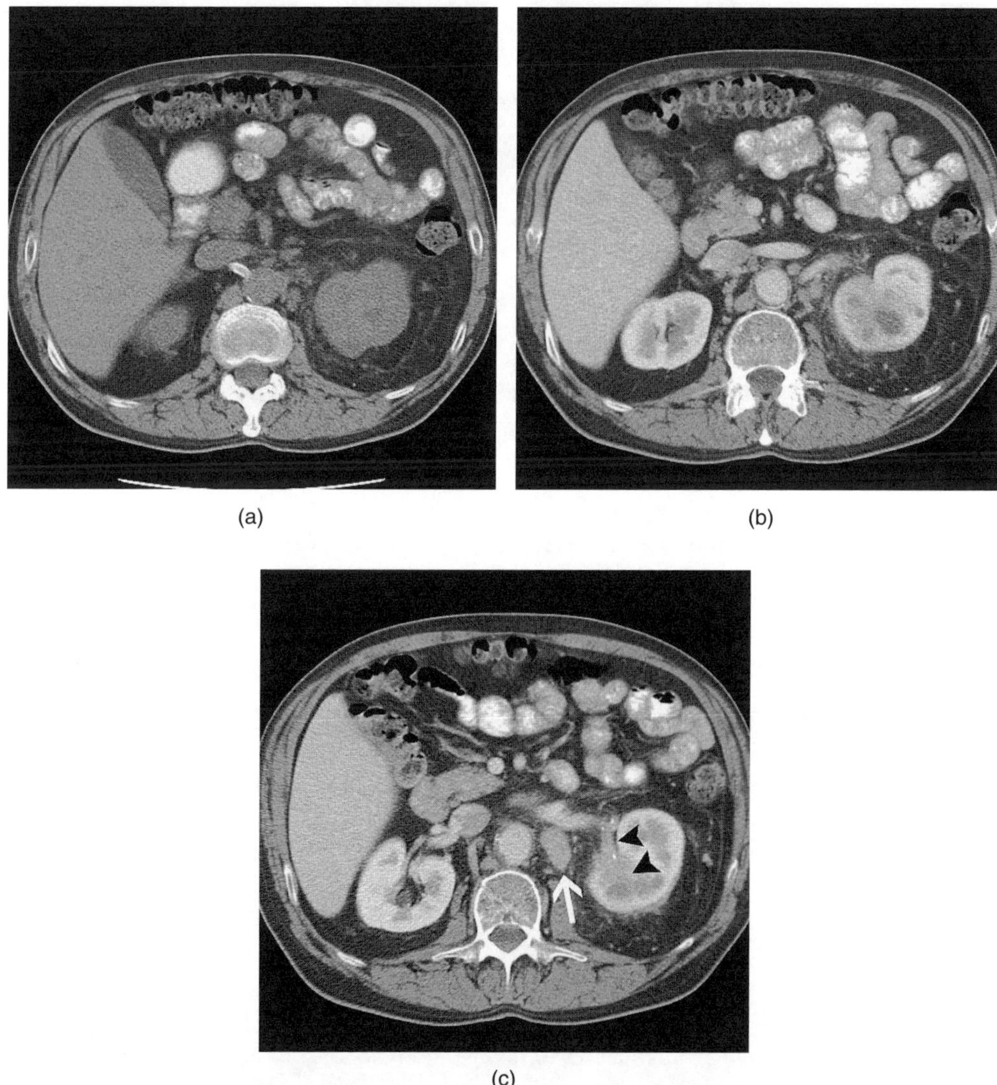

Figure 4.15 A patient with a history of intermittent hematuria over 2 years. (a) Unenhanced image shows enlargement of the upper pole of the left kidney (40 HU), with stranding and nodularity in retroperitoneum and perinephric space. (b) Heterogeneous enhancement after contrast (80HU) evident, with central location of mass. (c) More caudally, the mass involves collecting system (arrowheads) and enlarged nodes are present (arrow). This could represent either atypical RCC invading pelvis or TCC. Nephrectomy was carried out and revealed a 5 cm invasive urothelial tumor with positive nodes.

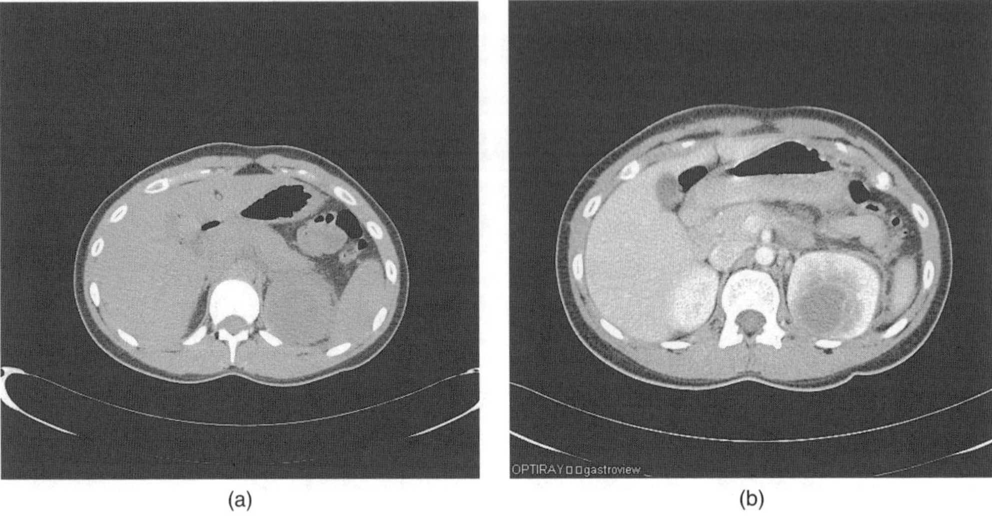

(a) (b)

Figure 4.16 A 19-year-old female with left flank pain and fever. (a) Unenhanced CT shows low attenuation mass left upper pole. (b) Enhanced CT shows non-enhancing center with enhancing rim, typical appearance of renal abscess. Percutaneous aspiration of the lesion produced pus, a drain was placed and abscess resolved on antibiotics.

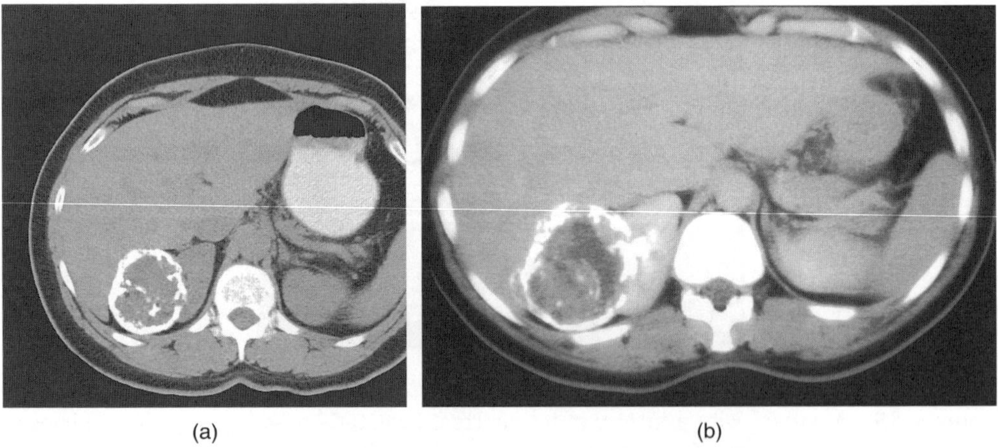

(a) (b)

Figure 4.17 Following motor vehicle collision, CT revealed a calcified renal mass. (a) Unenhanced image shows dense calcification in and on periphery of upper pole mass in the right kidney. (b) No internal enhancement shown on post-contrast image. Patient stated she was diagnosed with echinococcus many years ago and treated. Tuberculosis, old hematoma or pyogenic abscess might also cause similar appearance. Calcified renal carcinoma usually will show some area of enhancement.

- Can produce various signs and symptoms including hematuria.

- These lesions should be readily recognized on Doppler sonography or contrast enhanced CT or MRI, but can be misconstrued as a mass if seen on unenhanced studies (Fig. 4.18).

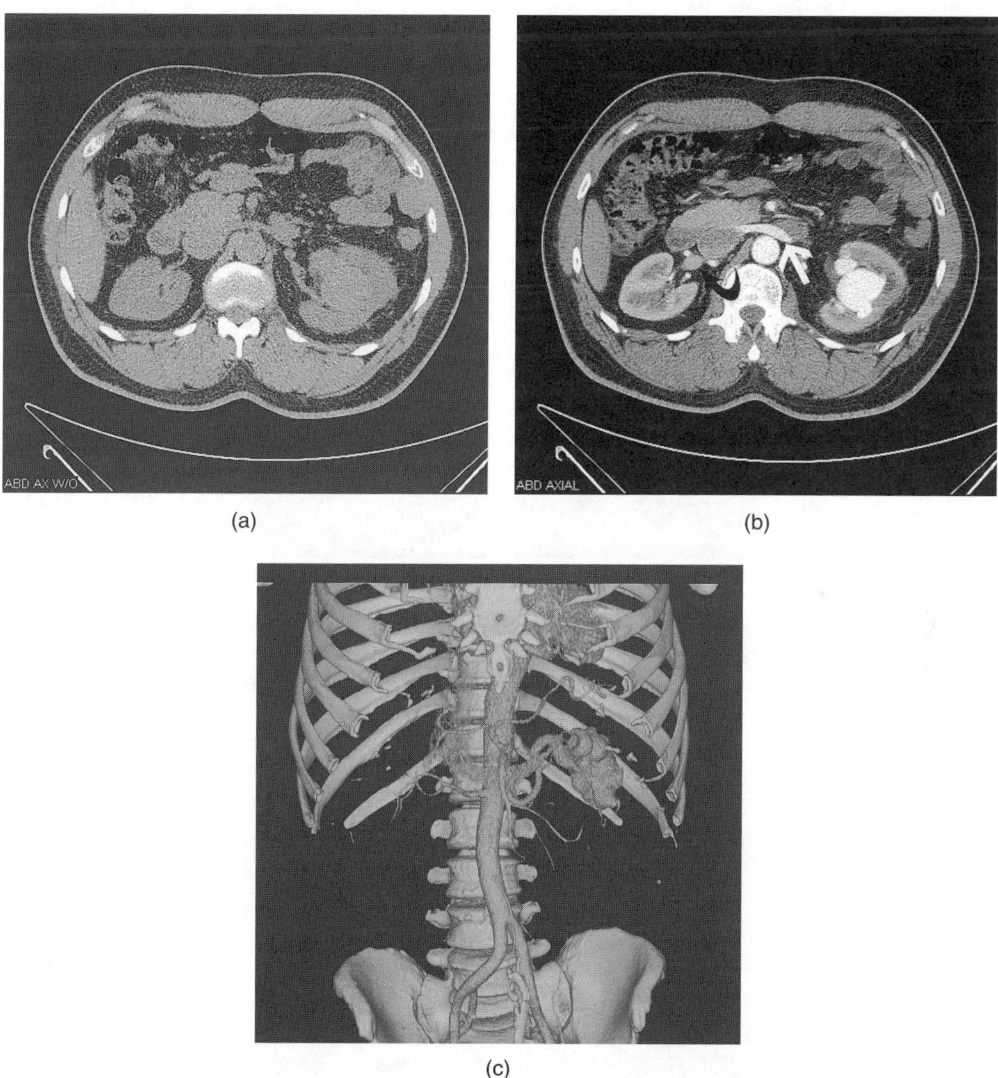

Figure 4.18 A 51-year-old male had a CT examination to investigate epigastric pain. (a) Unenhanced image shows a central mass of soft tissue attenuation in the left kidney suspicious of collecting system lesion. (b) Arterial phase image after contrast shows enhancement of the lesion similar to that of aorta; note brighter enhancement of left renal vein (arrow) compared to right (curved arrow) indicative of shunting. (c) Coronal reformatted 3D image displays the large central AVM. Without contrast and properly timed techniques such lesions may be misconstrued as neoplastic.

4.7 Renal mass in patients with cystic disease

- Patients with Von Hippel Lindau disease commonly develop multiple renal cysts as well as clearly increased incidence of RCC including cystic RCC. Other manifestations of the disease, pancreatic cyst, pheochromocytoma, can suggest the diagnosis.

- Tuberous sclerosis patients most commonly develop multiple AML's, which may become large and bleed, but renal cysts and RCC also can occur.

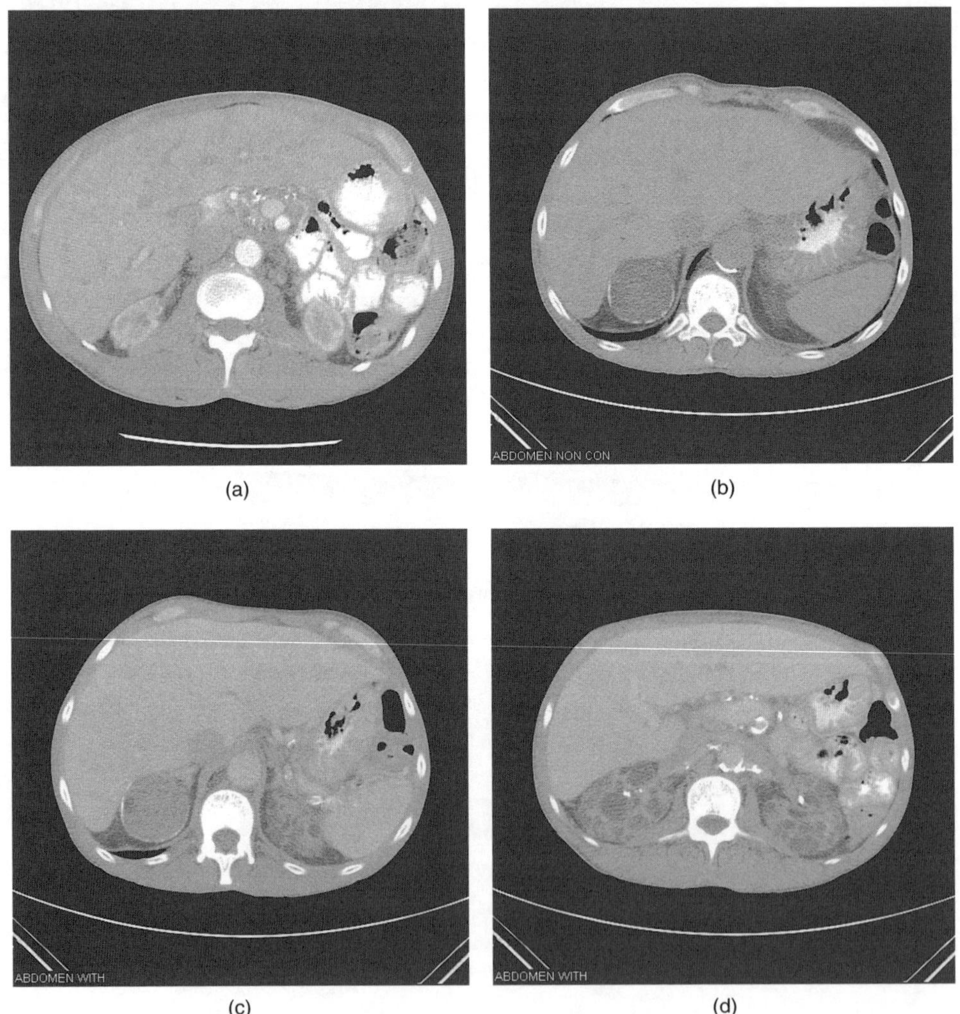

(a)   (b)

(c)   (d)

Figure 4.19 A 47-year-old male been on hemodialysis for 8 years previously. (a) Baseline CT 1999 shows atrophic kidneys with very tiny cysts. (b) Unenhanced CT 2007 shows right upper pole mass with calcified periphery, central attenuation 40 HU. (c) Following contrast, central attenuation 80HU. This enhancement excludes hemorrhagic cyst which otherwise might be considered. Peripheral calcification may occur in RCC. The right kidney was resected and presence of clear cell RCC was confirmed.

- Acquired cystic disease of the kidney, seen in patients after several years of dialysis have a clearly increased propensity to develop RCC (Fig. 4.19).

4.8 Treatment

- Resection with open nephrectomy holds out the best chance for cure of lower stage RCC.

- Recently, some new systemic therapies including angiogenesis inhibitors have shown promising results even in patients with widespread RCC.

- Patients with localized RCC and small tumors treated with a variety of nephron sparing techniques whether open or laparoscopic have shown excellent results.

- Non-surgical ablation with radiofrequency or cryotherapy is also appealing as a relatively non-invasive treatment, with results to date promising although very long term follow-up has not yet been reported.

- Given the aforementioned difficulty with diagnosing the nature of some lesions, non-malignant lesions may inadvertently be treated with non-surgical ablation if a patient is scheduled for ablation without prior biopsy (Fig. 4.9).

References

Beer, AJ, Dobritz M, Zantl N *et al.* (2006) Comparison of 16-MDCT and MRI for Chracterization of renal lesions. *AJR* **186**: 1639–1650.

Bosniak, MA (1986) The current radiological approach to renal cysts. *Radiology* **158**: 1–10.

Kang DE, White RL, Zuger JH *et al.* (2004) Clinical use of Fluorodeoxyglucose F 18 positron emission tomography for the detection of renal cell carcinoma. *J. Urol.* **171**: 1806–1809.

Logue LG, Acker RE, Sienko AE (2003) Angiomyolipomas in tuberous sclerosis. *Radiographics* **23**: 241–246.

Pantuck AJ, Zisman A, Belldegrun AS (2001) The changing natural history of renal cell carcinoma. *J. Urol.* **166**: 1611–1623.

Silverman SG, Gan YU, Mortele KJ *et al.* (2006) Renal masses in the adult patient: role of percutaneous biopsy. *Radiology* **240**: 6–22.

Tuncali K, vanSonnenberg E, Shankar S *et al.* (2004) Evaluation of patients referred for percutaneous ablation of renal tumors: importance of preprocedural diagnosis. *AJR* **183**: 575–582.

5
Non-neoplastic Renal Cystic Lesions

Sameh K. Morcos

Department of Diagnostic Imaging, Northern General Hospital, Sheffield

5.1 Introduction

The study of renal cystic disease has been made difficult by confused nomenclature, with a tendency to regard all forms of cystic change in the kidney as manifestations of what is vaguely referred to a 'multicystic' or 'polycystic' disease. This approach is unhelpful since the significance of renal cystic change varies from trivial to grave, and some forms are inherited whilst others are not. Accurate diagnosis is therefore vital both for clinical assessment and proper genetic counseling. Imaging of patients with cystic kidneys relies mainly on ultrasound scanning (US). Computed tomography (CT) and magnetic resonance imaging (MRI) also plays important role in diagnosing these lesions particularly if malignancy is suspected. In this chapter a simple classification of benign cystic renal lesions is offered. Clinical features, pathology and imaging findings of the different lesions are presented. Neoplastic cystic lesions of the kidneys are discussed elsewhere in the book.

5.2 Classification

In this chapter benign renal cystic diseases are classified according to the predominant anatomical location of the cystic changes within the kidney (Fig. 5.1). Conditions like caliectasis and hydronephrotic moiety of duplex collecting system are not considered renal cystic diseases and not included in this classification.

Urogenital Imaging: A Problem-oriented Approach   Edited by Sameh K. Morcos and Henrik S. Thomsen
© 2009 John Wiley & Sons, Ltd

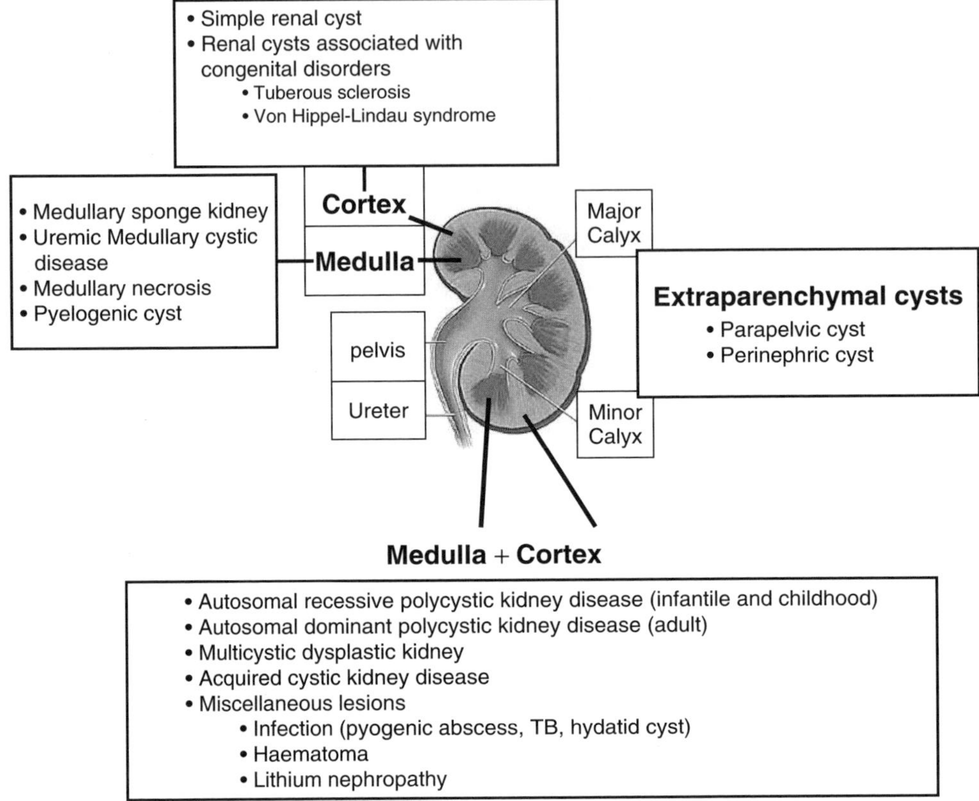

Figure 5.1   Classification of non-neoplastic renal cystic diseases.

5.3 Cystic lesions affecting renal cortex

Simple renal cyst

A simple renal cyst is the commonest benign cystic lesion of the kidney.

Clinical features

- Usually asymptomatic and associated with normal renal function.

- Commonly seen as an incidental finding in middle aged and elderly patients during cross sectional imaging of the abdomen.

- They are rare in children and young adults under the age of 30. A cyst in a child must be carefully differentiated from a cystic Wilms' tumor.

- May present as an abdominal mass causing some flank discomfort.

- Loin pain may occur due to cyst wall distension or spontaneous intracystic bleeding.

- Rarely may cause hematuria or polycythemia.

- They uncommonly become infected or traumatized, a large cyst may obstruct the collecting system or cause hypertension.

- Simple renal cysts can be associated with hereditary disorders such as tuberous sclerosis or Von Hippel Lindau syndrome.

Pathology

- Simple renal cysts are acquired lesions that probably arise from obstructed ducts or tubules.

- They Occur mainly in the renal cortex but occasionally seen in the renal medulla.

- They are usually unilocular, often multiple and vary in size. A few thin septa within the cyst are occasionally seen.

- They have thin fibrous wall and are lined by flattened epithelium.

- The cyst contains serous fluid and does not communicate with the collecting system.

Imaging

- Simple renal cysts are easily diagnosed by US, CT or MRI.

- The findings in intravenous urography are often non-specific.

- Renal angiography is rarely required these days to diagnose renal cysts with availability of modern cross sectional imaging techniques.

- Percutaneous needle aspiration under imaging guidance for cytological, bacteriological and biochemical analysis of the aspirate may occasionally be required in difficult cases to exclude the possibility of malignancy or infection.

Ultrasound

- Ultrasound represents the most cost efficient modality to confirm the presence of a simple cyst. When all the criteria for a benign simple cyst are present, further evaluation is not indicated.

  - Typical features of a simple cyst (Fig. 5.2):

    - a rounded homogeneous echolucent mass
    - a sharp interface with the surrounding renal parenchyma
    - acoustic enhancement posterior to the lesion.
    - A few thin septa may occasionally be seen within the lesion.

  - Tissue harmonic imaging improves the characterization of renal cysts.

  - Atypical features such as high echo content within the lesion, thick irregular wall or septa should raise the possibility of a neoplastic lesion and should be evaluated further by MRI or CT with contrast enhancement.

  - Bleeding in a simple cyst would produce internal echoes and these may be mobile. A decrease in the posterior acoustic enhancement may be observed.

  - A simple renal cyst is avascular on color or power Doppler US scanning.

  - It does not show enhancement after intravenous injection of an US contrast agent.

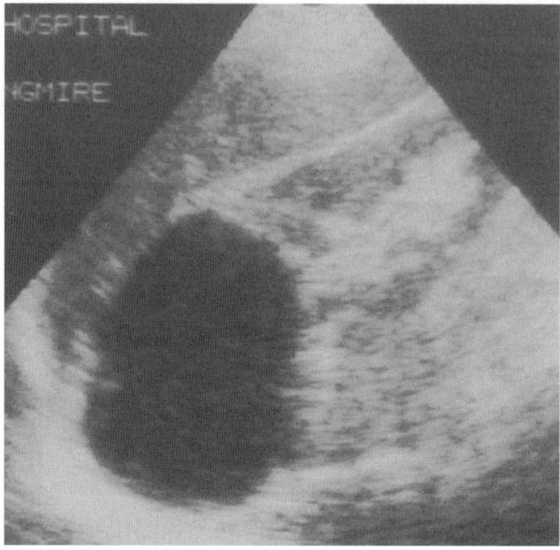

Figure 5.2 A large cyst at the upper pole of the right kidney shows the typical sonographic features of a simple cyst.

CT

- CT of the kidneys performed before and after the administration of intravenous contrast is used for characterizing renal lesions when US has been indeterminate or suspicious of a neoplastic lesion.

- It is extremely important to determine the presence or absence of contrast enhancement, to distinguish benign cysts from neoplasms. Typically, greater than 10 Hounsfield unit increase in density after contrast enhancement is only seen in neoplastic processes.

- *A simple renal cyst at plain CT*

   o Presents as a well defined lesion of water density (slightly lower in density in comparison to adjacent renal cortex).

   o Thin wall calcification is occasionally seen but more often encountered in neoplastic lesions.

   o May occasionally presents as a homogeneously high density well-defined lesion (Fig. 5.3a). This is due to bleeding within the cyst. A high density benign cyst does not show enhancement after contrast medium injection.

- *Post contrast, scanning* (nephrographic phase)

   o Well defined uniform water density.

   o The lesion is often in the cortex.

   o No septation, solid elements or enhancement.

   o Thin septa without contrast enhancement may occasionally be seen.

MRI

- Renal MRI can be used as an alternative to CT.

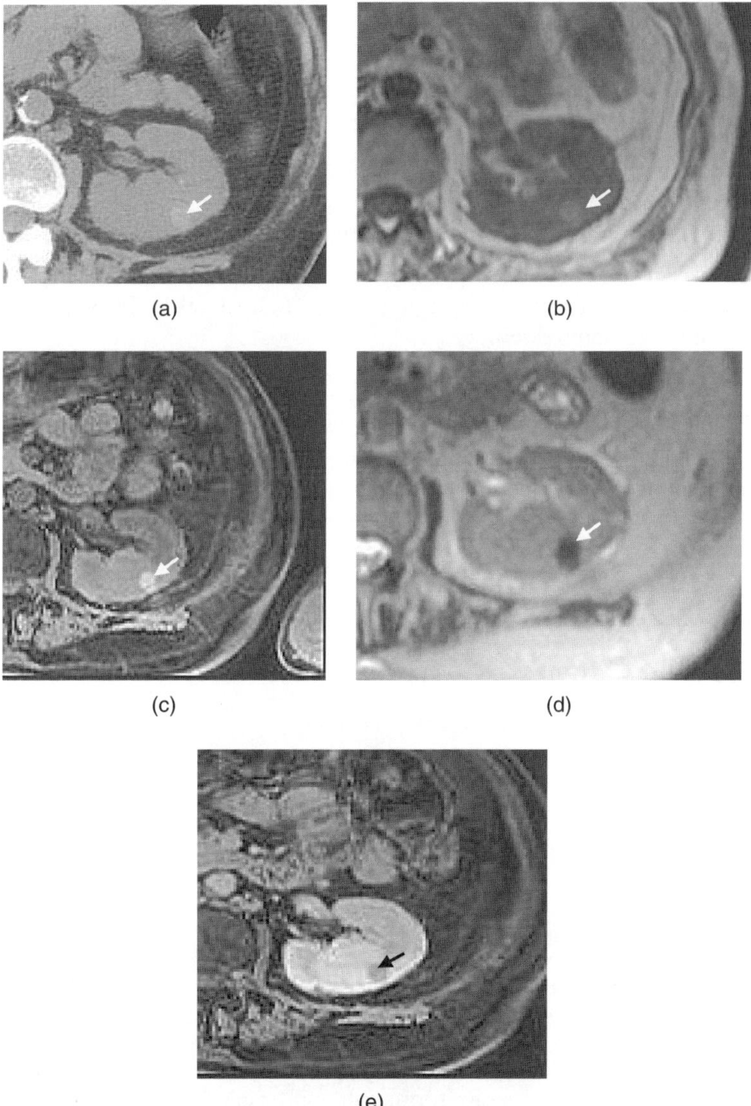

(a)

(b)

(c)

(d)

(e)

Figure 5.3   (a) Unenhanced CT shows a high density cyst in the left kidney (arrow) due to hemorrhage. (b) The same hemorrhagic cyst (arrow) at T1 MRI shows high signals due to presence of methemoglobin. (c) The hemorrhagic cyst (arrow) at T1 MRI with fat saturation shows obvious high signals. (d) The hemorrhagic cyst (arrow) at T2 MRI shows low signals due to presence of intracellular methemoglobin. (e) The hemorrhagic cyst (arrow) at T1 MRI, fat saturation after gadolium contrast injection shows no enhancement.

- A simple renal cyst will be of low signal intensity on T1, and very high signal intensity on T2-weighted images.
- It appears as a homogeneous rounded mass with a thin wall and sharp interface with the surrounding normal renal parenchyma.

- Appearance of the hemorrhagic cyst varies according to the time lapsed between the onset hemorrhage and the MRI examination.

  o Hemorrhage of less than 24 hours may cause low signal in T1 and high signal in T2 imaging due to intracellular oxyhemoglobin.

  o Hemorrhage between 1–3 days old may cause low signal in T1 and T2 imaging due to intracellular deoxyhemoglobin.

  o Hemorrhage between 3–7 days may cause high signal in T1 and low signal T2 imaging due to intracellular methemoglobin (Fig. 5.3b, c, d).

  o Hemorrhage between 7–14 days old may cause high signal in T1 and T2 imaging due to extracellular methemoglobin.

  o Hemorrhage of more than 14 days old may cause low signal in T1- and T2 imaging due to extracellular hemosiderin.

- No enhancement is seen in the wall or septa of a simple renal cyst on T1-weighted imaging after intravenous injection of extracellular gadolinium based contrast medium (Fig. 5.3e).

5.4 Cystic lesions of renal medulla

Medullary sponge kidney

- A developmental abnormality of unknown etiology.

- It occurs in the renal medulla and is characterized by cystic dilatation of the collecting tubules which may contain small stones.

- The disease can affect one or more renal pyramids in one or both kidneys. One of every 100 to 200 people have some form of this disease.

Clinical features

- Patients are usually asymptomatic and the disease is often discovered as an incidental finding at intravenous urography (IVU).

- Renal colic, flank pain, fever, and dysuria may be the presenting complaint in approximately 10% of patients due to stone formation and urinary tract infection.

- Medullary sponge kidneys have been associated with some congenital conditions such as hemihypertrophy, Ehlers-Danlos and Marfan syndrome.

Pathology

- The affected kidneys are usually normal in size or slightly enlarged.

- Dilated medullary collecting ducts (ducts of Bellini) near the tips of one, several or all renal papilla.

- The size of dilated ducts range from 1–6 mm in diameter.

- Calculi are frequently contained within the dilated ducts.

Imaging

Dilated collecting ducts in the renal medulla which contains small stones seen on IVU or CT urography (CTU) are the landmark of diagnosing medullary sponge kidneys.

- *Plain radiographs*

  o Multiple small rounded and linear densities might be observed in the renal area (Fig. 5.4a).

  o Ureteric and bladder stones may also be seen.

- *Intravenous urography (IVU)*

  o The kidneys and the pyramids might be enlarged.

  o In the excretory phase the characteristic feature is radial, linear striations in the papillae (papillary blush) or cystic collections of contrast material in ectatic collecting ducts (brush pattern) (Fig. 5.4b).

- *Ultrasound*

  o Hyperechoic medulla with or without shadowing can be observed.

  o The sonographic appearances of medullary sponge kidney are non-specific and can be observed with other conditions.

- *CT*

  o Plain CT would confirm the presence of medullary small stones in the kidneys.

  o At the excretory phase of CTU dilated collected ducts will be seen in the renal medulla.

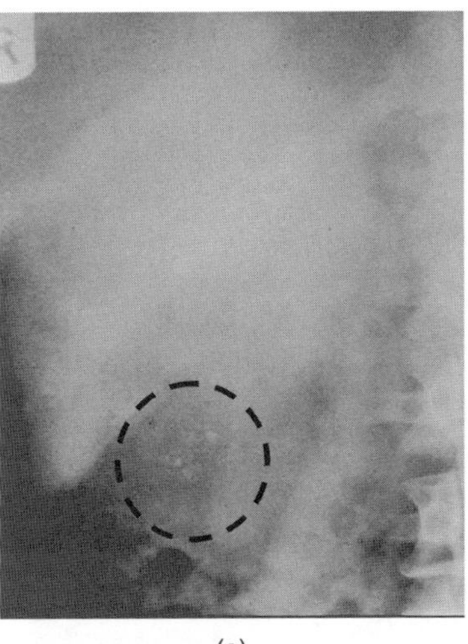 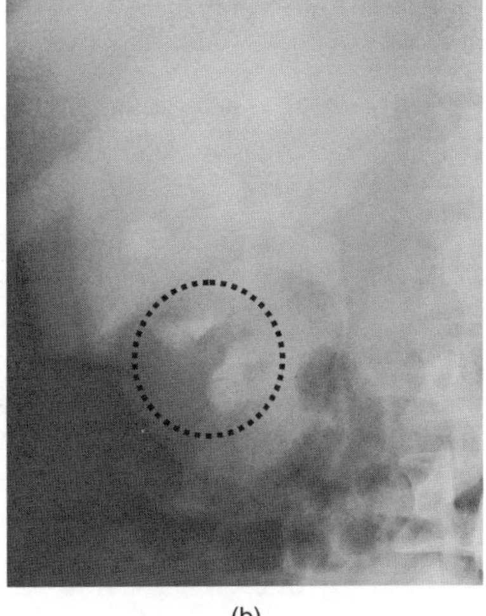

(a)   (b)

Figure 5.4   (a) Plain radiograph of the abdomen of a patient with medullary sponge kidneys shows multiple small stones in the right kidney (black ring). (b) Intravenous urogram of the same patient showing the filling of the dilated collecting ducts in the renal pyramids with contrast medium (black ring).

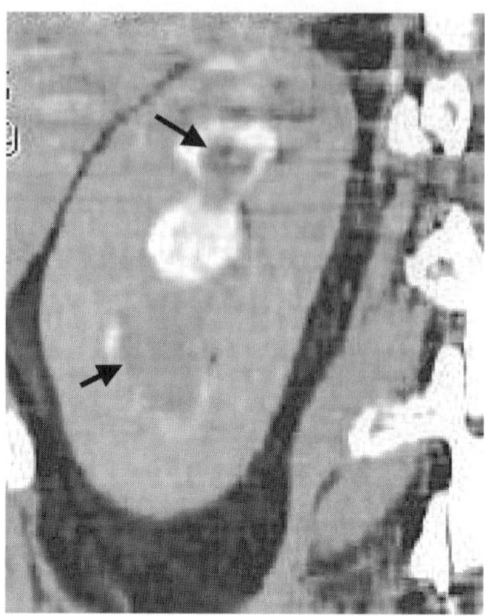

Figure 5.5 The excretory phase of a CT urography of a patient with medullary necrosis demonstrating sloughed papillae (arrows) within dilated calyces

- *MRI*

  - Excretory MR urography after intravenous injection of an extracellular gadolinium contrast agent and a small dose of diuretic is a useful alternative in patients who are allergic to iodinated contrast media.
  - Dilated collecting ducts might be seen in the renal medulla.
  - Stones would produce filling defects within the pelvicalyceal system but small medullary stones may not be detected.

Uremic medullary cystic disease (Juvenile Nephronophthisis)

- This is a hereditary condition. Both autosomal dominance and recessive inheritance has been described.

Clinical features

- Presents in children and young adults.
- Cases present either sporadic or show strong family history.
- Polyuria, polydipsia, salt craving and nocturia.
- Normochromic normocytic anemia.
- Renal impairment with elevated serum creatinine.
- The diagnosis is usually suggested by the clinical triad of

  - Anemia
  - Uremia
  - Salt wasting.

Pathology

- Bilateral small, smooth kidneys.

- Widespread interstitial fibrosis.

- The cysts are most prominent near the corticomedullary junction.

- The cysts vary from microscopic to several cm. in size.

Imaging

- The imaging findings are non-specific and relies mainly on ultrasound scanning.

- *Ultrasound*

  o Bilateral small kidneys.
  o Increase in the echogenicity of the renal parenchyma.
  o Individual cysts might be seen.

- *MRI*

  o Bilateral small kidneys.
  o Cysts at the corticomedullary junction may be observed on T2 imaging.

Medullary necrosis

- Expulsion of necrotic papilla into the calyx creates a cyst like cavity communicating with the calyx.

- Renal papillary necrosis could be due to analgesic abuse, diabetic nephropathy, sickle cell anemia, obstructive nephropathy or infection.

Clinical features

- The acute progressive form is rare and may result in death from septicemia and renal failure.

- The chronic form is more common and patients may remain asymptomatic.

- The symptomatic form manifests as fever caused by secondary infection.

- Acute ureteral obstruction from sloughed papillae manifests as flank pain and colic. Hematuria invariably is present. Tissue in the urine may be observed.

- Reduced glomerular filtration rate, salt wasting, an impaired ability to concentrate, and polyuria can be observed.

- Progression into end-stage renal failure may occur specially with analgesic abuse.

- The risk of urothelial cancer is increased in patients with analgesic abuse.

Pathology

- Never involves the entire medulla; the disease is always strictly limited to the inner, more distal zone of the medulla and the papilla.

- Renal papillary necrosis may simply affect a single papilla, or the entire kidney may be grossly involved.

- More often a bilateral process.

- Two pathologic forms of renal papillary necrosis, the medullary form and the papillary form.

- The medullary form is characterized by

  o intact fornices

  o discrete grain-sized necrotic areas, and later defects in the papillae

  o sinus tracts may be observed extruding from irregular medullary cavities.

- In the papillary form

  o the calyceal fornices and the entire papillary surface are destroyed, and sequestered;

  o necrosis in situ may occur without sloughing.

Imaging

- *Plain radiographs of the abdomen*

  o May demonstrate calcification in a sloughed papilla, which is characteristically ring shaped and may be the only abnormal imaging finding in necrosis in situ.

- *Intravenous urography*

  o Ulcerated papillae can be observed.

  o Contrast-containing rice-grain-sized cavities in the papilla, which are pathognomonic for the medullary form of renal papillary necrosis.

  o Streaking of contrast from the calyx into the papilla is almost diagnostic of renal papillary necrosis.

  o Sloughed papillae may produce filling defects in dilated calyces or causing ureteric obstruction and delayed excretion of contrast in the affected kidney.

  o Desquamated papilla in situ, demarcated by contrast material as a ring shadow, often in a triangular shape might be observed and commonly referred to as the ring sign.

- *Retrograde pyeloureterography*

  o Images may reveal a clubbed calyx or a filling defect in the ureter.

- *Ultrasound*

  o Non-specific.

  o Sloughed papillae can be revealed as echogenic material within the collecting system.

  o Hyperechoic pyramids might be observed.

- *CT*

  o Calcified papillae might be observed in plain CT of the abdomen.

  o Contrast-filled clefts in the renal parenchyma and filling defects produced by necrotic, detached papillae might be within medullary cavities, renal pelvis or ureters at CTU (Fig. 5.5).

- *MRI*

  - ○ Excretory MR urography may show abnormalities similar to those observed at IVU or CTU.

Pyelogenic cyst (calyceal diverticulum/cyst)

Congenital etiology is the most likely cause of this cystic lesion.

Clinical features

- Usually asymptomatic but may present with symptoms of urinary tract obstruction when complicated by calculi, or of infection.

- Stones in a pyelogenic cyst are important to identify as they are not suitable for extracorporal lithotripsy treatment.

Pathology

- Size varies from a few mm to several cm.

- Has a smooth wall lined with transitional epithelium.

- Connected by a thin channel to the adjacent calyx.

- May contain multiple small calculi and occasionally, milk of calcium may be present.

Imaging

- *Plain radiography of the abdomen*

  - ○ Multiple small stones localized in one area of the kidney might be observed.

- *Intravenous urography*

  - ○ A spherical collection of contrast medium adjacent to a calyx is seen. The connecting channel may be visualized but is often too narrow to be demonstrated (Fig. 5.6a).

- *Ultrasound*

  - ○ The distinction between a calyceal diverticulum, an obstructed calyx and a renal cyst may be difficult. Stones might be observed within the calyceal diverticum (Fig. 5.6b, c).

- *CT*

  - ○ *Pre-contrast*

    - A group of multiple small stones localized in one are in the kidney might be observed.

  - ○ *Post-contrast (excretory phase of CTU)*

    - A spherical cavity filled with contrast medium adjacent to a calyx would be seen.

    - A fluid level might be seen within the cavity between the opacified and non-opacified urine with the former accumulating in the dependent part of the diverticulum.

- *MRI*

  - ○ At T2-weighted imaging the diverticulum would present as a simple cyst adjacent to a calyx.

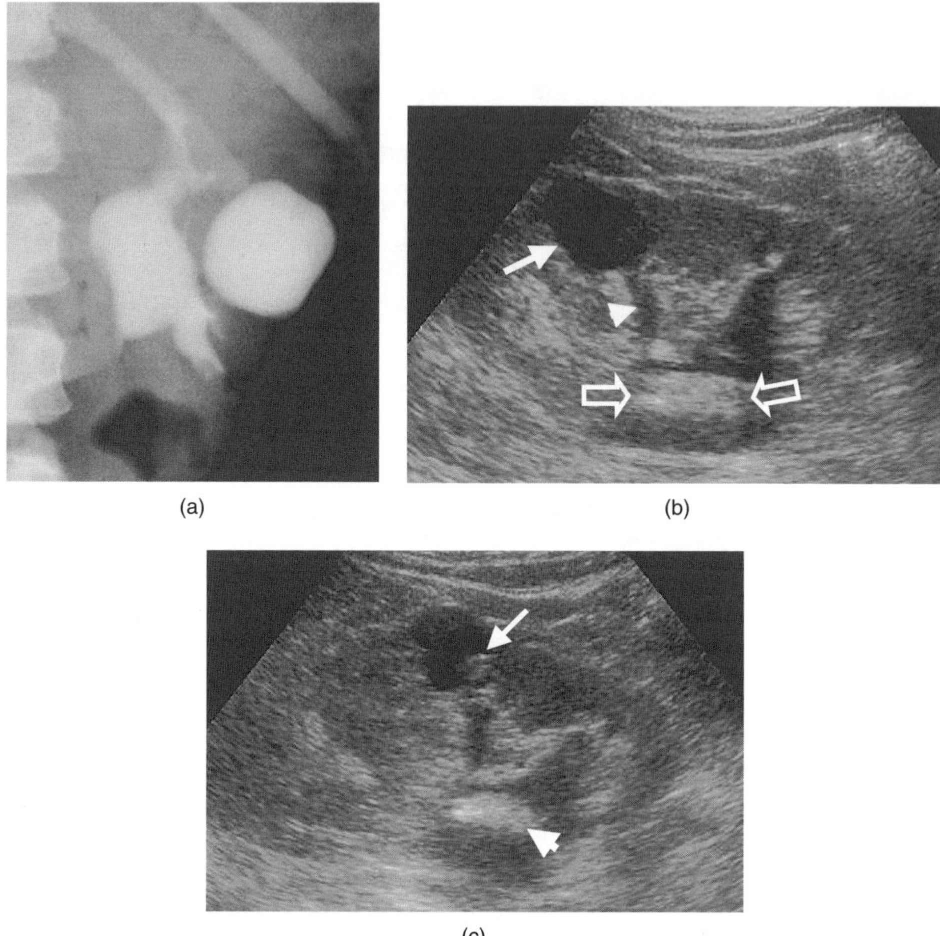

Figure 5.6 (a) Intravenous urogram demonstrates a pyelogenic cyst of the left kidney filled with contrast medium. (b) Ultrasound scan of a kidney with a pyelogenic cyst (arrow) in the upper pole. A calculus is present in the renal pelvis (open arrows). The major calyx of the upper pole (small arrow) is also demonstrated. (c) A small stone (arrow) is shown within the pyelogenic cyst, the stone in the renal pelvis (short arrow) is also shown.

- o At excretory MRU the diverticulum would be filled with contrast.
- o Stones within the diverticulum would cause filling defects at both T2 imaging and excretory MRU.

5.5 Cystic diseases affecting both the cortex and medulla

These include:

- Polycystic kidney diseases [autosomal recessive (infantile and childhood type).
- Autosomal dominant polycystic kidney diseases (adult type).

- Dysplastic multicystic kidney.

- Acquired renal cystic disease.

- Lithium nephropathy.

- Renal cystic lesions due to infection or hematoma.

Autosomal recessive polycystic kidney disease
The infantile type

- It is uncommon autosomal recessive polycystic kidney disease that occurs approximately one in 20 000 births.

- The gene responsible for this disease has been linked to the short arm of chromosome 6.

Clinical features

- Presents in the first days of life. The mother would had oligohydramnios due to decreased fetal urine out put.

- Most babies die in the first days mainly from renal failure.

- The infant may have Potter faces (Fig. 5.7).

- The kidneys are markedly enlarged. This may cause thoracic cage compression leading to pulmonary hypoplasia and respiratory distress. The large kidneys may also obstruct delivery.

- The liver is generally enlarged.

- Those who survive the first days develop progressive renal failure, hypertension and failure to thrive.

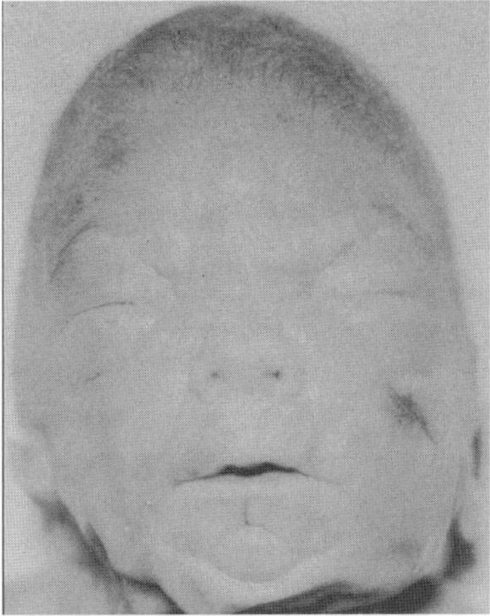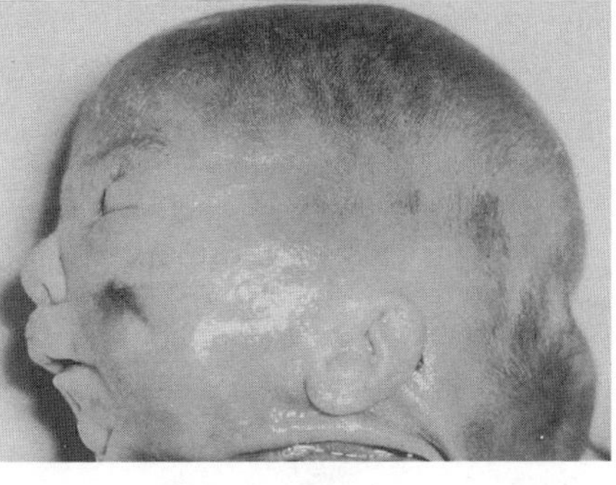

Figure 5.7 A stillborn infant with bilateral multicystic dysplastic kidneys shows typical features of Potter faces: wide set eyes; v-shaped epicanthic folds; flat nose; large, flaccid, low set ears.

Pathology

- Hyperplasia of the interstitial portions of the collecting ducts leads to saccular and cylindrical cystic enlargement of the collecting tubules.

- Fibrosis develops in the renal interstitium.

- The kidneys are enlarged and the cut surface has a spongy appearance.

- The pelvicalyceal system is normal in shape and the ureters are not dilated.

- The liver is enlarged and contains hepatic cysts with evidence of periportal fibrosis and dilated bile ducts.

Imaging

Ultrasound is the main imaging technique to assess these infants. It is also very useful for prenatal diagnosis of this condition.

Ultrasound

- Bilateral enlarged kidneys which are hyperechoic (Fig. 5.8). The increase in the echogenicity of the kidneys is secondary to the many interfaces caused by the multiple very small cysts beyond the resolution of the technique to be identified as cystic lesions.

- Loss of corticomedullary differentiation.

- Hepatic cysts may be observed.

CT

- Precontrast CT scan images show enlarged smooth kidneys with low attenuation.

- Renal calcifications might be observed.

Childhood type

This is similar to infantile polycystic disease except the renal involvement is less and the hepatic involvement is the predominant feature of the disease. This form of polycystic disease is also referred to as Caroli syndrome.

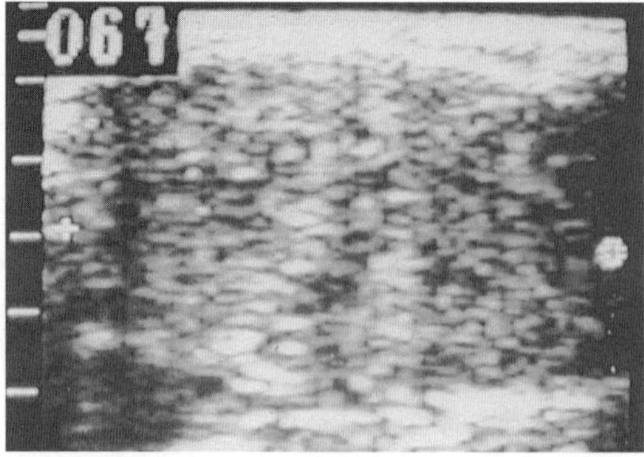

Figure 5.8 An ultrasound scan of a kidney with infantile recessive polycystic kidney disease shows generalize increase in the echogenicity of the kidney and loss of cortico-medullary differentiation.

Clinical features

- The disease is seen in children above the age of 3 years and in young adults.
- Hepatosplenomegaly is present.
- Patients may present with hematemesis from oesophageal varices secondary to portal hypertension.
- The renal impairment is usually mild but occasionally progressive renal failure may develop.

Pathology

- The cystic changes in the liver and kidneys are not striking.
- Hepatic periportal fibrosis is a predominant feature leading to portal hypertension.
- Sacular dilatation of the bile ducts can be observed.
- The renal involvement is not severe and the cystic dilatation of collecting ducts is seen in the medulla.

Imaging

The hepatic abnormalities are the predominant features. The renal findings are similar to those observed in medullary sponge kidneys.

Barium meal

- Esophageal and gastric varices due to portal hypertension.

Endoscopic retrograde cholangiopancreatography (ERCP)

- Effective in demonstrating the multiple localized cystic dilatations of the bile ducts (Fig. 5.9) but it is an invasive procedure.

Ultrasound

- Increase in the echogenicity of the portal tracts in the liver due to periportal fibrosis.
- Multiple cysts in the liver due to intrahepatic bile ducts dilatation.
- Splenomegaly secondary to portal hypertension.
- The kidneys often appear normal.

CT

May be used, particularly if a diagnostic US examination cannot be obtained.

- Rounded low density areas might be seen in liver due to intrahepatic bile ducts dilatation.
- Splenomegaly would be observed.
- Striated pattern of contrast material might be seen in the kidneys following intravenous contrast injection.

MRI

- MR cholangiography would provide excellent imaging of the cystic dilatation of the bile ducts.

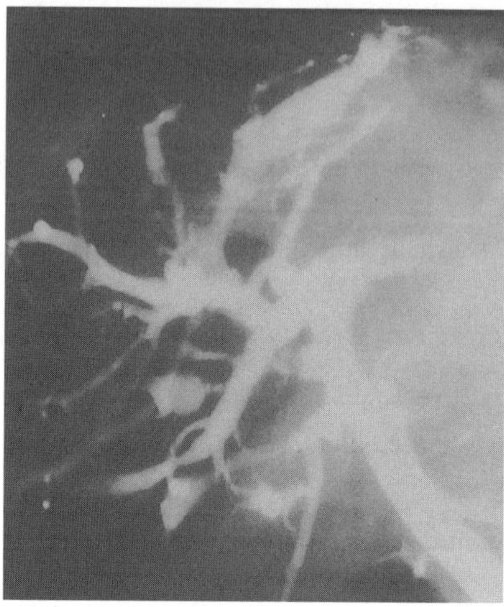

Figure 5.9 Endoscopic retrograde cholangiogram of a patient with the childhood form of recessive polycystic kidney disease (Caroli's syndrome) showing cystic dilatation of the intrahepatic bile ducts.

Autosomal dominant polycystic kidney disease (ADPKD)

- A hereditary disorder but some cases occur from spontaneous gene mutations.

- The pattern of inheritance is autosomal dominant that involves at least two genes.

- *PKD1* is located on chromosome16p and accounts for most ADPKD cases and *PKD2* is located on chromosome 4q and accounts for 15% of ADPKD cases.

- ADPKD1 is more severe than ADPKD2.

Clinical features

- Presents clinically by the third or fourth decade of life but ADPKD 2 may present later in life.

- The most common symptom is dull pain in the back and the sides which can be temporary or persistent, mild or severe.

- Hypertension is a common feature and develops before the onset of renal insufficiency.

- Approximately 45% of patients will have end-stage renal disease by the age of 60 years. Patients with ADPKD2 are older at the onset of renal insufficiency than patients with the ADPKD1.

- Substantial variability of severity of renal disease and other extrarenal manifestations occurs even within the same family.

- Patients with ADPKD can experience the following:
  - Urinary tract infections
  - Hematuria

o Intracranial aneurysms

o Subarachnoid hemorrhage

o Diverticulosis

o Mitral valve prolapse

o Dissection of the thoracic aorta.

Pathology

- Bilateral progressive cystic dilation of the renal tubules, affecting all segments of the nephrons. Less than 5% of nephrons become cystic. It is not known whether more nephrons are recruited into the cystic process over time or whether existing cyst simply enlarge.

- The kidneys become enlarged and full of cysts which vary considerably in size and appearance from a few millimetres to many centimetres in diameter and fluid content varies from clear to cloudy to chocolate-colored, suggestive of hemorrhage within the cysts.

- Cysts may rupture leading to subcapsular and perinephric hematoma.

- Infection of the cysts may also occur.

- Calcification may develop in the wall of the cysts or in the renal parenchyma between the cysts.

- There is increase in secretion of both rennin and erythropoietin.

- Vascular sclerosis and interstitial fibrosis occur in the kidneys. Hypertension is likely to play a part in the vascular changes.

- Cysts are commonly seen in the liver, but may also occur in ovary, pancreas and spleen.

- Cerebral aneurysms may occur in 4–10% of patients with ADPKD.

- Cardiac valvular abnormalities particularly mitral valve prolapse may occur.

- Colonic diverticulosis is common in patients with ADPKD.

Imaging

Ultrasound scanning is a very useful imaging technique for diagnosing ADPKD. Intravenous urography is no longer indicated for the diagnosis of the disease.

- **Ultrasound.**

  o Uncomplicated cysts are echolucent. Complicated cysts are seen in cases with cyst infection, hemorrhage or calcification.

  o Ultrasound can demonstrate perinephric or subcapsular hematom caused by rupture of a cyst.

  o It is useful in demonstrating cysts in other abdominal organs such as liver, spleen, pancreas and ovaries.

  o Echocardiography is useful to exclude mitral prolapse, which is often associated with ADPKD. Dilatation of the aortic root may also be observed.

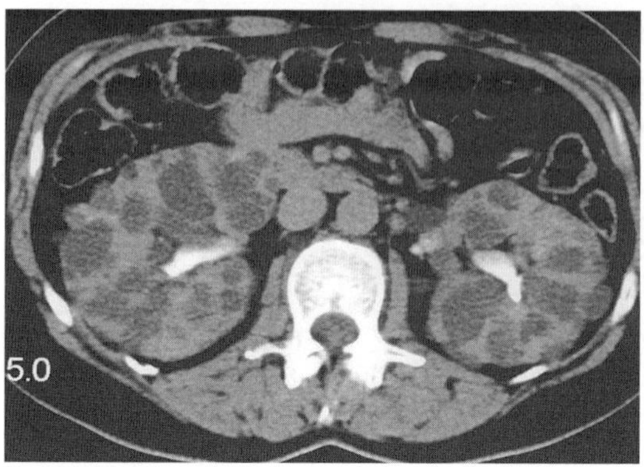

Figure 5.10 CT urography of a patient with autosomal dominant polycystic kidney disease showing bilateral large kidneys full of cysts.

- According to Ravine *et al.* (1994) diagnostic criteria for ADPKD1 are:
  - At least 2 cysts in one kidney or one cyst in each kidney in an at-risk patient younger than 30 years.
  - At least 2 cysts in each kidney in an at-risk patient aged 30–59 years.
  - At least 4 cysts in each kidney for an at-risk patient aged 60 years or older.

- *CT scan.*
  - CT urography (CTU) at the nephrographic phase using thin collimation is more sensitive than US in demonstrating small renal cysts and can be used to exclude ADPKD in patient above the age of 20 years.
  - On unenhanced CT scans hemorrhagic cysts are identified as well-defined masses with attenuation values ranging from 40 to 100 HU. No contrast enhancement would be seen in these cysts.
  - Calcification in hemorrhagic cysts might be seen in unenhanced CT scans.
  - CTU is useful in complicated cases or when malignancy is suspected providing there is no marked reduction in renal function (Fig. 5.10).

- *MRI.*
  - Hemorrhagic cysts may show varieties of signal intensities on T1 and T2-weighted images depending on how old is the hemorrhage.
  - MRI with contrast enhancement can be useful in identifying coexisting renal cell carcinoma.
  - MRI can be used to determine renal volume. New software has been developed to measure renal cystic volume. These measurements are useful for clinical trials testing new drugs that aimed to slow the progress of the cystic changes in the kidneys.
  - MR angiography is useful for diagnosing suspected intracranial aneurysm.

Multicystic dysplastic kidney

Multicystic dysplastic kidney (MCDK) is a rare condition that results from malformation of the kidney during fetal development.

Clinical features

- Typically a unilateral disorder.

- Bilateral MCDK is incompatible with extrauterine survival. Affected children are stillborn and features of Potter faces are usually present (Fig. 5.7).

- MCDK is often detected in utero during antenatal ultrasound screening. The abnormal kidney can be identified if the fetus is older than 15 weeks.

- MCDK can present as an abdominal mass in the newborn.

- MCDK is occasionally detected in older children or adults as an incidental imaging finding.

- In over 50% of cases, other urinary tract defects are detected. Ureteropelvic junction obstruction and vesicoureteral reflux (VUR) are the most common defects in the contralateral kidney.

- MCDK can be associated with cardiac and gastrointestinal tract anomalies. Associations with infection, hypertension, renal cell carcinoma and Wilm's tumor have also been reported.

Pathology

- The affected kidney is enlarged and consists of irregular cysts of varying sizes.

- The renal pelvis and calyces are absent or severely attenuated.

- The draining ureter is atretic.

- The renal artery is absent or very small.

- Histology:

  - Primitive ducts and glomeruli. No functional renal tissue is identifiable.

  - Metaplastic cartilage may be seen in the poorly differentiated mesenchymal stroma.

- The affected kidney involutes or decreases in size in 60–70% of cases. This process can take up to 20 years.

- Compensatory renal hypertrophy of the contralateral side is observed.

Imaging

- Sonography is the preferred initial examination.

- Currently with the use of prenatal ultrasound, most cases of MCDK are discovered prior to birth.

- Voiding cystourethrography is indicated in a child with MCDK to evaluate the urinary tract for other anomalies specifically the presence of vesico-ureteric reflux.

- *Ultrasound*

  - The kidney becomes replaced by cysts of variable sizes and shapes with minimal surrounding parenchyma (Fig. 5.11).

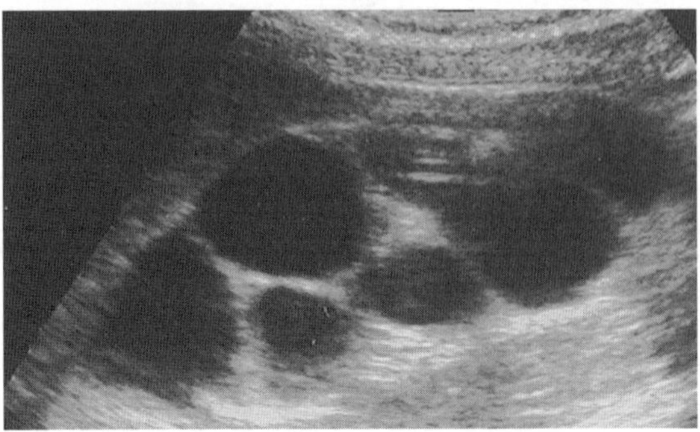

Figure 5.11 Ultrasound scan of a multicystic dysplastic kidney showing multiple cysts with no identifiable normal renal tissue.

- o Lack of communication between cysts.
- o The normal shape of the kidney tends to be lost.
- o Absence of an identifiable renal sinus.
- o The previously mentioned features are useful to differentiate MCDK from gross hydronephrosis with thin renal cortex. In hydronephrosis the dilated calyces communicate with the dilated central renal pelvis.
- o The contralateral kidney is mostly normal (bilateral disease is incompatible with life).

- **CT**
  - o Cyst wall calcification can be seen.
  - o Multicystic mass with little or no parenchyma replacing the kidney.
  - o If a contrast-enhanced CT is performed, there is poor enhancement with no excretion of contrast is seen.

- **MRI**
  - o Multicystic mass with little or no renal parenchyma.

Acquired cystic kidney disease (ACKD)

It refers to the development of multiple renal cysts in patients with chronic renal failure including those on long-term hemodialysis or peritoneal dialysis. By 10 years 90% of patients on dialysis develop ACKD.

Clinical features

- ACKD is often asymptomatic.
- Painless hematuria may occur.
- Abdominal or loin pain secondary to retroperitoneal hemorrhage may develop.
- Rising hemoglobin level can be observed.
- Most tumors in ACKD are clinically silent.

Pathology

- Hyperplasia of tubular epithelium leading to tubular blockage and cyst formation.

- The hyperplasia may progress to form tubular papillary adenomas that might culminate into clear cell or papillary cell renal cancer in equal proportions.

- The kidneys are usually small in size.

- The cysts vary in size from microscopic to several centimetres in diameter.

- Hemorrhage may occur in some of the cysts.

- The papillary adenomas tend to be small in size (<5 mm). Renal cancer may develop in some of these lesions.

- Approximately 2–7% of patients with ACKD ultimately develop renal cancers. Renal cell carcinoma in these patients is frequently multifocal and bilateral.

Imaging

- The diagnosis of ACKD is established if five or more cysts are present in each kidney in patients with end stage renal disease.

- Ultrasound, CT and MRI are capable of demonstrating the cystic changes in the kidneys (Fig. 5.12).

- CT or MRI with contrast enhancement should be considered when renal cancer is suspected.

- The value of routine screening to detect renal cancer remains contentious.
  - Screening can be beneficial for patients who have a good medical condition with life expectancy of 20 years or more.
  - In such patients annual sonography after five years of dialysis would be reasonable.
  - CT with contrast enhancement should be considered if the US examination is suspicious of a solid mass and prior to transplantation in patients who have been on dialysis for a substantial periods of time.

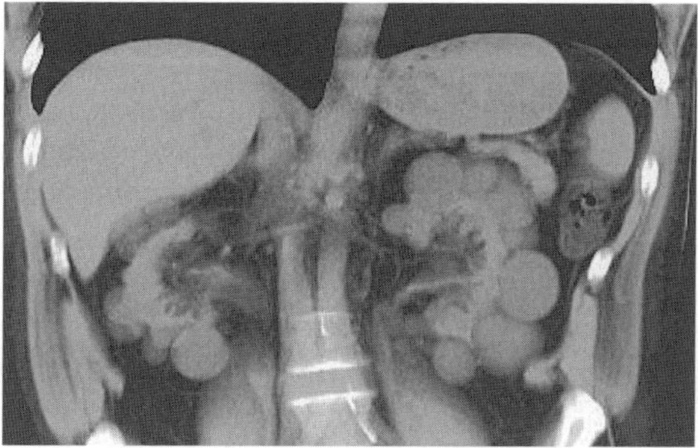

Figure 5.12 A coronal image produced by unenhanced multidetector CT scanning of the abdomen of a patient with acquired cystic disease of the kidneys showing bilateral small kidneys containing multiple simple cysts.

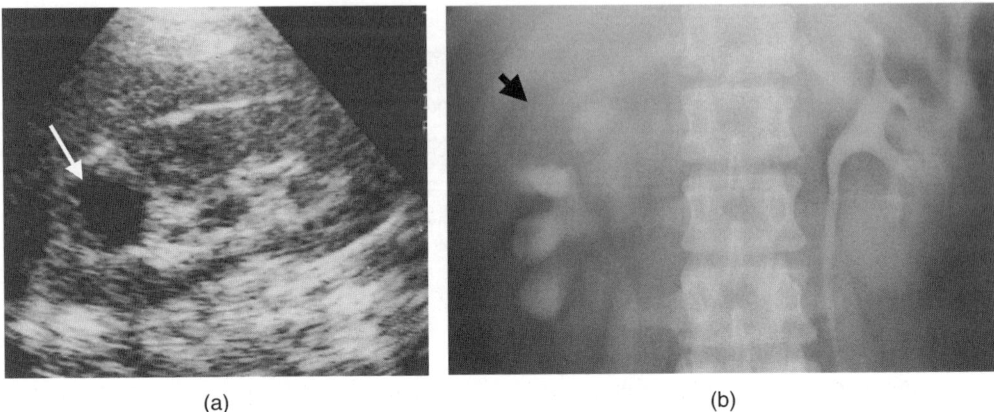

(a)   (b)

Figure 5.13   (a) Ultrasound scan of a 19-year-old patient with tuberculosis of the urinary tract showing a cystic lesion (arrow) in the upper pole of the right kidney caused by a tuberculous abscess. (b) A tomogram of intravenous urogram shows the abscess cavity in the right kidney (arrow). Dilated calyces of the right kidney is secondary to tuberculous stricture of the right ureter (not shown in this figure).

Miscellaneous acquired cystic lesions of the kidneys

- *Lithium nephropathy*
  Microcysts (1–2 mm in diameter) affect both kidneys.

  o Cysts are abundant, uniformly and symmetrically distributed with cortical predominance.

  o Patients with this condition been on long-standing lithium therapy and suffer from chronic renal insufficiency.

  o Polyuria and polydyspia occurs in about 40% of patients.

  o T2-weighted MRI are effective in demonstrating the cystic changes in the kidneys.

- *Cystic lesions secondary to infection or trauma.*

  o *Infection* [pyogenic, tuberculous (Fig. 5.13a, b), hydatid cyst].

  o Trauma causing *hematoma*.

  o Cross sectional imaging whether with US, CT or MRI are effective in detecting such lesions. The diagnosis is often made in association with clinical and laboratory findings.

Extraparenchymal renal cysts

They include *pericalyceal lymphangiectasia and urinoma*. Sonography, CT and MRI are effective in depicting these lesions. The type of the lesion is often determined according to the clinical context.

Pericalyceal lymphangiectasia (cystic hygroma, para pelvic cyst)

- Irregular multicystic mass of dilated lymphatic vessels which invests the renal pelvis.

- May cause pelvi-ureteric obstruction.

- Etiology:

  o Lymphatic obstruction.

  o Hamartomatous malformation.

Perinephric pseudocyst (urinoma)

- Urine collection in the perinephric space could be secondary to trauma or obstruction. This can give rise to a formation of a pseudocyst called *urinoma*.

References

Choyke PL (2000) Acquired cystic kidney disease. *Eur. Radiol.* **10**: 1716–1721.

Grantham JJ (1995) Polycystic kidney disease: etiology, pathogenesis and treatment. *Dis. Mon.* **41**: 693–765.

Lanergan GJ, Rice RR, Suarez ES (2000) Autosomal recessive polycystic kidney disease: radiologic-pathologic correlation. *Radiographics* **20**: 837–855.

Ravine D, Gibson RN, Walker RG, Sheffield LJ, Kincaid-Smith P, Danks DM (1994) Evaluation of ultrasonographic diagnostic criteria for autosomal dominant polycystic kidney disease 1. *Lancet* **343**: 824–827.

Thomsen HS, Levine E, Meilstrup JW, Van Sluke MA, Edgar KA, Barth JC, Hartman DS (1997) Renal cystic disease. *Eur. Radiol.* **7**: 1267–1275.

6

Urological and Vascular Complications Post-renal Transplantation

Tarek El-Diasty and Yasser Osman

Urology and Nephrology Center, Mansoura University

6.1 Introduction

- Renal transplantation is the preferred mode of renal replacement therapy in end-stage renal disease. Better comprehension of the rejection response, improved preservation of organs, better immunosuppressant, and specific protocols for the prevention and treatment of infection have all contributed to increased patient and graft survival rates after renal transplantation.

- Proper use of imaging modalities is crucial for the diagnosis and management of post-transplantation complications and preservation of the transplanted kidney function.

This chapter presents the clinical picture, pathology and imaging features of the different vascular and urological complications post-renal transplantation (Table 6.1).

6.2 Vascular complications

Thrombosis

- Incidence of vascular thrombosis following renal transplantation has ranged from 0.5% to 6% in most published series.

Urogenital Imaging: A Problem-oriented Approach   Edited by Sameh K. Morcos and Henrik S. Thomsen
© 2009 John Wiley & Sons, Ltd

Table 6.1 Summary of vascular and urological complications post-renal transplantation

Type of complication	Incidence	Clinical picture	Imaging techniques	Treatment
Vascular thrombosis	0.5–6%	Anuria Present few hours post-transplant	Doppler US MRA IA-DSA	Thrombectomy Graft nephrectomy
Renal artery stenosis	1–6%	Hypertension Impaired graft function	Doppler US MRA IA-DSA	Percutaneous transluminal angioplasty
Urinary leakage	1.2–9%	Urinary discharge through wound or drain Pelvic urinoma	Ultrasound MRI Antegrade pyelography	PCN ± stenting Redo operation
Ureteric stricture	1.3–10%	Incidental upon regular check up visits Recurrent UTIs	Ultrasound MRI Antegrade pyelography	PCN ± stenting Redo operation
Symptomatic lymphocele	1.5%	pressure effects → hydronephrosis Edema lower limb DVT	Ultrasound MRI CT	Aspiration ± sclerotherapy Marsupialization
Delayed Graft Function	8–50%	Need of dialysis during the first week post-trasplant	Ultrasound Radionuclide studies Functional MRI	Treatment of the cause
Post- transplant bladder cancer	1–3%	Irritative bladder symptoms Hematuria	Ultrasound MRI CT	Radical cystectomy and urinary diversion

- Treatment includes immediate exploration, thrombectomy with reperfusion of the graft.

- Graft nephrectomy is indicated in the case of late diagnosis or failed conservative management. Vascular thrombosis of transplanted kidneys carries usually a dismal prognosis with high rates of graft loss.

Clinical features

- Sudden anuria is the main presenting symptom.

- It usually occurs in the first few days following transplantation.

Pathology

- Develops secondary to intimal damage mostly due to vessel twist or kinking during graft placement and stream slowing resulting in the formation of intraluminal thrombus.

- Many predisposing factors were suggested such as pediatric transplantation, diabetic recipients, hypercoagulable states, pre-transplant peritoneal dialysis or impact of some immunosuppressive drugs such as OKT3 or cyclosporine.

Imaging findings
Ultrasound (US)

- Conventional color and power Doppler sonography can diagnose the type of vascular thrombosis whether arterial, venous or both.

  - In arterial thrombosis, no flow is demonstrated on color flow mapping within the main renal artery, intraparenchymal vessels and renal vein (Fig. 6.1a).

  - In acute renal vein thrombosis, spectral Doppler demonstrates sharp systolic peak and plateau-like reversed diastolic flow with complete absence of venous flow. This reversed diastolic flow is not specific to acute renal vein thrombosis as severe vascular rejection can result in retrograde diastolic flow and absent venous signals.

  - Large infarcts appear as wedge-shaped areas of increased reflectivity and show no color flow signals on both conventional and power Doppler modes (Fig. 6.2a).

- In cases of arterial thrombosis, the kidney will be diffusely enlarged and appears hypoechoic. Associated pathologies such as compressing hematoma or accumulating lymphocele can be detected.

MR angiography (MRA)

- MRA and dynamic enhanced MR imaging are useful for diagnosing both global and segmental infarctions, as it can depict total or segmental lack of perfusion. Thrombosis of the graft artery can also be demonstrated (Fig. 6.1b).

- MRA is particularly beneficial in cases with patchy perfusion of the graft by Doppler ultrasound as it can differentiate between severe rejection and vascular thrombosis.

- On Gd-enhanced MR imaging the infarcts appear as peripheral wedge-shaped hypointense non-enhancing segments (Fig. 6.2b).

Dynamic radionuclide studies

- A photopenic region may be seen. However, these findings are not specific since hyperacute or accelerated acute rejection may have similar features.

Intra-arterial digital subtraction angiography (IA-DSA)

- An invasive technique that is currently rarely indicated. It seldom provides extra diagnostic information over MRA. It is usually used in institutes lacking MRI facilities.

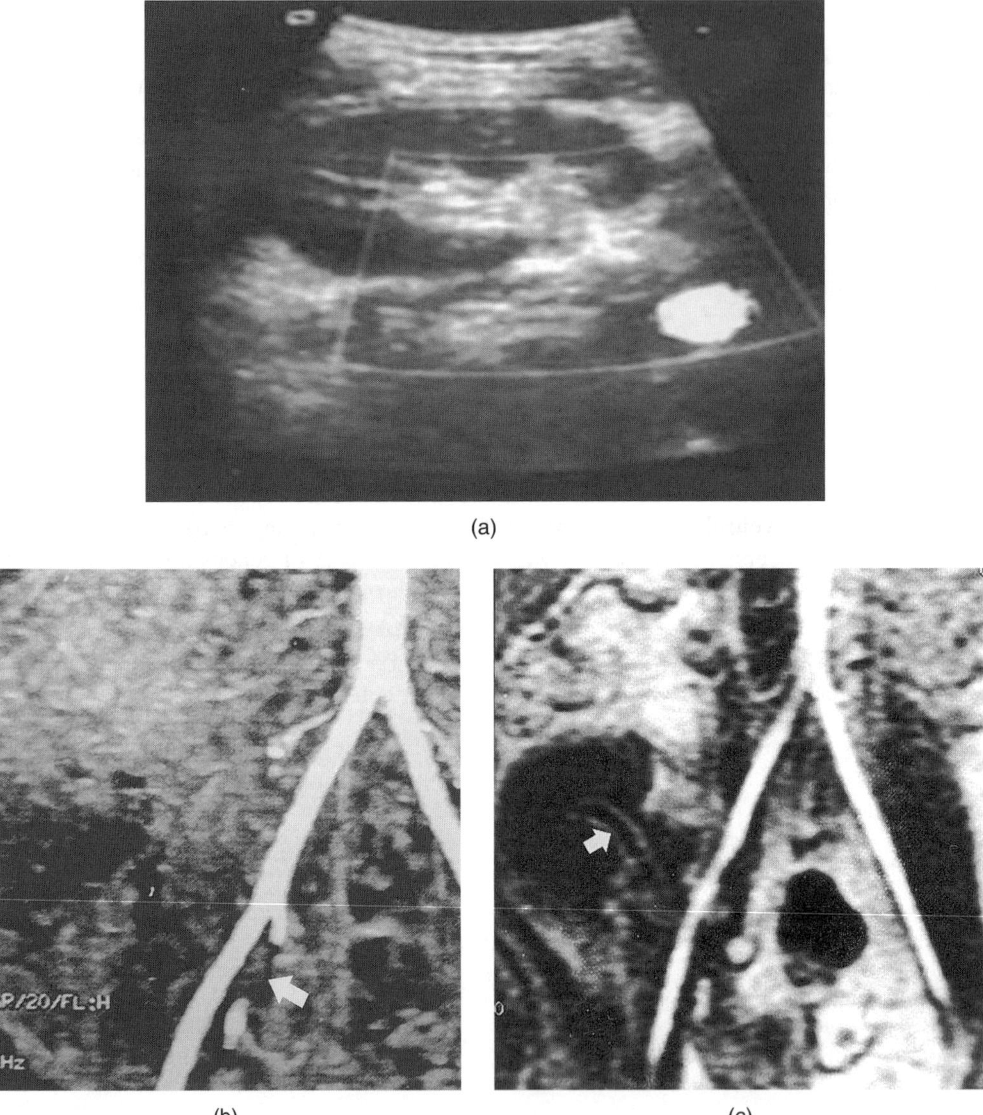

Figure 6.1 Thrombosis of a graft renal artery. (a) No flow is demonstrated within the main renal artery and intraparenchymal vessels on color Doppler sonography. (b) MIP image of MR angiography demonstrates complete occlusion of the graft renal artery at its origin (arrow) and (c) lack of cortical enhancement with hypointensity of the transplanted kidney and the renal artery (arrow). This appearance indicates total infarction of the kidney which was proved at surgery.

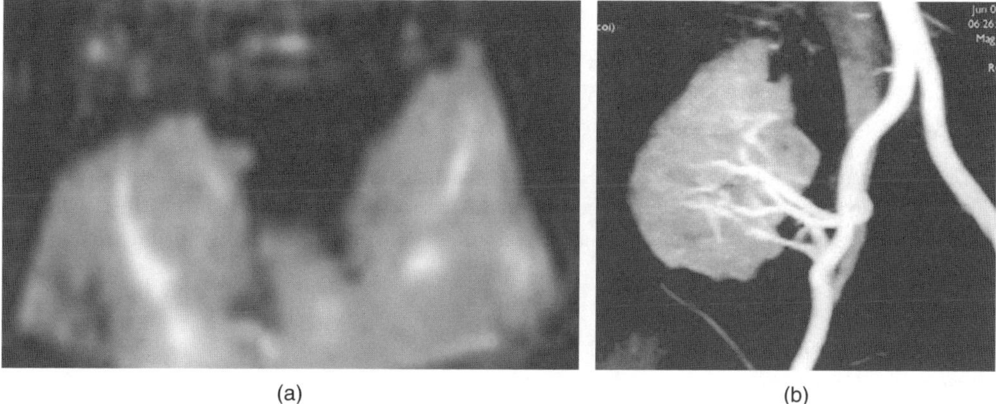

(a)   (b)

Figure 6.2   Segmental infarcts. (a) Anterior wedge-shaped subcapsular segment shows no color flow signals on power Doppler US due to infarction. (b) A total of four graft arteries were anastomosed to the iliac arteries. Thrombosis of the upper pole artery caused non filling of the artery with contrast and absence of contrast enhancement in the upper pole of the transplanted kidney at MR angiography.

Summary

- Vascular thrombosis is a rare event following renal transplantation that usually carries a dismal prognosis.

- Doppler ultrasound offers immediate bed-side diagnosis while MRA confirms the diagnosis.

- Nephrectomy is frequently inevitable.

Transplant renal artery stenosis

- Transplant renal artery stenosis (TRAS) is a potentially reversible cause of hypertension and graft loss.

- The reported incidence of TRAS is around 6%.

- Percutaneous transluminal angioplasty (PTA) is accepted as the initial treatment of choice with fair success rate while open surgical correction is rarely employed.

Clinical features

- Uncontrolled hypertension despite increasing the dose of anti-hypertensive therapy.

- Impaired graft function.

- An audible bruit over the graft.

- Recurrent acute rejection episodes refractory to immunotherapy is a rare presentation.

Pathology

- Although TRAS is mostly induced technically, many risk factors were suggested to be associated with this pathology such as long cold ischemia time, acute rejection episodes, end-to-end anastomosis, multiple vessels as well as atherosclerotic arteries.

- TRAS would result in a decrease in the pressure of the renal afferent arteriole with subsequent activation of the renin-angiotensin-aldosterone system resulting in rise in the levels of angiotensin II which induces systemic vasoconstriction causing an increase of the blood pressure.

Imaging findings
Ultrasound(US)

- Extrarenal Doppler criteria for significant TRAS:

  o velocity greater than 180 cm/s.

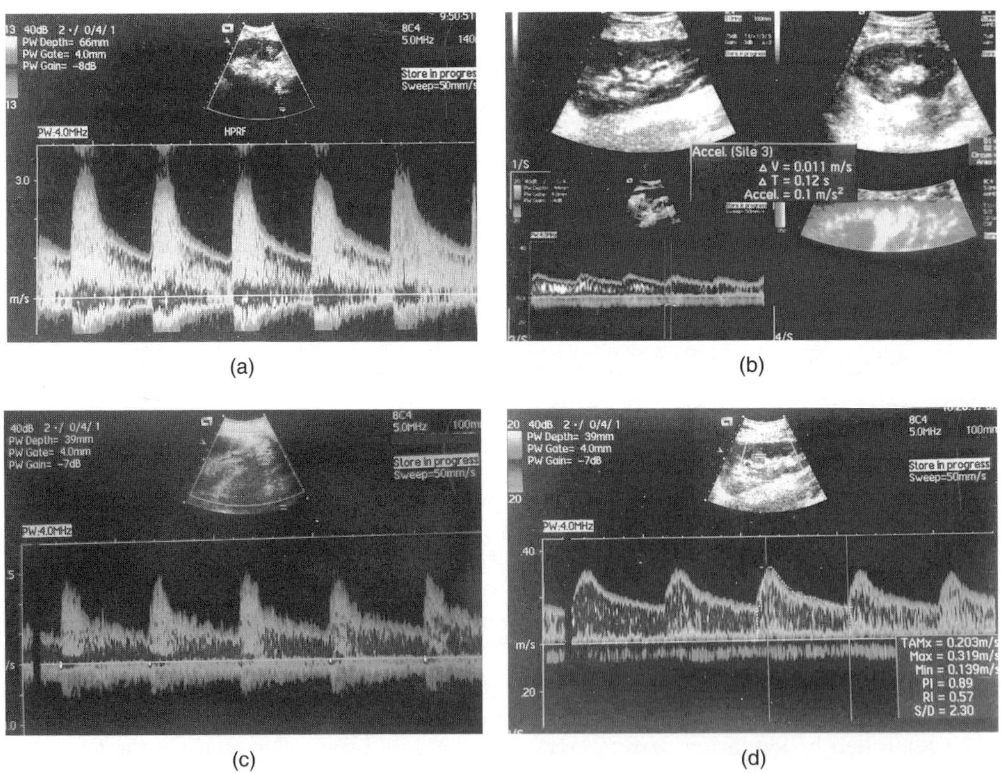

(a) (b)

(c) (d)

Figure 6.3 Transplant renal artery stenosis (TRAS). Doppler US findings before (a & b) and after angioplasty. (c & d). (a) Extrarenal criteria in the form of high peak systolic velocity (>3 m/s) and spectral broadening. (b) Intrarenal criteria are dampened wave form with prolonged acceleration time (0.12 s). Note normal grayscale pattern and preserved perfusion on power Doppler mode. (c) & (d) After angioplasty, normalization of the extrarenal spectral Doppler criteria (c) and the intrarenal wave form (d) was achieved.

- o marked spectral broadening.

- o velocity gradient between stenotic and prestenotic segments of more than 2:1.

- Distal Doppler criteria, in the renal parenchyma, are

  - o dampened waveform 'Tardus and Parvus abnormalities'.

  - o prolonged acceleration time of more than 0.07s (Fig. 6.3).

Magnetic resonance angiography (MRA)

- Gadolinium-enhanced MRA (Fig. 6.4) could be utilized to assess the arterial flow in suspected cases. It provides both anatomical and functional diagnosis.

Renal scintigraphy

- Demonstrates reduced perfusion in kidney transplant with RAS. This finding is non-specific as it can be seen with other causes of parenchymal failure.

IA-DSA

- Usually used as a routine basal step prior to definitive intervention with percutaneous transluminal angioplasty (PTA) (Fig. 6.5).

- PTA with or without stenting is the recommended method of treatment.

Summary

- Renal artery stenosis may result in uncontrolled hypertension with subsequent graft impairment and loss.

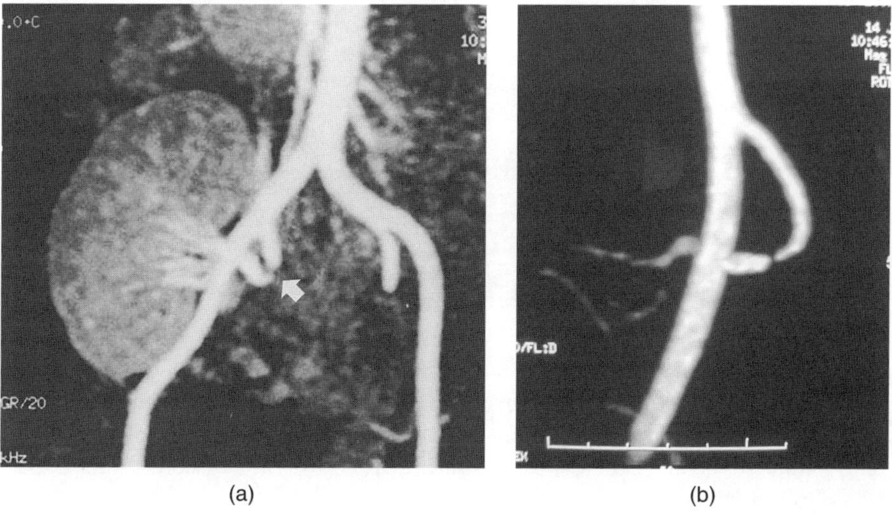

(a)   (b)

Figure 6.4 Transplant renal artery stenosis (TRAS). MRA findings. (a) MIP image of contrast enhanced MRA demonstrates stenosis (arrow) at the site of anastomosis between the graft renal artery and the recipient right internal iliac artery. (b) Reconstructed coronal oblique MIP image demonstrates the stenosis clearly.

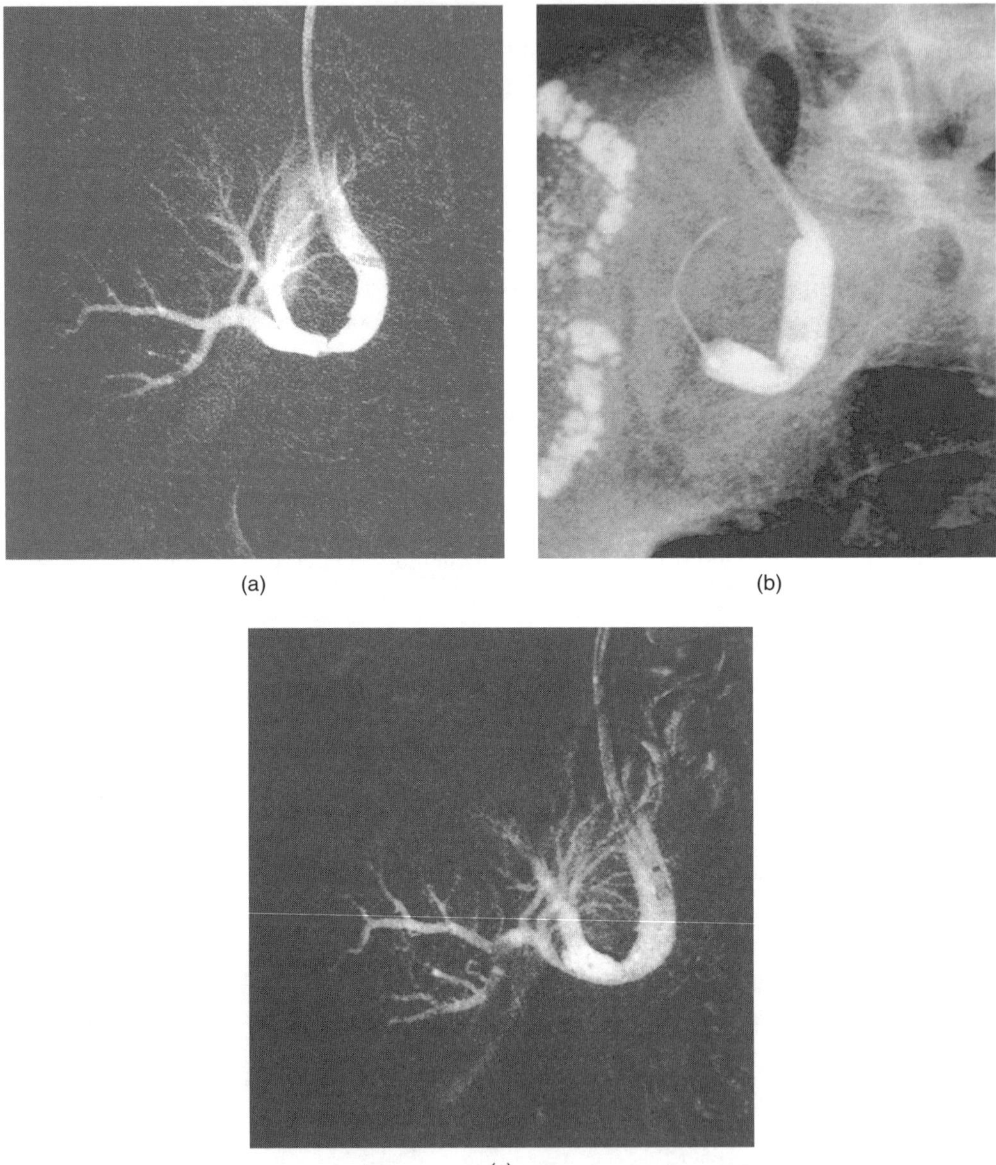

(a)

(b)

(c)

Figure 6.5 Percutaneous transluminal angioplasty (PTA) of TRAS. (a) Intraarterial digital subtraction angiography (IA-DSA) of the right internal iliac artery via contralateral femoral approach shows a localized post-anastomotic stenosis. (b) The balloon of the angioplasty catheter is inflated across the stenotic segment. (c) Post-PTA IA-DSA shows satisfactory dilatation of the stenosis.

- Doppler ultrasound, MRA and conventional angiography are the usual diagnostic imaging modalities.

- Percutaneous transluminal angioplasty is the recommended treatment with fair success rate.

6.3 Urological complications

Urinary leakage

- The reported incidence of urinary leak following renal transplantation has ranged from 1.2 to 8.9% in most published series.

- Endourologic management is the recommended initial therapy through percutaneous nephrostomy tube drainage with or without ureteral stent placement.

- Open surgical intervention can be used subsequently following failure of initial therapy.

Clinical features

- Urinary fistula is usually diagnosed in the early postoperative period following renal transplantation. Late presentation is exceptional.

- It is suggested by excessive fluid drainage through the drains or the wound. The diagnosis of urine leakage can be confirmed by creatinine estimation of the drained fluid.

- Rarely, pelvic urinoma may present with high grade fever, rising serum creatinine or oliguria.

- In neglected cases, significant complications such as perigraft abscess, burst abdomen or even fatal septicemia may develop.

Pathology

- Urinary leakage usually occur secondary to disruption of ureterovesical anastomosis.

- Factors on the recipient side include defunctionalized bladder as in anuric patients for more than one year or pathological bladder as in patients with neurogenic bladder dysfunction or bladder bilharziasis.

- Over-dissection of the ureter in the donor side during harvesting would result in ureteral ischemia and subsequent necrosis.

- Vesical leaks are uncommon in the current transplant era as most of the transplant surgeons are adopting the extravesical techniques of ureteral implantation.

- Calyceal fistulae secondary to significant polar vessel thrombosis or ligation is rare with current refinement of surgical techniques.

Imaging findings

Ultrasound

- US is the initial screening technique.

- A urine leak or urinoma appears as well-defined, anechoic fluid collection with no septation (Fig. 6.6).

- Aspiration may be performed with US guidance. The creatinine level of the aspirated fluid differentiates urine leak from a seroma or lymphocele.

- US can be used to guide antegrade pyelography and percutaneous nephrostomy (PCN) drainage with or without stent placement. This allows healing of the fistula in more than half of the patients.

Antegrade pyelography

- It is applied for most of the diagnosed cases with urinary fistula prior to definitive intervention (Fig. 6.7).

- It is necessary to provide detailed information about the site of origin of the urinoma in order to plan appropriate intervention.

Magnetic resonance imaging (MRI)

- Excretory MRU provides accurate non-invasive delineation of the leakage site as well as the extent of ureteral loss (Fig. 6.8).

- T2 MRU would also provide adequate and safe delineation of the collecting system in patients with renal impairment.

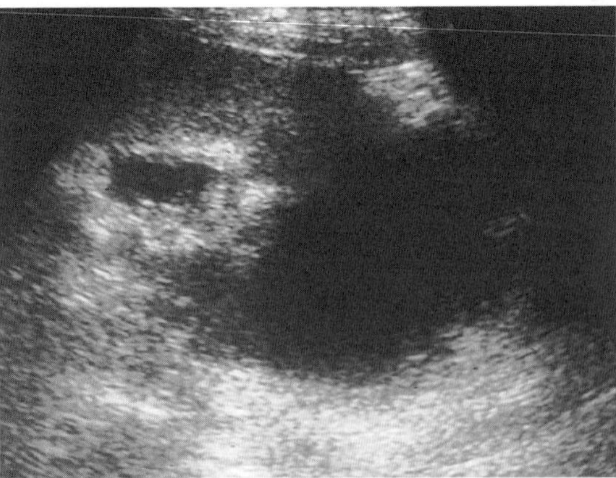

Figure 6.6 Urinary leakage. US findings. Longitudinal US scan demonstrates mild hydronephrosis secondary to a compressing urinoma which appears sonolucent and well circumscribed adjacent to the lower pole of the transplanted kidney.

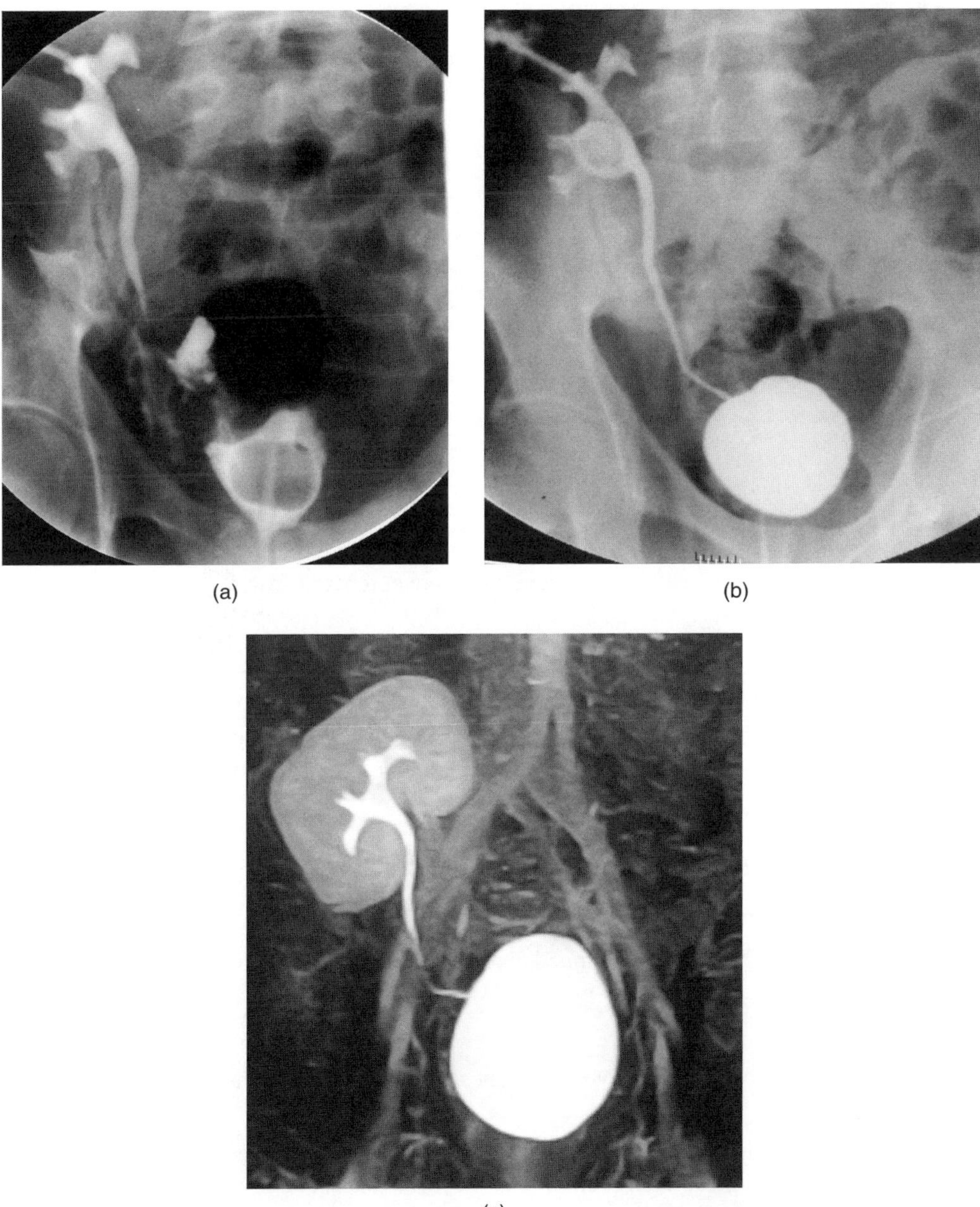

Figure 6.7 Percutaneous nephrostomy (PCN) in management of urinary leakage. (a) Antegrade pyelography prior to PCN identifies urinary leakage from the distal ureteric segment. (b) Antegrade pyelogram through the nephrostomy tube after 4 weeks demonstrates no further urine leakage with complete visualization of the ureter down to the urinary bladder. (c) Excretory MRU, after removal of the PCN tube confirms complete healing of the urinary fistula.

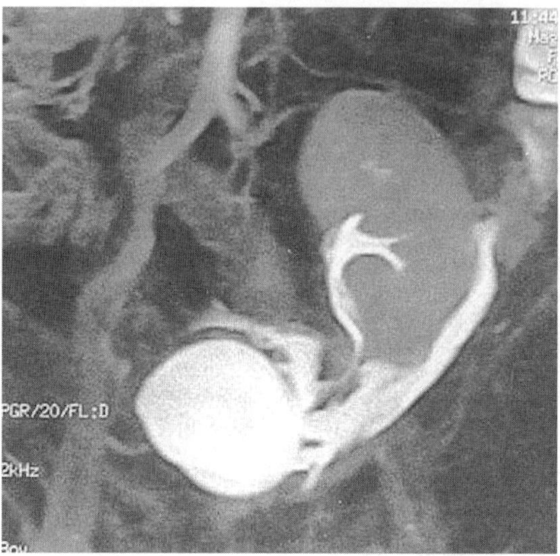

Figure 6.8   MRU in urinary leakage. Urine leakage (perivesical and perirenal) from a ureteric fistula is shown on excretory MRU in a patient with normal renal function.

Ascending cystography

- A routine diagnostic procedure in patients with urinary fistula to diagnose vesical leaks and assess its extent.

- Absence of abnormalities in ascending studies excludes vesical and distal ureteral pathologies.

Radionuclide studies

- Shows extravasation of radiotracer.

- Delayed scintigrams should be obtained since accumulation of radiotracer might be slow.

Summary

- US, antegrade pyelography and MRU are the main diagnostic tools used to establish the diagnosis

- Percutaneous techniques with or without ureteral stenting are the recommended initial treatment. Open surgical intervention can be used subsequently following failure of initial therapy

6.4 Ureteric strictures

- Reported incidence ranged from 1.3% to 10.2% in most published series.

- Percutaneous techniques are the recommended initial treatment with percutaneous nephrostomy tube placement to be followed by endoscopic dilatation with stent placement.

- Open surgical intervention can be used subsequently following failure of initial therapy.

Clinical features

- Ureteric strictures are usually asymptomatic because of complete graft denervation during harvesting.

- Rise of serum creatinine is observed.

- Rarely, anuria (oliguria) or high grade fever would be the presenting symptom.

- Recurrent urinary tract infection could be the leading clinical feature particularly in late and chronic obstruction.

Pathology

- Causes of ureteric strictures are mostly technical; overdissection of the ureter in the donor side during harvesting is a major cause of distal ureteral ischemia and subsequent fibrosis.

- Twisting of the implanted ureter on the recipient side is an implicating factor.

- Other possible risk factors include ureteritis secondary to acute rejection episodes or peri-ureteric fibrosis complicating urinary leakage.

Imaging findings
Ultrasound (US)

- Minor pelvicalyceal dilatation can be seen in the immediate postoperative period without obstruction (Fig. 6.9a).

- US demonstrates the degree of hydronephrosis as well as the level of obstruction based on the level of ureteral dilatation (Fig. 6.9b).

- The ultrasound will guide nephrostomy tube placement.

- US excludes other causes of hydronephrosis e.g. accumulating lymphocele.

- Doppler US shows high resistive index (RI) (Fig. 6.9c).

Magnetic resonance imaging (MRI)

- T2 MRU is safe and provides accurate information about the level and length of the ureteric stricture and degree of hydronephrosis particularly in patients with marked reduction in renal function (Fig. 6.10a).

Antegrade pyelography (Fig. 6.10b)

- It should be employed in almost all the cases with diagnosed ureteral strictures prior to definitive intervention.

- Insertion of PCN tube allows reduction of serum creatinine down to its basal level and permits definitive intervention to be carried out under improved clinical circumstances.

- It guides antegrade balloon dilatation ± stent placement. Early strictures are usually successfully managed by antegrade balloon dilatation and stent placement.

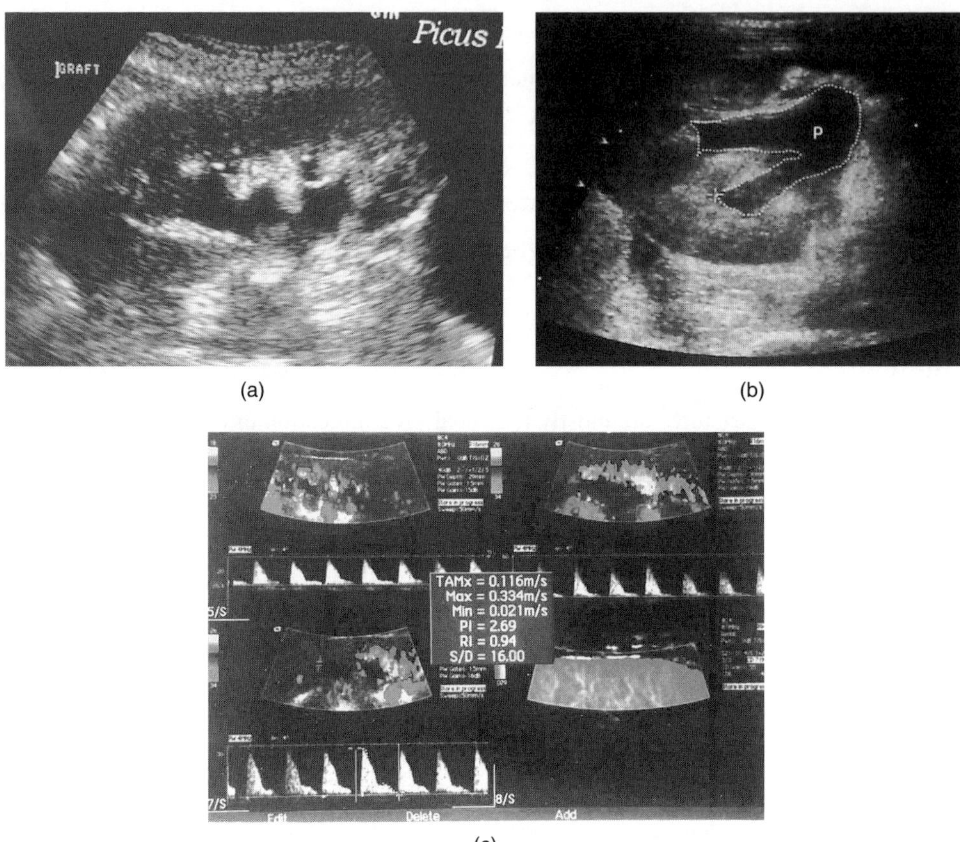

Figure 6.9 Post-transplant hydronephrosis. US findings. (a) Mild pelvicalyceal dilatation is frequently seen in the transplanted kidney without obstruction. (b) Moderate degree of hydronephrosis is shown on transverse US scan of a transplanted kidney secondary to ureteric stricture. (c) High RI (0.94) and preserved perfusion on color Doppler US (c) confirmed the diagnosis of obstructive uropathy.

Ascending cystography

- It should be performed if high grade reflux or infravesical obstruction was suspected as a possible cause of graft hydroureteronephrosis.

  - This should be considered in patients with ureteral dilatation down to the bladder, long standing urinary tract infections or possible prostatic enlargement.

  - Ascending cystogram would prove the possibility of reflux and diagnose significant post-voiding residual urine in cases of infravesical obstruction.

Summary

- Ultrasound, MRU and antegrade pyelography are the main diagnostic tools to establish the diagnosis of post-transplant ureteric strictures.

- Percutaneous techniques are the recommended initial treatment.

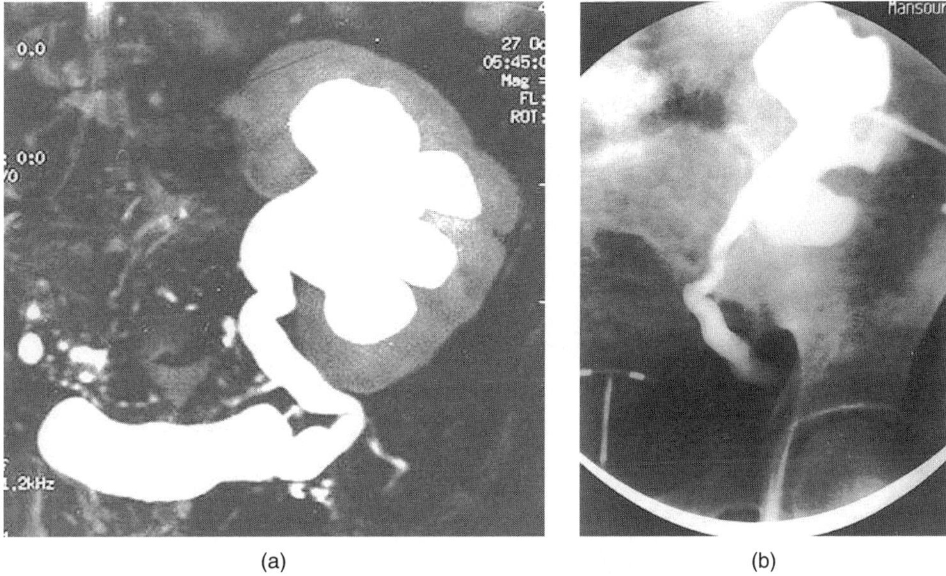

(a)   (b)

Figure 6.10   Post-transplant ureteric stricture. (a) T2 W MRU demonstrates hydronephrosis of the transplanted kidney and dilatation of the ureter secondary to stricture at the uretero-vesical junction developed 3 months postoperatively. (b) Antegrade pyelography demonstrates the dilatation of the ureter to the level of the stricture.

6.5 Post-transplant lymphocele

- The development of perigraft lymphatic collections is not uncommon. The incidence has been reported to be as high as 36% most of which were small and resolved spontaneously.

- Active management of lymphoceles is only indicated if they are large enough to become symptomatic or cause an obstruction of the ureter.

- Percutaneous drainage with sclerotherapy can be tried initially, but if these measures are not sufficient, marsupialization by an open or laparoscopic procedure is then necessary.

Clinical features

- The majority of lymphoceles are asymptomatic and discovered accidentally during routine ultrasound examination.

- Lymphocele can induce pressure upon the surrounding vital structures causing obstruction.

  o Pressure upon the graft ureter would result in graft hydronephrosis with rising of serum creatinine.

  o Less commonly, pressure on the iliac vein would induce venous stasis leading to deep venous thrombosis.

  o Rarely, huge lymphocele may cause reduction of the arterial flow in the graft artery inducing renal hypertension or even graft artery thrombosis.

Pathology

- Source of lymph production is either the perivascular lymphatics of the recipient or the renal allograft lymphatics of the donor.

- Technically, meticulous dissection and ligation of these lymphatics would minimize the possibility of developing such a complication.

- Risk factors for lymphocele formation including

  - Acute rejection episodes
  - Heparinization
  - Some immunosuppressive protocols, e.g. Rapamycin
  - Re-transplantation.

Imaging findings

Ultrasound

- US could diagnose small asymptomatic lymphoceles as well as large complicated collections.

- On US, lymphoceles are well-circumscribed, anechoic and may have septations (Fig.6.11a).

- US also diagnoses accurately any hydronephrotic changes in the graft.

- Ultrasound is very useful in guiding fluid needle aspiration to judge its chemical and bacteriological nature prior to intervention (Fig. 6.11b).

- Ultrasound is also very useful in follow up to diagnose re-collection.

Computed tomography (CT)

- Non-contrast CT represents the second line of diagnosis. It provides accurate delineation of the collection and its dimensions.

- Lymphoceles are usually sharply demarcated with attenuation values of those of water (Fig. 6.11c).

- The density of lymphoceles is less than that of recent hematoma and abscesses.

- In patients with normal kidney function CT urography (CTU) would depict clearly the pelvi-calyceal system as well as the relation of the lymphocele to the ureter and bladder (Fig. 6.11d).

Magnetic resonance imaging

- MRU provides accurate depiction of the lymphocele in relation to the transplanted kidney, ureter and urinary bladder. It also identifies any pressure effect leading to hydronephrosis (Fig. 6.11e).

Image-guided percutaneous drainage (PCD)

- Large lymphoceles usually cause secondary hydronephrosis and should be drained.

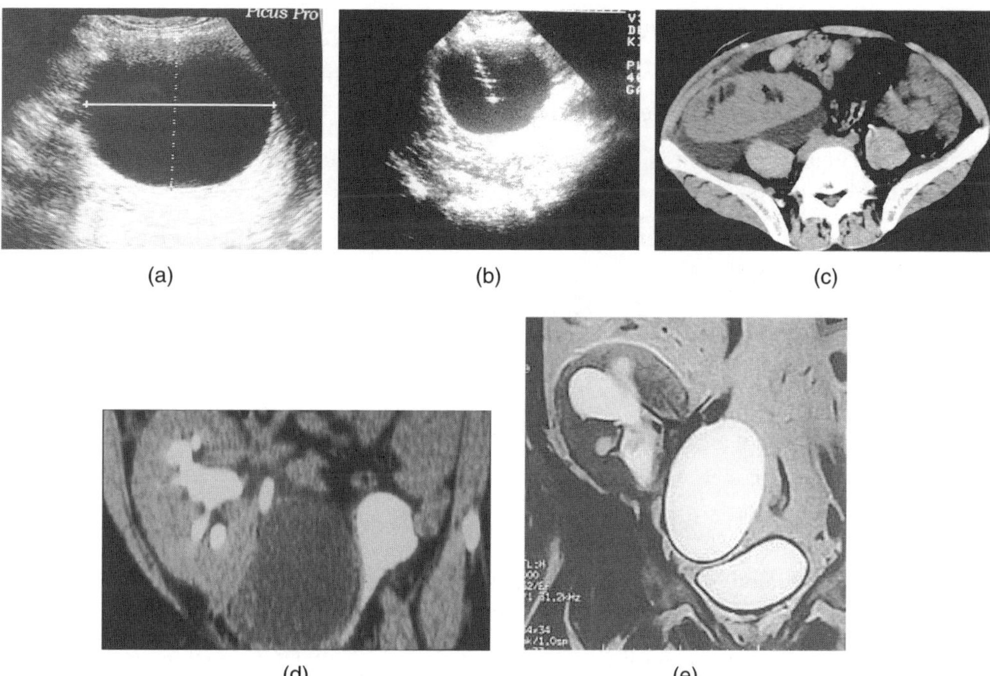

Figure 6.11 Lymphocele (a) An US scan of a lymphocele shows a well-circumscribed anechoic lesion with no septation and with posterior echo-enhancement. (b) US-guided aspiration of lymphocele fluid content. The echogenic shadow of the needle is well visualized. (c) A non-contrast axial CT image of right iliac transplanted kidney shows a well-defined hypodense collection posterior to the kidney due to a lymphocele. (d) A coronal image of CT urography of another patient demonstrates a hypointense lymphocele extends between the kidney and the urinary bladder which is compressed and outlined with contrast. No graft hydronephrosis is present in this case. (e) Coronal image of T2 MRU demonstrates graft hydronephrosis secondary to a large lymphocele extends between the kidney and the urinary bladder causing compression of the ureter.

- They commonly recur after simple percutaneous aspiration.

- Permanent resolution may require prolonged catheter drainage and transcatheter instillation of sclerosing agents such as povidine-iodine or doxycycline.

Summary

- Lymphocele is a frequent finding following renal transplantation that rarely induce obstruction of the surrounding vital structures.

- Ultrasound is the initial screening tool to diagnose such a pathology while MRI provides a safe detailed delineation of the collection and the graft.

- Percutaneous drainage with sclerotherapy would be tried initially with fair success rate with marsupialization to be employed in recurrent cases.

6.6 Delayed graft function (DGF)

- DGF is usually defined as the need of dialysis during the first 7 days after transplantation or the failure to improve pre-existing renal function.

- DGF of a kidney transplant is the most common allograft complication in the immediate post-transplant period.

- DGF represents a clinical dilemma with wide range of etiologies that include

  - acute tubular necrosis,
  - arterial occlusion,
  - venous thrombosis,
  - ureteral obstruction, and
  - severe rejection episodes.

Clinical features

- Vary from subtle slowing of the expected decline in the serum creatinine to prolonged oliguria requiring dialysis support for a number of days after transplantation.

- The presenting clinical symptom may suggest the cause of DGF, e.g. fever and tender graft is observed in rejection cases and hematuria in venous thrombosis.

Pathology

- DGF represents an irreversible loss of functioning nephron mass at time of transplantation leaving the patient with diminished functional reserve and more vulnerable to subsequent injury.

- It is associated with release of rich pro-inflammatory agonists including interferon, interleukin 2, transforming growth factor β and interleukin 4 which might stimulate non-antigen dependent inflammation and scarring.

- DGF secondary to acute tubular necrosis is associated with increased risk of acute rejection through up-regulation of adhesion molecules and HLA class II antigens.

Imaging findings

Ultrasound

- An ultrasound scan should be performed soon after surgery to be considered as baseline study.

- Ultrasound could reveal features suggestive of ureteric obstruction to be confirmed by further investigations as mentioned before.

- Doppler ultrasound could easily exclude vascular thrombosis.

- Differentiating acute rejection, acute tubular necrosis and cyclosporine toxicity are often difficult on US and is usually made by US-guided renal biopsy.

- The sonographic features that might be seen in acute rejection include:

  ○ Graft enlargement

  ○ Heterogeneity of renal cortex

  ○ Enlarged hypoechoic pyramids

  ○ Loss of corticomedullary differentiation

  ○ Hypoechogenic areas involving both cortex and medulla

  ○ Reduced renal sinus echoes

  ○ Thickening of the walls of collecting system.

- These features are non-specific and many of them are seldom seen. The kidney may even appear normal in many cases of acute rejection.

- Doppler US (Fig. 6.12) shows decreased diastolic flow with subsequent high resistive index (RI). This is also a non-specific finding. A high RI, more than 0.9 is relatively specific for acute rejection.

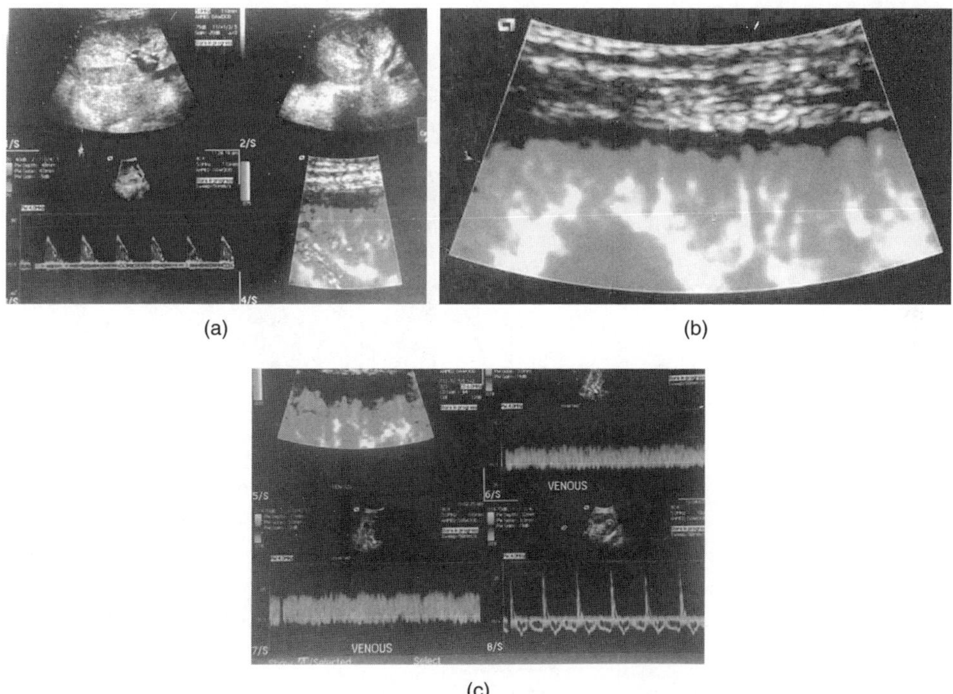

(a)   (b)

(c)

Figure 6.12 Acute rejection on Doppler US. (a) Increased echogenicity of renal cortex on grayscale US is associated with absent diastolic flow (RI equals 1) on spectral Doppler and mild hypoperfusion on power Doppler evidenced by absent color flow in the subcapsular zone. (b) Subcapsular hypoperfused zone on power Doppler mode in a transplanted kidney. Note hypoperfusion as a narrow subcapsular rim lacking of color flow on power Doppler mode. Biopsy revealed grade II acute rejection. (c) Significant subcapsular hypoperfusion on power Doppler US with reversed diastolic flow on spectral Doppler in a patient with early postoperative anuria. Preservation of venous flow excludes renal vein thrombosis. Acute vascular rejection (grade II) was confirmed histologically.

- Pulsatility index (PI) of more than 1.5 is relatively diagnostic.

- Power Doppler US asses the degree of perfusion reduction that is usually a feature of acute rejection, particularly the sever forms.

- The association of moderately preserved perfusion on power Doppler US, with elevated RI on Doppler sonography is highly suggestive of ATN (Fig. 6.13a).

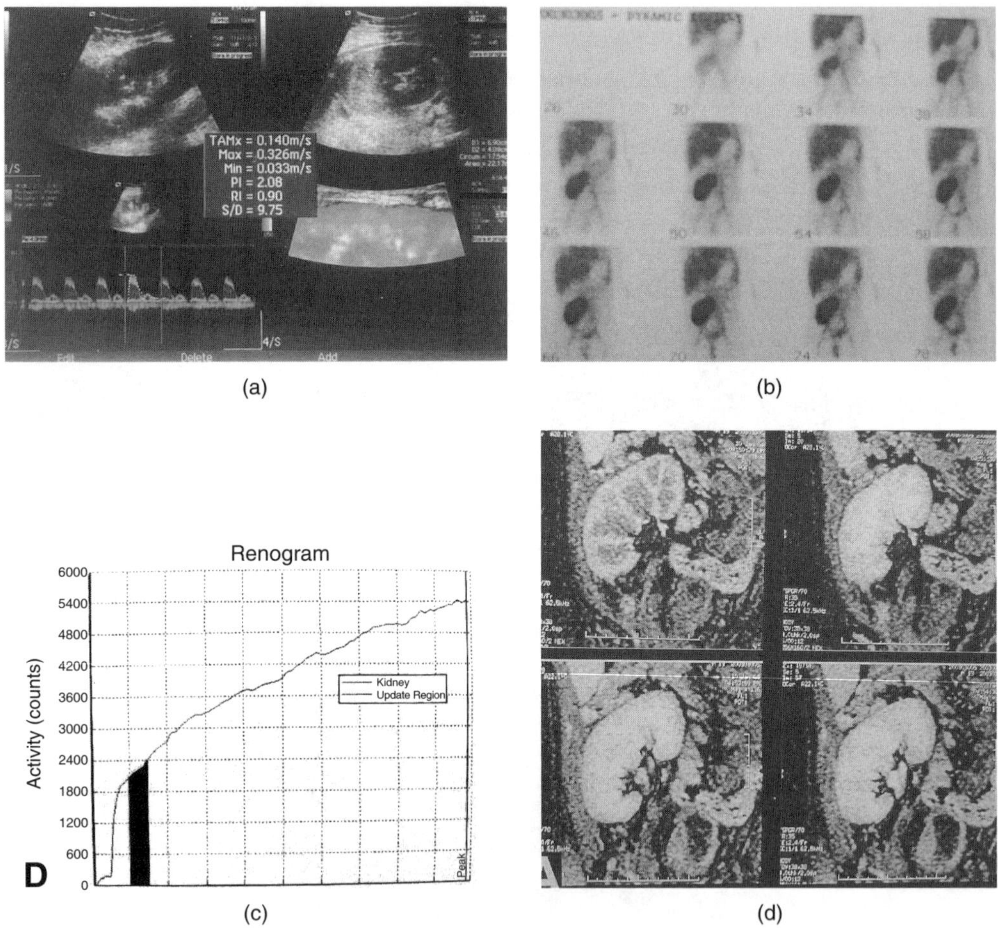

Figure 6.13 Acute Tubular Necrosis (ATN); Doppler US, radionuclide, and functional MRI findings. (a) Spectral Doppler analysis demonstrates absent end diastole with elevated RI (0.90). US-guided biopsy was performed and the final diagnosis was ATN (b) Radionuclide study showing the perfusion phase is relatively well maintained. Images of later phases show persistent isotope accumulation and slow washout. (c) Time-activity curve of a radionuclide study shows mildly diminished flow to the transplanted kidney with rising up curve due to delayed excretion of the radio-active agent. These features are similar to those seen with obstructive uropathy. (d) Dynamic MRI study shows moderately preserved perfusion of the transplanted kidney with progressive enhancement in nephrographic and excretory phases and with delayed excretion of contrast medium.

Radionuclide studies

- Show reduced renal perfusion with delay in the early vascular phase.

- Reduction of the early peak activity.

- Prolongation of the time between aortic and kidney peak activities.

- A baseline scintigraphic study is important.

- If an isotope study is normal in early postoperative phase and becomes abnormal subsequently, acute rejection should be suspected.

- In patients with cyclosporine nephrotoxicity, the perfusion phase is normal but there is prolonged clearance of 99m Tc MAG3. Measurement of blood cyclosporine level and renal biopsy are the confirmatory tests.

- In conditions where there is mildly diminished flow to the kidney with delayed excretion on radionuclide imaging (Fig. 6.13b, c), acute tubular necrosis (ATN) could be suspected.

Functional MRI (Fig. 6.13d)

- It could be used in evaluating glomerular filtration, tubular concentration, regional perfusion, water movement (diffusion), as well as oxygenation in addition to morphological information.

- Recent reports had confirmed the great ability of functional MRI in differentiating between various etiologies of DGF namely acute rejection and acute tubular necrosis.

- Non-enhanced techniques can provide important information without the potential risk of adverse effects of Gd contrast agents in kidney transplant patients with severe impairment of renal function.

Summary

- DGF is a common problem following renal transplantation.

- Ultrasound offers the initial imaging diagnostic modality to exclude ureteric obstruction and vascular crises. Although biopsy represents the gold standard modality to diagnose acute rejection or acute tubular necrosis.

- Functional MRI is a new promising non-invasive diagnostic modality.

6.7 Post-transplant bladder malignancy

- There is 6.9 fold increases in the incidence of bladder cancer among male and female patients compared with general population one year following renal transplantation.

Clinical features

- Irritative bladder symptoms:
  - Frequency, nocturia and urgency.

- Hematuria.

- Many of these patients have a poor prognosis due to delayed diagnosis and aggressive disease.

Pathology

- The enhanced emergence and progression of neoplasms among transplant patients may be explained by blockage of apoptosis (programmed cell death) as immunosuppressive agents may cause DNA damage and interfere with normal DNA repair mechanisms.

- These drugs may allow promotion of the synthesis of proneoplastic cytokines: transforming growth factor beta (TGF-β) and vascular endothelial growth factor (VEGF).

- A number of cancers were linked to viral infection but their role in development of urologic malignancy has to be more ascertained.

Imaging findings

The imaging findings of bladder cancer are covered elsewhere in the book.

Summary

- Malignant bladder tumor is a serious sequel following renal transplantation. Hematuria is the leading presenting symptom and diagnosis is established by endoscopic biopsy.

- Ultrasound offers the initial imaging diagnostic modality. Adequate staging could be achieved with CT or MRI.

- Superficial bladder tumors are managed by endoscopic resection and adjuvant intravesical instillation while invasive disease needs cystectomy and urinary diversion.

References

El-Mekresh M, Osman Y, Ali-El-Dein B, El-Diasty T, Ghoneim M (2001) Urologic complications after living-donor renal transplantation. *BJU Int.* **87**: 295–306.

Kasiske B, Snyder J, Gilbertson D, Wang C (2004) Cancer after kidney transplantation in the United States. *Am. J. Transplant.* **4**: 905–913.

Khauli R, Stoff J, Lovewell T, Ghavamian R, Baker S (1993) Post-transplant lymphoceles: A critical look into risk factors, pathophysiology and management. *J. Urol.* **150**: 22–26.

Osman Y, Shokeir A, Ali-El-Dein B, Tantawy M, Wafa E, Shehab-El-Dein A, Ghoneim M (2003) Vascular complications after living-donor renal transplantation: Study risk factors and effects on graft and patient survival. *J. Urol.* **169**: 859–862.

Pfaff W, Howard R, Patton P *et al.* (1998) Delayed graft function after renal transplantation. *Transplantation* **65**: 219.

Teh H, Ang E, Wong W *et al.* (2003) Magnetic resonance renography: an alternative to radionuclide renography *AJR* **181**: 441–445.

7
Urinary Tract Injuries

Elliott R. Friedman, Stanford M. Goldman and Tung Shu

University of Texas Health Science Center at Houston

7.1 Introduction

The management of genitourinary system trauma has evolved over time, with an increased trend towards conservative management. Generally accepted indications for urgent operative intervention are hemorrhage control and preservation of tissue and function. Frequently, penetrating and blunt trauma of the genitourinary tract is associated with other abdominal or pelvic injuries, and management of these concominant injuries influences approach to the genitourinary injury.

Contemporary radiographic evaluation and clinical management decisions of renal injuries represent a shift from traditional practices. The widespread availability and speed of CT scanners in most emergency departments has essentially replaced the intravenous urogram in the workup of renal trauma.

This chapter covers the different injuries that may affect the urinary tract including those affecting the adrenal gland and scrotum.

7.2 Renal trauma

Introduction

- Renal trauma occurs in approximately 3% of all trauma cases and in as many as 10% of abdominal trauma cases.

- Multiorgan involvement is estimated to occur in approximately 80% of patients with penetrating renal trauma and 75% of patients with blunt kidney trauma.

Urogenital Imaging: A Problem-oriented Approach   Edited by Sameh K. Morcos and Henrik S. Thomsen
© 2009 John Wiley & Sons, Ltd

- With the advent of improved radiographic imaging and awareness of clinical outcomes, most renal injuries are now managed expectantly.

- In severe cases, aggressive surgical management is still warranted in order to retain renal function, prevent significant hemorrhage, and avoid future complications.

Clinical presentation and evaluation

- Most blunt traumas are either from a sudden deceleration or a direct injury to the flank area.

- The majority of blunt renal injuries are low grade; however these injuries are not uncommonly seen in major trauma centers.

- For penetrating trauma, the entry and exit locations may suggest renal injury. Penetrating trauma is more likely to cause high grade renal injury.

  o In many penetrating injuries, concomitant injuries are likely and must be evaluated.

- Management of the renal injury can be affected by the management of concomitant injuries.

- Hematuria and hypotension are two of the most important indicators for significant renal trauma.

  o Significant hematuria is defined as gross hematuria or more than five cells per high power field as seen from the first collection of urine of a catheterized specimen.

  o There is a low correlation between the amount of hematuria and severity of renal trauma. For example, renal pedicle injuries often do not present with hematuria.

  o Hematuria is a relatively common sequela following blunt abdominal trauma, but major renal injury is much less commonly present.

Staging of renal injury (Table 7.1)

- A renal organ injury scale has been developed by the American Association for the Surgery of Trauma (AAST) (Table 7.1).

- The AAST renal injury scale has been prospectively validated and was found to correlate with the need for surgical management.

- The various radiological classifications are not universally accepted and make communication with surgeons and urologists difficult.

Imaging

Techniques

Computed tomography (CT)

- Early and delayed phase imaging through the kidneys is required.

- Scanning should begin at the dome of the diaphragm.

Table 7.1 American Association for Surgery of Trauma (AAST) organ injury severity scale for renal trauma

Grade	Clinical/Imaging Findings
I	Microscopic or gross hematuria without imaging abnormality.
	Contusion
	Non-expanding subcapsular hematoma without parenchymal laceration.
II	Non-expanding perirenal hematoma confined to retroperitoneum.
	Superficial cortical laceration <1 cm depth and not involving the collecting system.
III	Renal laceration >1 cm depth and not involving the collecting system.
IV	Deep parenchymal laceration involving the cortex, medulla, and collecting system
	Injury of the main renal artery and vein with contained hemorrhage.
	Expanding subcapsular hematoma which compresses the kidney.
V	Completely shattered kidney.
	Renal hilar avulsion with devascularization of the kidney.

Adapted from: Moore EE, Shackford SR, Pachter HL (1989) Organ injury scaling: spleen, liver, and kidney. *J. Trauma* **29**: 1664–1666.

- Early phase
  - approximately 70 s after intravenous contrast administration, of 150 cc of contrast (2.5–3 cc/sec)
  - allows evaluation of the kidneys during the late cortical or homogeneous nephrographic phases of enhancement.
  - allows optimal parenchymal enhancement so that major solid organ injuries such as hepatic or splenic laceration may be identified with greatest sensitivity.
- Excretory phase
  - scanning is performed at least 3 min following the intravenous contrast infusion covering the whole abdomen and pelvis to evaluate collecting system injury.
  - Multiplanar reformatted images provide helpful adjunctive assessment.

Intravenous urography (IVU)

- In trauma assessment is generally relegated to gross evaluation of renal function in
  - patients who are too hemodynamically unstable to undergo CT.
  - patients brought to the operating room before CT can be performed.
  - institutions where CT is not available 24 hours per day.
- An IVU is usually sufficient to screen for the presence of bilateral renal function and to identify major parenchymal and collecting system injury.
- Limited intravenous urography consists of a scout KUB followed by images obtained immediately following the intravenous infusion (2 cc/kg) or rapid bolus (100 cc) of contrast, as well as delayed images obtained 5–10 min later.

- Oblique projections and tomograms might are of value when CT is not readily available.

Ultrasound

- *Focused abdominal sonograph* is often performed in trauma centers to evaluate for hemoperitoneum.

- Ultrasound is less sensitive than CT, and serious injuries may be missed, especially renal arterial injury.

- Color and power Doppler techniques, technology which is not universally present in emergency rooms, can establish the presence of blood flow to the kidney.

- Ultrasound evaluation has certain limitations

  o It is operator dependent.

  o A dynamic ileus which is a frequent occurrence in trauma patients, may interfere with adequate imaging of the kidneys.

  o Does not provide information about renal function.

Magnetic Resonance Imaging (MRI)

- MRI has not been extensively studied in patients with renal trauma and generally conceded to be an adjunctive assessment tool as opposed to a primary imaging modality in most cases.

- Major impediments to the routine use of MRI as a primary imaging modality in suspected cases of renal trauma include the more widespread availability of CT scanners in most emergency departments, as well as increased cost and imaging time.

- MRI has the following advantages:

  o Can distinguish renal ischemia from infarction and accurately assess the viability of renal fragments.

  o Able to suggest the age of a hematoma based on differences in signal intensity associated with the evolution of hemoglobin and its metabolites.

  o Can accurately distinguish intrarenal from perirenal hematoma and depict laceration in cases complicated by additional abnormalities such as perirenal hematoma and renal infarction; a distinction not always reliably made by CT.

  o Does not require ionizing radiation or the routine administration of intravenous contrast.

Imaging findings

The majority (75–85%) of renal injuries are considered to be minor injuries (grade 1 and grade II injuries).

- *Contusions* may appear as a focal area of striation or persistent contrast staining on delayed imaging (Fig. 7.1a).

- *Small intrarenal hematomas* appear as round or ovoid areas of diminished attenuation on CT (Fig. 7.1b).

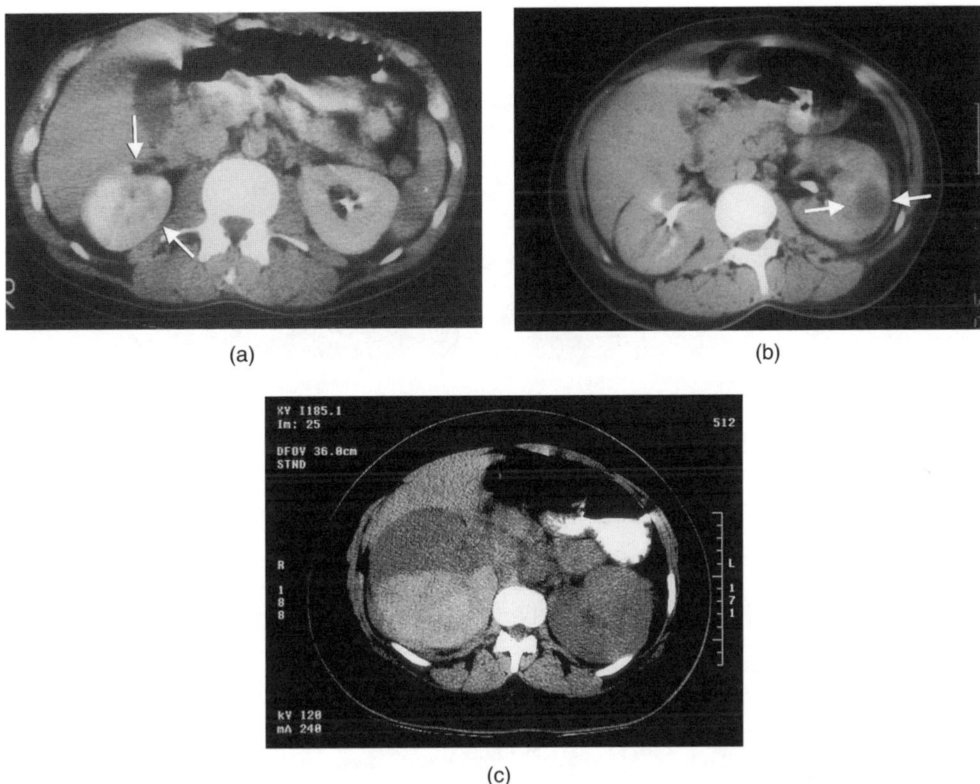

Figure 7.1 (a) Renal contusion (grade I) of the right kidney. Excretory Phase of CT shows normal left kidney with contrast in collecting system. On the right, a focal area of striated nephrogram (arrows) due to contusion of the kidney. (b) Small intrarenal hematomas appear as a rounded area of diminished attenuation (arrows) in the left kidney. (c) A subcapsular hematoma appears as an elliptical fluid collection flattening the contour of the right kidney.

- *A subcapsular hematoma* appears as a round or elliptical fluid collection indenting or flattening the renal contour (Fig. 7.1c).

- *A localized perinephric hematoma* confined between the renal capsule and the bridging septum may simulate a subcapsular hematoma. A high-attenuation value of the fluid (40–70 HU) is suggestive of acute clotted blood.

- *Lacerations*

  o Appear as linear parenchymal defects with associated perinephric hematoma (Fig. 7.2a).

  o The depth of the laceration and associated involvement of the collecting system or vascular structures determines the severity of the laceration (Fig. 7.2b).

  o Major renal lacerations may be associated with devascularization of the renal parenchyma or extension to the renal collecting system.

- *Parenchymal infarction* may be recognized as areas of diminished contrast enhancement without associated perinephric hematoma (Fig. 7.3). In distinction to contusions, which

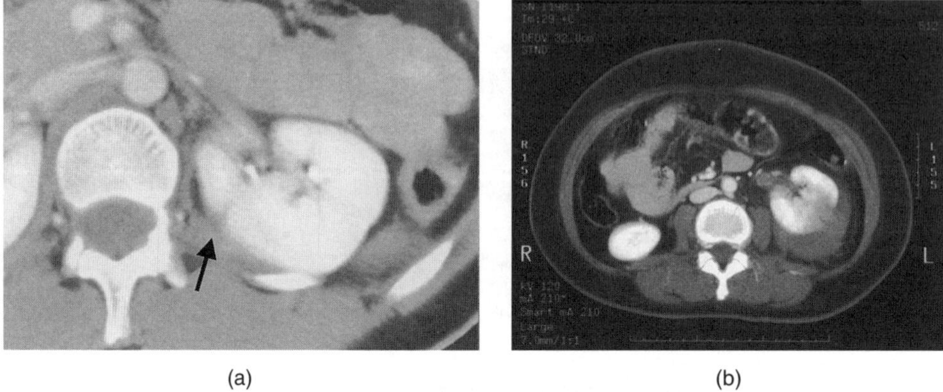

(a)   (b)

Figure 7.2   (a) A linear parenchymal laceration (arrow) associated with a small perinephric hematoma is shown in the left kidney. (b) A deep renal laceration extending from cortex into the pelvis of the left kidney with perinephric hematoma.

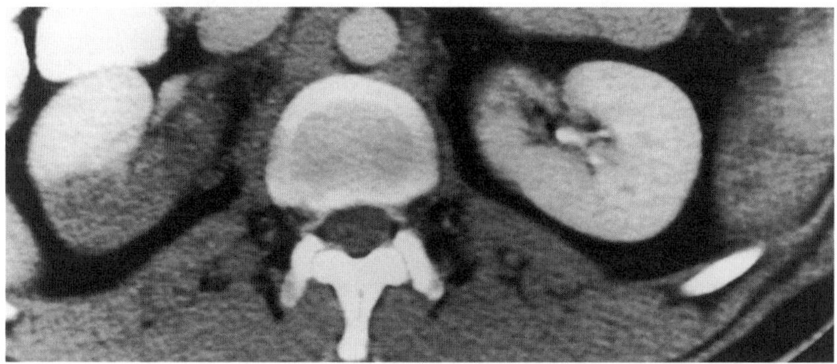

Figure 7.3   Parenchymal infarction of the right kidney appears as area of diminished contrast enhancement without associated perinephric hematoma.

may enhance to some degree on delayed imaging, areas of infarction remain hypoattenuated.

- ○ *Subsegmental infarcts* result from stretching or thrombosis of the accessory renal, capsular, or intrarenal segmental arteries and have a wedge shape.
- ○ *Segmental infarctions* result from occlusion of segmental renal arteries.

- • *Shattered kidney or renal rupture*

  - ○ Multiple severe renal lacerations, usually associated with one or multiple devitalized fragments (Fig. 7.4a).
  - ○ lacerations extending to the renal pelvis and collecting system.
  - ○ Severe compromise in the excretion of contrast material.
  - ○ Extensive hemorrhage, and active arterial bleeding.
  - ○ A devitalized segment may be difficult to distinguish when it is surrounded by a hematoma of similar attenuation to the devitalized segment.

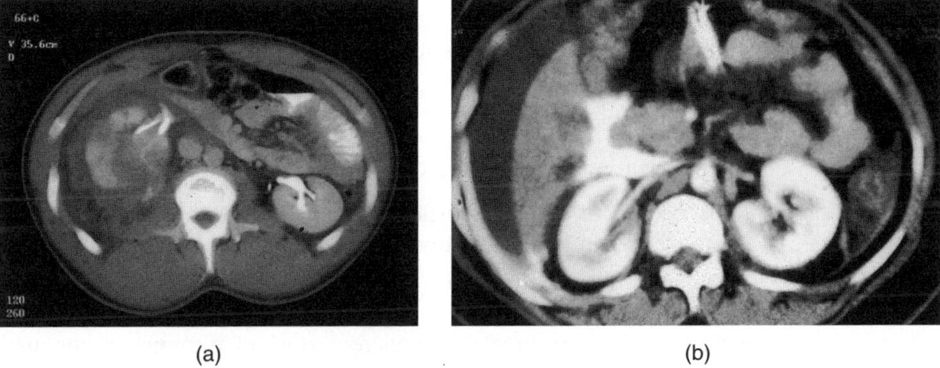

Figure 7.4 (a) Severe trauma causing shattering of the right kidney. (b) Active arterial extravasation of the right kidney on a CT scan immediately following contrast bolus administration shows contrast extravasation.

- o Active arterial extravasation is often best distinguished on CT scans immediately following contrast bolus administration as patchy areas of higher attenuation (85–370 HU, mean of 132 HU) within a less dense hematoma (Fig. 7.4b). Not infrequently, the delayed images provide the only clue of injury as evidenced by pooling of contrast near the site of arterial injury.

- o Urine extravasation may be detected on delayed scans, and urine leakage typically collects within the lateral perinephric space.

- **Occlusion of the main renal artery**

  - o Results as a consequence of intimal tearing and thrombus formation at the intimal flap following a rapid deceleration mechanism of injury.

  - o In most cases, contrast-enhanced CT is sufficient to confidently make the diagnosis of renal artery thrombosis.

    - ■ An abrupt termination of the renal artery distal to its origin with global renal infarction, with or without a cortical rim of enhancement (cortical rim sign).

    - ■ A small amount of hematoma may be present around the proximal renal artery.

    - ■ Arterial occlusion is characterized by the absence of a perinephric hematoma.

- **Renal artery avulsion**

  - o Caused by a laceration through the muscularis and adventitial layers

  - o CT demonstrates global infarction with extensive medial perirenal hematoma.

- **Renal vein thrombosis**

  - o Is a rare entity following blunt trauma.

  - o Pre-contrast CT

    - ■ Thrombus may appear as a high attenuation intraluminal mass.

    - ■ The renal vein may be distended.

- ○ Enhanced CT
  - ▪ May show findings of acute venous hypertension
    - nephromegaly
    - delayed and diminished nephrogram
    - decreased excretion of contrast into the collecting system.
  - ○ Venography may be needed in cases of suspected injury to the renal vein or inferior vena cava as venous laceration is not reliably detected by enhanced CT.

Commonly seen artifacts

- Patient motion during scanning can create an apparent zone of diminished attenuation along the surface of the kidney.
- *Pseudocapsular hematoma* is readily distinguishable because
  - ○ similar findings may be seen on the same image in the anterior abdominal wall, liver, spleen, and contralateral kidney.
  - ○ This artifact will be absent on adjacent images or repeat scans.
- A *renal pseudofracture* appears as a sharp cleft of the renal contour near the hilum, and unlike a true laceration, no perirenal hematoma is present.

Assessment of complications of renal injury

- CT and angiography are useful in detecting many of the possible urologic complications that may follow renal injury.
- Early complications generally occur within four weeks of injury and include urinary extravasation or urinoma formation, delayed bleeding, perinephric abscess or infected urinoma, sepsis, and arteriovenous fistula or pseudoaneurysm.
- Late complications include hypertension, hydronephrosis, calculus formation, and chronic pyelonephritis.
- The presence of devascularized segments are more often associated with delayed complications than are vascularized renal fragments.
- The combination of devascularized renal fragments and pancreatic or bowel injury places the patient at greater risk for infection and abscess formation.
- Selective renal angiography and renin sampling may effectively evaluate patients with suspected post-traumatic renovascular hypertension when vascular lesions are not depicted by CT angiography.
- Page kidney due to a post-traumatic subcapsular hematoma may appear as a subcapsular fluid collection or perirenal soft tissue thickening on CT with an asymmetrically delayed nephrogram in the affected kidney. The traumatic 'page' kidney is very rare and often resolves spontaneously.

Management

- In hemodynamically stable patients, most renal injuries may be managed non-surgically following full imaging evaluation.

- In a large series of close to 3000 blunt renal traumas, only a small number of patients (2.6%) required surgical exploration and there was a less than 1% nephrectomy rat.

- Most urinary extravasation can resolve with conservative management.

- A ureteral stent or a percutaneous nephrostomy tube may be required for complete healing.

- With Grade IV or V renal injury, particularly renal pedicle avulsion and shattered kidney, a nephrectomy may be required.

- Post-traumatic renovascular hypertension is an uncommon complication of renal injury. It is usually treated non-surgically unless there is cardiovascular instability.

Absolute indications for surgical management

- Persistent life threatening hemorrhage from renal injury.

- Avulsion of the renal pedicle or tear of the renal artery.

- Expanding or uncontained retroperitoneal hematoma.

The relative indications for surgical exploration

- Incomplete radiographic evaluation.

- Devitalized renal parenchyma.

- Vascular injury.

- Urinary extravasation.

Special circumstances

- In patients who present with severe shock, exploratory laparotomy should be performed without any delay and before radiographic studies can be obtained.

- IVU should be performed intra-operatively to demonstrate the extent of the renal injury and confirm the presence of a normal contralateral kidney.

- Renal arterial repair

  - reserved for solitary kidneys, bilateral injured kidneys and renal arterial injury that is detected early (within 6 h of injury).

  - Endovascular stenting has a limited role in renal arterial injury since other intra-abdominal injuries are typical associated and time may therefore be limited.

- Renal vein injury typically results in significant hemorrhage. Reconstruction is feasible for the main renal vein whereas segmental veins can be safely ligated.

- Complete transection of the ureteropelvic junction requires immediate surgical repair.

7.3 Adrenal trauma

Introduction

- Adrenal injuries are relatively uncommon sequelae of blunt abdominal trauma.

- The incidence of adrenal injury is estimated to be between 0.8–0.9% following blunt abdominal trauma.

Clinical presentation

- While adrenal injuries are by themselves rarely life-threatening, their presence generally indicates a high-energy mechanism of trauma.

- Adrenal hematomas following blunt trauma are nearly always associated with other visceral, skeletal, intracranial, or thoracic injuries.

- Adrenal injuries are more commonly unilateral, and most frequently right-sided.

- In the absence of significant hemorrhage, unilateral adrenal injuries are typically clinically silent.

Imaging

CT

- *Adrenal gland hematomas* (Fig. 7.5)

  - 2–4 cm ovoid or round hyperattenuating lesions with a mean attenuation of 52 HU on initial CT.

- *Focal adrenal hemorrhage*

  - A small high attenuation focus in an otherwise normal-sized adrenal
  - Typically less well defined than a hematoma.

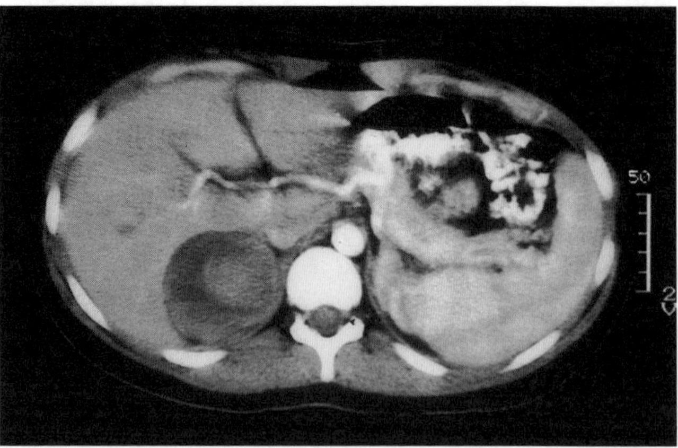

Figure 7.5 Post-traumatic hemorrhage of the right adrenal gland following a major trauma to the abdomen.

- *Other CT findings of adrenal trauma*

  - periadrenal fat stranding
  - retroperitoneal hemorrhage
  - diaphragmatic crural thickening
  - indistinct or enlarged adrenal gland
  - active contrast extravasation (rarely)

Points to remember

- Nearly all patients with adrenal hematomas have associated injuries:

  - Visceral injuries are frequent; the liver is most commonly involved.
  - 85% of cases have associated orthopedic trauma.
  - Intrathoracic injuries including pneumothorax and hemothorax are not infrequently seen.
  - Associated injuries are more commonly seen ipsilaterally.

- Focal adrenal injuries must be distinguished from non-traumatic adrenal pathology, the commonest is non functioning adenoma which has the following features:

  - less than 4 cm in size
  - less than 10 HU on non-contrast imaging
  - homogeneous enhancement after contrast injection.
  - In the absence of precontrast imaging, 15-min delayed images may be obtained. Hematomas should demonstrate no substantial change in attenuation while adenomas should demonstrate greater than 50% washout.

Clinical management

- The presence of adrenal injury should prompt a search for additional injuries.

- Operative intervention is usually only required for the associated injuries.

- Adrenal injuries may be a source of delayed hemorrhage or infection.

- Bilateral adrenal injuries may be associated with adrenal insufficiency, a potentially life-threatening condition requiring steroid replacement therapy.

7.4 Ureteral trauma

Introduction

Ureteral trauma may not be easily recognized, especially in patients who are critical ill and have sustained multiple injuries.

Clinical presentation

- Injuries to the ureter following blunt trauma typically occur at the ureteropelvic junction (UPJ), where acute flexion or extension can lacerate or avulse the ureter.

- While blunt trauma UPJ injuries were previously thought to occur exclusively in children, cases of partial and complete UPJ tears have been reported in adults.

- Nearly all ureteral injuries following blunt trauma are associated with injuries to other abdominal organs or a major blood vessel.

- Penetrating trauma can result in injury to the ureter at any location (Fig. 7.6a).

- The absence of hematuria does not preclude a complete ureteral tear. This is especially true with complete transection.

Imaging

- Imaging of suspected ureteral injuries should be performed using the most expeditious technique available (Fig. 7.6b).

- UPJ injuries are reliably demonstrated using an intravenous pyelogram. However, CT urography (CTU) at the excretory phase is an effective technique in evaluating the ureter.

- Contrast extravasation around the kidney defines a high ureteral laceration on imaging studies. This extravasation is often more profound medially.

- Contrast may be seen in the ureter with a partial laceration, however no contrast enters the ureter following a complete tear.

- If contrast extravasation is extensive, distinguishing contrast in the ureter from extravasate may be difficult.

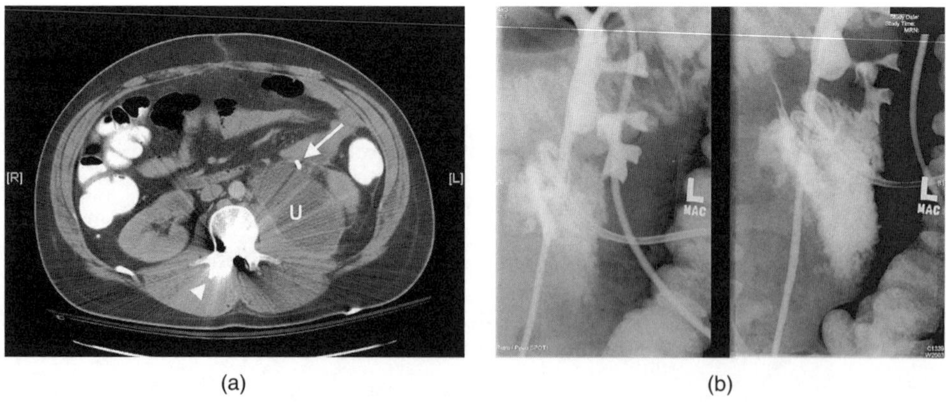

(a)   (b)

Figure 7.6 (a) Injured upper third of ureter secondary to bullet, which caused quadriplegia in a 21-year-old male. CT performed several days after injury shows development of an urinoma (U) around a ureteral stent (arrow). Arrowhead points to bullet lodged in the spine. (b) Progressive injection of contrast through the nephrostomy tube shows contrast extravasating through the rupture of the upper third of the left ureter. A stent is seen within the lumen of the ureter. A pig tail catheter draining the urinoma is shown.

- In cases of non-diagnostic IVP or CT, a retrograde or antegrade pyelogram may be performed to elucidate ureteral integrity.

Clinical management

- Ureteral injuries can be classified by location (upper, middle or lower), timing of presentation (immediate or delayed), cause (blunt or penetrating), and extent of injury.

- Injuries that are non-penetrating or minor may require no intervention.

- Controversy exists regarding the most appropriate management of ureteral injuries following penetrating trauma.

- Generally, primary repair of penetrating injuries is preferable, however the effect of concomitant abdominal injuries may preclude this.

- Surgical repair attempted more than 7 days following the injury may be difficult due to a marked inflammatory response.

- A retrograde or antegrade ureteral stent or percutaneous nephrostomy tube may be placed (Fig. 7.6c).

- In some cases, urinary diversion by nephrostomy or stent placement may be sufficient.

- Strictures can be managed endoscopically through balloon dilatation or endoureterotomy.

- Approximately 6–8 weeks are necessary prior to open surgical repair to allow for adequate healing and resolution of inflammation.

7.5 Bladder trauma

Introduction

- Bladder injuries may occur from penetrating or blunt trauma.
- Major bladder injury occurs in approximately 10% of patients with pelvic fractures.
- The susceptibility of the bladder to injury increases with its degree of distention.
    - In children, the bladder is intra-abdominal and therefore more vulnerable to injury at any capacity.

Clinical presentation

- Gross hematuria occurs in over 95% of bladder injuries.
- Other presentations may include microscopic hematuria, suprapubic tenderness, or urinary retention.

Classification of bladder injuries

- Type 1 – Bladder contusion
    - represents an incomplete tear of the bladder mucosa, and is generally conceded to be the most common type of bladder injury following blunt trauma (Fig. 7.7a).

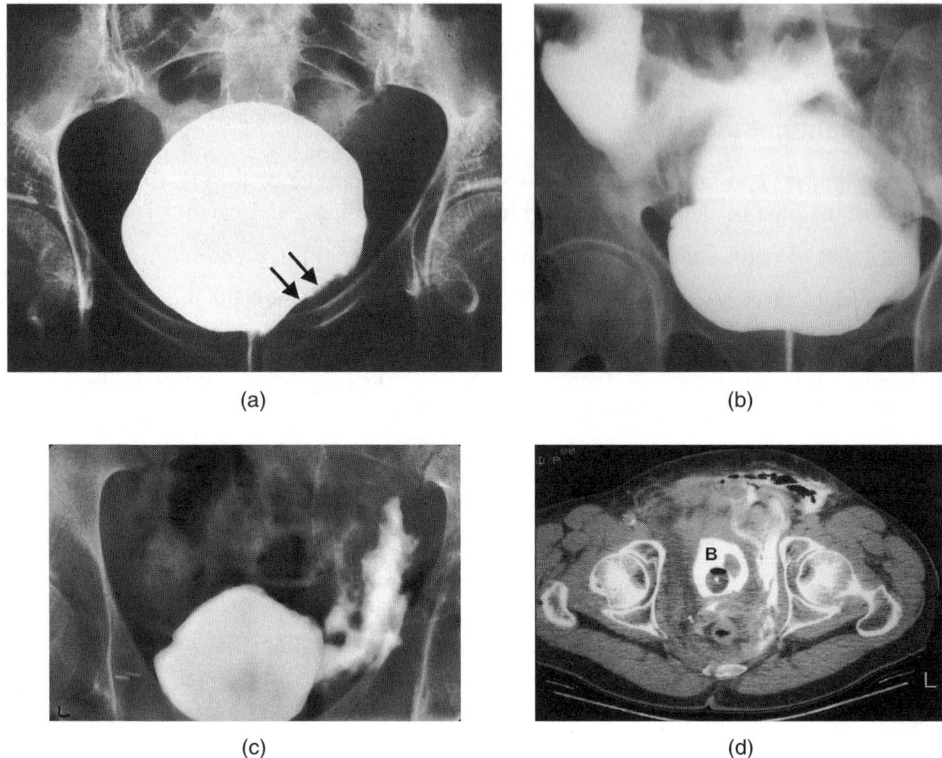

Figure 7.7 (a) Cystogram shows bladder contusion (arrows) following blunt trauma. (b) Cystogram shows contrast leaking into the peritoneal cavity secondary to intraperitoneal rupture of the bladder. (c) Cystogram shows extraperitoneal extravasation of contrast on left side. (d) CT shows extraperitoneal extravasation of contrast surrounding the bladder (B) and running along the lateral gutter into the anterior abdominal wall.

- Type 2 – Intraperitoneal rupture

  - accounts for approximately one-third of major bladder injuries, and approximately 25% of cases are not associated with a pelvic fracture (Fig. 7.7b).

- Type 3 – Interstitial bladder injury

  - is a rare injury representing an incomplete laceration of the bladder wall.

- Type 4 – Extraperitoneal rupture

  - is almost always seen in conjunction with pelvic fracture or diastasis of the pubic symphysis, and represents approximately 60% of major bladder injuries.

- Type 5 – Combined bladder injury

  - consisting of both intra and extraperitoneal rupture, represents approximately 5% of cases of major bladder injury.

Imaging

- The bladder can be initially evaluated at IVU or the excretory phase of CTU.

- A normal appearance of the bladder on IVU or at the excretory phase of CTU does not exclude a bladder injury.

- Static or CT cystography with retrograde filling of the bladder with contrast would be required to exclude bladder injury. Cystography is reported to be accurate in the assessment of bladder injury in 85–100% of cases.

- In male patients, a retrograde urethrogram must be performed before placement of a Foley catheter if there is clinical concern for a urethral injury.

- Static cystography consists of

  - a scout radiograph followed by the initial retrograde instillation of approximately 100 ml of 20–30% contrast material to assess for gross bladder extravasation.

  - Subsequently, an additional 200–250 ml of contrast is infused to completely fill the bladder.

  - A 14 × 17 inch radiograph of the entire abdomen will effectively demonstrate the pattern of extravasation.

  - A post-drainage radiograph is obtained after emptying the bladder to demonstrate contrast extravasation that may have been obscured by a distended bladder, an occurrence encountered in approximately 10% of cases of bladder rupture.

- CT cystography

  - The bladder is filled retrograde with at least 350 ml of dilute (3–5%) contrast material.

  - 10 mm contiguous axial sections are obtained through the pelvis.

- *Cystography findings*

  - *Bladder contusion*

    - Normal cystogram.

  - *Interstitial bladder injury*

    - A defect in the bladder wall representing an intramural hematoma is observed, however contrast extravasation is notably absent (Fig. 7.7a).

  - *Intraperitoneal rupture*

    - Contrast extravasation into the paracolic gutters and contrast outlining loops of small bowel is observed (Fig. 7.7b).

  - *Extraperitoneal rupture*

    - In *simple* extraperitoneal rupture, extravasation is limited to the pelvic extraperitoneal space (Fig. 7.7c).

    - In *complex* extraperitoneal rupture, contrast extends into the anterior abdominal wall, penis, scrotum, perineum, or down the leg (Fig. 7.7d).

- ○ *Combined bladder injury*
  - Features of both intra and extra peritoneal rupture are present.
- ○ *Penetrating injuries*
  - May result in intraperitoneal, extraperitoneal, or combined bladder ruptures.

Management

Contusion

- If hematuria is persistent and clots form, a urethral catheter should be placed until the urine is clear.
- Continuous bladder irrigation with a 3-way Foley catheter is discouraged since clot retention may occur and lead to bladder distention and possible rupture.

Intraperitoneal rupture

- Prior to repair, the bladder interior must be inspected.
- A two to three layer watertight repair with absorbable sutures is required.
- A urethral catheter is left to drainage.
- A suprapubic tube is not necessary.

Extraperitoneal rupture

- For purely extraperitoneal rupture, a Foley catheter left to drainage for 10 days typically allows the injury to heal without surgical repair.
- If the drainage is inadequate or surgical exploration is required, a two to three layer watertight repair with absorbable sutures should be performed.

7.6 Urethral trauma

Introduction

- Urethral injuries must be efficiently diagnosed and properly managed to prevent serious long-term outcomes.
- Management of urethral injuries depends on the location and degree of injury, the patient's clinical stability, and concomitant injuries.
- Most urethral injuries associated with blunt trauma are from either pelvic fractures or straddle injuries.
- Penetrating injuries, from gunshot or knife, mostly involve the anterior urethra.
- Injury of the female urethra is rare and generally associated with major pelvic ring disruption and concomitant vaginal laceration.

Clinical presentation

- Blunt trauma such as pelvic fracture, straddle injury, or blow to the perineum should increase the clinical suspicion for urethral injury.

- The typical clinical triad is

  o blood at the urethral meatus

  o inability to void

  o a palpable urinary bladder.

- Other clinical findings include

  o high riding prostate upon digital rectal examination

  o perineal hematoma.

Classification of urethral injuries

- Type I

  o *Posterior urethra intact but stretched* (Fig. 7.8a, b).

  o Uncommonly recognized injuries.

  o Occur when the puboprostatic ligaments are ruptured but the continuity of the urethra is preserved.

- Type II

  o *Pure posterior injury with tear of membranous urethra above the urogenital diaphragm – partial or complete.* (Fig. 7.8c, d).

  o The urogenital diaphragm remains intact.

  o This injury comprises 15% of urethral injuries resulting from pelvic fracture.

- Type III

  o *Combined anterior/posterior urethral injury with disruption of urogenital diaphragm – partial or complete.* (Fig. 7.8e–g).

  o The most common type of urethral injury, and represent a combined anterior/posterior urethral injury.

- Type IV

  o *Bladder neck injury with extension into the urethra.*(Fig. 7.8h, i).

  o The bladder neck laceration may damage the internal urethral sphincter.

- Type IVa

  o Pure injury of the base of the bladder with periurethral extravasation simulating a true type IV urethral injury (Fig. 7.8k–m).

- Type V

  o Pure anterior urethral injury – partial or complete. (Fig. 7.8n–p).

  o Typically occur following a straddle injury and are more often partial than complete.

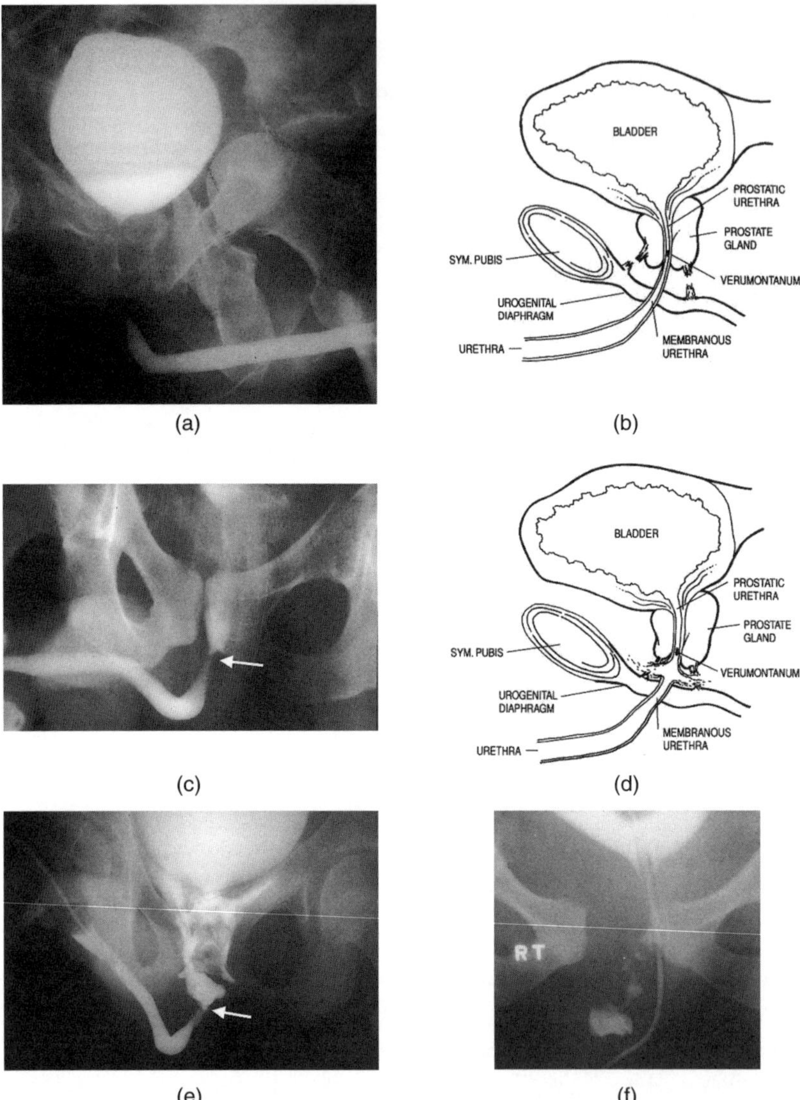

Figure 7.8 Urethral injuries *Type I urethral injury, posterior urethra intact but stretched* (a) Retrograde urethrogram shows posterior urethral stretching and narrowing. (b) Diagrammatic illustration reproduced from SM Goldman *et al., J. Urol.* **57**: 85–89, 1997 with permission. *Type II urethral injury, pure posterior injury with tear of membranous urethra above the urogenital diaphragm.* (c) Urethrogram shows contrast extending from UG diaphragm (arrow) and above. (d) Diagrammatic illustration reproduced from SM Goldman *et al., J. Urol.* **57**:85–89, 1997 with permission. *Type III urethral tear with complete disruption of UG diaphragm.* (e) Cystogram shows extensive extravasation above and below the UG diaphragm. (f) Note bladder base is elevated and symphysis pubis widened. Contrast is seen leaking below the symphysis pubis and therefore, represents a tear through the UG diaphragm.

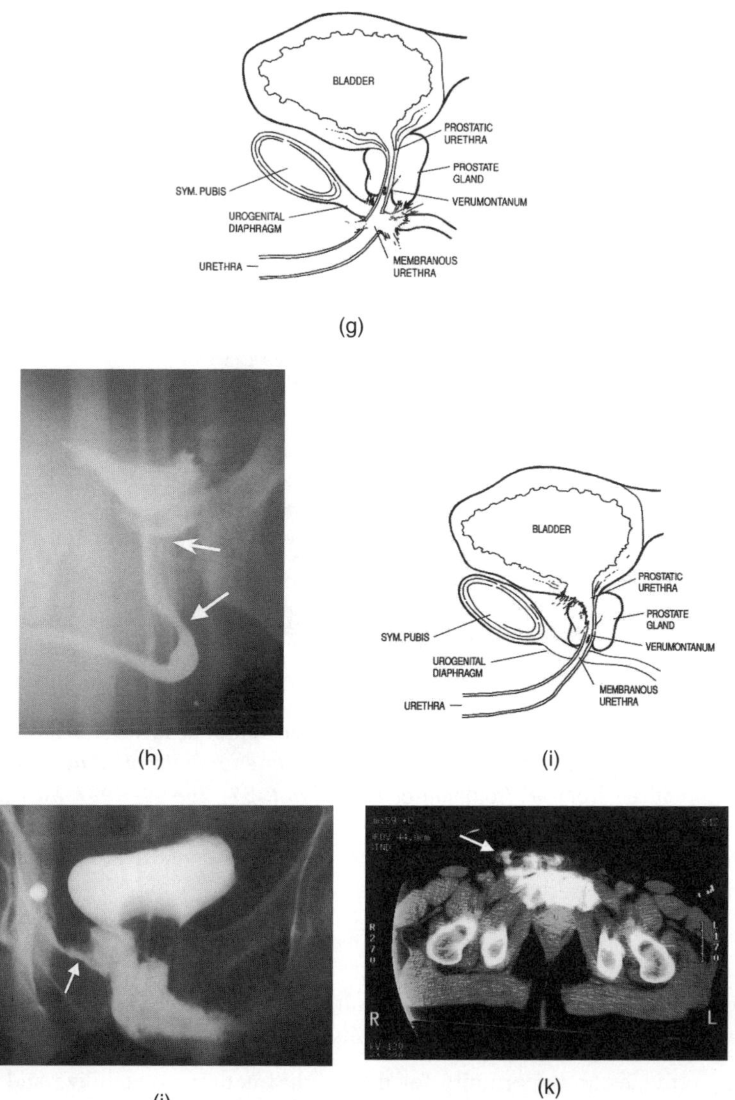

(g)

(h)   (i)

(j)   (k)

Figure 7.8 *(Continued)* (g) Diagrammatic illustration reproduced from SM Goldman *et al.*, *J. Urol.* **57**: 85–89, 1997 with permission. *Type IV urethral injury, bladder neck injury with extension into the urethra.* (h) Contrast noted at base of bladder extending along posterior urethra (upper arrow). Contrast 'clearly extends to the level of the membranous urethra, but not past the UG diaphragm (lower arrow). (i) Diagrammatic illustration reproduced from SM Goldman *et al,*. *J. Urol.* **57**: 85–89, 1997 with permission. *Type IVA urethral injury, pure injury of the base of the bladder with periurethral extravasation simulating a true type IV urethral injury.* (j) Retrograde urethrogram shows extravasation from bladder base (arrows) mimicking a high posterior urethral tear. (k) CT shows contrast extending along anterior abdominal wall muscles and subcutaneously (arrows).

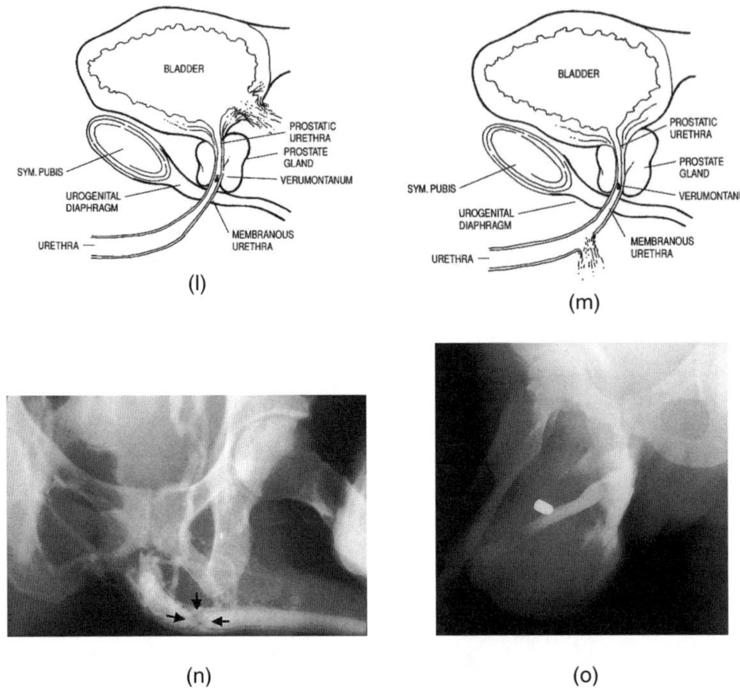

Figure 7.8 *(Continued)* (l) Diagrammatic illustration reproduced from SM Goldman *et al.*, *J. Urol.* **57**: 85–89, 1997 with permission. *Type V injury (anterior urethral injury)*. (m) Diagrammatic illustration reproduced from SM Goldman *et al.*, *J. Urol.* **57**: 85–89, 1997 with permission. (n) Retrograde urethrogram shows rupture of the anterior urethra (arrows) and extravasation of contrast from the urethra into the surrounding tissue and venous drainage. (o) Urethrogram shows tear of the urethra secondary to a bullet.

Outcome

- Complete type II and III lacerations result in complete urethral strictures, which are usually repaired on a delayed basis, typically six months after the initial injury.

- This delay provides an opportunity for the pelvic fractures to stabilize and for the pelvic hematoma to resolve so that the bladder has descended into the pelvis.

- In general, type II injuries result in shorter strictures that are easier to repair.

- Recognition of bladder neck injury (type IV and IVA) is important to prevent urinary incontinence.

Imaging

- Diagnosis is made by a retrograde urethrogram, which must be obtained prior to an attempt to place a urethral catheter.

- A Foley catheter is inserted into the penile urethra and its balloon is partially inflated within the fossa navicularis.

- No lubricant is used and an exposure is acquired during the active injection of 20–30 ml of a water soluble contrast medium (300 mgI/ml) so that the deep bulbar and prostatic urethras will be filled.

- Ideally this should be performed under fluoroscopic control but this is not always available in the accident and emergency department.

Findings at urethrogram of urethral injury

- Type 1 (Fig. 7.8a, b)

  - The posterior urethra is stretched as a hematoma forms in the prostatic fossa, displacing the bladder slightly upward.
  - Extrinsic compression of the posterior urethra by a periurethral hematoma without displacement of the bladder base is not considered a true type I injury.

- Type II (Fig. 7.8c, d)

  - Partial or complete laceration of the posterior urethra.
  - Extravasated contrast material is confined to the pelvic extraperitoneal space above the urogenital diaphragm.

- Type III (Fig. 7.8e–g)

  - Membranous urethral tear.
  - The tear extends into the proximal bulbous urethra.
  - Contrast will extravasate below the urogenital diaphragm into the perineum.

- Type IV (Fig. 7.8h, i)

  - Tear of the bladder neck that extends into the proximal urethra.

- Type IVA (Fig. 7.8j–m)

  - Radiographically indistinguishable from true Type IV injuries, as both demonstrate periurethral contrast extravasation.

- Type V (Fig. 7.8n–o)

  - Anterior urethral disruptions
    - If Buck's fascia (the deep fascia of the penis that binds the three cylindrical erectile bodies in the pendulous portion of the penis) remains intact, then the extravasation is confined to the space between Buck's fascia and the tunica albuginea [the thick connective tissue layer that surrounds the erectile tissue around the urethra (corpus spongiosum)].
    - If Buck's fascia is ruptured, extravasated contrast will be confined by Colle's fascia (a layer of superficial penile fascia invests the Buck's fascia).

Clinical management

- Repair of urethral injuries may be done in primary (soon after the injury) or in a delayed fashion.

- Primary reapproximation of the severed urethral stumps

  - Reserved for stable patients with a short urethral injury.
  - Associated injuries of bladder, bladder neck or rectum may dictate the need for immediate primary repair.
  - Not done routinely now due to the high rate of postoperative impotence and incontinence.
  - The stricture rate is low.

- Delayed repair

  - Initially only involves placing a suprapubic drainage catheter.
  - Urethral strictures are universally present because no initial attempt is made to repair the urethra.

- Primary realignment by endoscopic approach

  - Is now the preferred option.
  - Some cases may be accomplished with one flexible retrograde cystoscope.
  - Others may be realigned with two flexible cystoscopes introduced both retrograde and antegrade.
  - Once a wire can bridge the gap of injury, a urethral catheter is placed and maintained for 4 to 6 weeks to allow the urethra to heal.

- In the unstable or multi-organ trauma patient

  - A suprapubic catheter is placed to divert the urine during damage control and resuscitation.
  - Delayed realignment can be performed endoscopically a few days to two weeks later, once the patient is stable and resuscitated.
  - When a delayed realignment is not possible, a delayed open urethroplasty or urethrotomy is performed in 3 to 6 months.

- In isolated bladder neck injury, repair is needed but can be technically demanding, especially in unstable patients.

- Women with proximal urethral disruptions should immediately undergo exploration with realignment of the urethral ends or primary reanastomosis over a catheter.

- For women with distal urethral lacerations, a urethral catheterization with primary closure of the vaginal laceration is adequate.

7.7 Penile and scrotal trauma

Introduction

- The incidence is not well established.

- Ultrasound is the first-line imaging modality for evaluation of scrotal trauma and is crucial in determining appropriate clinical approach and management.

Clinical presentation

Injuries to the penis

- Divided into four categories:
  - Penile fracture
    - The erect penis is more prone to injury because the increased pressure within the penis makes it more susceptible to sudden blunt trauma or abrupt bending.
    - Approximately one-third of penile fractures occur during sexual intercourse, and embarrassment associated with the mechanism of injury may lead to delayed presentation.
    - A popping sound with acute pain followed by immediate detumescence of the penis is the typical presentation of penile fracture.
    - Penile fractures, usually limited to Buck's fascia, typically present with only swelling of the shaft and localized ecchymosis
    - When the blunt trauma involves the deep investing fascia, a perineal hematoma and/or scrotal hematoma may develop.
    - The disruption of the tunica albuginea can involve one or both corpora and concomitant injury to the urethra may occur.
    - The penile urethra is more likely to be involved when both corpora cavernosa are injured.
  - Amputation
    - Partial or complete severing of the penis.
  - Penetrating injury
    - Induced by gunshot or knife.
    - May involve the corpora, urethra, or penile soft tissue.
    - When penetrating trauma involves the deep investing fascia, a perineal hematoma and/or scrotal hematoma may develop.
  - Soft tissue injury
    - May be secondary to thermal or chemical burns or avulsion of the penile skin.

Injuries to the scrotum

- The laxity of the scrotal skin gives some measure of protection to the underlying contents.
- Injuries to the scrotum are divided into:
  - Blunt
    - most common, can be due to
      - athletic injury
      - motor vehicle collision
      - assault.
    - The right testis is injured more frequently than the left in blunt trauma, due to its greater tendency of being trapped against the pubis or inner thigh.

- Penetrating trauma, most commonly gun shot wounds.
- lacerations or avulsions
  - May not involve the testes or scrotal contents.
  - However, evaluation of the testes is mandatory with radiographic studies or surgical exploration.
  - Delayed diagnosis may result in decreased fertility, delayed orchiectomy, infection, ischemia or infarction, and atrophy.
- Thermal (rare).

Imaging

The penis
MRI

- MRI is the imaging technique that can most accurately define the presence, extent, and location of tunical tears, however it is often not available on an acute basis.
- Tunical tears appear as disruptions of the low signal intensity tunica albuginea on T1 and T2-weighted sequences.
- Injuries to the urethra and corpus spongiosum, as well as intracavernosal or extratunical hematomas may also be demonstrated.

Penile cavernosography

- reveals extravasation of contrast material from the corpora cavernosum into the penile soft tissues when the tunica albuginea is ruptured.
- Drawbacks
  - invasive
  - potential for complications.

Ultrasound

- Often demonstrates the site of the tunical tear, which is the most important initial issue that needs to be resolved for the urologist.
- Evaluation may be limited in the setting of severe penile pain, swelling, and hemorrhage.

The scrotum
Ultrasound (US)

- The first line imaging modality in scrotal trauma except for lacerating injuries.
- US findings in injury
  - *Fluid collections*
    - Hematoma
      - *Intratesticular hematoma (Fig. 7.9)*: Single or multiple focal collections that may be hyperechoic (acute bleed), hypoechoic (evolved hematoma), or heterogeneous (complex hematoma). There is no internal vascularity.

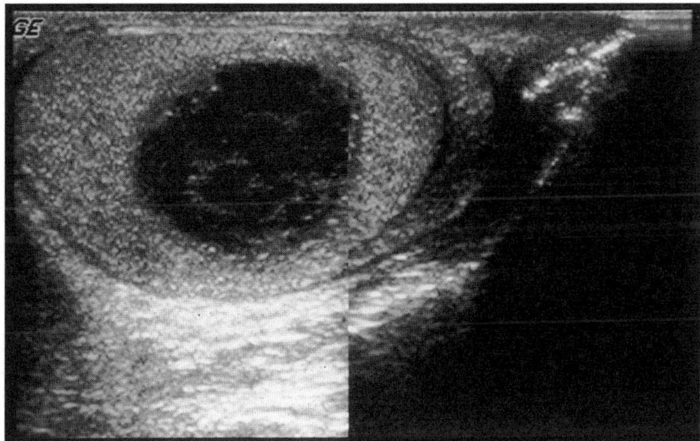

Figure 7.9 Ultrasound scan demonstrates intratesticular hematoma which was secondary to trauma.

- *Scrotal wall hematomas* may appear as focal thickening of the wall or an intramural fluid collection.
- Hydrocele
  - Anechoic fluid collections that collect in the potential space between the parietal and visceral layers of the tunica vaginalis.
  - Present in 25% of cases of major trauma.
  - Rupture of the bulbous urethra may result in extravasation of urine into the scrotum which may simulate a hydrocele.
- Hematoceles are
  - Acutely echogenic and become more hypoechoic and complex over time.
  - Subacute and chronic hematoceles may have fluid-fluid levels or internal debris.
- *Testicular injuries*
  - *Fracture* (a break in the testicular architecture)
    - A linear hypoechoic band extending across the testicular parenchyma without disruption of the tunica albuginea or alteration in testicular shape.
    - May be seen in association with a hematocele or testicular hematoma.
    - Doppler is useful to evaluate vascular integrity.
  - *Rupture* (hemorrhage and extrusion of testicular contents into the scrotal sac).
    - Discontinuity of the tunica albuginea is pathognomonic of testicular rupture and requires emergent surgery, especially when testicular tissue is seen protruding from the tear.
    - Tunical tears may be difficult to define on ultrasound because of the presence of severe intratesticular and extratesticular hematomas.
    - Extratesticular hematomas and herniation of testicular tissue may be difficult to differentiate.

- Poorly defined testicular margins and heterogeneous echotexture with areas of focal hyper and hypoechogenicity corresponding to areas of hemorrhage or infarction respectively are consistent with testicular rupture.
- Possible associated findings:
  - diminished or absent vascular flow
  - hematocele
  - scrotal wall thickening.

MRI

- MRI is certainly warranted when ultrasound findings are equivocal.
- MRI readily distinguishes intratesticular and extratesticular hematomas as well as tunical tears and scrotal wall thickening.
- Currently the cost, time constraints, and availability on an emergency basis limit the routine use of MRI.

Evaluation of penetrating trauma

- US may be used to determine vascular injury, or identify bullet fragments or other foreign bodies, in addition to findings seen in blunt trauma.
- As in blunt trauma, MRI provides superb definition of soft tissue anatomy.

Surgical management

Injuries to the penis

- The surgical goals for injuries to the penis are to restore function and appearance.
- Penile fracture
  - The injury almost always occurs just distal to the penile suspensory ligament.
  - By making a circumcision incision and degloving the penis, a complete examination of the urethra and corpora is available.
  - A defect in the tunica albuginea and penile hematoma are characteristics of both penile fracture and penetrating trauma.
  - After copious irrigation with normal saline to remove the hematoma, only minimal debridement is needed.
  - Primary closure of the corpora cavernosa, corpus spongiosum and the urethra is performed.
- Penile amputation
  - Meticulous repair of the urethra, cavernosa, neurovascular bundle, and skin is the key to recovery of penile function and appearance.
- Gross contamination or bit injuries to the penis may need to be closed within 6 to 12 h after antibiotic administration or allowed to granulate secondarily.
- Penile skin lacerations are typically closed primarily.

Injuries to the scrotum

- Testicular injuries are managed conservatively if the tunica albuginea is intact.

- Immediate surgical exploration is warranted if there is evidence of testicular rupture or equivocal US findings with high suspicion for rupture or non-perfusion of the testis.

- A ruptured testis can be salvaged by debridement and primary closure of the tunica albuginea.

- Following vascular transaction of the spermatic cord, a microscopic reanastomosis may be performed as long as the testis has been under warm ischemia for a minimal duration ($<30\,min$) or cold ischemia for less than $24\,h$.

- Surgical delay may decrease the salvage rate from 80–90% to 45–55% and thereby necessitate orchiectomy.

- Partial loss of the scrotal skin is repaired by debridement of devitalized tissue and primary approximation of the remaining scrotal skin. The scrotal skin has good vasculature, compliance and elasticity, allowing for excellent recovery.

- Testicular fracture and rupture due to penetrating injuries are managed similarly to injuries resulting from blunt trauma.

- Stab wounds and low velocity missiles are managed with a combined inguinal and scrotal approach to explore above and below the injury site.

- High velocity injuries cause more tissue loss and are associated with a higher propensity for vascular thrombosis.

- Adjacent tissues including the contralateral testis and penis must be evaluated.

- Epididymal injuries are managed conservatively unless associated with infertility.

References

Deurdulian C, Mittelstaedt CA, Chong WK, Fielding JR (2007) US of acute scrotal trauma: optimal technique, imaging findings, and management. *Radiographics* **27**: 357–369.

Goldman SM, Sandler CM (2004) Urogenital trauma: imaging upper GU trauma. *Eur. J. Radiol.* **50**: 84–95.

Kawashima A, Sandler CM, Corl FM *et al.* (2001) Imaging of renal trauma: a comprehensive review. *Radiographics* **21**: 557–574.

Kawashima A, Sandler CM, Wasserman NF *et al.* (2004) Imaging of urethral disease: a pictorial review. *Radiographics*, **24**: S195–S216.

Moon-Hae C, Kim B, Ryu J, Lee SW, Lee KS (2000) MR imaging of acute penile fracture. *Radiographics* **20**: 1397–1405.

Sandler CM, Goldman SM, Kawashima A (1998) Lower urinary tract trauma. *World J. Urol.* **16**: 69–75.

Sinelnikov AO, Abujudeh HH, Chan D, Novelline RA (2007) CT manifestations of adrenal trauma: experience with 73 cases. *Emerg. Radiol.* **13**: 313–318.

8
Urinary Tract Infections

Mikael Hellström[1], Ulf Jodal[2], Rune Sixt[3] and Eira Stokland[4]

[1] *Department of Radiology, Sahlgrenska University Hospital, Gothenburg, Sweden*
[2] *Department of Nephrology, The Queen Silvia Children's Hospital, Gothenburg, Sweden*
[3] *Department of Clinical Physiology, The Queen Silvia Children's Hospital, Gothenburg, Sweden*
[4] *Department of Radiology, The Queen Silvia Children's Hospital, Gothenburg, Sweden*

8.1 Symptomatic urinary tract infection in children

Introduction

Symptomatic urinary tract infection (UTI) is one of the most common bacterial infections in children, and at 7 years of age, the cumulative incidence is 8% in girls and 2% in boys. The peak incidence is below 1 year of age. The infection may be located mainly in the lower urinary tract (urethra, bladder; 'cystitis') or affect also the upper tract (ureter, renal pelvis, renal parenchyma; 'pyelonephritis'). Lower urinary tract infections may be painful but do not normally cause significant or long-term morbidity. On the other hand, bacterial infections of the upper tract carry a risk for permanent damage of the renal parenchyma with reduced renal function, hypertension and complications during pregnancy as potential long-term consequences.

In some infants (especially neonate boys) presenting with first time UTI, major renal damage is seen already at presentation of UTI, often together with severe malformations, gross vesicoureteral reflux (VUR) or urinary obstruction. Many of the children with congenital dysplasia have reduced renal function from birth and early identification is of importance to prevent further deterioration. Thus, the etiology is different from the acquired type typically seen after infection.

Urogenital Imaging: A Problem-oriented Approach   Edited by Sameh K. Morcos and Henrik S. Thomsen
© 2009 John Wiley & Sons, Ltd

A number of risk factors that increase the risk for permanent renal damage have been identified:

- *Delay of treatment* Antibiotics should be given promptly, as soon as adequate urine samples have been obtained.
- *Recurrent pyelonephritic episodes* Prompt treatment in case of recurrence is essential.
- *Pre-existing abnormalities of the urinary tract*, especially dilating VUR and obstructive uropathies.
- *Atypical bacteria* are more often found in children with malformations of the urinary tract, i.e. findings of uncommon bacteria strengthen the indication for imaging.

Clinical features

The symptoms depend upon the age of the patient and the level of infection (bladder or kidney involvement).

Pyelonephritis

Infants and young children

- unexplained fever (often the only symptom)
- irritability
- vomiting
- failure to thrive.

Newborns and neonates may present with other unspecific symptoms relating to septicemia.

- subnormal, normal or only slightly elevated temperature
- lethargy
- anorexia
- grayish color
- body tenderness.

Older children are able to report symptoms directing the suspicion of the level of infection towards the upper or lower urinary tract.

Signs of *pyelonephritis*

- high fever (38.5°C or more) or chills
- flank pain and tenderness along the costovertebral angle

Signs of *cystitis*

- dysuria

- frequency

- body temperature may be elevated (below 38.5°C).

Laboratory tests and findings

Urine sample

The urine sample is used

- for investigation of nitrite and pyuria

- for urine culture (mandatory for diagnosis)

  - the diagnostic threshold depends on the method of urine collection

  - suprapubic aspiration, catheterization, clean catch or bag sampling are techniques used to obtain urine, depending on the age of the patient.

Blood tests

Serum samples are obtained for

- C-reactive protein (CRP)

  - elevated CRP indicates renal involvement

- Serum creatinine - an indirect indicator of renal function

- Cystatine C – by some considered to be a better indicator of renal function than serum creatinine.

Pathology

Acute infection

- UTI is mainly an ascending infection with bacteria from the peri-urethral area colonizing the urinary tract.

- *Escherichia coli* accounts for >90% of first time infections in infants and children.

- Other organisms, usually less virulent, such as *Klebsiella, Enterobacter*, enterococci, staphylococci, *Proteus* and *Pseudomonas* are causative agents mainly in malformed or malfunctioning urinary tracts.

- Acute renal parenchymal infection is typically focal or multifocal, but may be more generalized.

- Bacterial invasion of the kidney causes oedema, swelling and focal impairment of renal function.

- If untreated, acute parenchymal infection may develop into renal abscess.

- Inflammation may spread outside the renal parenchyma, affecting the perirenal fatty tissue.

- Bacterial toxins may induce paralysis of smooth muscle in the walls of the ureter and pelvicaliceal system, causing dilatation of the upper urinary tract.

- The effects of infection are enhanced by obstruction of the urinary tract, which may promote bacterial spread to the bloodstream (septicemia).

Healing/scarring

- Healing may be complete and leave no detectable residue, or result in permanent renal damage.

- Permanent renal damage (post-pyelonephritic scarring) occurs mainly in young children, and is less commonly seen to develop in adolescents or adults with UTI.

- Post-pyelonephritic scarring is typically focal or multifocal.

- Scarring is due to fibrosis and contraction of parenchymal tissue, resulting in focal parenchymal thinning and deformation (clubbing) of adjacent calices.

- If combined with VUR, parenchymal thinning and caliceal deformation may be more uniform ('reflux nephropathy').

- Scarring may take several months to become fully developed.

- In severe cases, scarring may result in a small, contracted and non-functioning kidney (end-stage kidney).

Imaging findings

Uncomplicated *lower* UTI usually requires no imaging. For evaluation of children with suspected *upper* UTI (*pyelonephritis*), the following may serve as a guideline. Imaging after first UTI is controversial, however, and there is no consensus on how an imaging protocol should be designed. Local availability of imaging equipment, local tradition and local competence may motivate different routines.

The goal of imaging in children with UTI is to identify those who have renal damage and associated abnormalities, and to identify those at risk of having recurrent pyelonephritis and of developing progressive renal damage.

- Several important questions should be addressed

  - Is there renal parenchymal involvement or not?
  - If there is evidence of parenchymal involvement, is it due to acute infection or permanent damage?
  - Is there an underlying cause, such as urinary tract malformation, VUR, calculus or outflow obstruction?
  - Is there evidence of complications that need therapeutic intervention (percutaneous drainage, pyelostomy), such as renal abscess or acute obstruction?

For investigation of children with first time UTI, different combinations of ultrasound (US), DMSA scintigraphy and voiding cystourethrography (VCUG) may be used. As alternatives and for problem solving in complicated cases, computed tomography (CT), magnetic resonance imaging (MRI) and renography are usually employed. The use of urography in children with UTI has decreased markedly in recent years.

Most protocols focus on infants and small children in whom risk factors are most likely to be found.

- *Acute* investigations are indicated in children who
  - o present with atypical UTI
  - o have infection with non-*E. coli* bacteria
  - o fail to respond to adequate antibiotic treatment
  - o have poor urine flow
  - o have an abdominal mass
  - o have elevated serum creatinine.

Evaluation of the urinary tract

Ultrasonography (US)

Indication

US is the primary imaging modality for examining the urinary tract in most protocols dealing with young children with their first UTI

In the acute phase of febrile UTI

- The main indication for US is to detect an underlying malformation or obstruction (obstructive uropathy) (Fig. 8.1).

- Dilatation of the collecting system is indicative, but not confirmative, of VUR or urinary obstruction, and should be followed by confirmative tests.

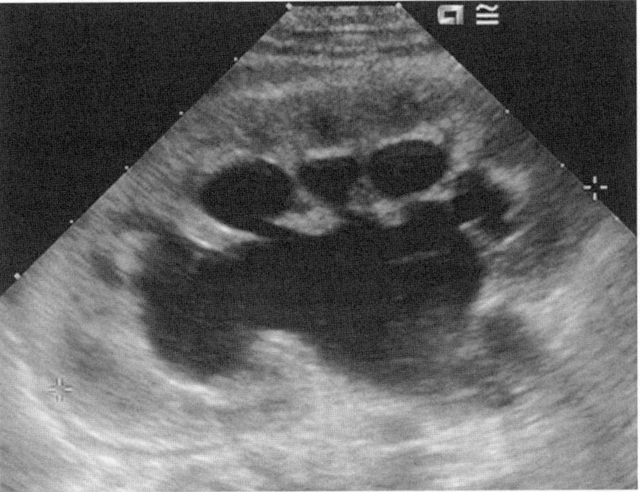

Figure 8.1   Ultrasonography demonstrating widening of the renal pelvis and calices (black) due to obstruction.

- When dilatation of the collecting system is found at US, voiding cystourethrography (VCUG) is recommended for exclusion of high grade VUR and posterior urethral valve (boys), while renography (MAG3 scintigraphy) can be used for evaluation of kidney function (split renal function) and to assess obstruction.

- In the majority of cases of acute pyelonephritis, the renal parenchyma appears normal at US.

- Acute pyelonephritis may cause swelling of the kidney, indicated at US by an increased renal length or volume.

- Other unspecific signs include loss of normal corticomedullary demarcation and areas of heterogeneous parenchymal echogenicity.

- Acute pyelitis or ureteritis may be suggested by mild dilatation of the urinary system, thickening of the renal pelvic wall (urothelium) and increased echogenicity of the renal sinus, but these are unspecific findings and may be difficult to evaluate.

- The sensitivity of US for detection of acute renal parenchymal involvement is lower than with DMSA scintigraphy, CT or MRI.

- US with power Doppler may somewhat improve the detection of acute pyelonephritis.

- Contrast-enhanced US (microbubbles, harmonic imaging) has shown promising results in detection of acute pyelonephritis in adults, but has not been adequately evaluated in children.

- Renal abscess is rare in children but can be suspected on US when a low-echogenic lesion surrounded by a thicker 'capsule' is seen.

  - In an early stage, enlargement of the kidney, and distortion of the normal renal contour or of the collecting system may be the only, and non-specific signs.

  - The appearance of an abscess changes with time and during treatment, and it may liquefy, with few internal echoes.

- CT or MRI with i.v contrast enhancement should be preferred for abscess imaging since these methods provide better anatomical overview, less observer dependence and more objective image documentation for treatment and follow-up, as compared with US.

- Pyonephrosis

  - refers to pus in a widened renal pelvis/ureter due to obstruction in combination with infection.

  - is a medical emergency that needs immediate treatment (antibiotics and decompression by percutaneous drainage) to avoid renal tissue destruction and septicemia.

  - may be indicated by thickened, echogenic urine content and layering of urine and debris in the renal pelvis at ultrasonography.

For follow-up

- US is considered insufficient for the detection of permanent renal damage (scarring), as compared with DMSA scintigraphy.

- At US renal scarring is seen as single or multiple cortical outline irregularities and thinning of parenchyma (usually polar), often in combination with reduced renal size.

- Normal renal lobulation (persisting foetal lobulation) should not be mistaken for renal scarring.

- For the evaluation of renal growth and renal damage, measurement of bipolar renal length must be included in the examination.

DMSA scanning – cortical scanning of the kidneys

Tc-99m DMSA slowly accumulates in proximal tubular cells after intravenous injection. Images of the uptake are taken two to three hours after injection of the radio-pharmaceutical.

In case of acute insult to the parenchyma, as in pyelonephritis, the uptake of DMSA is focally reduced and appears as one or more areas of reduced or absent uptake. Presently, DMSA scanning is the method of choice to look for inflammation of the renal parenchyma.

Also in the follow-up of children after acute febrile UTIs, the DMSA scan is considered to be the method of choice.

It should be remembered that less extensive renal involvement, acute or permanent, may be overlooked on DMSA scans due to poor resolution.

Indications

- In the acute phase of febrile UTI: to look for abnormal uptake pattern consistent with acute renal involvement (pyelonephritis)

  o *Key finding*: one or more focal areas of reduced or absent uptake in one or both kidneys, often with preserved renal outline (Fig. 8.2).

- In the follow-up: to search for signs of permanent renal damage

  o *Key finding*: focal uptake defect with indentation of the renal contour with or without reduced renal size (Fig. 8.3).

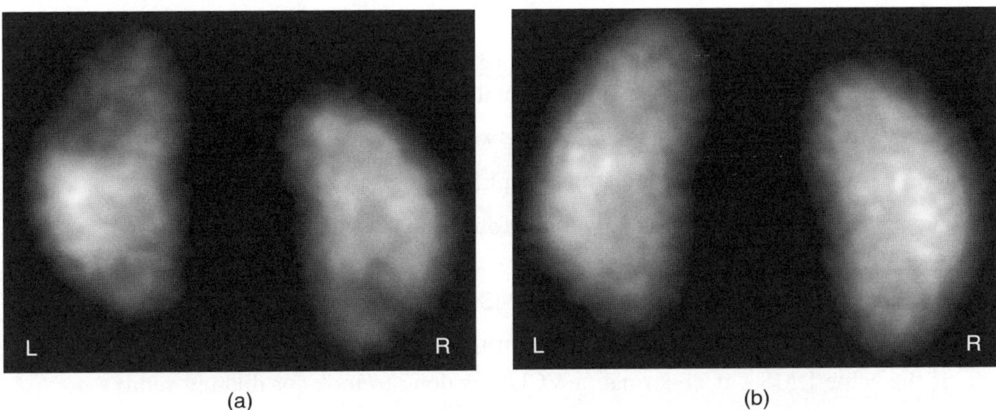

Figure 8.2 (a) Abnormal Tc-99m DMSA scan in a child, 11 months of age, during her first known febrile urinary tract infection. Areas of reduced uptake (darker areas) are seen in both kidneys indicating acute pyelonephritis. Split renal function is 52% for the right kidney and 48% for the left one. R = Right; L = Left (b) Follow up scan one year after the acute episode of pyelonephritis. The split function is unchanged (52% and 48%). The uptake defects are no longer discernible, indicating healing. R = Right; L = Left.

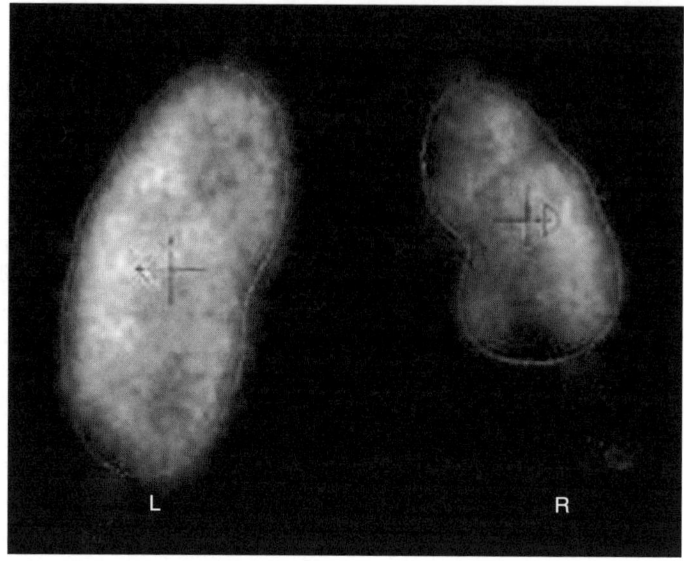

Figure 8.3   Permanent renal damage in a 9 year old girl with a history of several recurrences of febrile urinary tract infection. The DMSA scan shows a severely damaged right kidney with a split function corresponding to 28% of total. R = Right; L = Left.

Timing of investigation

- Acute UTI: scanning within 2–5 days of presentation.
- Follow up study: 6–12 months after the acute episode and only in those with abnormal acute scan.

Comments

- Antibiotic treatment of acute UTI should be initiated rapidly, on clinical grounds, and should not be withheld awaiting an abnormal DMSA scan.
- It is not always possible to differentiate between acute and permanent renal damage.
- There is usually only minor deviation of split function in the acute phase.
- Some perform DMSA scanning only in the follow up period to look for signs of permanent renal damage.
- Increasingly common is to perform the DMSA in the acute phase
  - if the acute DMSA scan is normal, no further imaging is done
  - if the acute DMSA is abnormal, a VCUG is done to look for dilating reflux.
- With a calibrated gamma camera a rough estimate of renal size can be obtained.

Renography

The renal uptake and excretion of a suitable radio-pharmaceutical is followed with 10 s frames during at least 20 min after the intravenous injection. In children it is often possible to include both the kidneys and the bladder in the field of view of the gamma camera.

During the early stage of acquisition it is possible to extract information about the intrarenal distribution of 'renal function' in a reframed image of the parenchyma, one to three minutes after the injection. By the use of regions of interest (ROI) on the acquired images, time-activity curves can be created and analysed in terms of split renal function and outflow characteristics.

In children, a tubular tracer, such as Tc-99m MAG3, with a rapid uptake and excretion should be used to get the best possible images of the urinary tract.

- The split function of the two moieties in duplex kidneys can be roughly evaluated.

- Renography is useful in case of suspected outflow obstruction

  o Poor drainage of activity from the renal pelvis is no proof of significant obstruction

  o Good drainage or increased drainage after voiding, gravity assisted drainage or administration of a diuretic makes significant obstruction less likely, as does a preserved split renal function.

- Renography is less suitable compared with DMSA scanning for focal evaluation of the parenchyma, both in the acute stage of UTI and during follow-up.

Urography

In the acute phase of UTI

- Urography has lost its place in the routine evaluation of acute pyelonephritis in children in many institutions, being replaced by US for detection of dilatation and by DMSA scintigraphy for evaluation of renal parenchymal involvement.

- Urography appears normal in most cases of uncomplicated acute pyelonephritis.

- Urography shows only unspecific signs of acute pyelonephritis (enlarged kidney, impaired nephrogram in severe cases).

- Urography adequately demonstrates the collecting system, including malformations and normal variations such as duplication (duplex) and ectopic kidneys, provided that the kidney is functionally normal and excretes contrast material.

- Urography reveals clinically significant obstruction and gross differences in function between right and left kidney (Fig. 8.4).

For follow-up

- Renal damage (scarring) at urography is indicated by focal or generalized caliceal deformation (clubbing) with a corresponding reduction of the adjacent parenchyma. (Fig. 8.5).

- It can take several months (up to two years) after infection before the renal damage is maximally demonstrable at urography.

- The sensitivity for detection of renal damage (scarring) is much lower at urography compared with DMSA scintigraphy. After one year, about 10% of children with first time UTI will show renal damage at urography, compared with 20–30% found at DMSA scintigraphy.

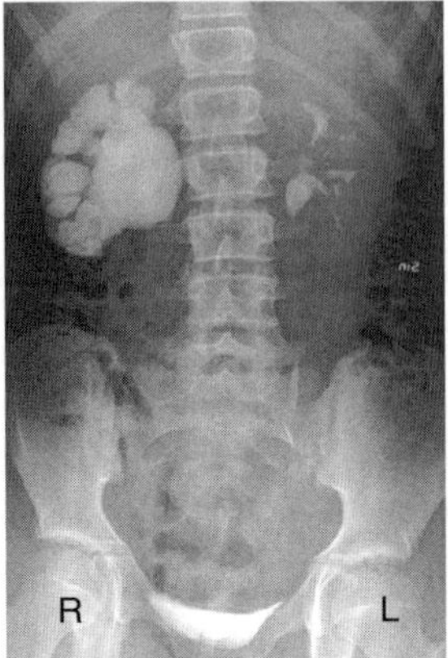

Figure 8.4 Intravenous urography may be useful to reveal the type and grade of urinary tract obstruction. On the right side, gross widening of the renal pelvis and calices is noted 20 minutes after contrast injection, suggesting obstruction at the level of the pelvo-ureteric junction (PUJ-stenosis). R = Right; L = Left.

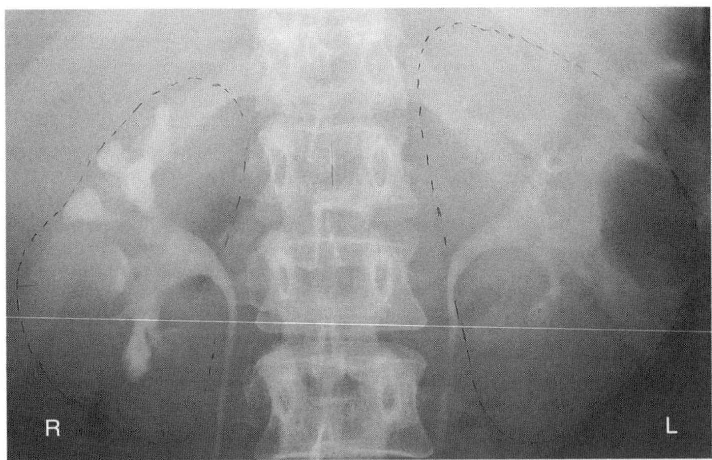

Figure 8.5 Intravenous urography in a patient with post-pyelonephritic renal scarring. The right kidney is markedly smaller than the left, normal kidney. On the right side, there is extensive parenchymal thinning in the upper pole, and there is deformation (clubbing) of the corresponding calices. Similar, less pronounced scarring is seen in the lower pole, while the intervening parenchyma and corresponding calices appear normal. The renal outlines have been outlined for clarity. R = Right; L = Left.

Computed tomography (CT)

In the acute phase of UTI

- CT (preferably multidetector-CT with multiplanar image reconstructions) is a very fast and efficient method for examining the urinary tract.

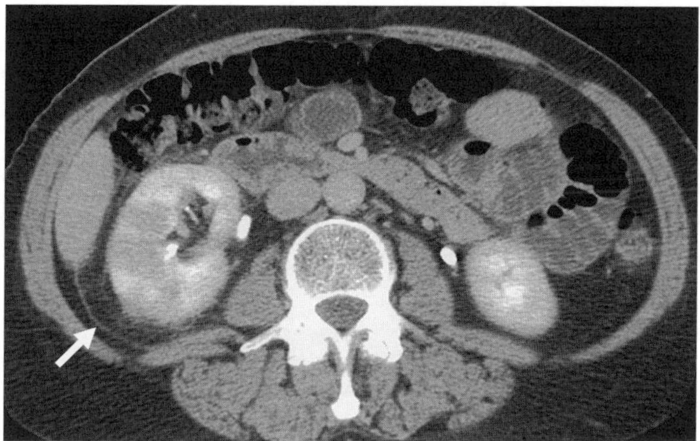

Figure 8.6 Contrast-enhanced CT in a patient with right-sided flank pain and high fever demonstrates areas of reduced contrast enhancement (darker areas) in the right kidney, compatible with acute pyelonephritis. Note also inflammatory infiltration (stranding) in the perirenal fat and slight thickening of the renal fascia (arrow).

- CT may be as efficient as DMSA scintigraphy in evaluation of renal involvement but is not routinely used for this purpose because of the higher radiation dose of CT.

- CT is reserved for complicated cases in children with UTI, e.g. evaluation of renal abscesses, calculi and complicated malformations.

- At contrast enhanced CT, acute pyelonephritis may be suggested by

  - triangular-shaped or ill defined areas of decreased enhancement corresponding to the involved parenchyma (Fig. 8.6)
  - enlargement of the kidney
  - thickening of the urothelium of the renal pelvis
  - infiltration (stranding) in the perirenal fatty tissue
  - a striated nephrogram on delayed imaging (see below 'Urinary tract infection in adults').

- Renal abscess

  - A mass with variable, low density, depending on the degree of necrosis (Fig. 8.7).
  - After i.v. contrast administration, a peripheral zone of higher attenuation is typically seen.
  - Any extension of abscess formation, e.g. into the perirenal space, is well depicted by CT.

- Multidetector-CT with multiplanar image reconstructions is especially useful for

  - evaluating complicated malformations, that may underlie UTI
  - presurgical evaluation.

- In children with renal impairment, i.v. contrast media should be administered with caution.

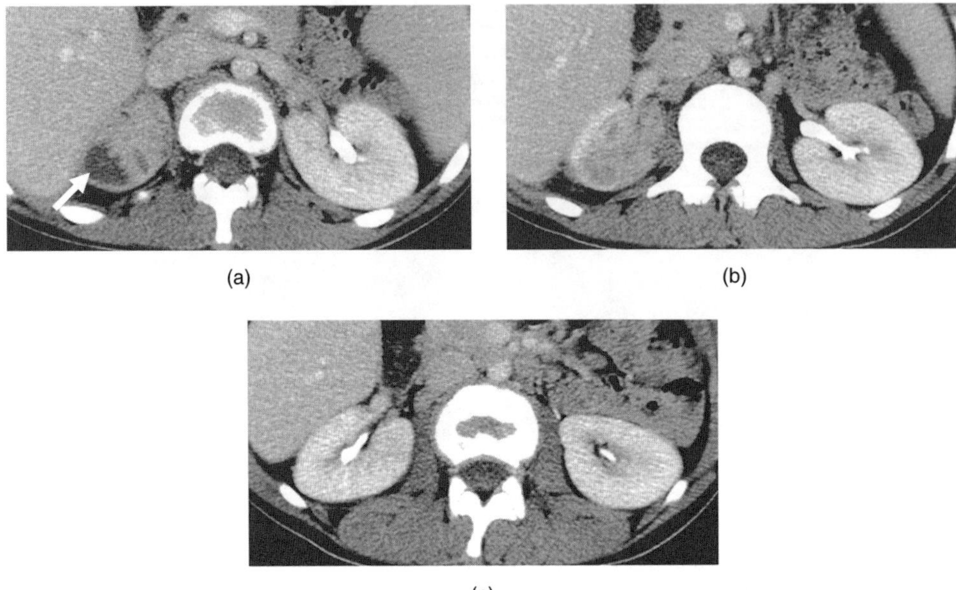

Figure 8.7   (a) Contrast-enhanced axial CT in a 15 year old girl with fever, bacteriuria and flank pain demonstrates a sharply demarcated lesion with fluid-like density posteriorly in the upper pole of the right kidney (arrow), compatible with necrosis in renal abscess. (b) CT-section at a slightly more caudal level demonstrates low attenuation and poor contrast enhancement of the renal parenchyma, compatible with pyelonephritic inflammatory changes. (c) CT-section in middle part of the kidney, showing normal contrast enhancement in non-affected parenchyma.

Follow-up

- Permanent renal damage is demonstrated as focal thinning and irregularity of the renal cortex and caliceal clubbing, usually in combination with reduced renal size.

- Reconstructed images (multiplanar reconstruction, MPR) in the coronal plane, including maximum intensity projections (MIP) allow visualization of the urinary tract in a way similar to that of urography, which may aid in the identification of caliceal clubbing and parenchymal reduction.

Magnetic resonance imaging
In the acute phase of UTI

- Typically, renal inflammation will show low signal at T1-weighted images and increased signal at T2-weighted images, together with a loss of normal corticomedullary differentiation.

- Depending on the MR-equipment used, several sequences have the potential to show inflammation. Additionally, gadolinium enhancement will improve the visualization of inflammatory changes.

- Indications for MRI in children with UTI are usually limited to complicated cases, such as renal abscess and anatomical mapping of complicated malformations (Fig. 8.8).

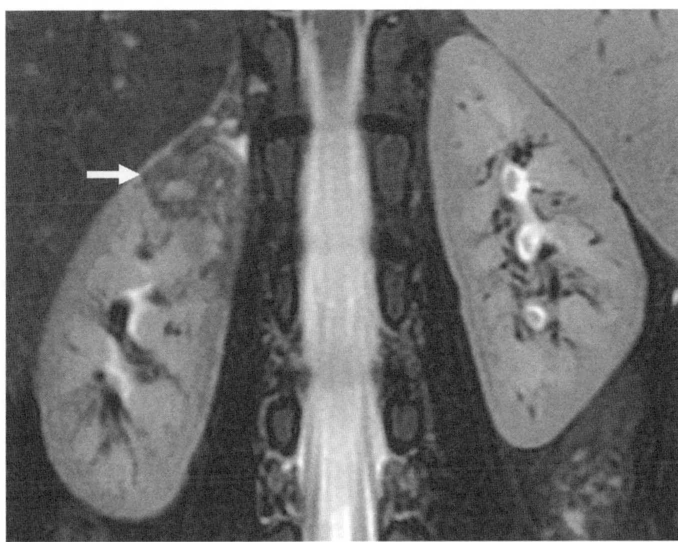

Figure 8.8 Same patient as in Figure 8.7. MRI of the kidneys 24 days after CT demonstrates residual low-signal intensity lesion (arrow) in the upper pole of the right kidney.

- Unlike CT, urography and DMSA scintigraphy, MRI does not utilize ionizing radiation.
- Limitations with MRI are the need for sedation or anesthesia when examining young children, the limited availability and the high cost.
- The anatomy of malformations of the urinary tract can be well visualized, regardless of the kidney function.
- Renal abscesses have low signal on T1-weighted images and increasing and often more heterogeneous signal on T2-weighted images.
  - The signal is depending on the relative content of fluid, protein and debris.
  - Gadolinium enhancement will usually show the abscess, including peripheral enhancement, more distinctly.
- Acute inflammation and permanent renal damage can usually be differentiated at MRI.
- In infants and in children with renal impairment, gadolinium contrast media should be avoided or administered with caution.

Follow-up

- MRI for detection of permanent renal damage in children has not been much evaluated. Renal damage is, however, well demonstrated at fat-saturated T1-weighted images, showing reduction in cortical thickness and indentation of contour often in association with reduced renal size (Fig. 8.9).

Cystography

The most important indication for cystography is identification of vesico-ureteral reflux (VUR) and of infravesical obstruction. Furthermore, grading of VUR is of clinical importance.

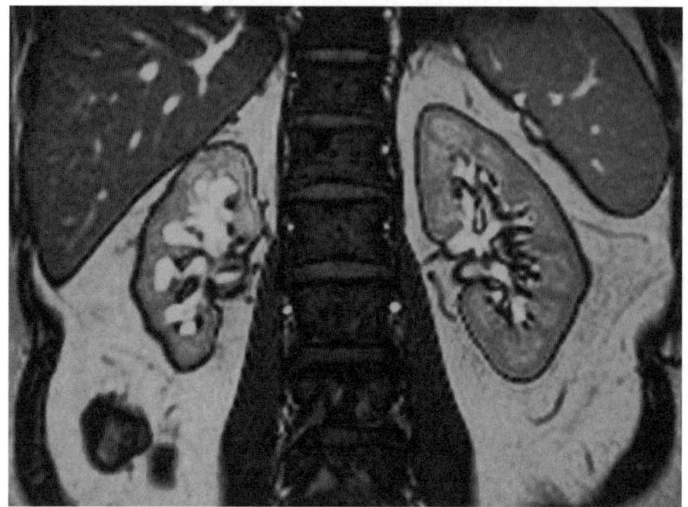

Figure 8.9 Coronal MRI of the kidneys, demonstrating caliceal deformation (clubbing) and irregular parenchymal reduction in the right kidney, which is smaller than the left one. The findings are compatible with post-pyelonephritic scarring.

Normally, the vesico-ureteral junction has a valve-like function to prevent urine (and bacteria) in the urinary bladder from leaking back (reflux) to the ureter and kidney. Due to maldevelopment or late 'maturation' of this valve, urine may re-enter the ureter, especially during voiding. In most cases, VUR is of low grade (no dilatation) and disappears spontaneously with time. Focus is therefore primarily on detection of dilating VUR, which in some cases may require surgical intervention

- VUR can only be identified with high sensitivity by cystography.

- VUR with dilatation of the upper urinary tract (grades 3–5) is a risk factor for recurrent pyelonephritis and permanent renal damage.

- Children with low grade VUR (grades 1–2) run a similar risk of renal damage as children without VUR.

- VUR may occur intermittently, i.e. it is not always demonstrable on imaging examinations.

- VUR in itself rarely causes symptoms.

Voiding cystourethrography (VCUG)

In young children, voiding cystourethrography (VCUG) is usually the preferred type of cystography, since it has the ability to reveal VUR as well as infravesical obstruction, especially posterior urethral valves in boys.

- The bladder is catheterized through the urethra, and filled with water soluble radiographic contrast medium by gravity.

- Fluoroscopy and digital radiographs are used to document bladder anatomy, bladder emptying, urethral anatomy (Figs. 8.10 and 8.11) and VUR that may occur during bladder filling or voiding.

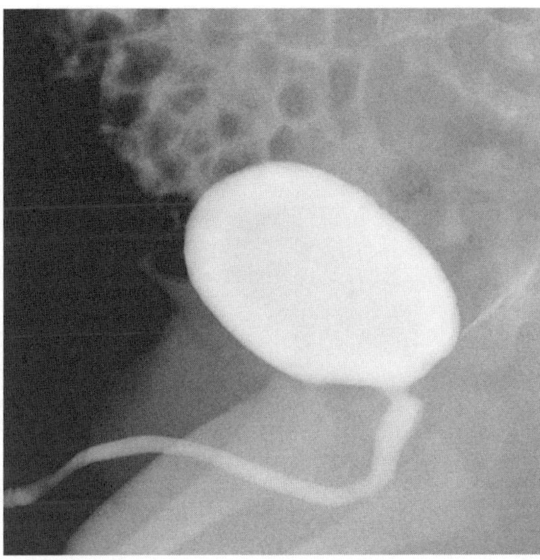

Figure 8.10 Normal voiding cysto-urethrography (VCUG) in a 6 weeks old boy, lateral view. The urethra has a normal appearance, and there is no evidence of urethral outflow obstruction or reflux (back-flow) of contrast material from the bladder to the ureters.

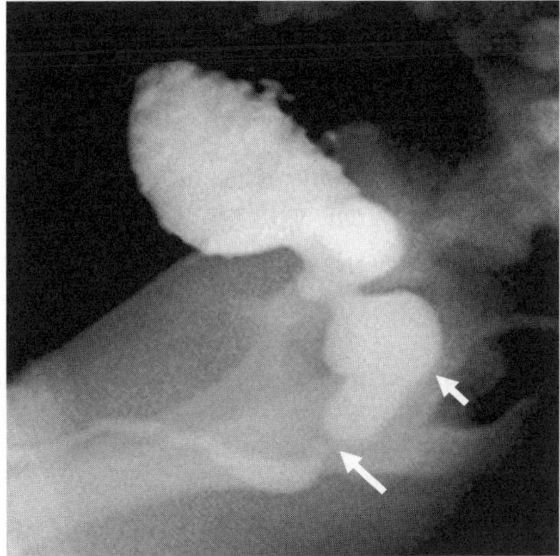

Figure 8.11 Voiding cysto-urethrography (VCUG) in a young boy demonstrating a urethral valve (long arrow), which causes urinary obstruction with marked widening of the proximal urethra (short arrow).

- In order to minimize the ionising radiation dose, fluoroscopy should be intermittent.

- VUR is graded 1–5, according to the recommendations of the International Reflux Study in Children (IRSC) (Fig. 8.12).

- From a practical point of view it is convenient to perform the VCUG when the clinical symptoms have diminished or disappeared.

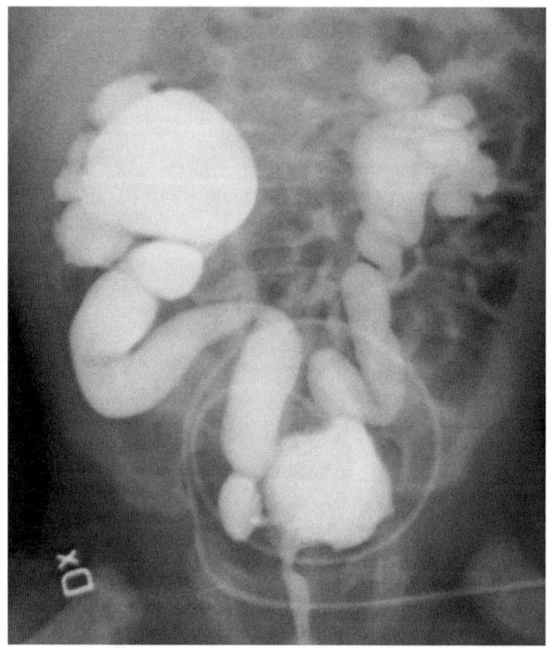

Figure 8.12 Voiding cysto-urethrography (VCUG) in a 2.5 months old boy, demonstrating bilateral gross (grade 4-5) vesico-ureteral reflux, i.e. back-flow of urine/contrast material from the bladder to the ureters. Image obtained during voiding (the bladder was filled with contrast material through a suprapubic catheter in this case).

- VCUG is invasive (requires bladder catheterization) and associated with a considerable radiation dose, and repeated VCUGs should therefore be limited or replaced by techniques with less radiation.

Radionuclide cystography

Direct radionuclide cystography (DRC) is the nuclear medicine equivalent of VCUG. After placing a catheter in the bladder, a weak radio-active solution is slowly infused till bladder capacity. The child voids with the kidneys and the bladder in the field of view of the gamma camera. DRC reveals VUR with about the same sensitivity as VCUG.

Drawbacks

- the need for bladder catheterization
- the lack of generally accepted VUR grading system
- the urethra can not be evaluated (in boys)

Advantages

- low radiation burden

Indirect radionuclide cystography (IRC) is done following a renographic study when the radionuclide, e.g. MAG3, has accumulated in the bladder. The child is allowed to void,

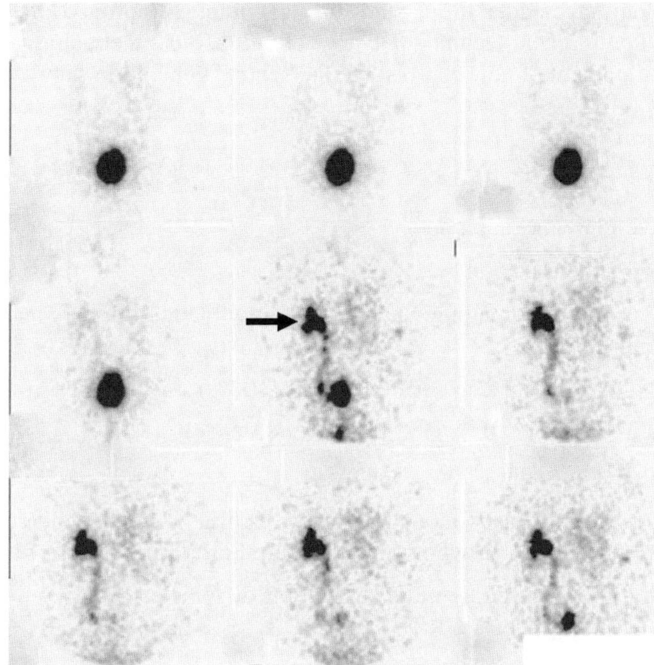

Figure 8.13   Indirect radionuclide cystography (7 secs/frame). Unilateral reflux reaching the renal pelvis (arrow) corresponding to at least grade II according to the International Reflux Study grading system. Note the empty bladder at the end of voiding, followed by refilling of the bladder by emptying of refluxed urine to the bladder on the last image.

usually sitting or standing in front of the gamma camera with the kidneys and the bladder in the field of view (Fig. 8.13).

Drawbacks

- the child needs to be toilet trained, i.e. at least 2–3 years old

- the lack of generally accepted reflux grading system

- less sensitive than VCUG and direct radionuclide cystography

Advantages

- no need for bladder catheterization

- less artificial voiding situation than in techniques requiring bladder catheterization.

Ultrasound (US) cystography

US cystography (voiding urosonography, VUS) is gaining increasing popularity as an alternative to radiographic VCUG or radionuclide cystography. It requires bladder catheterization for the introduction to the bladder of an US contrast medium (mixed with saline) that creates increased echogenicity in the bladder and in the ureter and renal pelvis, if the contrast medium is refluxing from the bladder. It requires US scanning over the bladder, ureters and renal pelvis during bladder filling and during voiding. Improved diagnostic accuracy has been obtained with recent technical advances in ultrasound technology (tissue harmonic imaging) and development of new contrast media (second generation stabilized micro-bubble contrast agents).

US cystography

- does not involve ionizing radiation

- requires bladder catheterization

- does not allow panoramic imaging, i.e. can not show bladder, ureters and kidneys simultaneously during voiding

- demonstrates VUR with varying sensitivity (67–100%)

- does not allow as accurate VUR grading as does VCUG

- does not visualize the urethra

- should not be used as primary modality for evaluating VUR in children with first time UTI, especially not in boys in whom posterior urethral valves should be ruled out

- may be used for special groups, i.e. examination of females, follow up of known VUR and screening of siblings for VUR.

Summary

- UTI involving the kidneys carries a risk for permanent renal damage and long-term complications such as hypertension, complications during pregnancy and renal failure.

- It has since long been considered good practice to investigate and follow children with UTI, particularly those with febrile infections (pyelonephritis). Although UTI is one of the most common infections in childhood there is no general (evidence based) agreement on how, and to which extent, these children should be investigated and followed up.

- Risk factors associated with permanent renal damage, such as obstruction, malformations and VUR, can be identified with different imaging modalities.

  - US is an excellent and non-invasive method for evaluation of kidney size, dilatation of the urinary tract and anatomical abnormalities, but of little value for detection of VUR.

  - Detection of VUR with high sensitivity requires cystography: radiological (VCUG), radionuclide (DRC or IRC) or with US (VUS).

  - Visualization of the urethra to reveal urethral valves in boys requires VCUG.

- DMSA scintigraphy is the preferred method to show renal parenchymal lesions.

  - The investigation can be done acutely during the UTI to show renal inflammation or after three or more months to show permanent renal damage.

  - Children with a normal DMSA scan in the acute stage of infection rarely have dilating VUR.

- There is an ongoing debate whether children with *first* time UTI should be investigated by imaging or not. Opinions vary from performing extensive imaging with ultrasound, cystography and DMSA scintigraphy to no imaging at all. The policies furthermore vary with patient age, with the most frequent use of imaging in infants. Less controversial is the use of imaging in children with risk factors for renal damage, such as an inadequate response to antibacterial treatment, UTI caused by non-*E. coli* bacteria or known abnormality of the urinary tract from prenatal US.

8.2 Symptomatic upper urinary tract infection in adults

Introduction

As in children, most symptomatic upper urinary tract infections in adults are ascending from the lower urinary tract, due to contamination from the fecal flora, mostly by *E. coli*. Other bacteria, such as *Enterobacter, Klebsiella, Proteus, Pseudomonas* and enterococci may also occur, but are more common in patients with recurrent or complicated UTI or as a result of antibiotic treatment.

UTI in adults is over-represented in certain patient groups

- sexually active and pregnant women, diabetics, elderly and those with indwelling bladder catheters.

- patients with urinary obstruction from e.g. prostate hyperplasia, ureteral stones, malignant pelvic tumors, spinal injuries or iatrogenic ureteral injuries, e.g. after gynecological or rectal surgery.

- Vesicoureteral reflux (VUR) may play a role in transportation of bacteria from the bladder to the upper tract, but is rarely documented as a causal factor in adults with pyelonephritis. Secondary VUR may appear in adults due to neoplastic or inflammatory processes in the bladder wall, or from bladder surgery.

Patients with obstructive abnormalities are at increased risk of serious complications, such as septicemia (uro-sepsis) or abscess formation. Hence, imaging in UTI in adults focuses more on the detection of complications, and less on the identification of risk factors for future renal damage, since clinically significant scarring is only rarely seen to develop in adults. Imaging of the urinary tract in adults is usually considered only after repeated UTI episodes or if a complication is suspected. Also, VUR is not routinely searched for in adults. Finally, ionizing radiation is less of an issue in adults, at least in the middle-aged or elderly. All these factors are reflected in the choice of imaging protocols in adult UTI. With the recent advancements in CT technology, multidetector CT is rapidly taking over as the imaging modality of choice in adult UTI.

Clinical features

Symptoms may differ from those in children, and underlying or complicating factors are relatively frequent.

Symptoms

- Fever $>38°$C

- Flank pain, tenderness on palpation over kidney area

- Malaise, nausea and vomiting may occur

- Frequency and dysuria

- Focal urinary tract symptoms may be absent, especially in elderly

- Hypotension, tachypnea and deteriorating clinical status may signal septicemia.

Laboratory tests and findings

- Urinary dip stick sensitive for nitrite and granulocyte-esterase is positive

- Significant bacteriuria, pyuria and sometimes hematuria

- Urinary culture positive (definition of bacterial type and antibacterial resistance pattern is mandatory)

- Blood culture should be obtained if septicemia is suspected

- Elevated C-reactive protein (CRP), sometimes elevated serum creatinine.

Long-term effects

- Renal scarring, usually developing in early childhood, may result in

  - hypertension
  - complications during pregnancy
  - reduced renal function (if scarring is bilateral and severe).

Pathology

- Patho-anatomic changes in the kidney parenchyma, collecting system and perirenal tissues are similar to those described for children.

- Distribution of infection in the renal parenchyma is usually patchy with spared areas, but may be more generalized.

- Focal vasospasm, tubular obstruction and interstitial oedema are factors underlying the CT-finding of low attenuation in affected parts of the parenchyma.

- UTI with certain ureas-producing bacteria, such as *Proteus mirabilis*, may induce stone formation.

- Renal scarring due to UTI occurs mainly in young children, and is rarely documented in adults, although it may occasionally be shown after pyelonephritis associated with obstruction or abscess formation.

Imaging findings

Females with acute, febrile UTI who respond promptly to antibacterial treatment need no radiological imaging. However, if an adult female has 2–3 UTI episodes in one year, imaging is motivated. UTI is less common in men, and recommendations vary. Some claim that imaging should always follow upper UTI in men, while others suggest imaging only after recurrent infection. In patients with diabetes or immunosuppression, early imaging should be considered.

Indications for imaging in adults with febrile UTI/pyelonephritis are:

- acute, febrile UTI with suspicion of concomitant urinary tract obstruction, e.g. ureteral stone (needs acute imaging).

- acute, febrile UTI that does not respond to antibacterial treatment (needs acute imaging).

- repeated febrile UTI/pyelonephritis episodes in men and women.

Imaging may confirm inflammation of the kidney, but the main purpose is to:

- detect underlying urinary tract obstruction, that may require acute treatment by, e.g. percutaneous pyelostomy (nephrostomy).

- detect renal or perirenal abscess formation, that may require drainage.

The most effective imaging method in adult UTI is multidetector CT, which has replaced urography in many institutions. Ultrasonography may show dilatation of the upper urinary tract, but is not sufficient by itself for detection or assessment of the full extent of renal and perirenal inflammation, obstruction or ureteral stones.

Computed tomography (CT)

The CT examination

- should include a non-enhanced scan including the entire urinary tract (kidneys, ureters, bladder)

- should include an early contrast-enhanced scan, obtained in the nephrographic phase (60–100 s after start of contrast medium injection)

- should include a late scan in the excretory phase (6–8 min after start of contrast injection), to allow visualization of the collecting system and ureters

- the two contrast-enhanced scans can be combined by first injecting half the volume of contrast medium, wait for 8 min and then inject the other half of contrast medium volume, followed by scanning 60–100 s after the start of the second contrast medium injection.

Non-contrast-enhanced CT may demonstrate

- inflammatory swelling of the affected kidney.

- slight reduction in parenchymal attenuation in areas of focal edema.

- inflammatory reaction in the perirenal fat (perinephric stranding) (Fig. 8.14a, b), (similar changes occur with obstruction, trauma, vascular disorders).

- spread of inflammatory reaction to Gerota's fascia (thickening) and pararenal space.

- dilatation of the renal pelvis (hydronephrosis) and ureter (hydroureter) (Fig. 8.14b, c).

- underlying urinary stones, including those that are 'non-opaque' at plain radiography (kidneys-ureters-bladder, KUB) (Fig. 8.14c).

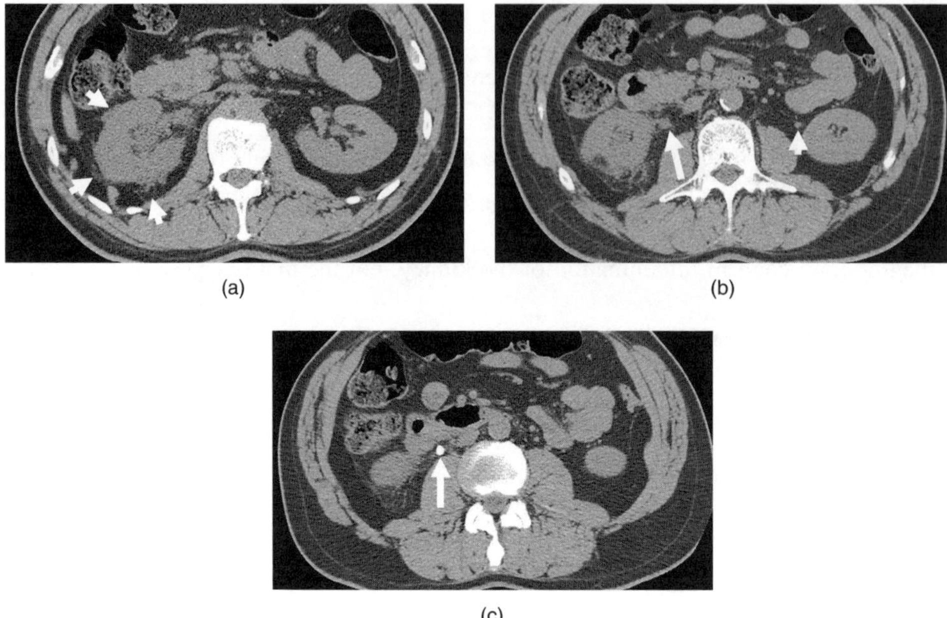

Figure 8.14   Non-enhanced CT of the urinary tract in an adult patient with fever and right-sided flank pain. (a) Swelling of the right kidney is noted, as compared to the left one, and there is fullness of the renal pelvis. Increased linear and patchy densities, so called stranding (arrows) are seen in the fatty tissue surrounding the kidney, indicating inflammation and/or urinary stasis. (b) CT section at a more caudal level demonstrates marked perirenal stranding and widening of the proximal part of the right ureter (long arrow). Note normal ureteral diameter (short arrow) and absence of perirenal stranding on the left side. (c) CT section at a more caudal level demonstrates a stone (arrow) in the ureter, causing hydroureter and hydronephrosis. Ureteral obstruction combined with fever indicates pyonephrosis, a medical emergency that requires antibiotics and percutaneous drainage.

- gas in the renal parenchyma, collecting system or perirenal tissues (see 'Emphysematous pyelonephritis' below).

Contrast-enhanced CT may demonstrate

- decreased parenchymal attenuation
  - Typically, sharply or diffusely demarcated, unifocal or multifocal wedge-shaped or rounded low-attenuating areas, extending from the papilla to the renal cortex, corresponding to poorly functioning parenchyma, are seen.
  - Occasionally, the entire kidney is diffusely involved, resulting in renal enlargement, poor enhancement and reduced contrast excretion.
  - Other infiltrative processes with decreased parenchymal attenuation should be kept in mind, such as renal infarct or neoplasia (e.g. renal or transitional cell carcinoma, myeloma, leukemia).
- reduced corticomedullary differentiation.

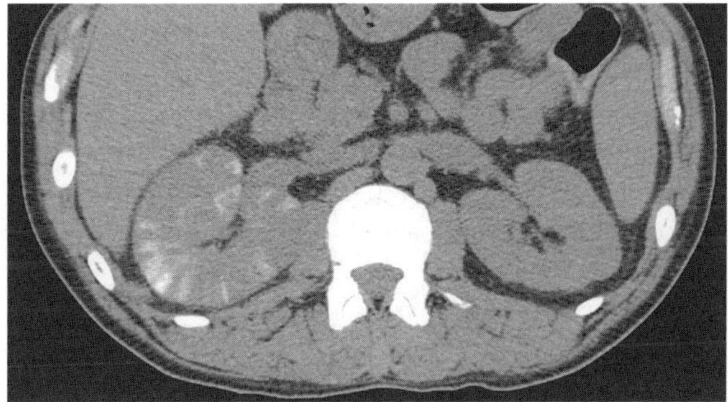

Figure 8.15 Delayed imaging after contrast-enhanced CT of the kidneys in a patient with acute, right-sided pyelonephritis. Retained contrast material is noted in the right kidney due to impaired tubular function, causing a striated pattern (striation). Note that contrast material has cleared from the left kidney and the collecting system at this time-point.

- delayed nephrogram (contrast enhancement) in affected parts of the kidney.

- striated nephrogram, i.e. alternating thin bands of high and low attenuation in the affected parenchyma, that

  - is due to obstructed tubules alternating with intervening normal tubules
  - may persist over time (persistent nephrogram), while non-affected parenchyma has been cleared of contrast material (Fig. 8.15)
  - may also be due to e.g. obstruction, renal vein thrombosis or renal contusion.

- inflammatory thickening of the renal pelvis wall (urothelium).

- abscess formations and spread to the surrounding tissues (Fig. 8.7).

- occurrence and degree of urinary obstruction, provided that late imaging in the excretory phase is performed.

Ultrasonography

- is widely available, easy for the patient and involves no harmful radiation

- is operator-dependent (skill and experience) and patient-dependent (more difficult in obese or large patients)

- may show hypo- or hyperechogenic areas, renal enlargement and loss of corticomedullary differentiation, but does often not show full extent of renal and perirenal inflammation

- Doppler and i.v. contrast material may improve detection of pyelonephritis

- may show inflammatory thickening of the renal pelvis wall (urothelium)

- demonstrates dilatation of the renal pelvis (hydronephrosis) with high accuracy, but can not confirm or rule out obstruction

- may demonstrate pyonephrosis, i.e. pus in a widened renal pelvis/ureter, by showing thick echogenic content and layering of debris/urine

- does not show underlying ureteral stones sufficiently well

- should not be used as single imaging modality in adult UTI

- can be used in pregnant women or otherwise when ionizing radiation is an issue, if necessary combined with single plain radiographs to improve detection of stones

- in pregnant women, dilatation of the collecting system and ureters may be caused by physiological hormonal changes, mechanical obstruction from the enlarged uterus, UTI, or a combination of these factors.

Urography

- is largely being replaced by multidetector computed tomography (CT)

- may show inflammatory swelling of the affected kidney, but this is an unreliable sign since there is considerable normal variation in size of the two kidneys

- may show impaired parenchymal contrast enhancement of the affected kidney, but in most cases (75%) urography appears normal in UTI

- demonstrates most, but far from all, urinary stones on pre-contrast (plain) radiographs (KUB)

- demonstrates occurrence, grade and location of urinary tract obstruction and hydronephrosis/hydroureter on images obtained after i.v. contrast medium injection. This may require delayed imaging after 30 min. up to several hours

- may be useful in demonstrating papillary necrosis and medullary sponge kidney (tubular ectasia).

MRI

- is less widely available than CT but involves no harmful radiation

- Intravenous contrast media (gadolinium) should be used with caution in patients with reduced renal function (risk of nephrogenic systemic fibrosis)

- is able to show renal and perirenal inflammation, abscesses, hydronephrosis and obstruction with high accuracy

- may be useful in assessing the extent of renal and perirenal inflammation (e.g. gadolinium-enhanced 3D FLASH sequences), as well as in assessing the collecting system (e.g. MR urography with HASTE-sequences)

- is less accurate than CT in identifying urinary stones

- is usually not routinely employed for acute or non-acute imaging in adult UTI

- may be useful for problem solving in individual cases

- may be useful for imaging children, young adults or pregnant women, when ionising radiation is an issue.

Radionuclide studies

- Renography may be employed for estimation of renal function and assessment of obstruction (see above, UTI in children)

- DMSA scintigraphy may demonstrate acute renal inflammatory involvement in UTI, but does not give information on underlying causes or complications, and is therefore usually not routinely employed in adults

- As in children, DMSA scintigraphy is very sensitive in revealing post-pyelonephritic scarring, but it is not routinely employed in adults.

Voiding cystourethrography (VCUG)

- is not routinely performed in adults with UTI

- VUR may persist into adulthood or occur secondary to bladder pathology, and may occasionally contribute to UTI and, rarely, flank pain.

Summary

- Adults with uncomplicated febrile UTI/acute pyelonephritis who respond promptly to antibacterial treatment need no radiological imaging.

- Imaging in UTI/acute pyelonephritis should be considered in patients with diabetes and those with growth of uncommon infecting bacteria.

- Adults with *repeated* episodes of febrile UTI/pyelonephritis should have imaging of the urinary tract performed, in order to reveal any underlying cause.

- Patients with febrile UTI/acute pyelonephritis, who do not respond to antibacterial treatment, and patients suspected of having complications (obstruction, uncommon bacteria), should have *acute* imaging of the urinary tract.

- Febrile UTI/pyelonephritis in combination with urinary obstruction is an emergency, that should initiate *immediate* imaging and treatment (antibiotics and percutaneous drainage), in order to reduce the risk of potentially life-threatening septicemia.

- Multidetector-CT without and with i.v. contrast medium is the preferred method to demonstrate the extent of inflammation and any underlying cause of the UTI, such as ureteral stone and/or obstruction, and to reveal complications, such as abscess formation.

8.3 Emphysematous pyelonephritis

Introduction

Emphysematous pyelonephritis is a serious complication of pyelonephritis with gas-forming bacteria, primarily (90% or more) affecting diabetics and patients with urinary obstruction. It requires systemic antibiotics, emergency nephrectomy or percutaneous drainage.

Clinical features

- More common in females than in males.

- Severe, sometimes life-threatening, necrotizing infection.

- Symptoms may be as described for severe acute pyelonephritis
  - rapid onset of fever, chills, flank pain
  - lethargy, fatigue
  - palpable flank mass with crepitations may occasionally be found
  - rapid progression to septic chock may occur.
- Mortality up to 50% has been described.

Pathology

- Unilateral infection with gas-forming bacteria (mostly *E. coli*), causing destruction of renal parenchyma and collections of gas within the parenchyma.
- Gas distribution may be focal or diffuse, and may spread to the perirenal tissues.
- The gas-forming bacteria may also reside in the collecting system (emphysematous pyelitis).

Imaging findings

- CT is the method of choice, since it is very sensitive in the detection of even very small amounts of gas.
- CT shows collections of gas within the parenchyma (focal or widespread), in combination with signs of inflammation (renal swelling, irregular, reduced contrast-enhancement and perirenal stranding).
- Urography may show gas, but is less sensitive than CT
- US may show highly reflective (echogenic) gas, but is less sensitive than CT.

Summary

- The demonstration by any imaging method of gas in the renal parenchyma, the collecting system or perirenal tissues in the clinical setting of UTI should raise the suspicion of emphysematous pyelonephritis.
- Emphysematous pyelonephritis is potentially life-threatening and requires immediate treatment.
- CT is the most sensitive imaging method to demonstrate abnormal gas collections.

8.4 Xanthogranulomatous pyelonephritis

Introduction

Xanthogranulomatous pyelonephritis (XGP) is a rare variant of chronic renal infection, caused by bacteriuria in combination with long-standing urinary obstruction. It may affect the entire kidney or be localized to one part of the kidney

Clinical features

- Female preponderance, mostly middle-aged or elderly, but may affect men and children.

- History of chronic or recurrent acute urinary tract infection.

- Unilateral flank pain and/or palpable mass.

- 10–30% of patients are diabetics.

- Anorexia, malaise, fever, weight loss, sometimes suggesting malignancy.

- Erythrocyte sedimentation rate is nearly always elevated.

- Leukocytosis, pyuria, anemia, hematuria and positive urine culture is commonly encountered.

- Liver enzymes may be elevated, probably due to renal tissue destruction.

Pathology

- Long-standing infection, usually with *Proteus* or *E. coli* bacteria, promoted by urinary obstruction due to stone in most cases.

- The lesion may be localized, but is more often diffuse and extensive, causing renal enlargement and functional deterioration.

- Chronic infection causes replacement of renal tissue by lipid-rich macrophages (xanthoma cells) and inflammatory cells.

- The granulomatous inflammation leads to necrosis of renal tissue, causing cavities.

- Inflammatory reaction spreading to the perirenal space and surrounding tissues.

Imaging findings

- Renal enlargement that may be difficult to differentiate from renal cell carcinoma.

- Central stones in the collecting system, often of stag-horn type.

- Poor or no function of the affected kidney.

- Urography may demonstrate a large kidney, central calculus and poor or no function, but the findings are not specific for XGP (Fig. 8.16).

- Ultrasonography may show renal enlargement, high-echogenic central structures with posterior shadowing representing renal stone, and multiple low-echogenic lesions in the parenchyma, but the full extent of disease is better shown by CT.

- CT is the best method to show all components of the disease. It is excellent to show the calculi and demonstrates low-density, cyst-like or necrotic areas, delineated by a slightly enhancing peripheral rim (granulation tissue) after i.v. contrast administration (Fig. 8.17).

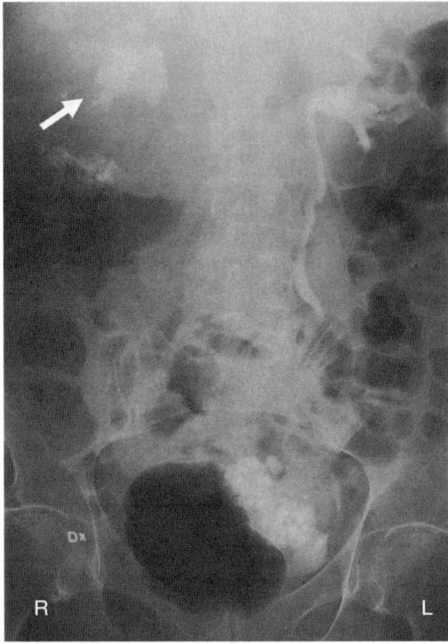

Figure 8.16 Intravenous urography in a 70 year old woman, demonstrating manifestations of xanthogranulomatous pyelonephritis on the right side. There is a central stag-horn calculus (arrow) and additional calcifications more peripherally. No contrast excretion was seen from the right kidney. There is normal excretion on the left side. Calcified myoma of the uterus was incidentally found in the pelvic region. R = Right; L = Left.

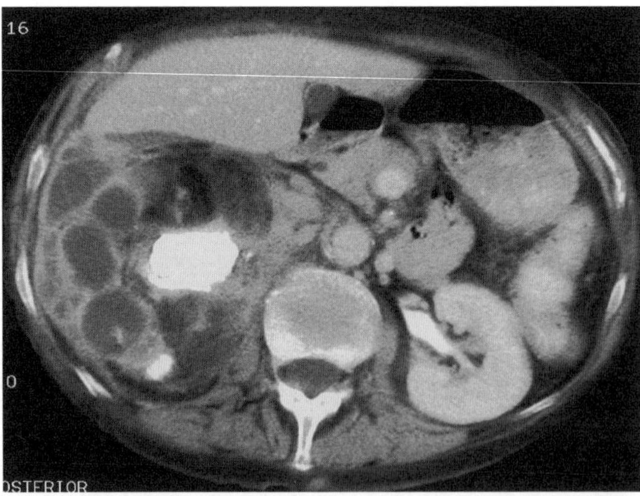

Figure 8.17 Same patient as in Figure 8.16. Contrast-enhanced CT demonstrates grossly enlarged right kidney with large stag-horn calculus in the renal pelvis and multiple peripheral renal calcifications. Multiple low-density lesions are noted in the renal parenchyma, representing xanthogranulomatous inflammatory degeneration. There was extension of inflammatory changes into the right perirenal space. Left kidney has normal appearance.

- Evidence of perirenal inflammatory process, i.e. infiltration of the perirenal fatty tissue (stranding) or extension along other contiguous structures, best shown at CT.

- 'Fractured stone' sign, i.e. breaking off part of a calculus in the collecting system due to pressure from the expanding abnormal renal parenchyma.

- MRI is not ideal for demonstration of calculi, and is therefore not the method of choice. It is otherwise capable of demonstrating all the pathological changes mentioned above.

Summary

- XGP is a severe chronic granulomatous infection of the kidney, usually associated with chronic UTI, calculi and obstruction leading to functional deterioration.

- XGP is associated with unilateral renal enlargement, central calculus (often stag-horn), multifocal parenchymal destructions, usually with evidence of perirenal inflammation.

- CT is the method of choice to show the full extent of XGP, including low-density parenchymal lesions with peripheral contrast enhancement.

- The combination of CT findings may be suggestive of XGP, but it can be difficult to differentiate XGP from renal neoplasia, and sometimes the diagnosis can only be made after nephrectomy.

- Since there is usually no or little renal function at detection, nephrectomy is often the only treatment option.

8.5 Urinary tract infection in the immunocompromised patient

Introduction

Patients with immunosuppression, as in AIDS and those treated with immunosuppressive drugs, e.g. after organ transplantation, are predisposed to infections of the urinary tract with uncommon bacteria, fungi, parasites and viruses. Malignancies are overrepresented in patients with HIV/AIDS.

Clinical features

Infections of the urinary tract in immunocompromised patients may involve several organs:

- Urethritis.

- Prostatitis, with lower urinary tract symptoms, fever, urinary retention and perineal pain. If untreated, abscess formation may occur.

- Epididymitis/orchitis, which may be severe, recurrent or resistant to therapy. Swelling, pain and tenderness over the affected part of the scrotum.

- Cystitis, with urgency, frequency and painful micturition.

- Pyelonephritis, with flank pain, fever, malaise and other symptoms described previously.

Pathology

The genito-urinary pathology is mainly related to the immunocompromised state of the patient.

- Inflammation due to unusual bacteria, fungi, parasites and viruses (tuberculosis is described separately, see below).

- Destruction of renal parenchyma leading to abscess formation.

- Recurrent cystitis may result in bladder malacoplakia, a granulomatous tumor-like inflammation of the bladder wall due to defective immune response to *E. coli*.

- Malacoplakia may rarely occur also in the ureter, renal pelvis and kidney.

Imaging findings

Imaging findings in the urinary tract are similar to those in other patients with infectious disorders of the urogenital organs. However, some findings that are more specifically related to immunodeficiency and HIV/AIDS should be noted.

- Abscess formation in the affected organs is more likely to occur due to the reduced immune response.

- Urinary tract infection with fungi (*Candida albicans* or *Aspergillus*) may produce radiolucent debris or 'fungus balls', i.e. masses of fungi that appear as filling defects in the collecting system at urography and contrast-enhanced CT. Fungus debris may take the shape of the collecting system and may be outlined by the excreted contrast material. Fungal debris or balls may cause obstruction and hydronephrosis, detectable also at US.

- Indinavir, a protease inhibitor, is used in the treatment of HIV/AIDS. It may precipitate in the urine and cause indinavir 'calculi', which may obstruct the urinary tract. These 'calculi' are radiolucent, even on CT. Indinavir 'calculi' may also act as a nidus for calcified stone formation.

- Malacoplakia of the bladder and collecting system causes tumor-like filling defects on radiographic examinations.

Summary

- Immunosuppression from AIDS, immunosuppressive treatment or other causes predisposes to urinary tract infection with unusual agents.

- Symptoms and imaging findings may be different from those usually encountered. Frequent abscess formation, fungus balls, indinavir 'calculi' and development of malacoplakia are such examples.

8.6 Tuberculosis

Introduction

Tuberculosis is a common disease, affecting several million people yearly. Parallel with the increase in AIDS, tuberculosis has increased in frequency. Other risk patients are those subjected to organ transplantation or dialysis, and e.g. rheumatology patients with anti-cytokine treatment.

Most commonly, tuberculosis affects the lungs. Genitourinary tuberculosis is the third most common site to be affected, after lungs and lymph nodes. Kidneys, ureters, bladder, prostate and epididymis are frequently involved. The severity of disease depends on the infectious site, the virulence of the bacteria and the immune response of the host. Urogenital tuberculosis is characterized by unspecific clinical presentation and varying radiological manifestations.

Clinical features

Clinical findings

- Most patients have a history of tuberculosis, mainly of the lungs, but it may be many years back, suggesting re-activation of infection.

- Renal tuberculosis is often asymptomatic and easily overlooked.

- Symptoms may be non-specific.

- Initial symptoms may be those of conventional cystitis with urgency, frequency, suprapubic pain, pyuria and hematuria, while focal signs of upper UTI and flank pain are less common as initial symptoms.

- Tuberculous cystitis is usually preceded by tuberculosis in the upper urinary tract.

- Typically, the symptoms of lower or upper UTI do not respond to standard antibiotic treatment.

- General symptoms like weight loss, fever and malaise occur occasionally.

Laboratory tests

- Pyuria together with negative urine culture using standard media should raise suspicion of tuberculosis.

- Diagnosis can be made by microscopic analysis showing acid-fast bacilli, or by PCR.

- A microbiological diagnosis is made by isolation of the organism from urine or biopsy specimen.

Pathology

- Tuberculosis of the kidney and urinary tract is nearly always caused by *Mycobacterium tuberculosis*. Rarely, in immunocompromised patients, other mycobacteria (*M. avis, M. bovis*) may be causative.

- Renal tuberculosis may be part of generalized (miliary) blood-borne tuberculosis, but is more commonly localized, following embolic hematogenous spread from lung tuberculosis.

- Initially, small granulomata, with or without caseation, form in the renal cortex, and with sufficient host immunity these may be stable for a long period of time.

- The infection may be dormant for many years following initial infection.

- Reactivation may result in renal papillary necrosis and severe renal parenchymal destruction, with subsequent direct spread to the perirenal tissues, collecting system, ureters and bladder.

- Scarring in the renal parenchyma results in tissue contraction and calcifications of variable appearances, including renal and ureteric stones. If extensive, the renal lesions may lead to autonephrectomy.

- Scarring in the caliceal system (infundibular narrowing) leads to focal strictures that may be 'amputation'-like and lead to obstruction and hydrocalicosis, while focal irregular strictures of the ureter lead to segmental hydroureter and hydronephrosis.

- Collecting system strictures may continue to develop during otherwise successful treatment.

- Tuberculous insterstitial nephritis is an atypical form of renal tuberculosis with equally sized smooth kidneys, leading to advanced renal failure.

- Extrarenal spread of the infection may lead to a tumor-like peri-renal mass, and retroperitoneal tuberculous abscesses along the psoas muscle, with or without fistula-formations, may ensue.

- Infection of the bladder usually occurs through direct spread from the upper tract. Bladder wall fibrosis and thickening may lead to impaired ureteral drainage, vesico-ureteral reflux and reduced bladder capacity.

- Calcifications of the bladder wall may occur, but is more typical of schistosomiasis.

- Bladder tuberculosis may simulate neoplasia.

- Tuberculous prostatitis occurs through spread from the urinary tract.

- Tuberculous epididymitis is thought to be mainly blood-borne, since it can occur without urinary tract infection.

- In women, tuberculosis may affect e.g. the fallopian tubes (tuberculous salpingitis), but there is no clear association with urinary tract tuberculosis.

Imaging findings

Urography

- Plain films may show calcifications that can attain characteristics ranging from small patchy, curvilinear or amorphous calcifications to extensive calcifications in the collecting system ('putty' kidney).

- Single or multiple widened calices, due to infundibular caliceal strictures, together with irregular parenchymal scarring, may be suggestive of tuberculosis.

- Segmental widening of the affected ureter, with corresponding irregular ureteral strictures are commonly seen.

- A thick-walled bladder may sometimes be discernible, indicating involvement of the bladder, often with impaired ureteral emptying.

- In late stages, a small, calcified, irregularly contracted kidney with poor function may be found.

- Extrarenal manifestations can not be reliably assessed.

Ultrasound

- Hydronephrosis and hydrocalicosis are easily detected, while segmental ureteral dilatation may be difficult to assess.

- Calcifications in the kidney and urinary tract can be seen, but may be underestimated.

- Extrarenal manifestations such as perirenal infection and psoas abscesses may be detected, but the full extent of extrarenal disease is better evaluated with CT.

- Involvement of the epididymis, testicle and scrotum can be assessed in detail by scrotal US using high frequency transducers.

- Involvement of the female genital organs is best assessed by transvaginal US, although abdominal US and CT of the pelvis may give complementary over-view in case of extensive and widespread disease.

CT

CT, and particularly CT urography without and with iv contrast administration, is the method of choice for detecting and assessing urinary tract tuberculosis and its complications. In case of suspected tuberculosis, the scanning should always extend from the top of the kidneys (or from the diaphragm) through the entire pelvic region, since complicating extrarenal tuberculosis may extend into the retroperitoneal space down to the inguinal or even scrotal region.

- Parenchymal and urinary tract calcifications are easily detected and can be accurately characterized by non-enhanced CT.

- Bladder wall calcifications may occur but are more typical for schistosomiasis.

- Regional renal functional abnormalities can be reliably assessed on contrast-enhanced series.

- Focal parenchymal scars can readily be assessed.

- Caliceal and ureteral dilatations and strictures can be assessed by delayed imaging in the excretory phase, allowing the collecting system and ureters to fill with contrast medium.

- Renal and peri-renal abscesses and other extrarenal manifestations are well depicted.

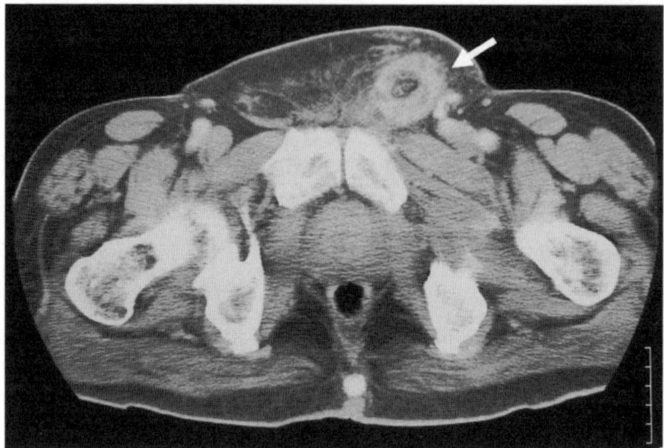

Figure 8.18   Adult male with tuberculosis (TB) of the epididymis. CT reveals a tubular soft tissue swelling (arrow) extending cranially from the left epididymis, compatible with spread of the TB infection to the spermatic cord and adjacent tissues.

- The bladder wall, prostate, epididymis and female genital organs can be assessed by extending the scanning from the diaphragm to below the pubic symphysis (Fig. 8.18).

MRI

- MRI is capable of demonstrating all changes associated with urogenital tuberculosis, except calcifications which are better displayed by non-enhanced CT (Figs. 8.19 and 8.20).

- MRI should therefore be reserved for children, young adults and other patients in whom the radiation dose is an issue. In such cases, plain radiography may be helpful to help assess renal and urinary tract calcifications.

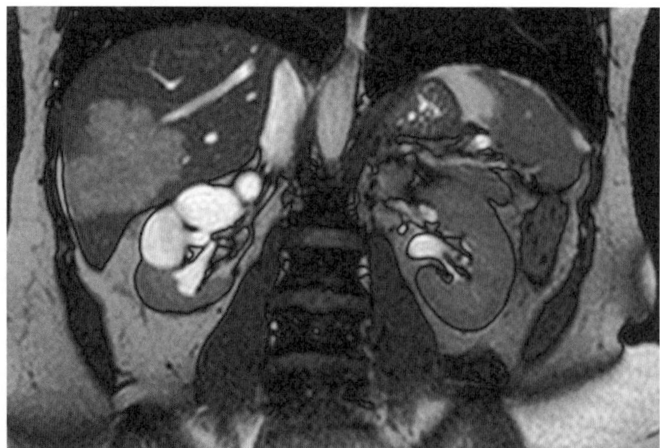

Figure 8.19   Coronal MRI of the kidneys in a 47 year old woman demonstrates gross widening of the calices due to multiple strictures of the caliceal infundibulae on the right side, from urinary tract tuberculosis. The lesion in the liver is an incidentally detected hemangioma.

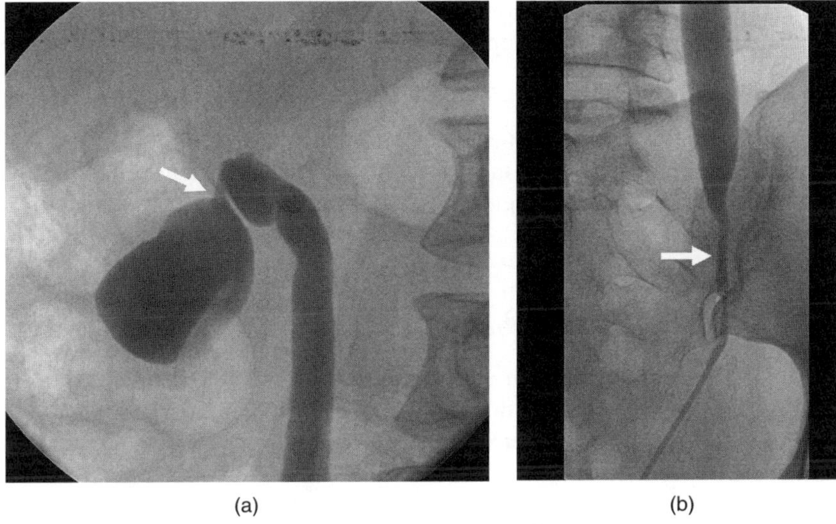

(a)   (b)

Figure 8.20 (a) Same patient as in Figure 8.19. Retrograde pyelography confirms marked widening of the lower calyx, due to stricture of the caliceal infundibulum (arrow). No passage of contrast medium to the middle and upper calices could be obtained. The findings are compatible with strictures due to urinary tract tuberculosis. (b) After retraction of the ureteral catheter to a more caudal position, another stricture (arrow), located in the lower part of the ureter is noted, causing widening of the proximal ureter.

Summary

- Tuberculosis damages the kidney in two ways
  - destructive parenchymal infection and scarring
  - obstructive damage due to strictures of calices, renal pelvis and ureters.

- Urinary tract tuberculosis has been called 'The great imitator', referring to its variable radiological appearance.

- Multidetector CT without and with intravenous contrast medium (CT urography) is the most effective imaging modality to detect and assess tuberculosis of the kidneys and urinary tract, although no single finding is pathognomonic for tuberculosis.

- The most important issue in revealing urinary tract tuberculosis is to keep tuberculosis in mind as a differential diagnosis.

- Since there may be a long time interval from the date of the initial tuberculosis infection to the presentation of urinary tract symptoms, obtaining a thorough patient history is essential.

8.7 Schistosomiasis

Introduction

Schistosomiasis (Bilharziasis) is a parasitic disease, caused by the trematode (flatworm) schistosoma. Several species of schistosoma can affect humans, primarily *S. haematobium,*

S. mansoni and *S. japonicum*. Infection with *S. mansoni* and *S. japonicum* mainly cause hepatobiliary and gastrointestinal symptoms, while *S. haematobium* typically affects the urinary tract. Urinary schistosomiasis is endemic in Africa, the Eastern Mediterranean and the Middle East.

Considering the increasing migration from endemic areas to other parts of the world and the fact that signs and symptoms may occur several years after infection, awareness of clinical symptoms and radiological signs of schistosomiasis also in non-endemic countries is of increasing importance.

Clinical features – *S. haematobium*

- An estimated 70 million persons in sub-Saharan Africa are reported to have hematuria related to *S. haematobium*, 32 million have dysuria, 18 million have ultrasonographic evidence of major bladder wall pathology and 10 million have major hydronephrosis. Mortality due to obstructive nephropathy is estimated to 150 000 per year.

- All ages may be affected, but peak morbidity is often in children aged 7–14 years.

- Individuals without prior exposure may feel ill and notice a skin rash a couple of days after exposure to infected fresh water. Three to four weeks later, flu-like symptoms may occur, including cough, malaise, lymphadenopathy, hepatosplenomegaly and eosinophilia. In some cases, severe neurological and abdominal symptoms may occur. In chronic carriers, symptoms may be mild or absent.

- Hematuria (mostly macroscopic, but sometimes only microscopic) and signs of cystitis, e.g. dysuria, frequency and urgency, are the most common initial urinary tract symptoms, occurring three months or more after infection. Hematuria is attributed to the bladder pathology.

- Ova in the urine, serological tests and biopsy from the bladder wall, rectum or vagina confirm the diagnosis.

- Long-term effects include calcifications and dysfunction of the bladder, vesico-ureteral reflux, and calcifications and strictures of the ureters, resulting in renal outflow obstruction.

- The prostate, seminal vesicles, vas deferens, testes and the female genital organs may become involved. Hemospermia may indicate genital schistosomiasis. Genital schistosomiasis may mimic neoplasms of the testicles, uterus and adnexa.

- Growth retardation, reduced physical fitness and impaired cognitive development may follow the more specific symptoms.

- Praziquantel treatment is effective in reducing prevalence and severity of pathology, but re-infection often leads to reappearance of lesions within one or two years, especially in children. Periodic treatment of populations at risk prevents severe late-stage morbidity.

- Squamous cell carcinoma of the bladder is over-represented in chronic schistosomiasis.

- Mortality due to *S. haematobium* is mainly due to kidney failure and bladder cancer.

Pathology

- Schistosomiasis commonly affects children (e.g. from swimming) and those engaged in e.g. fishing, irrigation, agriculture and domestic water contact.

- The infection requires contact with fresh water containing snails (intermediate host) that produce cercariae (larval forms of the parasite) which penetrate the human skin.

- The cercariae reach the human circulation and migrate to portal blood in the liver and mature into adult worms, migrating to mesenteric venules of bowel and rectum (*S. mansoni* and *S. japonicum*) or venous plexa of the urinary bladder and ureters (*S. haematobium*).

- Eggs penetrate from venules to bowel lumen and urinary bladder and are excreted in feces and urine, respectively.

- *S. haematobium* eggs initiate granuloma formation and arteritis in the bladder wall and ureters, resulting in oedema and subsequent fibrosis with tissue thickening.

- Tumor-like papillomas of the bladder may develop.

- Calcifications in the bladder and ureteral walls are typical, caused by dead, calcified eggs in the submucosa.

- The testes, seminal vesicles and prostate, as well as the female internal genital organs, may be infected, resulting in granulomas and calcifications.

Imaging findings of urinary tract – *S. haematobium*

- Changes in the urinary bladder and distal ureters precede renal changes.

- Early findings may be nodular filling defects in the bladder at bladder ultrasonography, urography or contrast-enhanced CT.

- Fibrosis, scarring and strictures add to narrowing of the ureters, leading to prolonged ureteral contrast medium filling and widening of the distal ureters at urography (Fig. 8.21).

- Thickening and irregularities of the bladder wall and ureters may be seen on ultrasonography, CT or MRI.

- With progressive disease, urinary outflow obstruction with bilateral but asymmetric hydronephrosis, evident on ultrasonography, urography, contrast-enhanced CT and MRI, will follow.

- Calcifications of the urinary bladder wall and lower thirds of the ureteral walls are almost pathognomonic findings of schistosomiasis.

  o Calcifications may be seen at KUB and urography, but are best seen at non-enhanced CT.

  o Calcifications may be punctate, granular, thick, irregular, linear or circumferential (Fig. 8.22) and may involve also the prostate, seminal vesicles and rectum (Fig. 8.23).

  o The calcified eggs may be shed, resulting in diminished radiographic calcifications over time.

- Involvement of the vesico-ureteral junction may lead to vesico-ureteral reflux.

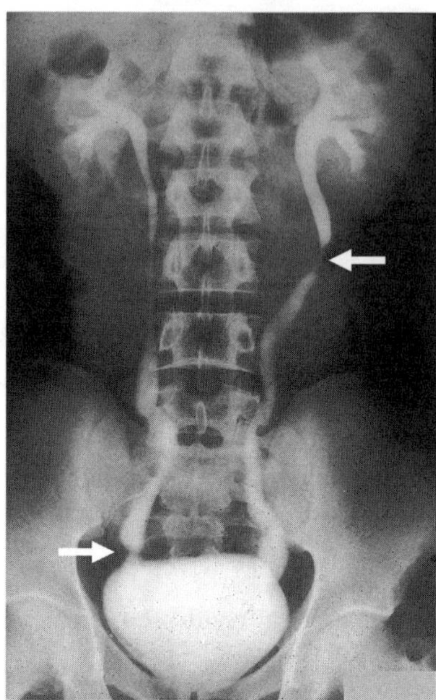

Figure 8.21 Intravenous urography in a patient with documented schistosomiasis. There is adequate renal function but segmental widening of the ureters is noted, due to luminal narrowings (arrows) from schistosomiasis infestation. (Courtesy of associate professor Håkan Jorulf, Uppsala, Sweden)

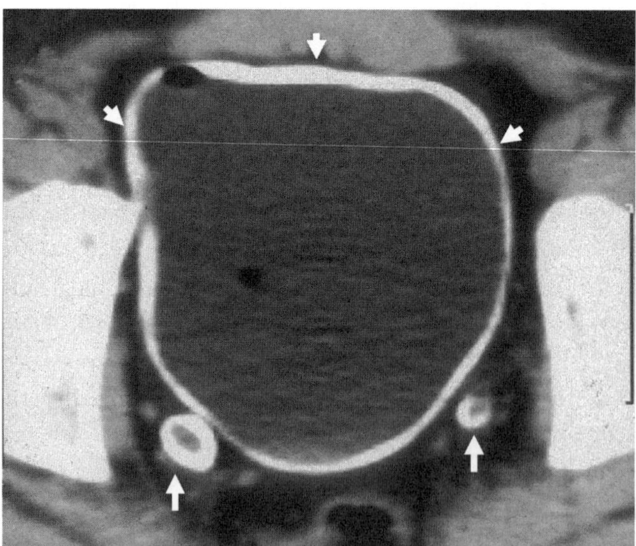

Figure 8.22 25-year old male with diagnosis of schistosomiasis. CT demonstrates circumferential bladder wall calcification (arrowheads), and calcifications of the distal parts of both ureters (arrows), characteristic for schistosomiasis. The bladder had been filled with lipid-containing contrast medium through a bladder catheter. An air bubble (black) is seen in anterior part of the bladder. (Courtesy of associate professor Håkan Jorulf, Uppsala, Sweden)

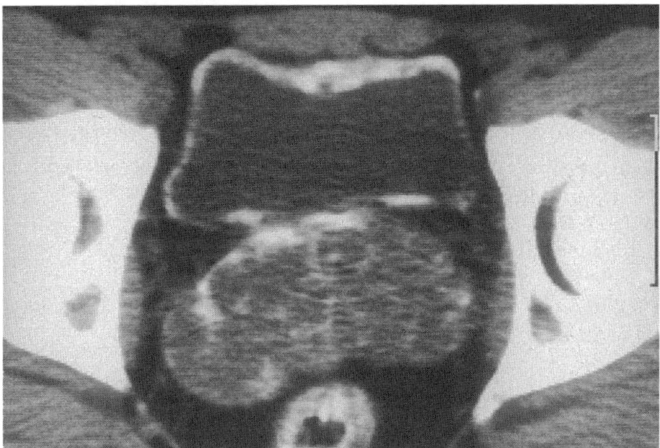

Figure 8.23 32 year old male with schistosomiasis. CT demonstrates extensive calcifications (white) of the urinary bladder wall, prostate, seminal vesicles and the rectum. (Courtesy of associate professor Håkan Jorulf, Uppsala, Sweden)

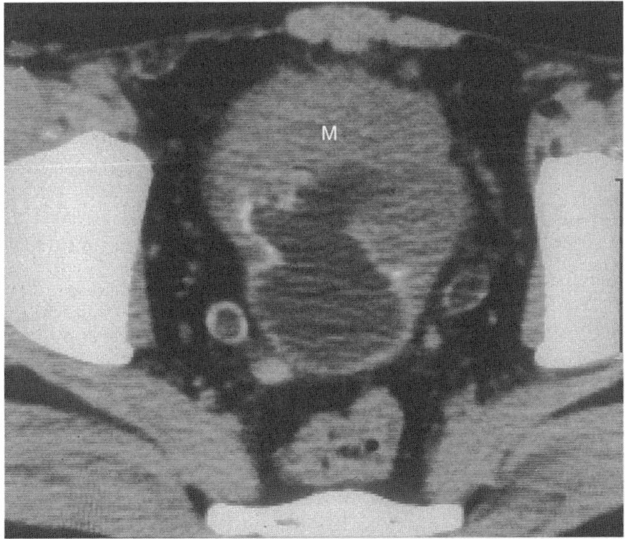

Figure 8.24 41 year old male presenting with hematuria. CT reveals calcifications of the bladder wall and distal ureters, typical of schistosomiasis, which was clinically confirmed. In addition, a large soft tissue mass (M) is noted in the anterior and left lateral parts of the bladder wall. Biopsy confirmed squamous cell carcinoma. (Courtesy of associate professor Håkan Jorulf, Uppsala, Sweden)

- Impaired bladder and ureteral function predisposes to pyelonephritis, urinary obstruction and calculus formation.

- Late in the course, urinary obstruction may lead to reduced renal function.

- Bladder cancer, associated with schistosomiasis, may appear as a soft tissue mass on CT of the bladder (Fig. 8.24).

- Ultrasonography is widely used in endemic areas in control programs for detection, monitoring of disease severity and treatment follow up.

- Ultrasound control programs at community level and in field studies include evaluation of the urinary bladder (wall calcifications, wall thickness, wall irregularities, bladder masses, pseudopolyps and residual urine), ureters (grade of dilatation) and kidneys (grade of hydronephrosis, parenchymal thickness).

- Differential diagnoses include tuberculosis of the urinary tract

  - tuberculosis usually starts in the kidney and progresses to lower urinary tract, while schistosomiasis starts in the bladder and spreads cranially.

  - calcifications are mainly proximal in tuberculosis, while they primarily affect the bladder and distal ureters in schistosomiasis.

Summary

- *Schistosoma haematobium* infection of the urinary tract affects very large numbers of individuals, especially in Africa.

- Hematuria is the dominant symptom, while fibrosis of the bladder and distal ureters leads to hydronephrosis and impaired renal function.

- Calcifications of the bladder wall or distal ureters are almost pathognomonic for schistosomiasis.

- In individual cases, CT is best suited to document disease spread and severity, while ultrasonography is widely used in mass screening and treatment follow-up in endemic areas.

8.8 Hydatid disease (echinococcosis)

Introduction

Hydatid disease (hydatidosis, echinococcosis) is a worldwide zoonosis, i.e. an infectious disease that is transmitted from animals to humans. It is most frequent in sheep- and cattle-raising areas. It is caused by the larval stage of the *Echinococcus* tapeworm. There are two main variants affecting humans. The most common type is *Echinococcus granulosus* that causes unilocular or cystic echinococcosis, while *Echinococcus multilocularis*, which causes multilocular or alveolar echinococcosis, is less frequent and rarely affects the urinary tract. The definite host of *E. granulosus* is usually a dog or other carnivore, harbouring the adult worm in the proximal small bowel. Eggs reach the intestine and are excreted in the feces of the definite host. Animals grazing on contaminated grounds, especially sheep, cattle or pigs, act as intermediate hosts. They ingest the ova, which penetrate the intestinal wall and reach the portal circulation, causing cystic formations primarily in the liver. The cycle may be closed by, e.g. dogs, eating infected meat, containing cyst-containing organs. Humans get infected by ingesting ova-containing water, food or soil, or by contact with dogs or sheep.

Clinical features

- Hydatid disease primarily affects the liver (75% of cases) and lungs (15%) while the kidneys are affected in approximately 3% of cases.

- Hydatid cysts develop slowly, and it may take months or years before symptoms occur.

- Symptoms are mainly related to the pressure exerted by the cysts on neighbouring organs, such as biliary obstruction in case of liver cysts or hydronephrosis in case of renal cysts.

- In most cases, symptoms of hydatid disease in other organs precede urinary tract symptoms, although isolated hydatid disease of the kidneys occasionally occurs.

- Hydatid disease of the kidneys may remain asymptomatic for many years.

- Specific signs of renal hydatid disease include a flank mass, flank pain and dysuria.

- Cyst rupture into the collecting system may lead to acute renal colic, obstruction and passing of hydatid scolices, hooklets or fragments of parasitic membranes.

- Cyst rupture outside the urinary tract may lead to disseminated cysts in the abdominal cavity or retroperitoneum and spread to other organs.

- Eosinophilia is commonly encountered.

- Puncture of a hydatid cyst may lead to leakage and spread of cyst material and life-threatening hypersensitivity reactions – it should therefore be avoided or performed with great caution.

- Diagnosis is established by microscopic examination of cyst content, antibodies in the blood and radiological imaging.

Pathology

- Eggs swallowed by humans hatch in the duodenum and so called oncospheres penetrate the mucosa to reach the mesenteric venules, portal system and lymphatics.

- The oncospheres primarily reach the liver, but may be spread to lungs or any organs.

- At the site where they are trapped, tiny cysts filled with clear fluid develop.

- The cysts grow at a rate of 1–5 cm per year, depending on the type of target organ and the host defence.

- The hydatid cysts consist of three layers:

  o An outer pericyst consisting of host adventitial cells forming a dense fibrous layer

  o An acellular laminated layer (ectocyst)

  o An inner germinal layer (endocyst) responsible for the growth of the cyst.

- Daughter cysts commonly develop within mother cysts and may grow through the wall of the mother cyst.

- Secondary changes in the hydatid cysts include infection, hemorrhage, rupture or necrosis.

- Cysts may perforate and spread to neighbouring organs, abdominal cavity or chest cavity.

Imaging findings (hydatid of the urinary tract)

- Plain radiography and urography may show a flank mass that may be 10 cm or more in size, but is otherwise inconclusive.

- Curvilinear or ring-like calcifications are seen at radiography in 20–30% of cases.

- If renal hydatid cysts have ruptured into the collecting system, ureteral filling defects and obstruction with hydronephrosis may be shown at urography, CT or MRI.

- A hydatid cyst in the earliest stage of development may resemble a simple cyst, i.e. rounded or oval shaped, well defined anechoic lesions with a thin wall.

- At a later stage ultrasonography typically shows a well defined, rounded or oval shaped fluid-containing lesion with low echogenicity and a well defined wall exhibiting the 'double line sign' or 'parallel stripes' (laminated membrane and pericyst).

- Echogenicity may be higher than in simple cysts due to internal echoes from small, dense, mobile echoes from hydatid constituents, often called 'hydatid sand'. At repositioning of the patient, hydatid sand is mobile, creating a 'snow-storm' or 'snow-flake' appearance at ultrasonography.

- Daughter cysts, i.e. smaller cysts within a larger cyst (multiseptated cyst appearance), are characteristic findings at ultrasonography, sometimes arranged in a 'spoke-wheel' or honeycomb pattern.

- In case the parasitic membrane has collapsed and been detached, it may be seen as a floating membrane inside the fluid filled cyst ('water-lily sign').

- If secondary changes such as cyst rupture, infection, hemorrhage or necrosis occur, the diagnosis is less clear, the hydatid cysts may appear as complex masses, even simulating malignancy.

- CT and MRI clearly show the cystic lesions, including wall thickening and daughter cysts, but ultrasonography is more sensitive in detecting septa, membranes and hydatid sand.

- In case of complications or disseminated disease, the full extent of lesions is best shown by CT or MRI.

- WHO has presented an ultrasound classifications system for hydatid disease for clinical and field study settings, grading cystic echinococcosis as CE1–CE5.

Summary

- Hydatid disease of the urinary tract should be suspected when a patient presents with unusual cystic changes, including cysts within larger cysts, laminated cyst walls and sand-like cyst content.

- The characteristics of the cystic changes are best demonstrated by ultrasonography, while the full distribution of cystic changes in perirenal and other tissues is best demonstrated by CT.

8.9 Urethritis

Introduction

Acute infection of the urethra (urethritis) is usually sexually transmitted, and in the acute phase imaging is rarely required. If untreated, acute urethritis in the male, especially gonococcal infection, may lead to long-term complications, typically post-inflammatory strictures. These occasionally require radiological imaging, as a complement to clinical evaluation, urine flow measurement and urethroscopy.

Clinical features

- Acute infectious urethritis causes dysuria and urethral discharge, but can be asymptomatic.

- The infection may spread from the urethra to the prostate, seminal vesicles and epididymis.

- Symptoms of post-inflammatory urethral stricture develop slowly (often years) after the initial infection.

  Symptoms of stricture include gradually increasing dysuria, impaired urinary flow and incomplete urethral emptying.

Pathology

- Primary infectious agent are usually gonococci or chlamydia. Rarely, tuberculosis of the urinary tract is a cause.

- The primary sites of infection are the periurethral glands (Littré's glands), which are most abundant in the bulbar part of the urethra.

- The infection may spread to the adjacent spongious tissue (spongiitis), causing local venous thrombosis, granulation tissue deposition, fibrosis and mucosal hyperplasia, resulting in scarring, urethral narrowing and stricturing.

- Urethral stricture development is slow but progressive and primarily affects the bulbar part of the urethra.

- Post-infectious strictures may be short or several centimetres and tend to be multiple and serial.

Imaging findings

Imaging in acute urethritis

- In the acute phase, there is usually no indication for imaging, unless a foreign body or urethral stone is suspected and transurethral endoscopic examination is insufficient.

- Instrumentation and retrograde injection of radiographic contrast media should be avoided in the acute phase due to the risk of spreading the infection.

- Acute urethritis may develop into an abscess. CT, MRI or ultrasonography may localize periurethral inflammatory tissue swelling and localized collections of thick fluid, similar to abscess formation elsewhere in the body.

Imaging of long-term complications

- The purpose of imaging of urethral *strictures* is to define the number, location, width and length of the strictures (Fig. 8.25).
- Urethrography is an adjunct to urethroscopy for visualization of urethral strictures.
- *Retrograde* urethrography
  - Technique
    - Retrograde injection of water soluble contrast material from the tip of the urethra through a thin Foley catheter with its small balloon placed in the fossa navicularis, which is a local widening of the urethral lumen just inside the urethral opening.
    - Alternatively, an instrument with a cone-shaped rubber tip placed in the distal urethra, held in place by two arms around the penis proximal to the glans, is used.
    - Radiographs of the urethra are obtained during retrograde injection of water-soluble contrast material.
  - Imaging
    - The anterior urethra is well visualized by retrograde urethrography.
    - It may show abnormal filling of Littré's periurethral glands, i.e. small multiple contrast filled cavities in the bulbar part of the urethra.
    - Urethral strictures may be short or several centimetres long, often multiple and serial.
    - Since the external urethral sphincter is not relaxed during retrograde contrast injection, optimal visualization of the urethra proximal to the sphincter is difficult to achieve.

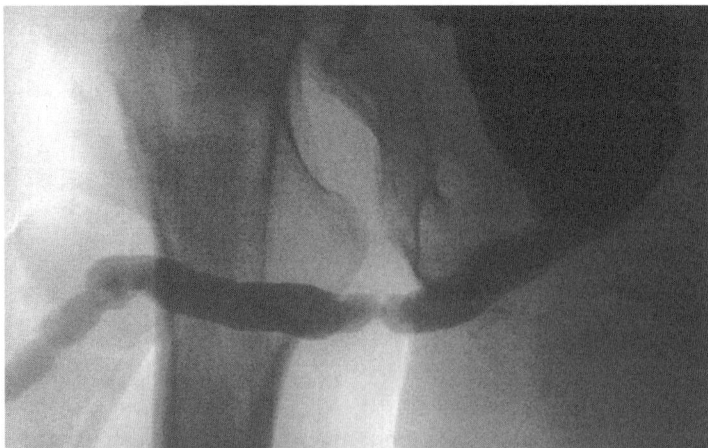

Figure 8.25 Antegrade urethrography (images obtained during voiding) demonstrating multiple short strictures of the urethra. The patient had a history of gonococcal infection.

- *Antegrade* urethrography

  - Technique

    - The bladder may be (slowly) filled by retrograde contrast injection, by urethral bladder catheterization or by a suprapubic bladder catheter.

    - Radiographs of the urethra are obtained during voiding.

  - Imaging

    - The posterior urethra is well visualized by antegrade urethrography, and opening of the external sphincter allows visualization also of the anterior urethra.

    - More proximal strictures, pre-stenotic dilatation and functional obstruction may be evaluated.

    - A combination of retrograde and antegrade contrast filling of the urethra usually allows visualization of the entire urethra.

- *Ultrasonography* is sometimes used to assess the extent and elasticity of urethral strictures. It requires that the urethra is distended by retrograde administration of saline or gel, and it is limited to the anterior urethra.

Summary

- Imaging in *acute* urethritis is limited to assessment of abscesses and foreign bodies.

- *Strictures* tend to develop in the male urethra following acute urethritis.

- Retrograde and antegrade urethrography are used as a complements to urethroscopy for visualization of post-infectious strictures.

References

Hansson S, Jodal U. (2004) Urinary tract infection. In Avner ED, Harmon WE, Niaudit P (eds) *Pediatric Nephrology*, 5th edn. Lippincott Williams & Wilkins, Philadelphia, pp. 1007–1025.

National Institute for Health and Clinical Excellence (NICE) (2007) Guidelines on childhood UTI. C654 www.nice.org.uk/guidance.

Biassoni, L, Chippington S (2008) Imaging in urinary tract infections: current strategies and new trends. *Sem. Nuclear Med.* **38**(1): 56–66.

Piepsz A, Ham H (2006) Pediatric applications of renal nuclear medicine. *Sem. Nuclear Med.* **36**(1): 16–35.

Paterson A (2004) Urinary tract infection: an update on imaging strategies. *Eur. Radiol.* **14** (Suppl 4): L89–100.

Browne RFJ, Zwirewich C, Torreggiani, WC (2004) Imaging of urinary tract infection in the adult. *Eur. Radiol.* **14**: E168–E183.

Stunell H, Buckley O, Feeney J, Geoghegan T, Browne RFJ, Torreggiani WC (2007) Imaging of acute pyelonephritis in the adult. *Eur. Radiol.* **17**: 1820–1828.

Van Der Molen AJ, Cowan NC, Mueller-Lisse UG, Nolte-Ernsting CC, Takahashi S, Cohan RH; CT Urography Working Group of the European Society of Urogenital Radiology (ESUR) (2007) CT urography: definition, indications and techniques. A guideline for clinical practice. *Eur. Radiol.* Nov 1, e-publication ahead of print

Eastwood JB, Corbishely CM, Grange JM (2001) Tuberculosis and the kidney. *J. Am. Nephrol.* **12**: 1307–1314.

www.who.int/tdr/diseases/schisto/diseaseinfo.htm

van der Werf MJ, de Vlas SJ, Brooker S, Looman CWN, Nagelkerke NJD, Habbema JDF, Engels D (2003) Quantification of clinical morbidity associated with schistosome infection in sub-Saharan Africa. *Acta Tropica* **86**: 125–139.

Richter J, Hatz C, Campagne G, Bergquist NR, Jenkins JM (1996) Ultrasound in schistosomiasis. A practical guide to the standardised use of ultrasonography for the assessment of schistosomiasis-related morbidity. Second International Workshop October 22–26, 1996, Niamey, Niger. World Health Organisation, Special programme for research and training in tropical diseases (TDR).

WHO Informal Working Group (2003) International classification of ultrasound images in cystic echinococcosis for application in clinical and field epidemiological settings. *Acta Tropica* **85**: 253–261.

Pavlica P, Barozzi L, Menchi I (2003) Imaging of male urethra. *Eur. Radiol.* **13**: 1583–1596.

Kawashima A, Sandler CM, Wasserman NF, Le Roy AJ, King BF, Goldman AM (2004) Imaging of urethral disease: a pictorial review. *Radiographics* **24**: S195–S216.

9
Imaging of the Genitourinary System – Urolithiasis

Sami A Moussa[1] and Paramananthan Mariappan[2]

[1] *Department of Radiology and Scottish Lithotriptor Centre, Western General Hospital, Edinburgh*
[2] *Department of Urology, Western General Hospital, Edinburgh*

9.1 Introduction

Urolithiasis and complications of stone disease form a large proportion of contemporary urological and uro-radiological workload. As the vast majority of patients require minimally invasive treatment, accurate imaging plays a pivotal role in management and follow-up of these patients.

Recent advances in imaging techniques in particular the widespread use of Multi-Detector CT (MDCT) scanning have changed the established imaging strategy of diagnosis of stone disease.

9.2 Pathology

- *Pathogenesis*

  - The formation of stones in the urinary tract is a complex process.
  - It begins with the formation of a crystal which grows and then gets retained within the urinary tract (Fig. 9.1).
  - Urinary pH dependent supersaturation of salts within the urine is thought to precede and result in crystal nucleus formation.
  - Urine also contains naturally occurring modifiers of crystal formation, i.e. promoters and inhibitors of crystal formation.

Urogenital Imaging: A Problem-oriented Approach   Edited by Sameh K. Morcos and Henrik S. Thomsen
© 2009 John Wiley & Sons, Ltd

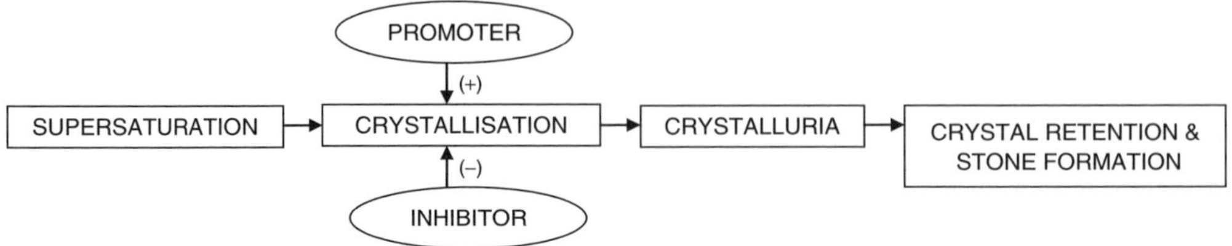

Figure 9.1   Pathogenesis of urinary stone formation.

o Inhibitors which suppress the rate of crystal formation include citrate, magnesium, pyrophosphate and glycosaminoglycans.

o Promoters stimulate crystal growth include matrix substance A and uromucoid.

o Growing crystals passing through renal tubules may get trapped within the tubules simply by becoming 'jammed' (free-particle theory) or become adherent to the epithelial lining of the tubules (fixed-particle theory) – either of these mechanisms result in crystal retention and subsequent stone formation (Fig. 9.1).

- *Types and causes of urinary stones (Table 9.1)*

  o Calcium oxalate stones. These can occur as a result of:

    ▪ Hypercalciuria – this is idiopathic in the majority of patients.

    ▪ Hypocitraturia – citrate is an inhibitor of calcium salt formation by forming a soluble complex with calcium.

    ▪ Hyperuricosuria – In conditions of hyperuricosuria (high dietary purine intake or chronic diarrheal diseases), uric acid crystals may act as a nidus for the nucleation of calcium oxalate crystals.

    ▪ Hyperoxaluria – oxalate forms an insoluble complex with calcium resulting in crystal formation and is often a result of increased dietary intake of oxalate.

  o Uric acid stones – urinary uric acid exists in an insoluble form at acidic pH < 5.5 and forms crystals. Uric acid crystals also occur when the concentration of uric acid is high or when the urine volume is low.

  o Struvite/triple phosphate/infection stones

    ▪ Composed of calcium-magnesium-ammonium-phosphate

Table 9.1   Types of urinary stones

Stone type	Proportion of all stones all stones	Radiology (typical appearance)
Calcium oxalate	75–80%	Radio-opaque
Uric acid	4–15%	Radiolucent
Struvite/triple phosphate	4–12%	Radio-opaque
Calcium phosphate	1–3%	Radio-opaque
Cystine		Radio-opaque
Xanthine		Radiolucent

- Caused by urease-producing organisms (e.g. *Proteus mirabilis*) which breakdown urea to ammonia and result in alkaline pH.
- o Calcium phosphate stones
  - Occurs at pH > 7.5
  - Associated with renal tubular acidosis (RTA) and hyperparathyroidism.
- o Cystine stones
  - Autosomal recessive disorder resulting in impaired renal tubular reabsorption of cystine.
- o Congenital and anatomical abnormalities resulting in stone disease
  - PUJ obstruction
  - Medullary sponge kidney
  - Horseshoe kidney
  - Urinary diversion
  - Bladder outflow obstruction.
- o Drugs causing stones
  - Calcium and vitamin D
  - Acetazolamide
  - Indinavir (protease inhibitor of HIV)

9.3 Clinical features

Symptoms are related to the location of the stone whether in the kidney, ureter or bladder and also on the presence of complications. Patients with stone disease may present with:

1. *Pain*

   - o Renal colic typically radiates from the loin to groin and is often associated with nausea, vomiting and sweating.

2. *Hematuria*

   - o Often microscopic and detected on urine dipstick analysis.

3. *Dysuria, urinary frequency and urgency* may occur when the stone has moved into the bladder or vesico-ureteric junction.

4. *Urinary tract infection (UTI)*

   - o Patients may have a history of recurrent UTI. Infective complications such as pyonephrosis or perinephric abscess are often a result of obstructive uropathy.

5. *Acute renal failure (ARF)*

   - o ARF can occur when a patient with a single kidney develops an acute ureteric obstruction from a stone or rarely, when there are bilateral ureteric calculi causing obstruction.

6. *Chronic renal impairment (CRF)*

   o May follow long-standing obstruction or bilateral large (staghorn) renal calculi.

7. *Incidental finding* of stones on imaging of adjacent viscera.

9.4 Evaluation of patients with suspected urinary stones

- A complete medical history and physical examination must be carried out and vital signs recorded.

- Differential diagnoses of acute renal colic include urinary tract infection (UTI), acute appendicitis, ectopic pregnancy and diverticular disease.

- Urinalysis.

- Urine culture and sensitivity.

- Full blood count.

- Renal biochemistry.

- Imaging.

9.5 Treatment

A. *Treatment of symptoms and complications*

   o NSAIDs for pain relief

   o Treat infection and drain infected system with nephrostomy

   o Decompress with stents or nephrostomy in presence of persistent ureteric obstruction

B. *Specific treatment of stones (aiming for complete stone clearance) depends on symptoms, location and size of the stone.*

   o *Symptomatic renal stones*

   - Stone <2 cm with normal renal anatomy

     • Extracorporeal Shock Wave Lithotripsy (ESWL)

   - Stone <2 cm with abnormal renal anatomy or located within lower pole calyx with long, narrow infundibulum with acute infundibulo-pelvic angle

     • Percutaneous Nephrolithotomy (PCNL)

   - Stone <2 cm after failed ESWL

     • PCNL

   - Stone >2 cm or staghorn stone

     • PCNL

   - Cystine stones

     • PCNL

- *Asymptotic renal stones*
  - Small asymptomatic stones do not require treatment unless movement of this stone could potentially result in serious consequences, e.g. in an airline pilot.
- *Ureteric stones*
  - Stone ≤ 4 mm
    - Conservative management. Stones ≤ 4 mm will pass spontaneously in 80% of patients.
  - Proximal ureteric stone <1 cm
    - ESWL
  - Proximal ureteric stone >1 cm
    - Ureterorenoscopy (URS) and laser fragmentation
  - Distal ureteric stone <1 cm
    - URS and laser or ESWL
  - Distal ureteric stone >1 cm
    - URS and laser fragmentation
- *Bladder stones*
  - Cystolitholapaxy

C. *Reduce the risk of recurrence:*
- Fluid intake >2000 ml/day
- Reduce oxalate rich food (tea/spinach/rhubarb/ nuts)
- Reduce urate rich food (liver/calf thymus/anchovies/ herring)
- Increase fibre in diet

9.6 Imaging

- CT scanning has become the main diagnostic modality in detecting renal and ureteric calculi in the acute and elective set-up.

- Ultrasound, the plain radiograph of the abdomen (KUB), intravenous urography (IVU) and other contrast studies of the urinary tract continue to have important role in the decision making process for the treatment, follow-up and management of urinary stones.

- Imaging should provide the following information:
  - Stone size
  - Stone site
  - Calyceal anatomy
  - Evidence of obstruction
  - Functional information
  - Stone density

The role of different imaging techniques in the evaluation of urinary stones (Table 9.2)

- *The plain radiograph of the abdomen (KUB)*

  o The majority (85%) of urinary stones are radio-opaque and can be visible on the KUB (Figs 9.2 to 9.8).

  o KUB has a low sensitivity varying between 45–60% in detection of urinary stones.

  o Factors affecting the KUB sensitivity:

    - Patient size/body habitus.

    - Stone density

    - Renal parenchymal calcification

Table 9.2   Imaging modalities that can be used in the diagnosis and management of urinary stones

Modality	Advantages	Disadvantages
Plain films KUB	Widely available Vital for choice of management Accurate assessment of stone size Accurate assessment of fragmentation Follow-up	Low sensitivity, radiolucent stones not seen Technical factors affect diagnostic value often requiring tomography Calyceal anatomy not assessed *Radiation*
Intravenous urography IVU	Widely available Excellent demonstration of calyceal anatomy	Low accuracy compared with CT Use of IV contrast *Radiation*
Ultrasound	Widely available Low cost Most stone visualized Identify hydronephrosis Identify ureteric jets Image guidance for renal puncture Useful for follow-up	Low sensitivity Small stones difficult to identify Inaccurate stone configuration Poor assessment of fragmentation after ESWL Inaccurate localization of stones Inability to visualize pelvicalyceal anatomy
Computed tomography CT including CTU	Highly accurate All stone visualized Assess obstruction Assess calyceal anatomy Plan renal access	High radiation Relatively limited availability Often requires other modalities for management and follow-up
Magnetic resonance MRI	No radiation and often no IV contrast Useful in specific situations	Relatively limited availability Stone seen as signal void, small stones missed

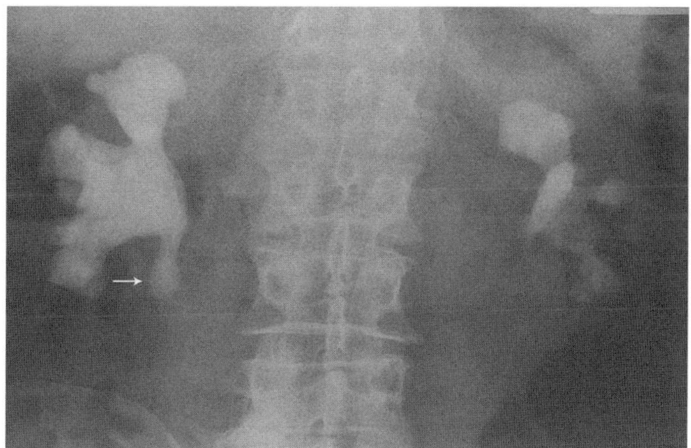

Figure 9.2 Bilateral Staghorn calculi. Arrow shows extension of calculus into right upper ureter.

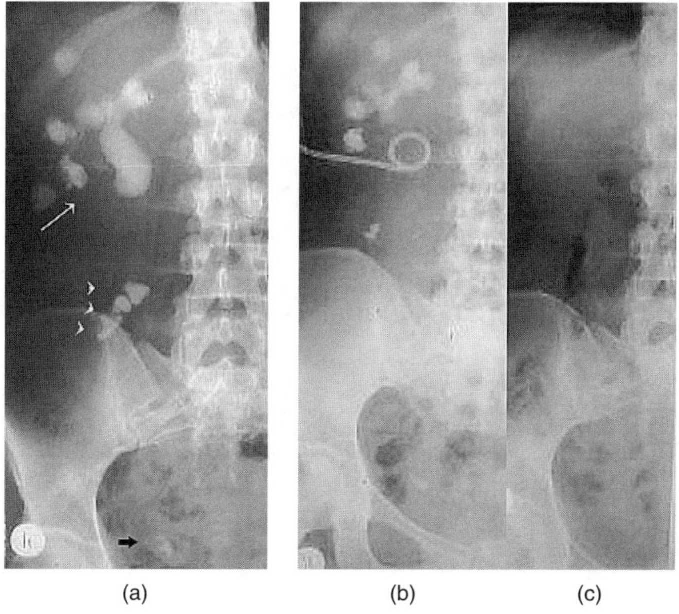

(a)   (b)   (c)

Figure 9.3 Complex stones: (a) Multiple stones in the right renal pelvis and calyces (white arrow), multiple stones in mid-ureter (white arrow heads) and stones at right vesico-ureteric junction (black arrow). (b) Partial clearance after initial ureteroscopy and PCNL. (c) Stone free after further sessions of PCNL and ESWL.

- Overlying bowel gas

- Constipation

- Extrarenal calcifications such as gallstones, costal cartilage calcification, calcified lymph nodes, vascular calcifications and phleboliths

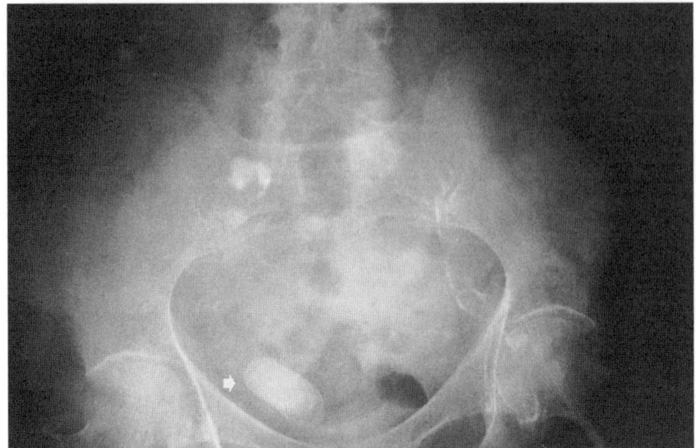

Figure 9.4   Laminated bladder calculus (arrow).

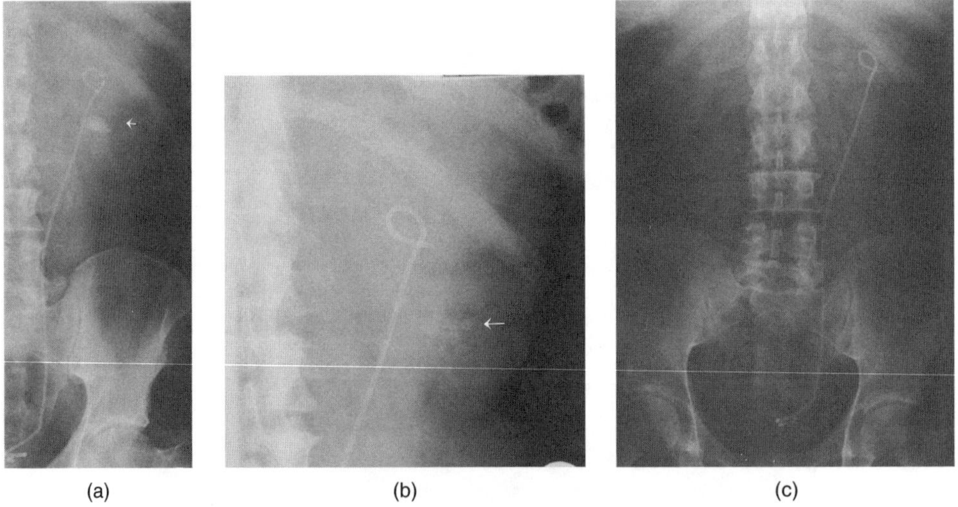

(a)   (b)   (c)

Figure 9.5   Calculus in left renal pelvis with JJ stent *in situ*, (a) Before ESWL (arrow) (b) After two sessions of ESWL the stone is fragmented (arrow) (c) Stone free 2 weeks after last session of ESWL.

- ○ KUB is helpful in:
    - ■ The initial management and choice of treatment modality particularly in planning fluoroscopically guided ESWL.
    - ■ Accurate assessment of stone size and configuration.
    - ■ Assess fragmentation after ESWL (Fig. 9.5).
    - ■ Follow-up after ESWL and PCNL to detect residual calculi and monitor the progress of stone fragments (Figs 9.3, 9.5 and 9.6).
    - ■ Long-term surveillance of patients with known small stones managed conservatively and known stone formers.

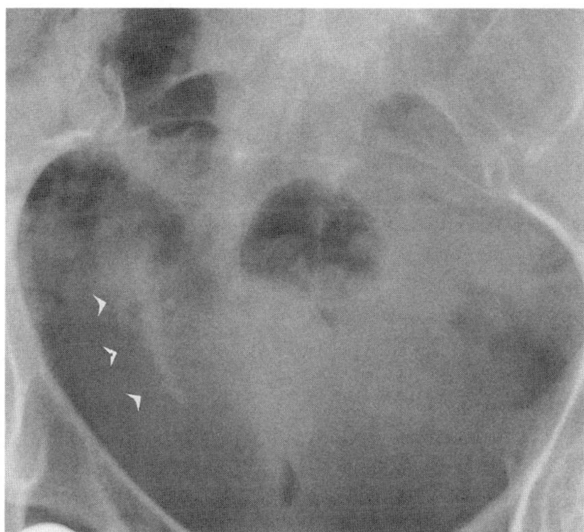

Figure 9.6 Steinstrasse. A row of multiple small stones (arrowheads) is seen in lower right ureter following ESWL for a right renal calculus.

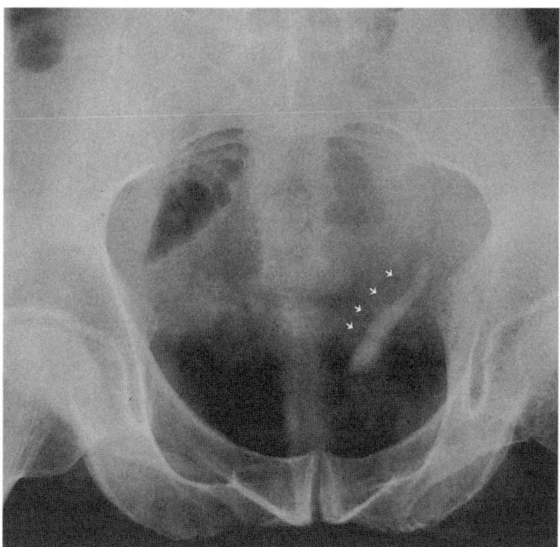

Figure 9.7 A left lower ureteric calculus forming cast of the lower segment of the ureter (small arrows).

- *Intravenous Urography (IVU)*

  - Accurately demonstrates the anatomical details of the calyces, renal pelvis and ureters. It also provides some functional information of the kidneys (Fig. 9.9).
  - Widely available and easy to perform.
  - Relatively safe (low radiation dose of approximately 1.5 mSv).
  - Accurate localization of stones within the collecting system.

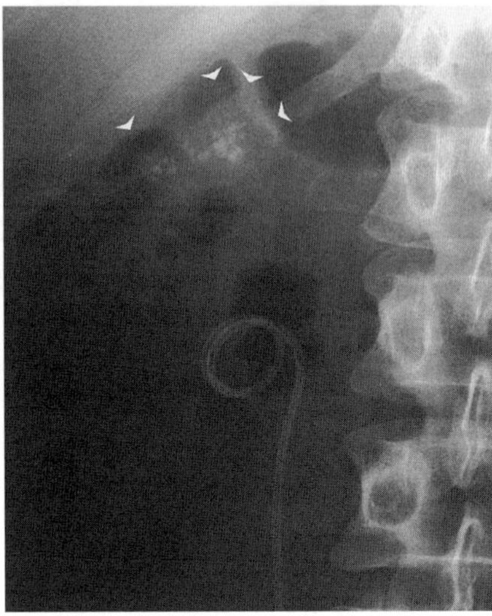

Figure 9.8 Medullary sponge kidney (MSK). Typical clusters of calcifications (arrowheads) in the upper calyceal papillae are shown.

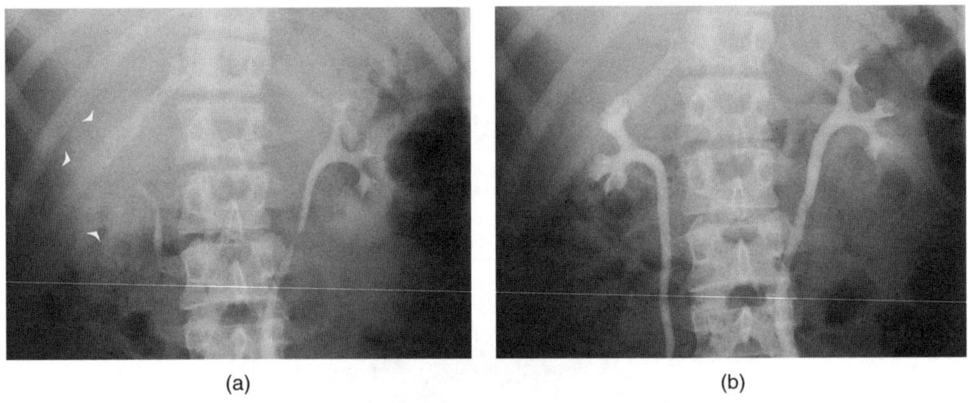

(a)   (b)

Figure 9.9 Intravenous urogram (IVU). (a) 5 min after contrast show poor filling of right pelvicalyceal system (white arrowheads). (b) Film at 15 min with compression showing good filling and distension of both upper tracts.

- o Accurate demonstration of obstruction including the demonstration of the level of obstruction (Fig. 9.10).
- o Accurate demonstration of congenital anomalies such as calyceal diverticula, duplication of collecting system, horseshoe kidneys and ectopias (Figs 9.11 to 9.13).
- o Pre planning of puncture site for PCNL.
- o The IVU limitations:
  - Low diagnostic accuracy compared with CT
  - Use of IV contrast media
  - Same technical limitation as KUB.

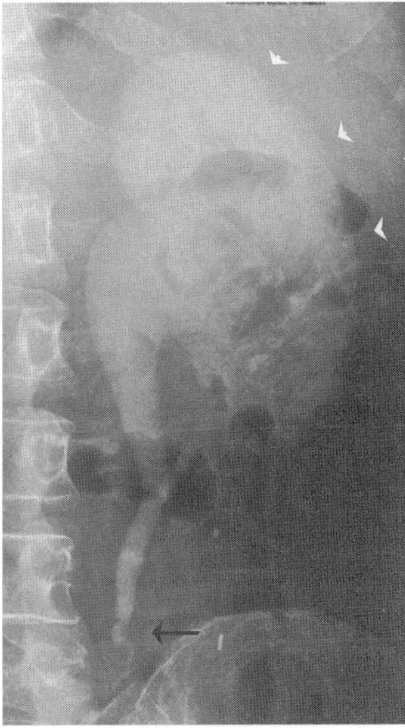

Figure 9.10 Late film from IVU series showing calculus (black arrow) obstruction of left mid-ureter, dilated proximal ureter and collecting system and a persistent nephrogram (white arrowheads).

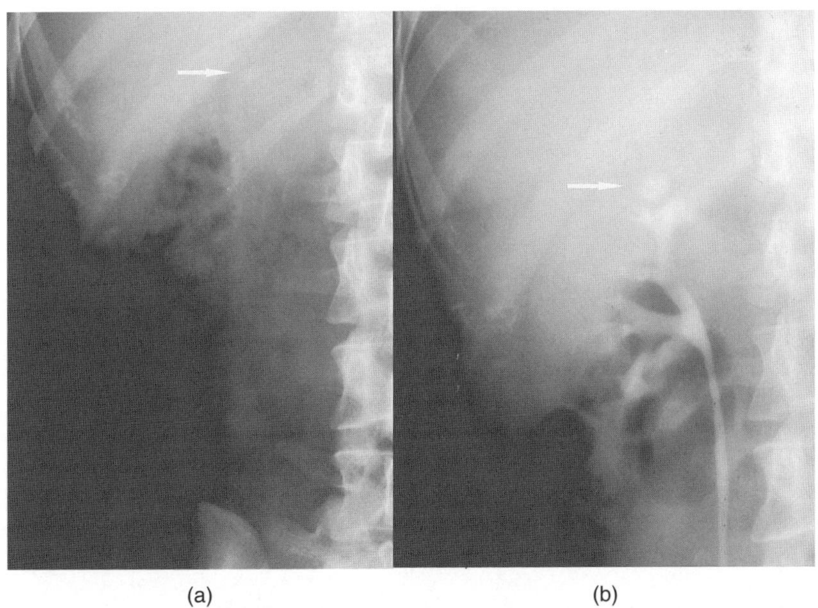

(a)   (b)

Figure 9.11 Calculi in a calyceal diverticulum. (a) Control film with small cluster of calcification in upper pole of right kidney. (b) 15 min film with compression showing calyceal diverticulum filled with contrast and containing the calculi.

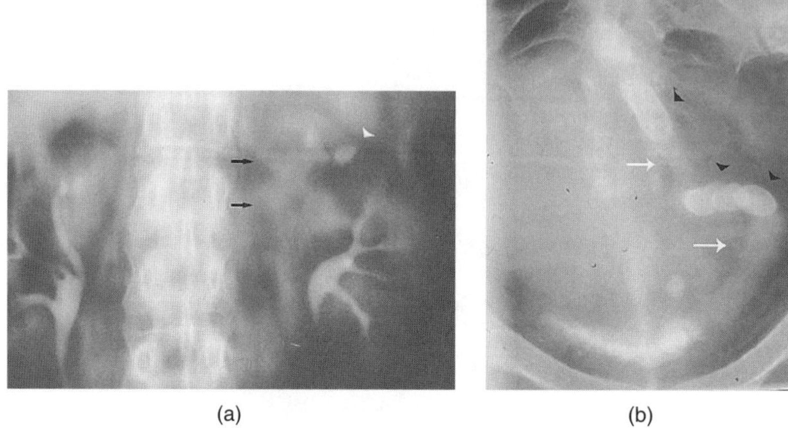

(a)   (b)

Figure 9.12 Left duplex collecting system with ureteric calculi. (a) Poorly functioning hydronephrotic upper moiety (black arrows) and stones (white arrowheads) are shown. (b) Late post-micturition film showing multiple large stones (black arrowheads) in the distended ectopic ureter (white arrows). The ectopic ureter communicated with the vaginal vault.

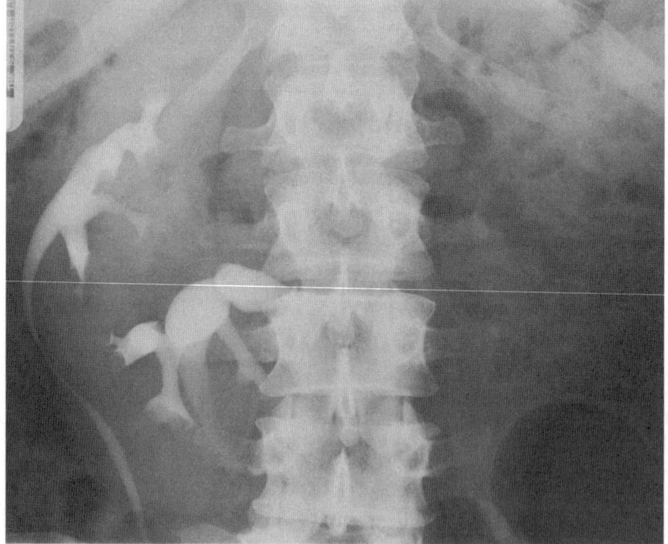

Figure 9.13 Crossed fused renal ectopia.

- *Ultrasound*

  - The sensitivity in detection of urinary stones is low ranging from 37–64%.
  - Ureteric stones are difficult to detect except in a dilated upper ureter or in the intramural segment of the distal ureter at the vesico-ureteric junction (VUJ).
  - Typically stone are recognized as echogenic foci usually casting acoustic shadows (Figs 9.14 to 9.17).

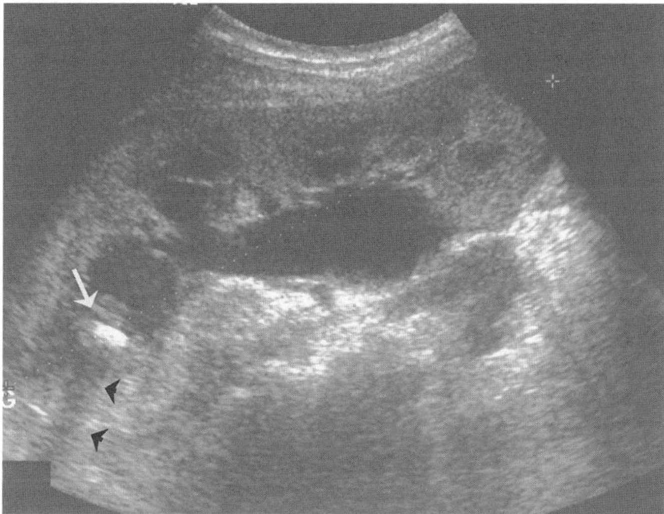

Figure 9.14 Renal ultrasound. Typical appearances of a calculus, echogenic focus (white arrow) and acoustic shadow(black arrowheads) is shown. The collecting system is also dilated (hydronephrosis).

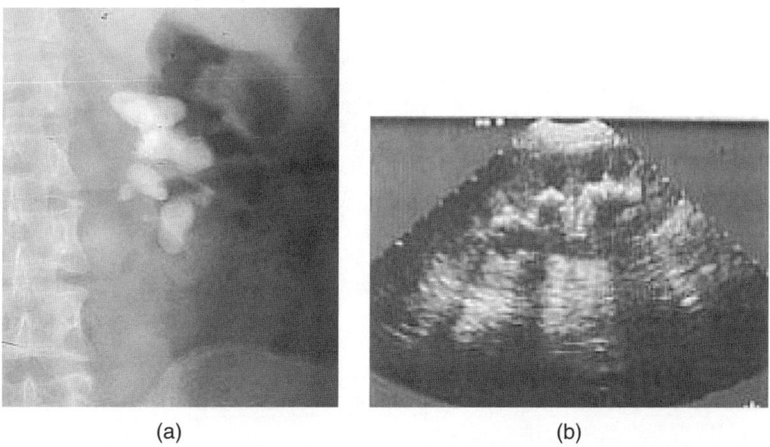

(a) (b)

Figure 9.15 Staghorn calculus. (a) Plain film, (b) Ultrasound appearances of multiple calculi.

- Small renal calculi are difficult to identify or differentiate from other echogenic foci within the kidney.
- Exact stone localization within the collecting system is difficult.
- Large stag horn calculi appear as multiple calculi (Fig. 9.15)
- Stone size measurement is not accurate.
- Advantages of ultrasound:
  - Easy to perform, low cost and widely available.
  - Easily identify hydronephrosis and perinephric fluid collection.

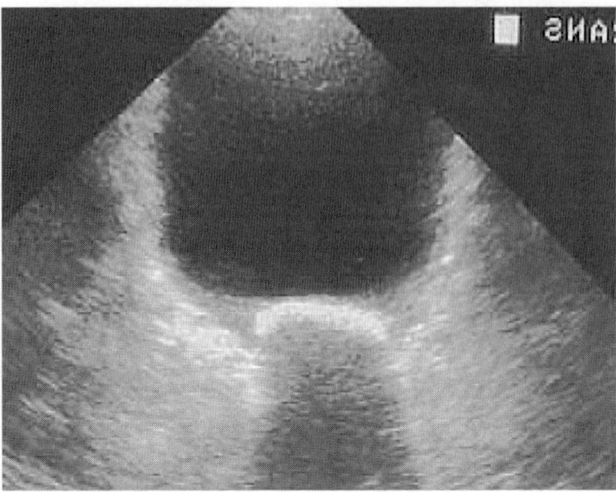

Figure 9.16   Ultrasound: bladder calculus.

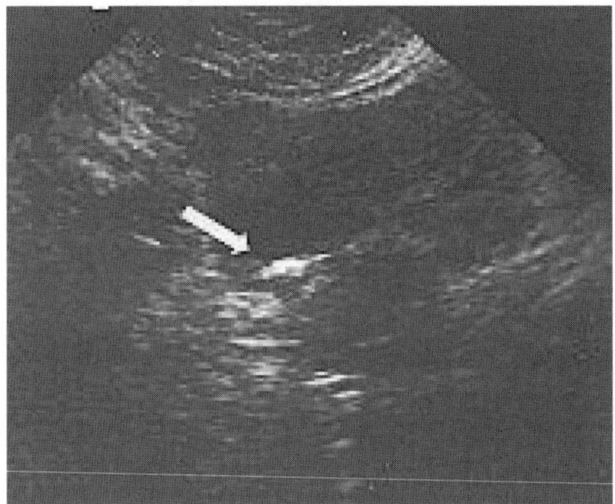

Figure 9.17   Calculus at right vesico-ureteric junction (white arrow).

- Identify ureteric jets in the urinary bladder which exclude ureteric obstruction.
- Image guidance for renal puncture, to relieve obstruction but often less useful for PCNL.
- Useful follow-up tool.

- *Unenhanced CT*

  - Non-contrast helical CT scanning (NCHCT) is now the gold standard in diagnosing renal tract calculi.
  - It does not require any preparation of the patient.
  - Not time-consuming.
  - May detect other causes of abdominal pain such as:
    - Appendicitis
    - Diverticulitis

- Gall stones
- Intra-abdominal/retroperitoneal collections.
- Over 99% of stones are visualized (Figs 9.18 to 9.25) with the exception of:
  - Indinavir stones (Indinavir crystals are iso-dense on CT)
  - Pure matrix stones (matrix stones have a pasty or gelatinous consistency and often contain little or no calcium giving the appearance of soft density in the collecting system making them difficult to visualize).
- Features of obstruction in acute renal colic (Fig. 9.18)
  - Dilated collecting system (hydronephrosis)
  - Dilated ureter
  - Enlarged kidney (nephromegaly)
  - Perinephric and periureteric stranding.
- In complex stones it can offer 3D reconstruction to plan renal access
- CT guided renal puncture in complex renal anatomy and ectopic kidneys
- Difficulties may be caused by
  - Phlebolith
  - Arterial calcification
  - Calcified lymph nodes
  - Renal parenchymal calcification.
- Main disadvantage is high radiation dose.

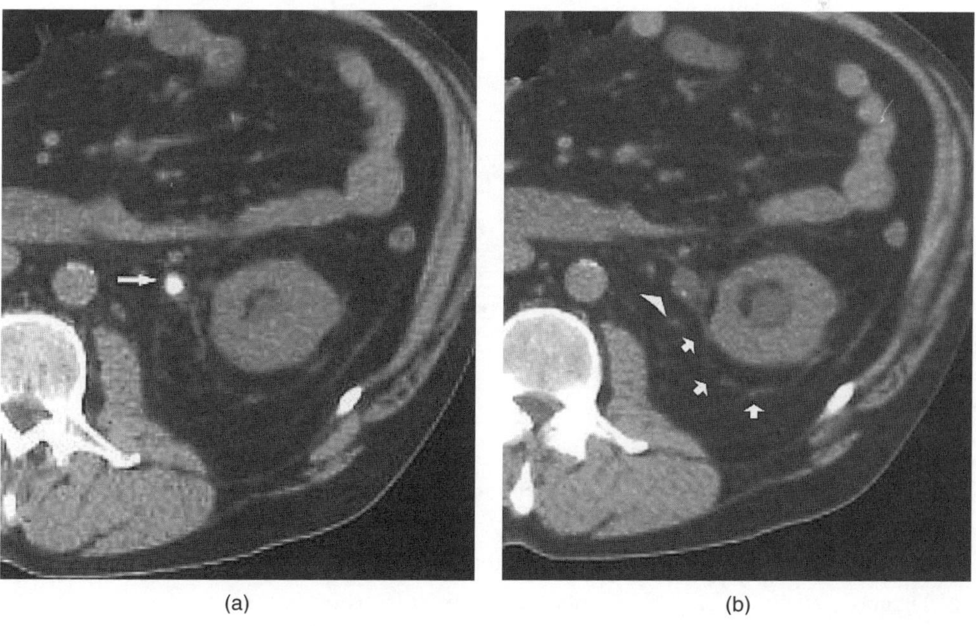

(a)   (b)

Figure 9.18 Non-contrast helical CT (NCHCT). (a) Left ureteric calculus (arrow) with typical rim sign, (b) dilated proximal ureter (arrowhead) and collecting system as well as perinepheric stranding (small arrows).

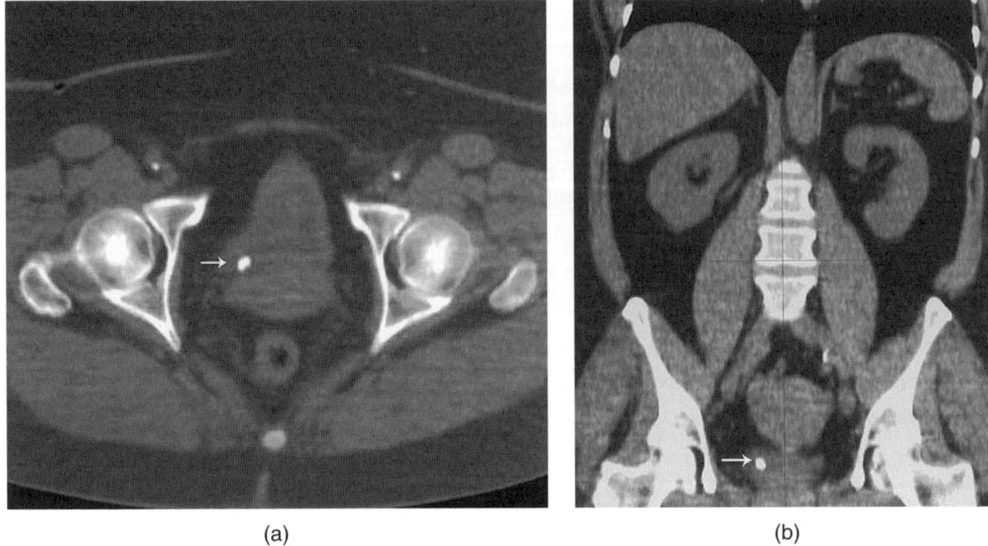

(a)   (b)

Figure 9.19   NCHCT, stone at right vesico-ureteric junction, (a) axial and (b) coronal reconstruction.

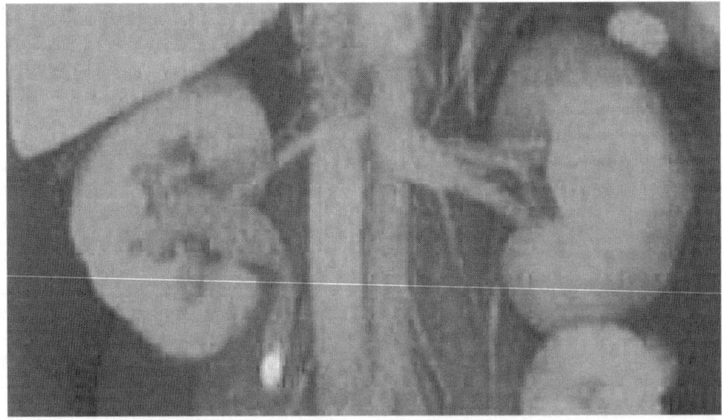

Figure 9.20   NCHCT, volume rendering; a stone in the right upper ureter with proximal hydronephrosis.

- *CT urography (CTU)*

  o Superior replacement of the IVU.

  o Visualize calyceal anatomy particularly associated with renal anomalies such as horseshoe kidneys, renal fusion and ectopic pelvic kidneys (Fig. 9.26).

  o Confirm the position of a stone within the collecting system.

  o Diagnose stones in calyceal or bladder diverticulae (Fig. 9.27).

  o Assist with planning renal access for percutaneous nephrolithotomy (PCNL) especially when combined with 3D reconstructions (Fig. 9.25).

  o Main disadvantage is high radiation dose.

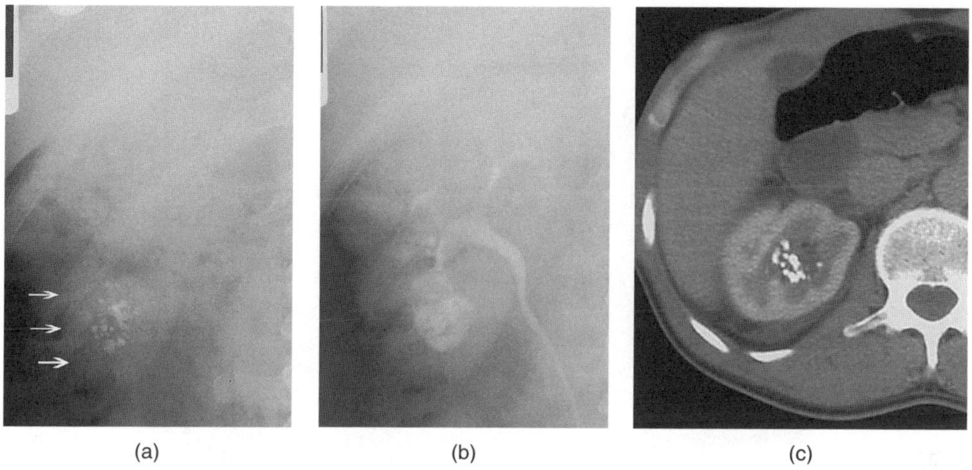

Figure 9.21 Medullary sponge kidney; (a) typical calcification on plain radiography, (b) appearances of duct ectasia in intravenous urogram, (c) characteristic appearances on CT.

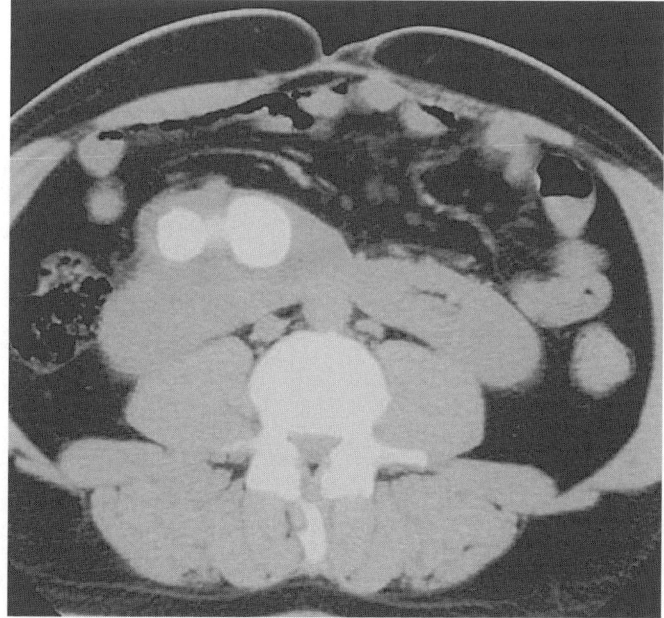

Figure 9.22 Horseshoe kidney with large stones in the right side.

- *Assessment of stone density*
  - Since the advent of ESWL attempts have been made to use stone density on plain radiographs and later CT (Hounsfield units) to predict stone composition or stone fragility.
  - Recent research suggests that the Hounsfield numbers are not reliable but more important is the internal structure of some stones.

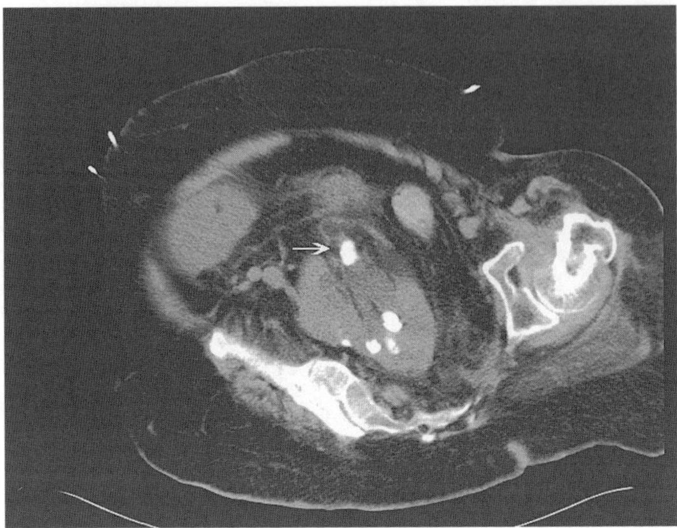

Figure 9.23   Multiple stones are present in a pelvic kidney of a spina bifida patient with severe spinal deformity. Stone obstructing the pelvi-ureteric junction is shown (arrow).

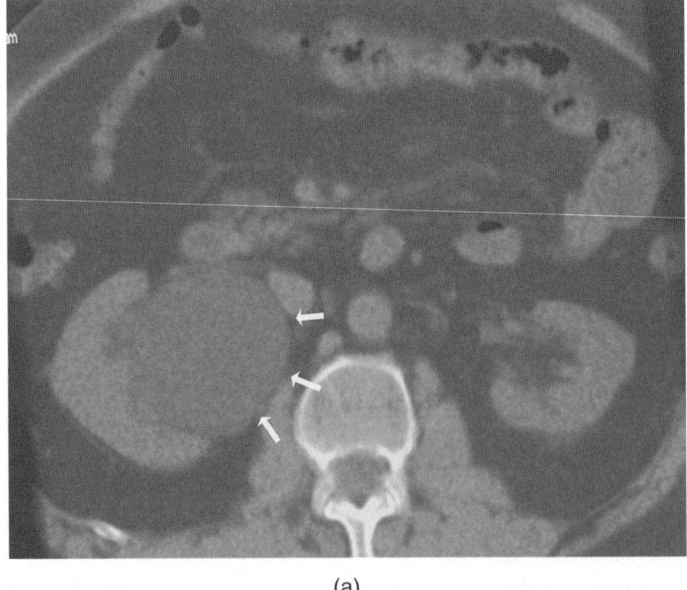

(a)

Figure 9.24   A large para-pelvic cyst minimicking hydronephrosis was seen on NCHCT (a) axial image (arrows), (b) coronal reconstruction: calculus in lower calyx (black arrow), (c) Intravenous urogram demonstrated displacement of the collecting system around the cyst and a calculus in the lower pole calyces (arrow).

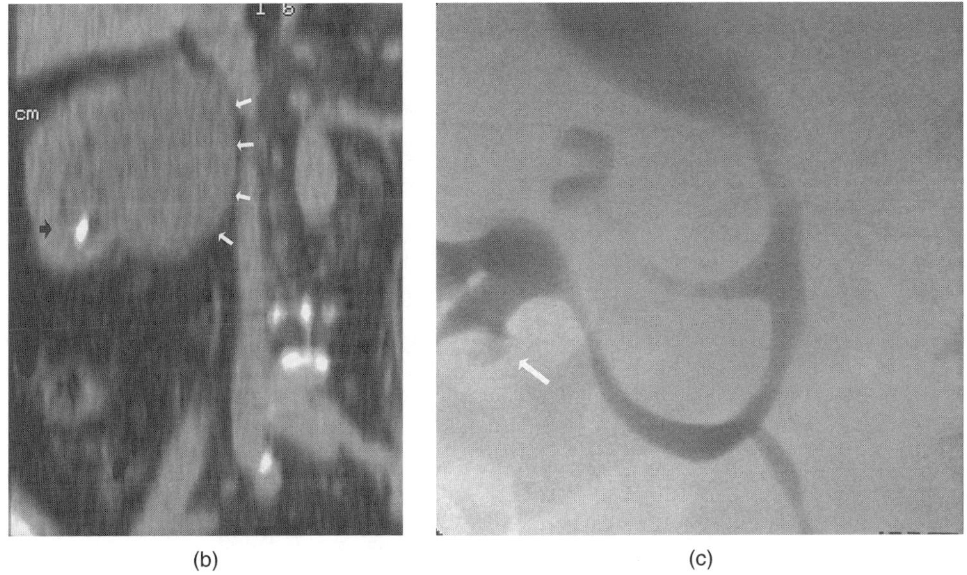

(b)   (c)

Figure 9.24 *(Continued)*

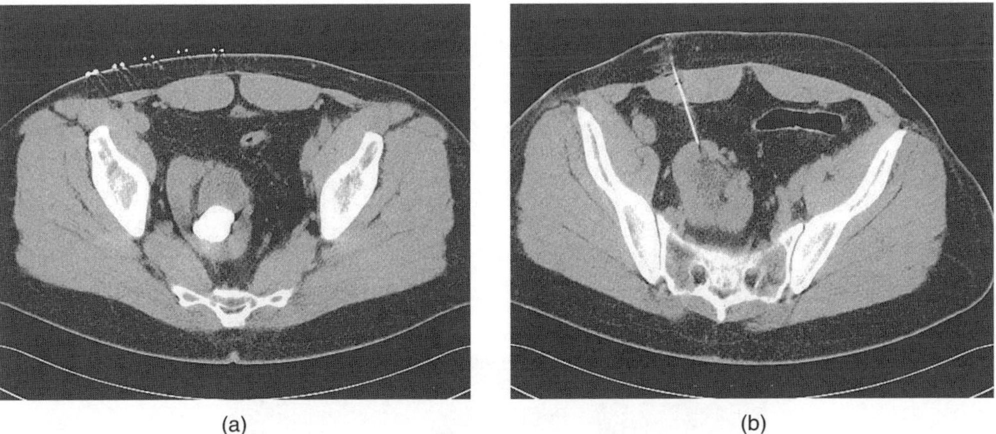

(a)   (b)

Figure 9.25 CT-guided puncture. (a) pelvic kidney containing large calculus, marker on skin anteriorly to plan puncture, (b) needle *in situ* entering upper pole calyx.

- **Radiation dose**
  - There has been growing concern regarding the radiation dose associated with CT examinations in general and in the diagnosis and management of stone disease in particular.
  - Scans are carried out on younger patients including children for a benign condition.
  - A 3 film IVU gives an average dose of 1.5 mSv, this can increase significantly with the use of tomography and larger number of films.
  - Early experience with NCHCT resulted in a dose of approx 4.5 mSv.

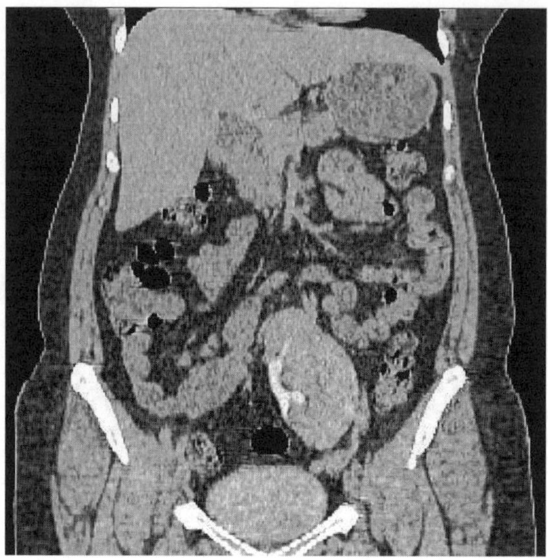

Figure 9.26 A coronal image of a CT urography showing a pelvic left kidney (courtesy of Professor SK Morcos, Sheffield, UK).

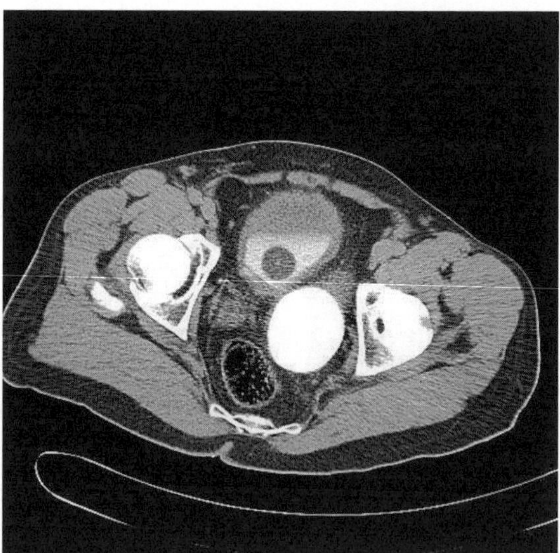

Figure 9.27 An axial image of CT urography demonstrating a calculus filling a large bladder diverticulum. The balloon of a folly's catheter is seen within the urinary bladder (courtesy of Professor SK Morcos, Sheffield, UK).

- o Low dose protocols (reducing mA from 220 to 100) have been shown to be diagnostically effective with a lower radiation dose.

- o Reducing the number of phases studied can reduce the high radiations dose associated with CT urography.

○ Factor affecting radiation dose:

- kV

- mA

- Pitch

- Patient build

- **Magnetic Resonance Imaging (MRI)**

  ○ **T2 MR urography (T2 MRU)** should be considered in:

    - Patients with poor renal function.

    - Imaging grossly dilated collecting system (Fig. 9.28).

    - Contraindication to contrast administration or use of ionizing radiation.

  ○ Technique

    - Stationary fluid in this technique produces high signals which are used to image the urinary tract.

  ○ Advantages:

    - Non-invasive

    - No ionizing radiation

    - No contrast media administration is required

    - Excellent display of the upper urinary tract in multiple plans including 3D images

    - Stones are recognized as areas of signal void (Fig. 9.28)

    - High accuracy in demonstrating secondary features of acute ureteric obstruction:

      • Perirenal fluid

      • Ureteric dilatation.

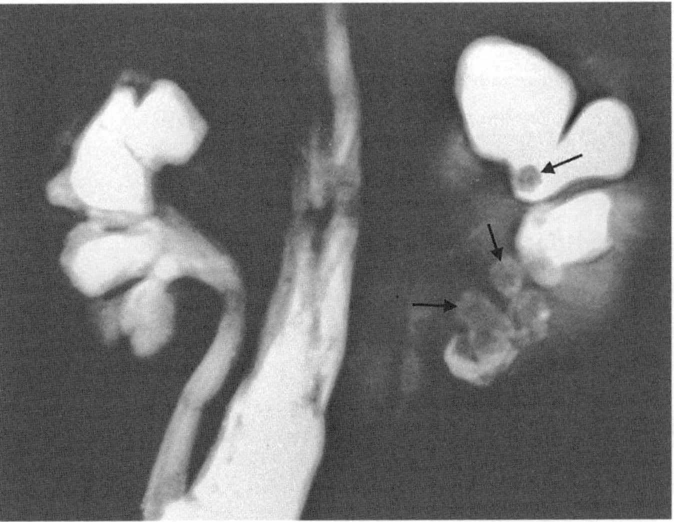

Figure 9.28 A coronal image of T2 MRU demonstrating bilateral hydronephrosis with multiple stones (arrows) in the left kidney (courtesy of Professor SK Morcos, Sheffield, UK).

- Disadvantages:
  - No functional information
  - Mucosal lesions, blood clots, debris can mimic calculi
  - Flow artefacts and tips of renal papillae can be confused with stones
  - Small stones may not be detected
  - Can not be used in presence of contraindications to MRI.
- *Excretory MRU*
- Evaluation of non dilated urinary tract when there is contraindication to administration of iodinated contrast media or use of ionizing radiation and absence of marked reduction of renal function (sr creatinine ≤ 170 micromol/l (1.9 mg/dL)).
- Technique
  - T1-weighted imaging
  - IV injection of gadolinium based contrast agent (0.1 mmol/kg)
  - IV injection of frusemide (10 mg) which is important for:
    - Dilution of the contrast medium avoiding T2 effect.
    - Uniform distribution of contrast.
    - Distension of collecting system.
- Advantages
  - Good visualization of the urinary tract particularly in absence of dilatation
  - Stones are recognized as areas of signal void.
  - Higher accuracy in detecting ureteral calculi in comparison to T2-MRU
  - Provides functional information.
- Disadvantages
  - Requires injection of contrast
  - Mucosal lesions, blood clots, debris can mimic calculi.
  - Cannot be used in presence of contraindications to MRI.

Summary

- MRU is accurate and suitable alternative to CT in selected patients
- The accuracy of MRU combined with KUB is comparable to CT
- Demonstration of small stones (≤ 5 mm) is higher with CT

Other contrast studies

- *Nephrostogram*
- *Loopogram*
- *Retrograde pyelography*

These additional studies are used as complementary techniques either in the initial assessment of renal and ureteric calculi or during follow-up after PCNL or ureteroscopy to demonstrate the presence of residual stone fragments in the kidneys or ureters.

Percutaneous renal access

- Intra-operative imaging is essential for patients undergoing percutaneous nephrolithotomy (PCNL).

- Imaging guides the renal puncture as well as confirms adequate clearance of stones.

- Fluoroscopy usually after contrast administration through a retrograde catheter (Fig. 9.29) remains the mainstay imaging modality, although ultrasound can often be used in the initial puncture.

- In complex cases access is achieved initially under CT guidance (Fig. 9.25).

Nuclear medicine

- In selected cases functional information is important to decide if a patient should undergo procedures to remove the stones.

- In cases of congenital ureteropelvic junction (UPJ) obstruction, istope functional information is important to plan surgical management whether to perform pyeloplasty or endopyelotomy to improve the drainage of the kidney or offering the patient nephrectomy when renal function is severely impaired.

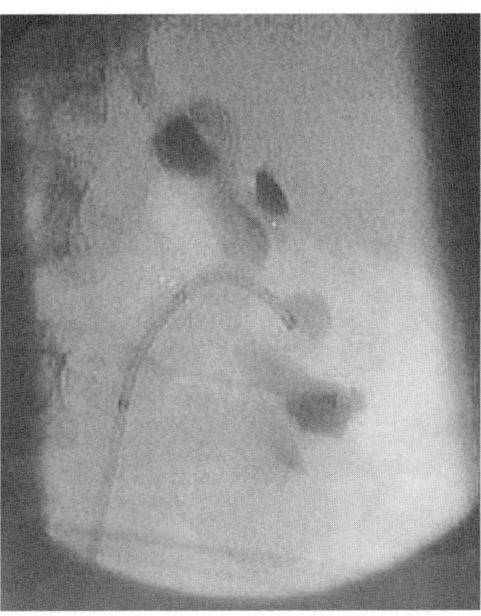

Figure 9.29 Retrograde pyelography combined with flexible ureteroscopy. Tip of ureteroscope is shown in left middle calyx.

Imaging strategies

Renal colic

- Most patients will be referred for NCHCT, if positive for stones in the ureter or kidneys a concurrent plain KUB is recommended:
  - ○ to assess stone lucency
  - ○ for planning the best treatment modality
  - ○ follow-up
- If CT not available: IVU
- MRU to be considered in selected cases

Renal calculi

- IVU or low dose CTU is recommended:
  - ○ Define calyceal anatomy
  - ○ Detect complicating factor (e.g. dilated lower pole calyx, calyceal diverticulum, etc.)
  - ○ Plan puncture
- NCHCT or CTU
  - ○ Patients with complex anatomy (spina bifida, spinal fusion, skeletal anomalies)
  - ○ Complex renal anatomy (horseshoe kidneys, renal ectopia)
  - ○ Large complex calculi

References

European Association of Urology Guidelines (2006) *Guidelines on Urolithiasis*. ISBN 13: 978-90-70 244-59-0

Galvin DJ, Pearle MS (2006) The contemporary management of renal and ureteric calculi. *Br. J. Urol. Int. (BJUI)* **98**: 1283–1288.

Heneghan JP, McGuire KA, Leder RA *et al.* (2003) Helical CT for Nephrolithiasis and ureterolithiasis: comparison of conventional and reduced radiation-dose techniques. *Radiology* **229**: 575–580.

Park S, Pearle MS (2006) Imaging for percutaneous renal access and management of renal calculi. *Urol. Clin. N. Am.* **33**(3): 353–364.

Sandhu C, Anson KM, Patel U (2003) Urinary tract stones – Part I: role of radiological imaging in diagnosis and treatment planning. *Clin. Rad.* **58**: 415–421.

Robertson WG (2004) The scientific basis of urinary stone formation, Chapter 10, *The Scientific Basis of Urology*, 2nd edn, 2004. ISBN 1-90186-513-4

10
Hematuria

Thomas Bretlau[1], Kirstine L. Hermann[1], Jørgen Nordling[2] and Henrik S. Thomsen[1]

[1]*Department of Diagnostic Radiology, Copenhagen University Hospital, Herlev*
[2]*Department of Urology, Copenhagen University Hospital, Herlev*

10.1 Definition

Hematuria is the term for presence of an abnormal amount of blood in the urine. Subgroups:

1. Visible hematuria (macroscopic hematuria or gross hematuria) or

2. Invisible hematuria (microscopic hematuria) – only visible by microscopy.

10.2 Clinical considerations

- Hematuria may be a symptom of an underlying serious disease.

- Most patients with hematuria, in particular microscopic hematuria, have no abnormalities following extensive investigations.

- Urine can be colored red by blood, hemo-myoglobinuria, paroxysmal nocturnal hematuria, porphyria, drugs like nitrofurantoin and intake of beetroots.

- The possibility of a distinction between nephrological and urological causes is important to allow correct specialist referral at an early stage.

- The aim of management should be prompt detection and treatment of serious underlying causes of hematuria, whilst minimizing the number of tests conducted in patients with benign causes.

Urogenital Imaging: A Problem-oriented Approach   Edited by Sameh K. Morcos and Henrik S. Thomsen
© 2009 John Wiley & Sons, Ltd

10.3 Diagnosis of hematuria

- The degree of hematuria can be measured in different ways. The three most important methods are:

  - Quantitatively by determining the number of Red Blood Cells (RBCs) per milliliter urine (chamber count).
  - Directly by examination of the centrifuged urinary sediment (sediment count).
  - Indirectly by dipstick examination of the urine.

- Determining the number of RBCs per milliliter urine (chamber count) is the most accurate technique, but time consuming. The analysis should be performed on a freshly voided, clean-catch, midstream urine specimen. Urine sample is also useful for:

  - Microscopy to distinguish between glomerular or non-glomerular origin; in practice this is often determined by the presence or absence of proteinuria.
  - Culture to rule out infection.
  - Cytology to detect urothelial cancers.
  - Measurement of tumor markers. However, the American Urological Association found that the available data are insufficient to recommend routinely use of these tests.

- Direct examination of the centrifuged urinary sediment (sediment count). It has the following limitations:

  - The number of erythrocytes depends on urine volume and handling of specimen.
  - The time between sampling and investigation affects the result.
  - Magnification and counting are not standardized.
  - There is a lack of consensus regarding the pathologic concentration.

- Indirectly by dipstick examination of the urine. In general it is moderately useful in establishing the presence of hematuria, but cannot be used to rule it out. It has several limitations:

  - A disposable collecting device must be used to avoid false positive reading.
  - Visual reading has poor reproducibility.
  - There is variation between manufacturers.
  - The presence of myo- and hemoglobin results in positive tests.
  - No consensus regarding pathologic values including number of positive tests.
  - Has high sensitivity (91–100%) but limited specificity (65–99%) for 2 to 5 RBCs per high-power microscopic field.

10.4 Epidemiology

Macroscopic hematuria

- When it occurs as a single symptom, the patient is usually alarmed, and the time between first observation and primary examination is often short.

- A full diagnostic investigation is necessary to determine its cause.

- It is associated with a higher prevalence of underlying pathology than microscopic hematuria.

- For any nephrological or urological pathology the prevalence is around 40% and for pure urological malignancies it is around 20%.

Microscopic hematuria

- Often an incidental finding, detected in primary care settings usually in connection with a routine health check and the dipstick method is most frequently used.

- There is huge controversy regarding the diagnosis, etiology and evaluation of asymptomatic microscopic hematuria as red blood cells in the urine are not always a sign of pathology.

- Exercise, trauma or sexual activity can transiently induce hematuria.

- Between 9% and 18% of apparently normal individuals have some degree of hematuria.

- Both in unselected, population-based and in screening studies the prevalence of asymptomatic microscopic hematuria has been estimated to vary between 0.2% and 21%.

- Such wide variations reflect the differences in age and sex of the population screened, the amount of follow-up, and the number of screening studies per patient.

- For any nephrological or urological pathology, the prevalence is around 20% and for pure urological malignancies it is around 10% in patients above 40 years of age, and much lower in patients below 40 years of age.

- Another important characteristic of microscopic hematuria is the possibility to be intermittent.

- Thus, a negative repeated urine analysis in a patient who has previously had a positive test. may not be sufficient to rule out a significant disease.

- If microscopic hematuria is diagnosed, and further investigation is considered, its important to remember that with direct microscopy or detection of proteinuria, it is possible to distinguish between nephrological and urological hematuria.

Hematuria secondary to malignancy in adults below 40 years of age is infrequent.

In patients with microscopic hematuria one should look for:

- Age over 40.
- History of macroscopic hematuria.
- History of urological disease.
- History of urinary tract infection.
- History of pelvic irradiation.
- Chemical exposure.
- Smoking.
- Analgesic abuse (Phenacetin).

Table 10.1 Causes of hematuria

Anatomical location:

Nephrological/ glomerular	Nephritis	Active glomerular nephritis Acute interstitial nephritis Progressive glomerular nephritis Thin membrane disease Hereditary nephritis (Alports syndrome)
	Other nephrological causes	IgA nephropathy Schönlein-Henoch's purpura Haematuria syndrome Renal atrophy
	Other	Hypertension Treatment with anticoagulation drugs
Urological/renal causes	Nephrolithiasis	Hypercalciuria Hyperuricosuria
	Infection	Pyelonefritis Renal tuberculosis
	Tumor	Renal-cell cancer Pelvis or ureteral transitional-cell cancer Wilm's tumor Haemangioma renis Metastases Lymphoma/leukemia Benign cyst
	Vascular	Renal infarction Papillary necrosis Arteriovenous malformation
	Trauma	
	Polycystic kidney disease	
	Medullary sponge kidney	
Lower urinary tract causes	Infection	Cystitis Prostatitis Urethritis Schistosoma haematobium
	Tumor	Benign bladder and ureteral papillomas and tumors Bladder cancer Prostate cancer
	Other	Benign prostatic hyperplasia Ureterocele

Presence of one or more of these risk factors increases the prevalence of significant underlying pathology. Causes of hematuria are presented in Table 10.1.

10.5 Distribution of malignancy in patients with hematuria

Each time you have a patient with a tumor in the upper two-thirds of the ureter, you should find:

- 2 patients with tumors in the lower third of the ureter

- 9 patients with tumors in the pelvic cavity

- 108 patients with renal tumors

- 228 patients with bladder tumors

- 812 patients with no tumors.

10.6 Imaging

For patients with monosymptomatic hematuria the diagnostic pathway shown in Figure 10.1 is recommended.

- If the hematuria is not monosymptomatic, one should always consider changing the diagnostic pathway guided by the other symptom(s).

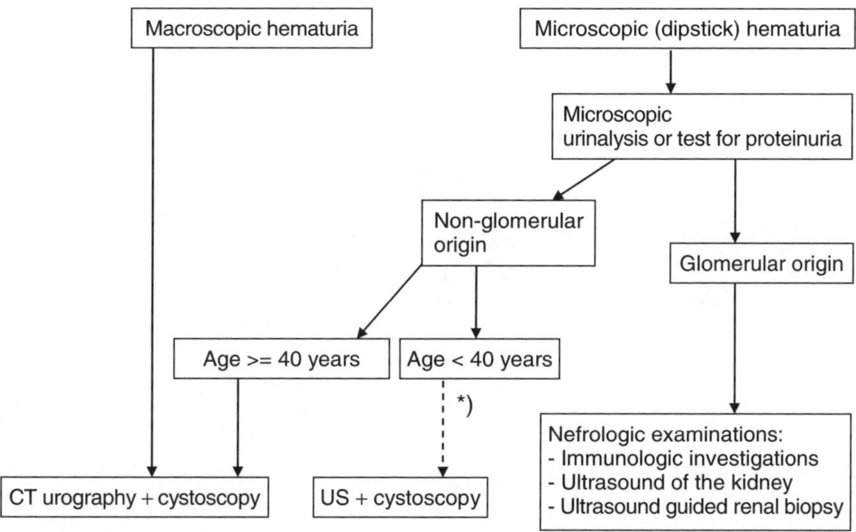

Figure 10.1 Diagnostic pathway.

- Because the majority of patients with hematuria have no abnormalities, it is important to minimize the radiation dose.

- On the other hand it is important to perform an examination that detects important pathology. Refined imaging, e.g. MRI of a kidney or the bladder, can be done subsequently.

CT urography

- CT urography is today the state-of-the-art radiological examination for investigation of monosymptomatic hematuria. We use a split bolus protocol with two runs in order to obtain maximal information with minimal radiation, but other protocols may also be sufficient. The split bolus technique offers simultaneously both high parenchymal concentration of contrast medium (nephrographic) and contrast medium in the upper urinary tract and bladder (excretory).

- Compared with intravenous urography complete luminal opacification is no longer important as the pathology in the wall will opacify.

- Most tumors are visible in a bladder full with contrast. The sensitivity is much lower in patients with an empty or only half full bladder.

- The contrast excretion may be so dense that small polyps can be hidden in the standard abdominal W/L-setting. Therefore, one should always use broad W/L-setting to assess the collecting system and the urinary bladder.

Recommended protocol for CT urography

- A low-dose unenhanced CT scanning from the top of the kidneys to the bottom of the bladder to look for stones (Fig. 10.2) and a basis measurement of changes in enhancement after contrast administration.

- 35 ml of 350–400 mg I/ml intravenous non-ionic contrast media.

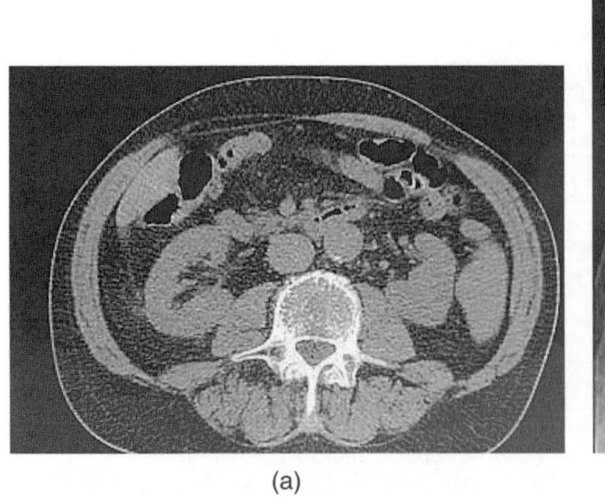
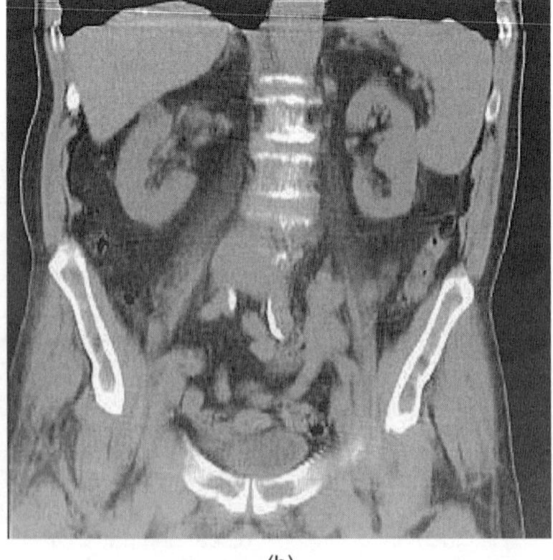

(a)   (b)

Figure 10.2   Unenhanced normal CT urography.

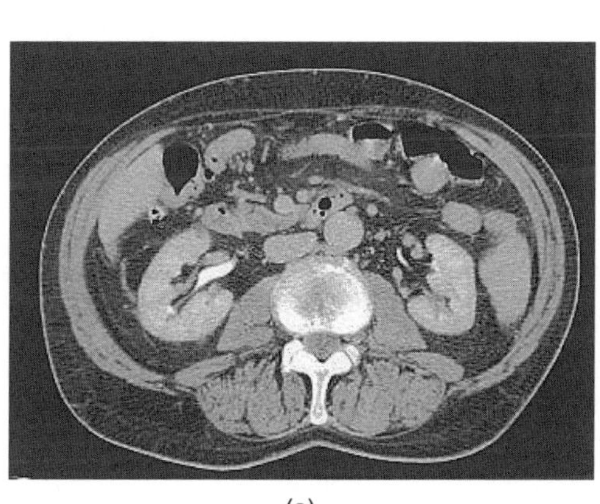 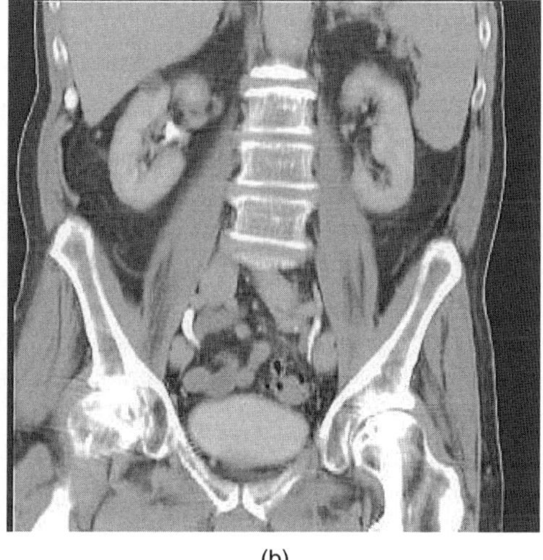

(a)   (b)

Figure 10.3 Enhanced normal CT urography.

- Let the patient move around.

- 8 min later 50 ml of 350–400 mg I/ml non-ionic intravenous contrast media.

- After 80 s another CT scanning from the top of the kidneys to the bottom of the bladder (Fig. 10.3).

- If delayed excretion or no bladder opacification, a third run is done 15 min later.

Cystoscopy

- CT urography and cystoscopy today complement each other for the evaluation of the upper and lower urinary tract respectively.

- In the future the standard CT urography may be optimized such that this examination also may be valid to rule out or detect malignancy in the bladder.

Intravenous urography

- Intravenous urography may be the examination of choice if CT urography is not available.

- It does not provide the same information about renal parenchyma, ureters, bladder and the surrounding structures as CT urography.

- Intravenous urography does not detect renal parenchymal lesions below 3 cm in diameter and 15% of those above. Only 60% of the bladder tumors are detected by intravenous urography.

Retrograde pyelography

- It is rarely necessary after CT urography, as significant pathology in the wall of the collecting system is often detected.

- If the CT urography/intravenous urography has been inconclusive for the evaluation of the renal pelvis or ureter, retrograde pyelography should be considered.

Ultrasound

- First line of imaging in young low-risk patients (<40 years).

- Useful in patients with reduced renal function.

- Ultrasound of the prostate with subsequent biopsy may be considered if prostatic hyperplasia or prostatic cancer is suspected, especially if there is an elevated PSA blood sample. For details see Chapter 13.

MRI

- MR urography is not a standard procedure at present, but might be used if there is a history of prior allergy to iodinated contrast media as well as detailed follow up of unclear findings at CT urography.

- MR urography can be an alternative to CT urography, when there is contraindication to the use of ionizing radiation, as in pregnancy.

Imaging of hematuria

- *Benign causes*

- Urinary stones

- Renal atrophy

- Tuberculosis and pyelonephritis. For details and examples see Chapter 8

- Ureterocele (Fig. 10.4)

- Renal infarction (Fig. 10.5)

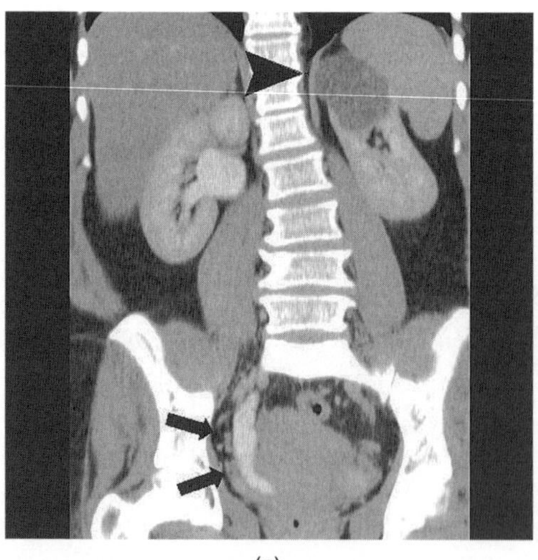
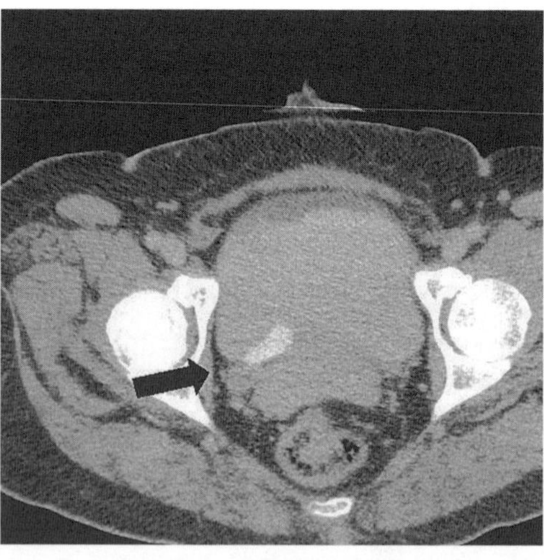

(a)   (b)

Figure 10.4   (a) and (b) Ureterocele. Incidental finding in a 44-year-old female referred for a better characterization of complex cysts in the upper left pole, found at a prior ultrasound examination. Ureterocele at the distal right ureter (arrow), cyst in the left upper pole (arrowhead). Figure 10.4a coronal, Figure 10.4b Axial.

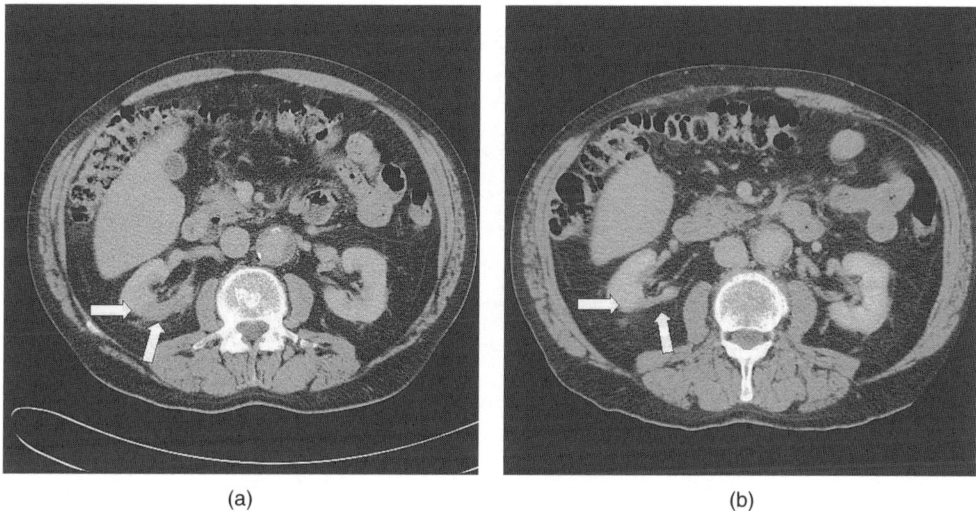

(a)   (b)

Figure 10.5 (a) and (b) Renal infarction. An area with a low density in the right kidney (arrow), found at a unenhanced CT in a 64-year-old female with right flank pain. Figure 10.5b shows follow-up CT six months later.

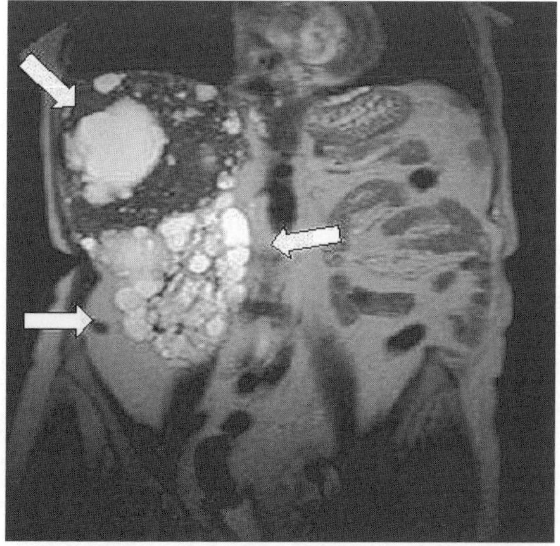

Figure 10.6 Polycystic kidney disease. A T2-weighted MRI of a male with only the right kidney, which is converted into at polycystic organ (arrow).

- Arteriovenous malformation
- Renal trauma
- Polycystic kidney disease (Fig. 10.6)
- Medullary sponge kidney
- *Malignant lesions*

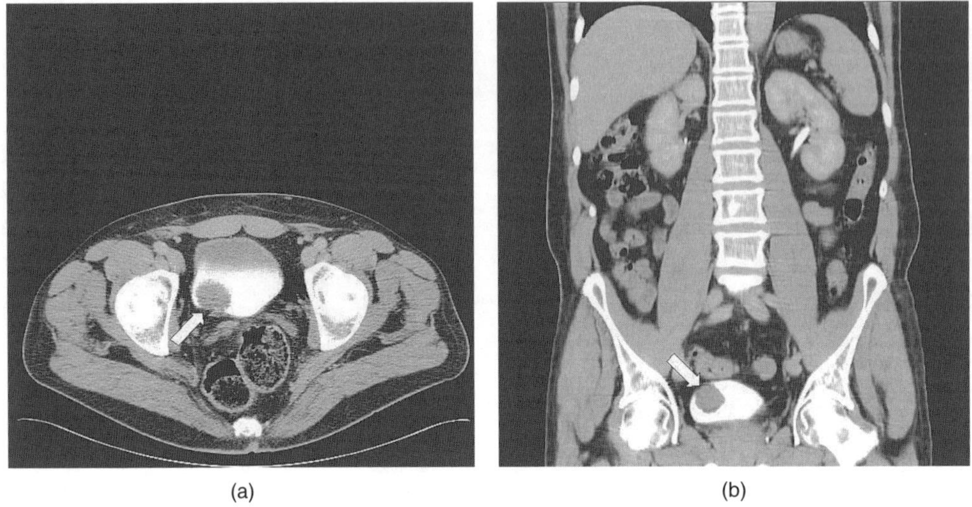

Figure 10.7   (a) and (b) Bladder papilloma. 53-year-old male referred for monosymptomatic macroscopic hematuria. Axial and coronal CT urography images (Fig. 10.7a+b) shows a filling defect in the bladder (arrow).

- Bladder tumors (Figs. 10.7, 10.13 and 10.14). For details and other examples see Chapter 11.

- Renal masses (Figs. 10.8 and 10.15). For details and other examples see Chapter 4.

- Pelvic tumors (Figs. 10.9 and 10.12)

- Ureter tumors (Figs. 10.10 and 10.11)

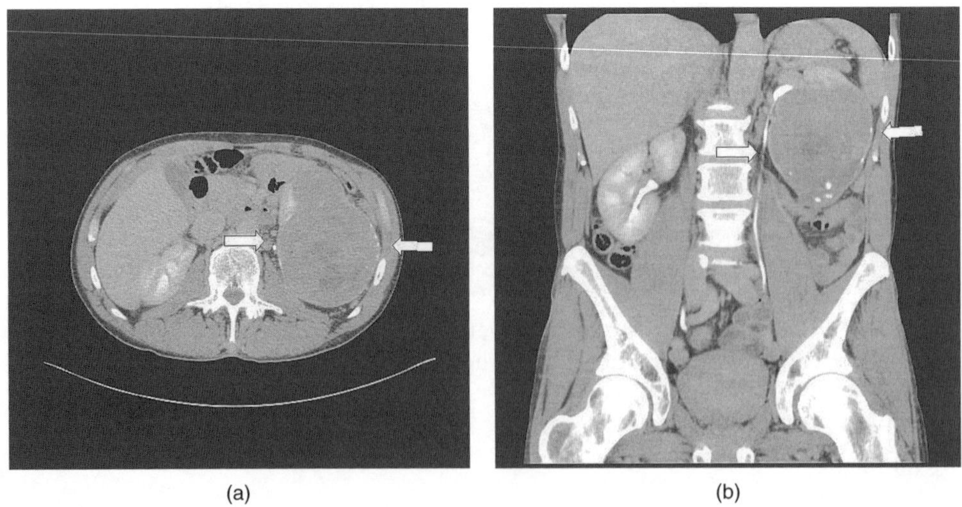

Figure 10.8   (a), (b) and (c) Renal cell carcinoma. 58-year-old male with flank pain, hematuria and weight loss. CT urography axial and coronal (Fig. 10.8a and b) a corresponding Ultrasound image (Fig. 10.8c).

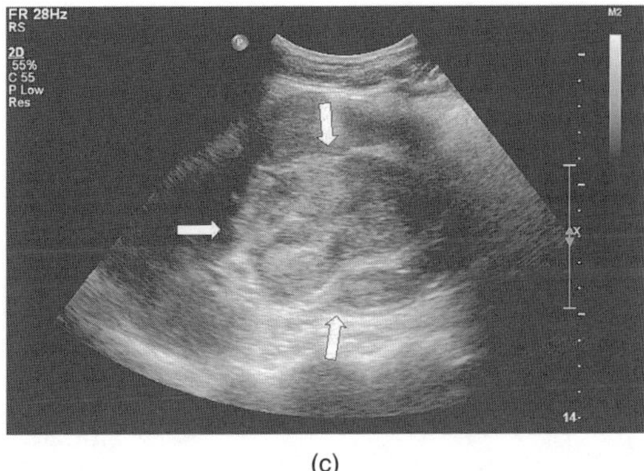

(c)

Figure 10.8 (a), (b) and (c) Renal cell carcinoma. 58-year-old male with flank pain, hematuria and weight loss. CT urography axial and coronal (Fig. 10.8a and b) a corresponding Ultrasound image (Fig. 10.8c).

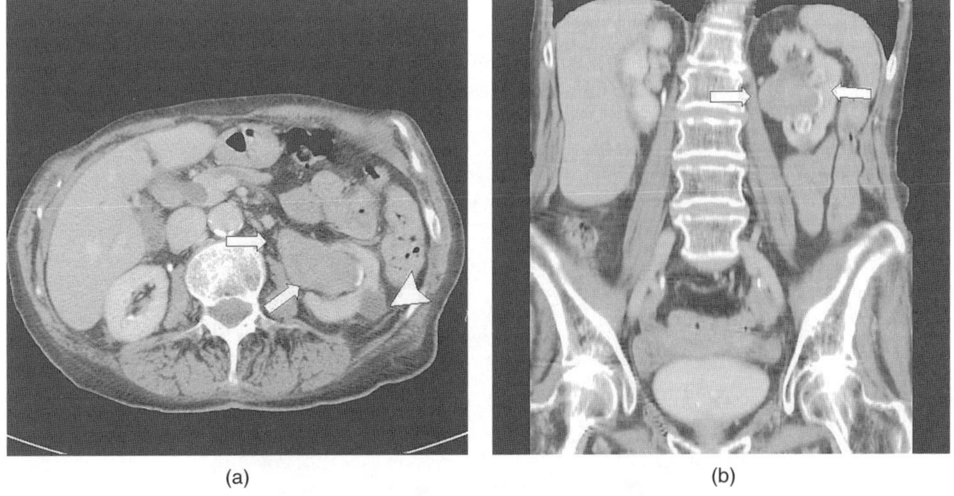

(a)   (b)

Figure 10.9 (a) and (b) Transitional cell tumor of the pelvis. 73-year-old female referred for monosymptomatic macroscopic hematuria. A CT urography shows a large mass in the pelvis (arrow). On axial scan (Fig. 10.9a) a simple cyst is also identified (arrowhead).

- Metastases
- Lymphoma/leukemia

Diseases which cannot be diagnosed by imaging

- Hemorrhagic cystitis (diffuse thickening of the bladder wall might be observed)
- IgA nephritis and other nephrological causes
- Treatment with anticoagulation drugs
- Intensive exercise

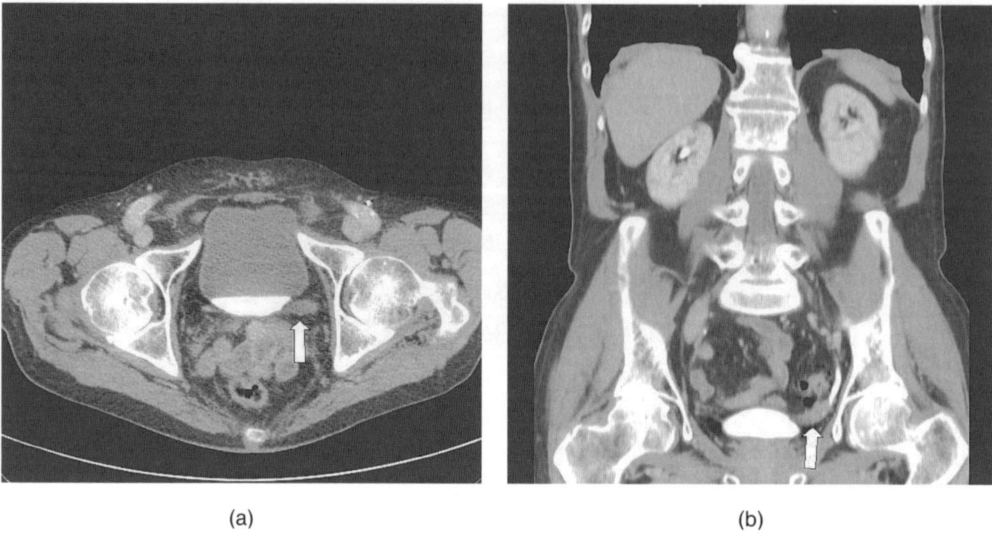

(a)   (b)

Figure 10.10 Transitional cell tumor of the distal ureter. 75-year-old male referred for monosymptomatic macroscopic hematuria. Prior history of bladder papillomas. CT urography shows on enhanced images a filling defect and a thickening of the distal left ureter (arrow).

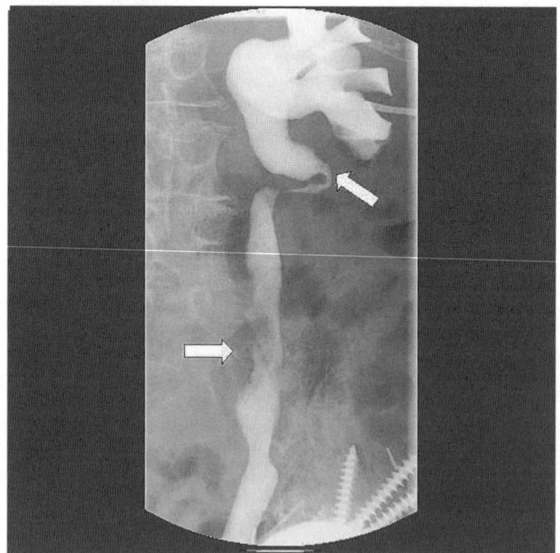

Figure 10.11 Papilloma of the pelvis and ureter. An antegrade pyelography shows filling defects at the pelvis and upper ureter.

10.7 Summary

- Microscopic hematuria is often an incidental finding possibly reflecting an entirely benign cause such as vigorous exercise, but may also be due to a malignant, possibly lethal cause such as cancer.

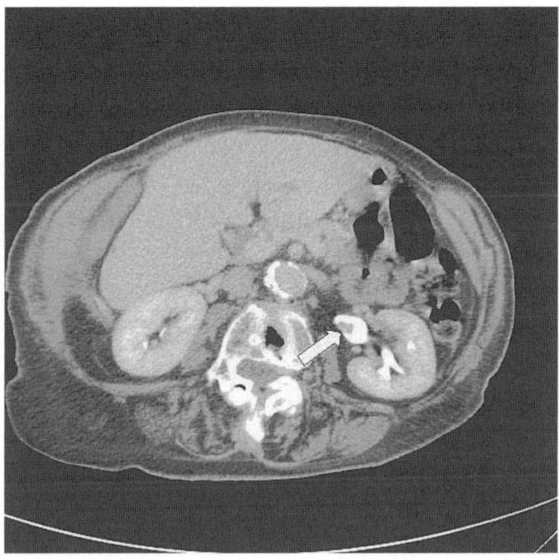

Figure 10.12 Papilloma of the pelvis. 78-year-old female referred for multiple times of cystitis. CT urography shows a papilloma of the pelvis (arrow).

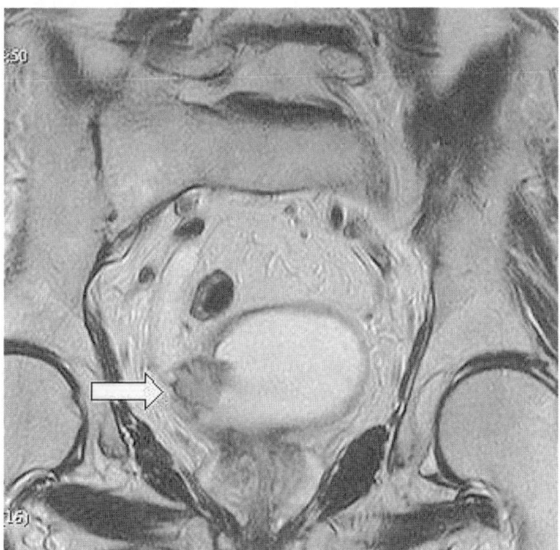

Figure 10.13 Bladder tumor. MRI shows a tumor in the right side of the bladder.

- Discrimination between glomerular or urologic origin of hematuria is essential.

- CT urography can accurately detect malignant lesions and stones of the urinary tract. It is more accurate than intravenous urography and currently is the preferred imaging tool for the evaluation of the urinary tract.

- Cystoscopy remains essential for excluding bladder lesions.

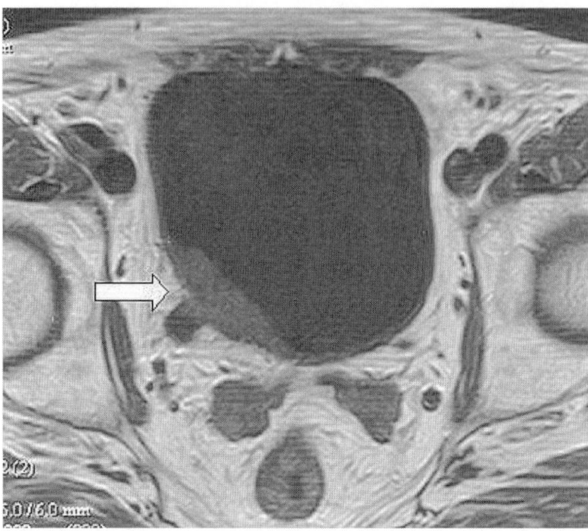

Figure 10.14 Bladder tumor. MRI shows a tumor in the right side of the bladder, involving the right ostium (arrow).

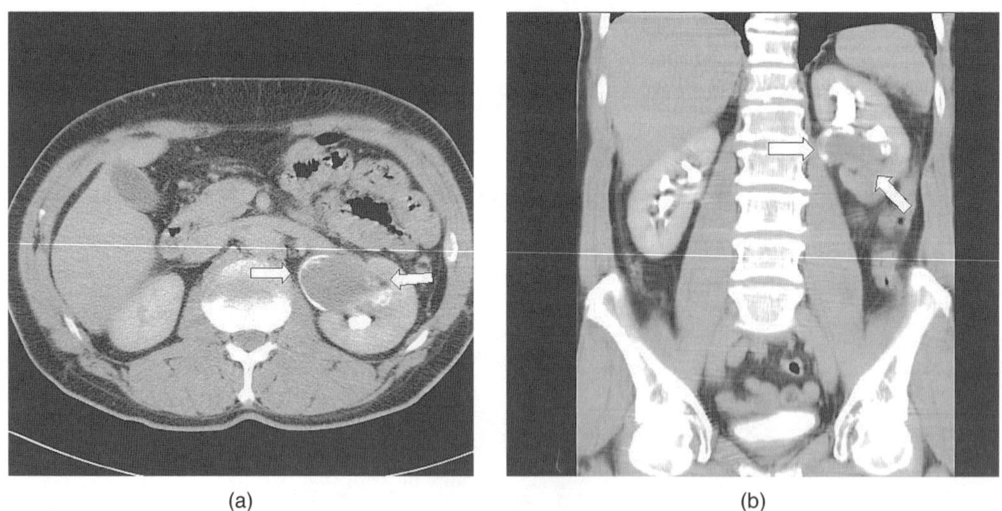

(a)   (b)

Figure 10.15 (a) and (b) Renal cell carcinoma. 75-year-old male with hematuria. CT urography shows an expanding mass, mainly growing in the pelvis.

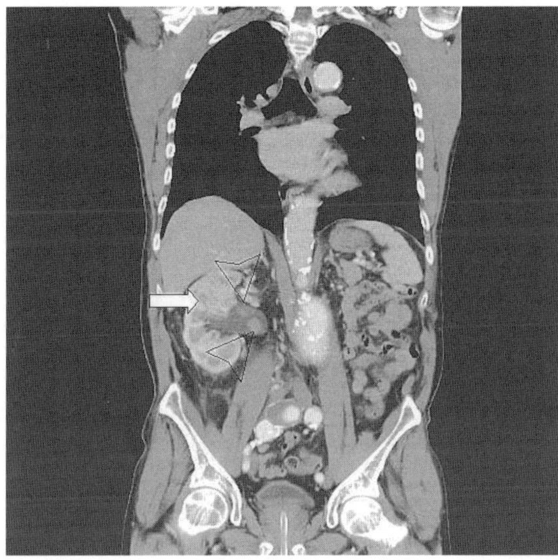

Figure 10.16 Renal cell carcinoma with bleeding in pelvis. 67-year-old male initially referred for macroscopic hematuria and right flank pain. CT urography shows a mass in the upper right pole (arrow) and blood cloths in the pelvis (arrowhead).

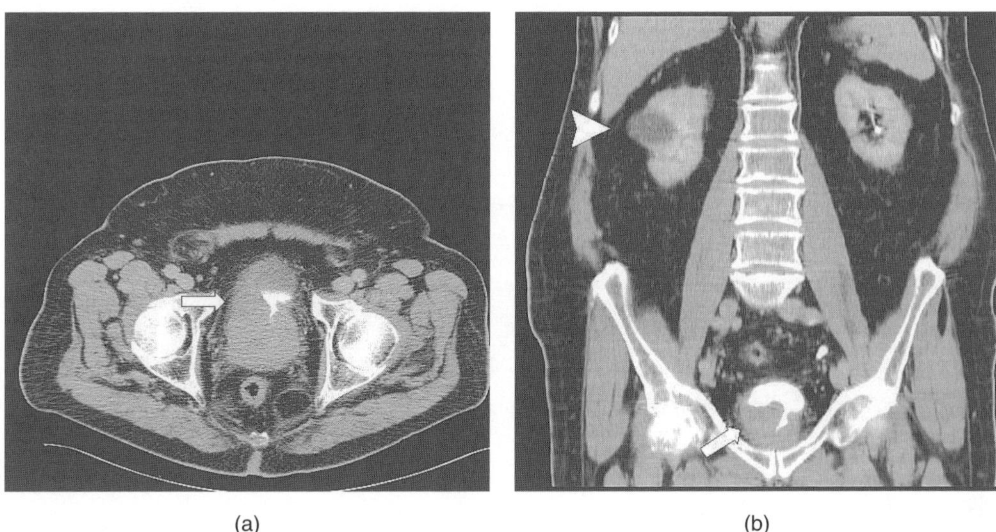

(a)   (b)

Figure 10.17 Prostate tumor. 76-year-old man with secondary carcinoma in situ in the bladder, referred for CT urography for investigation of the upper urinary tract. Fig 10.17a and b Tumor protruding into the bladder (arrow). On Fig 10.17b a simple cyst in the right kidney (arrowhead).

References

Cohen RA, Brown RS (2003) Clinical practice. Microscopic hematuria. *N. Engl. J. Med.* **348**(23): 2330–2338.

Grossfeld G D, Litwin M S, Wolf J J, Hricah H, Shuler C L, Agerler D C, Caroll P R (2001) Evaluation of asymptomatic microscopic hematuria in adults: the American Urological Association best practice policy – part I: definition, detection, prevalence, and etiology. *Urology* **57**(4): 599–603.

Grossfeld G D, Litwin M S, Wolf J S Jr, Hricah H, Shuler C L, Agerler D C, Caroll P R (2001) Evaluation of asymptomatic microscopic hematuria in adults: the American Urological Association best practice policy – part II: patient evaluation, cytology, voided markers, imaging, cystoscopy, nephrology evaluation, and follow-up. *Urology* **57**(4): 604–610.

Nabi G, Greene DR, O'Donnell, M (2003) How important is urinary cytology in the diagnosis of urological malignancies? *Eur. Urol.* **43**(6): 632–636.

Rodgers M, Nixon J, Hempel S, Aho T, Kelly J, Neal D, Duffy S, Ritchie G, Kleijnen J, Westwood M (2006) Diagnostic tests and algorithms used in the investigation of hematuria: systematic reviews and economic evaluation. *Health Technol. Assess.* **10**(18): iii–259.

11
Bladder Cancer

G. Heinz-Peer[1] and C. Kratzik[2]

[1] *Department of Radiology, Medical University of Vienna*
[2] *Department of Urology, Medical University of Vienna*

11.1 Introduction

Tumors involving the urinary bladder are most commonly of malignant character (>98%). Most benign bladder tumors are mesenchymal in origin and include leiomyomas, neurofibromas, hemangiomas, and pheochromocytomas (Fig. 11.1).

Malignant neoplasms are classified as primary or secondary. Primary tumors develop in the muscle wall or urothelium. Tumors of the urothelium are by far the most common bladder malignancies, comprising approximately 95% of all such lesions.

Bladder cancer represents 2% to 4% of all malignancies. It is a disease of later life with a peak incidence during the seventh decade. Bladder cancer is three times more common in men than women, and it affects twice as many Whites as Blacks.

The most well documented risk factor of bladder cancer is cigarette smoking. Up to 45% of urothelial cancers seem to be attributed to abuse of nicotine. Other agents possibly inducing bladder cancer include chemical carcinogens (such as aniline, benzidine, aromatic amines, and azo dyes) as well as exposure to asbestos. Analgesic abuse and urine stasis from structural abnormalities, such as horseshoe kidneys, are also associated with an increased incidence of these tumors. Other risk factors include chronic bladder infection or inflammation, bladder calculus, pelvic irradiation, and treatment with cyclophosphamide. A genetic propensity to develop bladder cancer has also been observed. *Schistosoma haematobium* infection is strongly associated with squamous cell carcinoma of the bladder and accounts for 40% of epithelial tumors in endemic areas. In this chapter we provide an overview of the clinical features, pathology, and imaging findings of bladder cancer.

Urogenital Imaging: A Problem-oriented Approach   Edited by Sameh K. Morcos and Henrik S. Thomsen
© 2009 John Wiley & Sons, Ltd

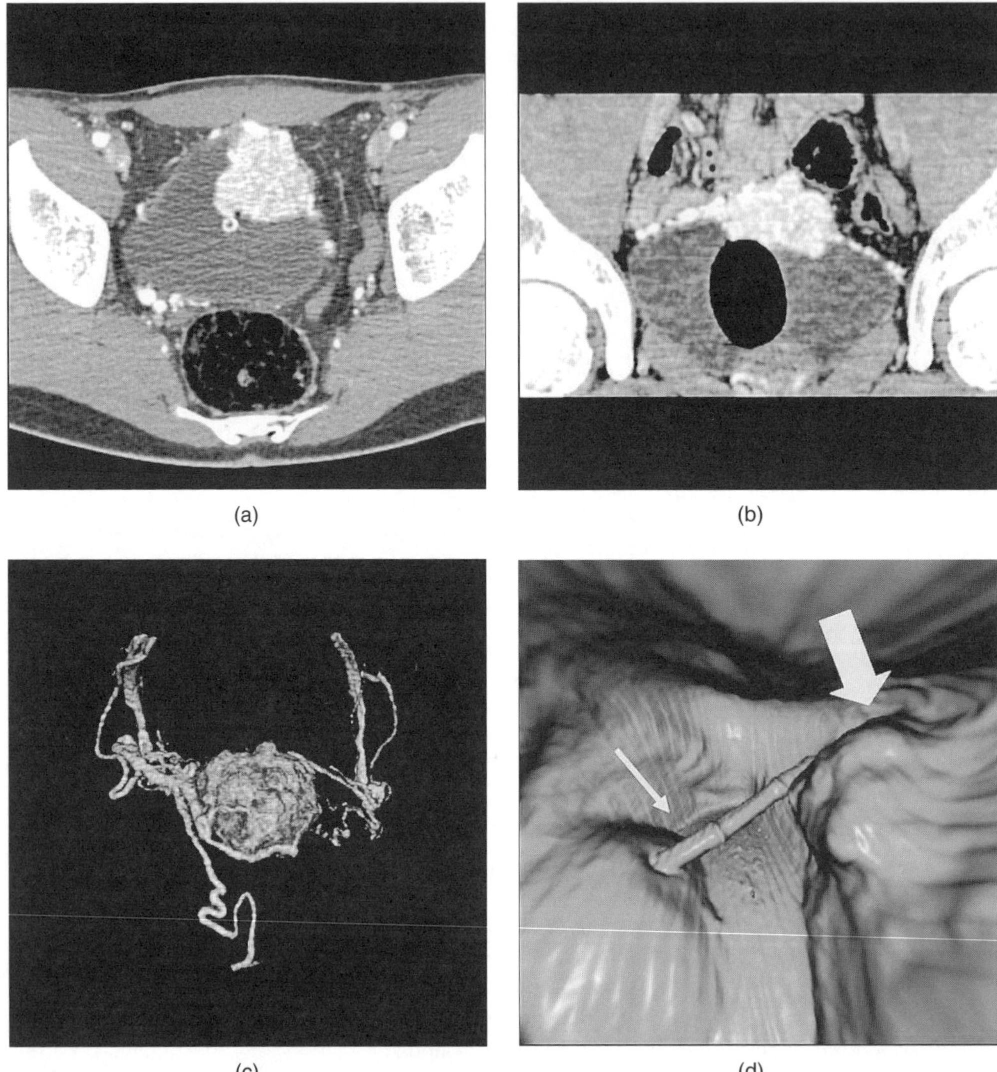

Figure 11.1 MDCT imaging of pheochromocytoma of the urinary bladder. 17-year-old man with history of intermittent hypertensive crisis especially during and after voiding. (a) Contrast-enhanced CT performed during the arterial phase shows a hypervascular broad-based lesion on the bladder wall. (b) On coronal reconstruction the lesion proves to be on the bladder dome. (c) 3D reconstruction of the lesion using volume rendering technique the vasculature of this lesion is nicely depicted. (d) Virtual endoscopic view of the urinary bladder shows intraluminary bulging of the bladder wall, however, the surface of the bladder remains very smooth.

11.2 Clinical features

- Patients most commonly present with painless hematuria, either gross or microscopic.

- The bleeding may be intermittent.

- A sense of false security may arise by the spontaneous disappearance of bleeding.

- Carcinoma in situ lesions may be associated with irritative voiding symptoms (increased frequency, urgency, and dysuria).

- With the later constellation of symptoms, differential diagnosis also includes benign entities, such as urinary tract infection, prostatism, and prostatitis.

- Locally advanced tumors present with pelvic or abdominal pain due to ureteric obstruction, pelvic side wall muscle invasion, or invasion of adjacent organs.

- Historical information acquired should include

  - Duration of hematuria
  - Presence of other coexistent symptoms – dysuria, flank pain
  - Prior abdominal, pelvic, or genital trauma
  - Interventional procedures or placement of transurethral catheters
  - Medication history (in particular anticoagulant or antiplatelet therapy)
  - Sexual history
  - Travel history (with emphasis on travel to geographic regions endemic for mycobacterial and bilharzial infections)
  - Severe hypertension
  - Bleeding diathesis
  - Occupation.

- Physical examination should include evaluation of

  - Blood pressure
  - Kidneys/pelvis/genital organs.

- Laboratory testing should include

  - Urinalysis and urine culture (to exclude infection)
  - Visual analysis (gross or microscopic hematuria)
  - Urine cytology
  - Microbiological testing for infectious organisms
  - Serum coagulation panel (in case of anticoagulant or antiplatelet therapy)
  - Complete blood count.

- When a clinical diagnosis of bladder tumor is suspected initial investigation includes lower urinary tract endoscopy (Fig. 11.2).

  - Flexible cystourethroscopy allows diagnostic endoscopy to be performed safely in an office setting with improved patient comfort.

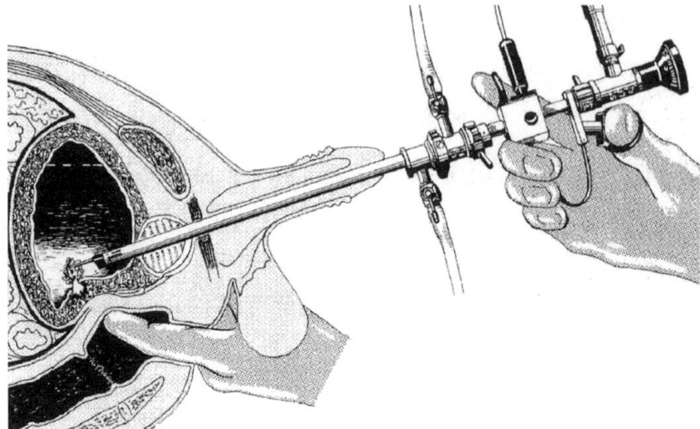

Figure 11.2 Schematic drawing of conventional cystoscopy with a flexible cystoscope.

- o It enables thorough endoscopic assessment of the entire urethra, including the prostatic urethra in men, and the entire urinary bladder.
- o Papillary and well circumscribed bladder tumors are easily recognized.
- o Areas of CIS may appear only as red areas on the mucosa.
- o Photodynamic diagnostics with 5-ALA may further improve detection of CIS and non-invasive bladder cancer (Fig. 11.3).

- After endoscopic visualization of a bladder tumor, the histopathologic diagnosis and initial treatment are achieved by TUR (transurethral resection) of the tumor.

  - o Complete endoscopic resection of the tumor using a loop diathermy electrode is attempted, unless there is obvious extravesical extension.

  - o Areas of abnormal appearing mucosa are biopsied.

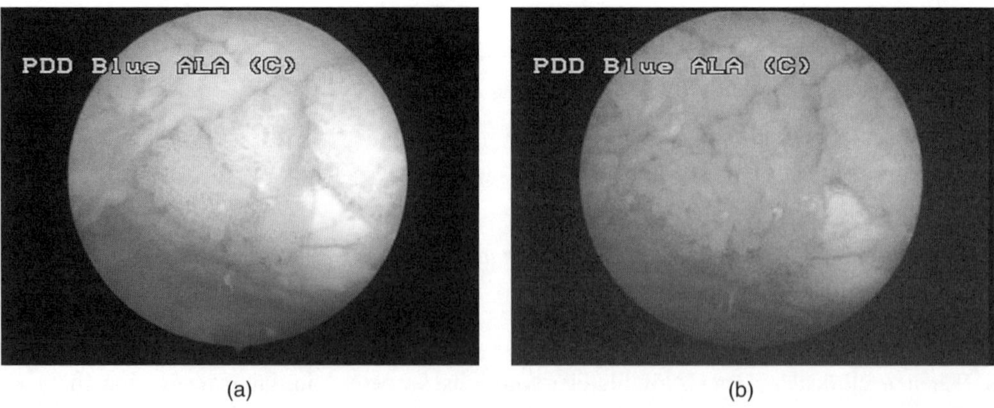

(a)   (b)

Figure 11.3 Multifocal papillary lesions in a 77-year-old patient with painless hematuria. (a) Standard light cystoscopy shows multifocal papillary lesions. (b) On fluorescence cystoscopy with 5-ALA these lesions are better demarcated by showing red color.

- Limitations of conventional cystoscopy include

  - diminished visualization of areas such as the mucosa of the bladder neck and within diverticula
  - technical difficulties in patients with urinary diversion
  - it is an invasive procedure and may be uncomfortable, time consuming, and expensive
  - it is contraindicated in patients with bacteriuria, acute cystitis, urethritis, prostatitis, obstructive prostatic hypertrophy, and stricture or rupture of the urethra.

- In rare cases complications like iatrogenic injury to the urethra and bladder as well as urinary sepsis may occur due to cystoscopy.

11.3 Pathology

- Most bladder tumors arise from the urothelium including

  - Transitional cell carcinomas (TCC) (90% to 95%)
  - Squamous cell carcinomas (SCC) or mixed transitional and squamous cell tumors (4% to 8%)
  - Adenocarcinomas and undifferentiated lesions (1% to 2%).

- Rare malignant bladder tumors not arising from the urothelium include

  - Malignant mesenchymal tumors of bladder muscle
  - Lymphoma
  - Secondary bladder tumors.

- Cellular grading is a histologic assessment of malignant change.

- Bladder cancer can be classified into three grades: well-differentiated (grade 1), moderately differentiated (grade 2), and poorly differentiated (grade 3).

- Tumor grade correlates with the natural history of the disease.

- Grade III tumors invading muscle have a significantly worse prognosis than those with grade I or II superficial lesions.

- Grading of bladder carcinoma usually correlates well with staging: 80% of grade 3 lesions are invasive into muscle, compared with 50% of grade 2 lesions, and 10% of grade 1.

- Grade I lesions are well differentiated tumors and are usually papillary, whereas grade III lesions are poorly differentiated and frequently show an infiltrating pattern of growth.

- Staging of bladder carcinoma is an attempted assessment of the extent of the tumor spread, in particular the degree of the bladder wall penetration.

- The Jewett–Strong–Marshall (ABCD) classification has been replaced by the tumor, nodes, metastases (TNM) staging classification.

- Figure 11.4 shows both, TNM and ABCD classification.

- Both are based on the involvement by tumor of the various layers of the bladder wall, perivesical fat, and more distant organs.

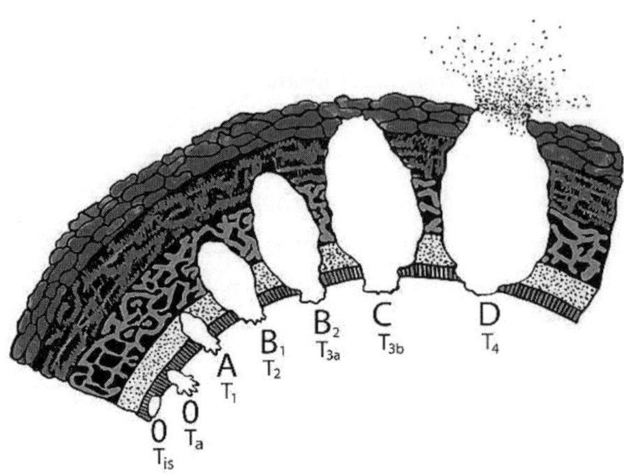

Figure 11.4 Depth of tumor penetration according to TNM system and ABCD system of staging transitional cell carcinoma of the urinary bladder. Layers of the bladder wall are as follows: 1, mucosa; 2, submucosa; 3, superficial muscle; 4, deep muscle; 5, perivesical fat; 6, denoting adjacent organs or distant metastases.

- There is a correlation between T-stage and the risk of recurrence, progression, and metastasis.

- Once the tumor has penetrated the basement membrane (T1) or muscle (T2–T4), there is an increased likelihood of distant metastases.

- Both staging and grading should be considered in the management of bladder carcinoma.

- Approximately one-third of patients present with muscle invasive disease at the time of initial diagnosis.

- Approximately 12% of patients with carcinoma in situ develop invasive carcinoma.

Transitional cell carcinoma

- TCC has a well known association with chemical carcinogens (aromatic amines, nitrosamines, aldehydes).

- The latent period between occupational exposure and the development of cancer varies from 15 to 40 years.

- Other causes of TCC include smoking and treatment of cyclophosphamide.

- Recent studies indicate genetic factors.

- TCC can occur anywhere in the urinary tract where urothelium is present, most commonly it occurs in the bladder.

- TCC is most commonly found on the lateral walls (47%) or in the region of the trigone (21%) and bladder dome.

- Approximately 30% of TCC patients present with multifocal disease in the bladder and sometimes widespread areas of squamous metaplasia and carcinoma in situ.

- TCC spreads by invading through the bladder wall into the perivesical lymphatics and capillaries.

- Involvement of pelvic lymph nodes is common in TCC.

- Synchronous upper urinary tract urothelial tumors occur in 2–5% of patients.

- 11% to 13% of patients who initially present with upper urinary tract lesions will develop additional upper tract neoplasms and 50% will develop metachronous tumors in the urinary bladder.

- Hematogeneous spread is most frequent to liver and lungs, and in a small percentage of cases to bones (lytic bone metastases).

- Direct extension can occur into prostatic urethra and seminal vesicals in men and into the vagina in women.

- TCC of the prostate is present in approximately 40% of men with invasive bladder cancer.

- Coexistent adenocarcinoma of the prostate is present in 40% of men undergoing cystoprostatectomy for invasive TCC.

Squamous cell carcinoma

- SCC is often associated with chronic and recurrent bladder infections, bladder calculi, or both.

- Patients with schistosomiasis are at increased risk for SCC.

- The incidence of SCC is higher in bladder diverticula than in the bladder lumen

- SCCs are multifocal in 25% of patients and tend to be poorly differentiated and invasive.

- The 5-year survival rate of patients with SCC is around 10%.

- Radiographically, SCC cannot be differentiated from other urothelial tumors.

Adenocarcinoma

- Typically associated with metaplastic change in extrophic bladders.

- It may be a result of malignant transformation in patients with cystitis glandularis.

- Adenocarcinoma usually arises in the region of the trigone.

- However, can be occasionally seen as exophytic growth arising at the bladder dome and originating from a persistent urachus.

Urachal carcinoma

- The urachus is a musculofibrous band 5 to 6 cm long extending from the umbilicus to the anterosuperior surface of the bladder.

- It represents a vestigial remnant of the obliterated umbilical arteries and the allantois.

- Its minute lumen is lined by transitional epithelium in 70% of adults.

- Numerous anomalies of the urachal closure may occur (patent urachus, urachal cyst, urachal sinus, urachal diverticulum).

- Transitional epithelium lining the urachus may undergo metaplasia to glandular epithelium that can produce mucin.

- Malignant change in urachal epithelium includes mucin-producing adenocarcinomas (70%), non-mucin-producing adenocarcinomas (15%), TCC, SCC, or sarcomas.

- Urachal sarcomas usually occur in patients younger than 20 years of age.

- SCC may be associated with urachal cysts and calculi in urachal diverticula.

- Urachal carcinomas occur in patients between 40 and 70 years of age and have a male preponderance.

- The prognosis is poor, the 5-year survival rate is less than 15%.

Malignant mesenchymal tumors of bladder muscle

- These are rare tumors, the most common being leiomyosarcoma and rhabdomyosarcoma.

- Leiomyosarcomas have a tendency to grow quite large and ulcerate.

- If undifferentiated, they may be difficult to be distinguished from rhabdomyosarcoma.

- Rhabdomyosarcomas have a biphasic age distribution. In adults, rhabdomyosarcomas and leiomyosarcomas tend to occur in the older age groups; the embryonal variety occurs during the first few years of life.

- Because of the lobulated appearance resembling a cluster of grapes, the term 'sarcoma botryoides' has been created.

- The prognosis is very poor even after radical exstirpative surgery.

Lymphoma

- Lymphoma may mimic urothelial carcinoma.

- It is rare and secondary, as there is no lymphoid tissue in the bladder.

- Lymphoma may show diffuse, albeit sometimes asymmetric thickening and enhancement of the bladder wall.

- Homogeneous appearance.

- Definite diagnosis generally requires biopsy.

Secondary bladder tumors

- Constitute approximately 1% of all malignant vesical lesions.

- 3% to 4% of patients with terminal carcinomatosis show involvement of the bladder.

- The bladder may be involved in malignant melanoma, carcinomas of the stomach, colon, pancreas, ovary, breast, kidney, and lung.

- Infiltration of the bladder by malignant tumors of adjacent organs is more common (prostate, sigmoid, cervical cancer).

- With the history of a primary tumor elsewhere, the diagnosis of a secondary spread should be suspected.

- However, never discard a primary tumor without biopsy.

11.4 Imaging findings

- **Imaging techniques**

  - **Computed tomography (CT)**

    - Imaging modality of choice for the work up of patients presenting with hematuria.

    - Indicated in patients with high-grade bladder cancer raising suspicion for muscle invasion.

    - Routine contrast-enhanced CT examinations are useful for detecting metastases.

    - On CT the bladder has a clearly delineated wall of soft tissue density.

    - When the bladder is distended the thickness of the wall is less than 5 mm.

    - If scanning is undertaken with an empty bladder the wall may be as thick as 5 mm.

    - The bladder wall enhances uniformly following a bolus injection of intravenous contrast medium.

    - Delayed scans (after 10 min) show opacification of the bladder lumen and sometimes the lower ureters as well.

    - Bladder tumors appear on CT as soft tissue density lesions arising from the bladder wall.

    - The tumor may be papillary, sessile or pedunculated, infiltrating or mixed (Figs 11.5–11.7).

    - In some cases the only abnormality seen is focal asymmetric bladder wall thickening (Fig. 11.8).

    - Retraction of the bladder wall may be present.

    - Urothelial carcinomas demonstrate increased vascularity on contrast-enhanced CT.

    - Tumors often enhance to a greater degree than the normal bladder wall following injection of intravenous contrast medium.

    - In the pre-MDCT era the accuracy of CT study in local staging of bladder neoplasm has varied between 68% and 85%.

    - Additionally, CT has failed in staging early tumors (TIS–T3a).

    - In patients with suspected perivesical spread and more advanced disease, the usefulness of CT has been reported.

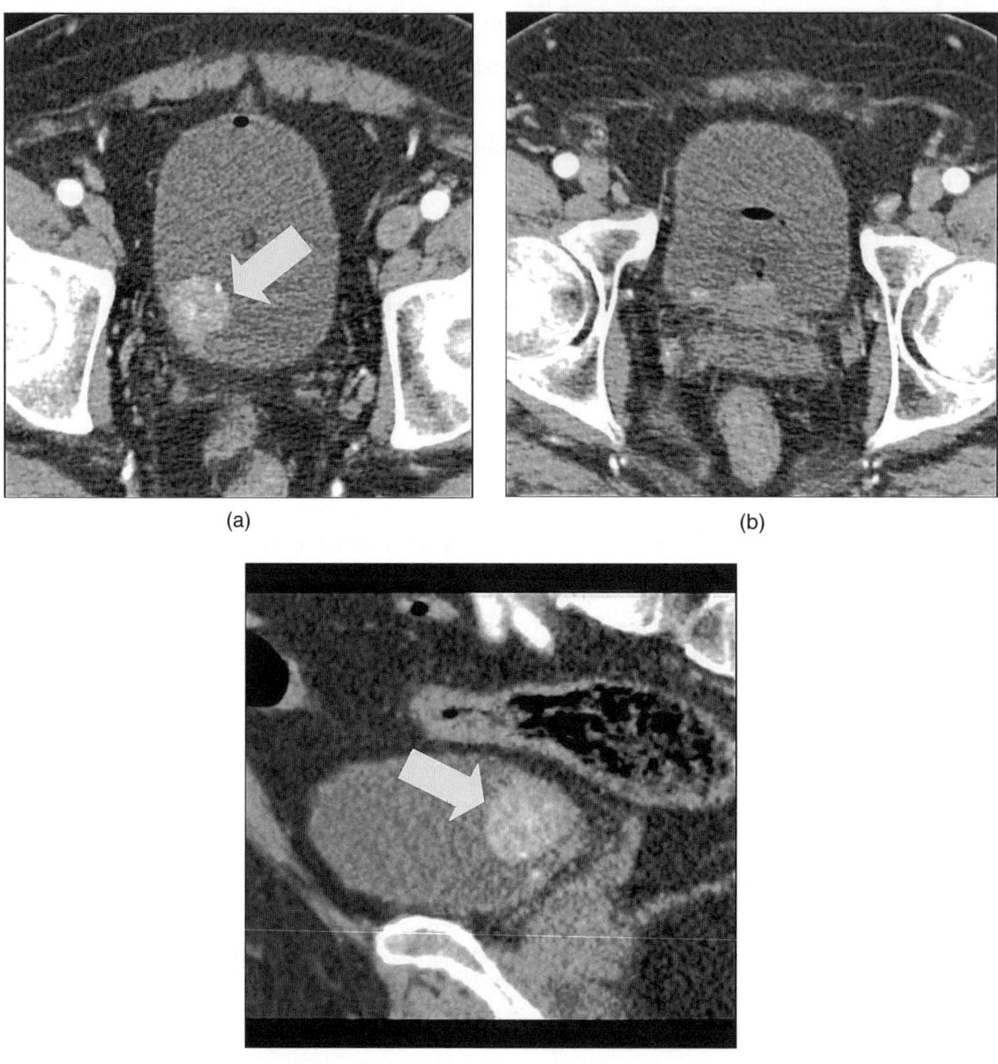

(a)

(b)

(c)

Figure 11.5　Contrast-enhanced MDCT of the urinary bladder in a 56-year-old heavily smoking female patient with one episode of hematuria and histologically proven Ta and T1 bladder cancer. (a) On the axial images a very small (<5 mm) hypervascular papillary lesion and a sessile hypervascular larger lesion are depicted. (b) On the reconstructed sagittal view both lesions can be shown in one plane.

- Overall in the pre-MDCT era CT has been regarded as inferior to MRI for staging bladder cancer, but as similar in evaluation of extravesical disease.

- Multidetector CT offers new possibilities.

- Using thin collimation, near isotropic imaging of the urinary tract is possible and provides high quality multiplanar reformations and 3D reconstructions of the organ including virtual cystoscopic views.

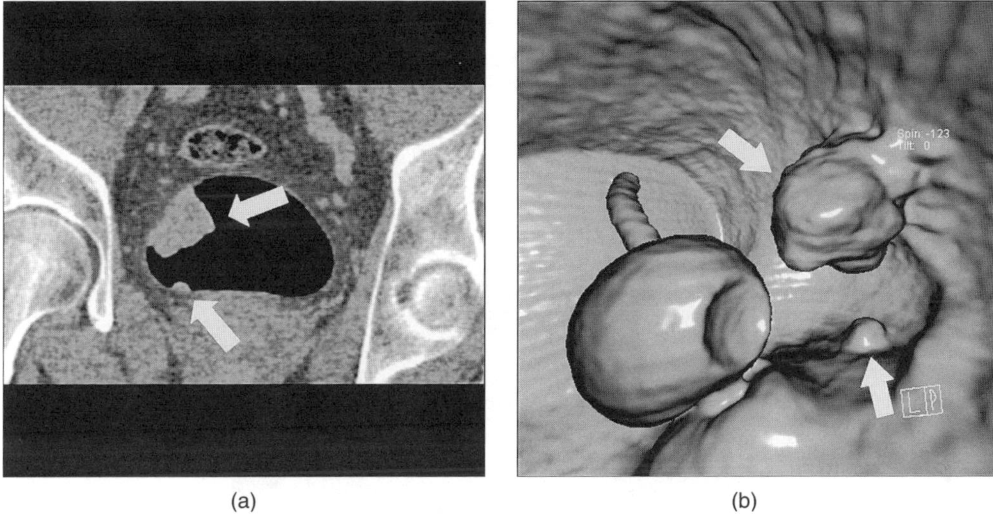

(a)   (b)

Figure 11.6 MDCT of the urinary bladder and virtual cystoscopy in a 65-year-old male patient presenting with painless hematuria. (a) On coronal reconstructed MDCT image of the air-filled urinary bladder a small papillary and an additional larger lesion that looks sessile can be depicted. (b) Virtual endoscopic view nicely shows the peduncular morphology of the larger bladder lesion.

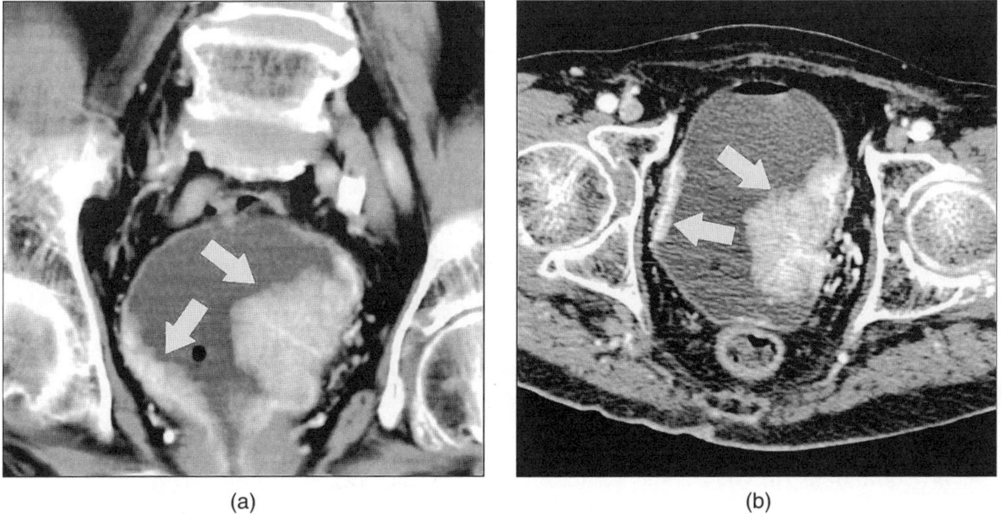

(a)   (b)

Figure 11.7 MDCT of the bladder in a 72-year-old patient with multiple episodes of painless hematuria during the last year. (a) Coronal MIP reconstruction of contrast enhanced MDCT of the fluid filled bladder shows a large muscle invasive TCC on the left lateral aspect of the bladder wall. Additionally, a very flat muscle invasive tumor is seen on the right lateral aspect of bladder. (b) On the axial image infiltration of the perivesical fat especially on the left side is demarcated.

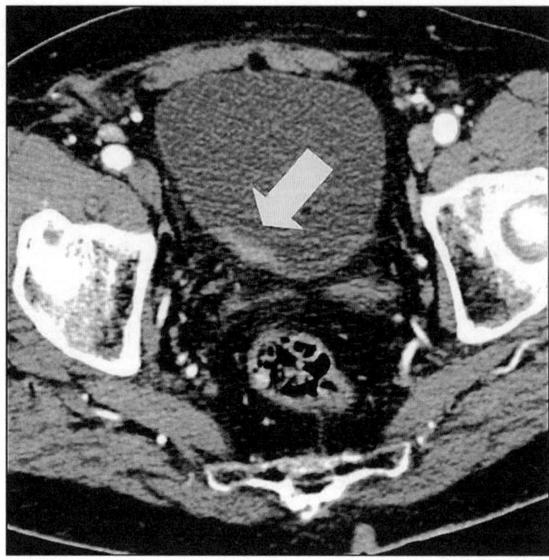

Figure 11.8 CE-MDCT in a 69-year-old female patient performed for staging of melanoma revealed focal asymmetric contrast enhancement and bladder wall thickening. Cystoscopy and TUR was performed. Histology showed a T1 lesion.

- Preliminary results of various studies show excellent detection rates, including lesions <5 mm and also accurate staging of bladder tumors by combined evaluation of source data and virtual cystoscopy (Fig. 11.9).

- Transverse and virtual views are complementary in lesion detection and characterization.

- Imaging of the urinary bladder in the prone and supine position is necessary for visualization of the entire mucosal surface without obscurity caused by residual urine (Fig. 11.10).

- Several examination techniques exists for virtual cystoscopy.

- The bladder can be filled through a Foley catheter either with iodinated contrast media as a positive contrast agent or with room air (CO_2 respectively) as a negative contrast agent.

- In case of bladder distension with negative contrast agent, the urinary bladder should be drained of residual urine with a Foley catheter first.

- 300–550 mL of room air or CO_2 is usually tolerated by patients.

- Limitations of MDCT and virtual cystoscopy include

  - inability to depict flat lesions (carcinoma in situ)
  - inability different mucosal thickening secondary to fibrosis from neoplasm
  - MDCT and virtual endoscopy cannot provide tissue for histologic evaluation.

- The accuracy of CT for detecting lymph node deposits in pelvic cancers ranges from 70% to 92%.

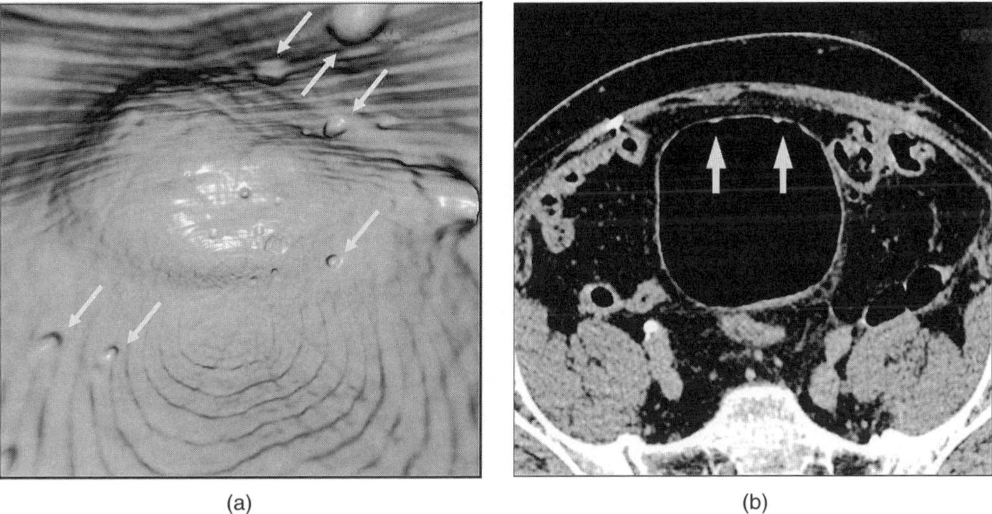

(a)   (b)

Figure 11.9 MDCT and virtual endoscopy was performed in a 63-year-old male patient with suspected bladder tumor. (a) virtual cystoscopy revealed multiple tiny papillary bladder lesions, most of them <5 mm which were overlooked at the initial read of the 2D images. (b) with knowledge of the virtual endoscopy findings these lesions were also detected on 2D images of the air-distended bladder.

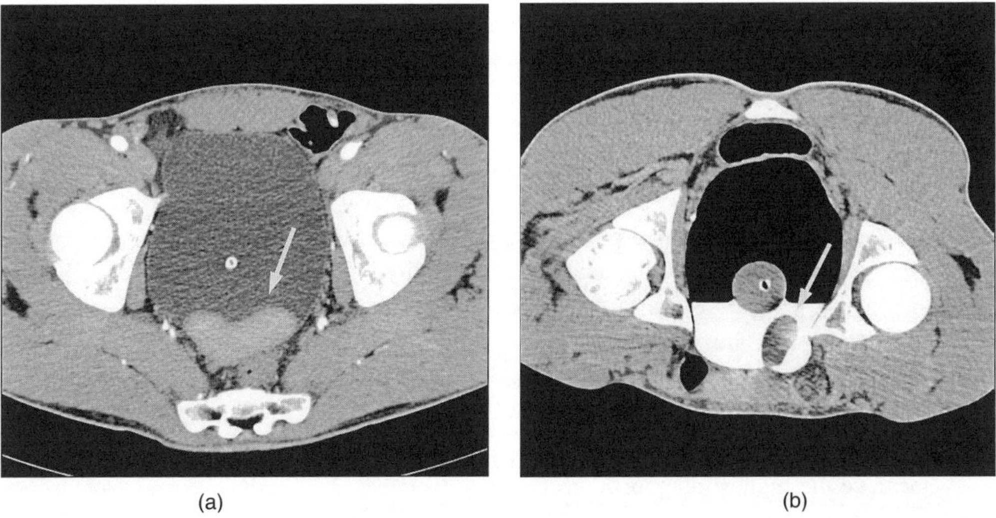

(a)   (b)

Figure 11.10 Hemorrhage may obscure visualization in conventional cystoscopy. (a), (b), imaging of the urinary bladder in the supine and prone position is necessary for visualization of the entire mucosal surface without obscurity caused by residual urine and to avoid that a blood clot is misinterpreted as a tumor (arrows).

- The sensitivity is generally lower than the specificity because of the inability to identify microscopic nodal deposits in normal or minimally enlarged nodes.
- False-negative rates as high as 40% have been recorded.

o **CT Urography (CTU)**

- In the setting of hematuria CTU can be used as a one-stop shop examination to evaluate the entire urinary tract.
- It may evaluate the various causes of hematuria such as urolithiasis, renal parenchymal lesions and urothelial neoplasms.
- In terms of cancer staging, CTU can detect direct perirenal, periureteral, and extravesical tumor spread, as well as lymphadenopathy and distant metastases.
- CTU protocols differ among institutions.
- Precontrast imaging are essential for evaluating urinary calculi.
- They also provide a baseline attenuation measurement for evaluating any incidentally identified lesions of the urinary tract.
- Postcontrast images during the renal parenchymal phase are helpful in the identification of enhancing urothelial lesions, renal cortical masses, and other abdominal/pelvic abnormalities.
- The excretory phase images (achieved with a scan delay of 10 min and more) provide information on enhancing lesions and in demonstrating filling defects caused by tumor.
- Additional delayed images may be performed if the urinary tract is not well distended and opacified.
- Putting the patient in the prone position, applying abdominal compression, or both, may help distend the urinary collecting system.
- The excretory phase images are reconstructed into thin overlapping sections which can be used for three-dimensional post-processing.
- Numerous different image post-processing algorithms are available for CTU (volume rendering, thick slab averaging, or maximum intensity projections).
- The major role of post-processed images is to provide a general overview of the anatomy and accentuate the areas of abnormality.
- Any abnormality visualized on the post-processed images need to be confirmed on the axial source images.
- Three-dimensional images alone have a suboptimal sensitivity in detecting upper tract lesions.
- Axial source images should be viewed with both bone and soft tissue windows to achieve the highest diagnostic accuracy.
- Upper tract TCC most commonly presents as a focal nodular, typically sessile, enhancing lesion (Fig. 11.11)
- Persisting as a filling defect on excretory phase images, or segmental urothelial thickening with enhancement and luminal narrowing (Figs 11.12 and 11.13).
- It can be associated with varying degrees of obstruction.

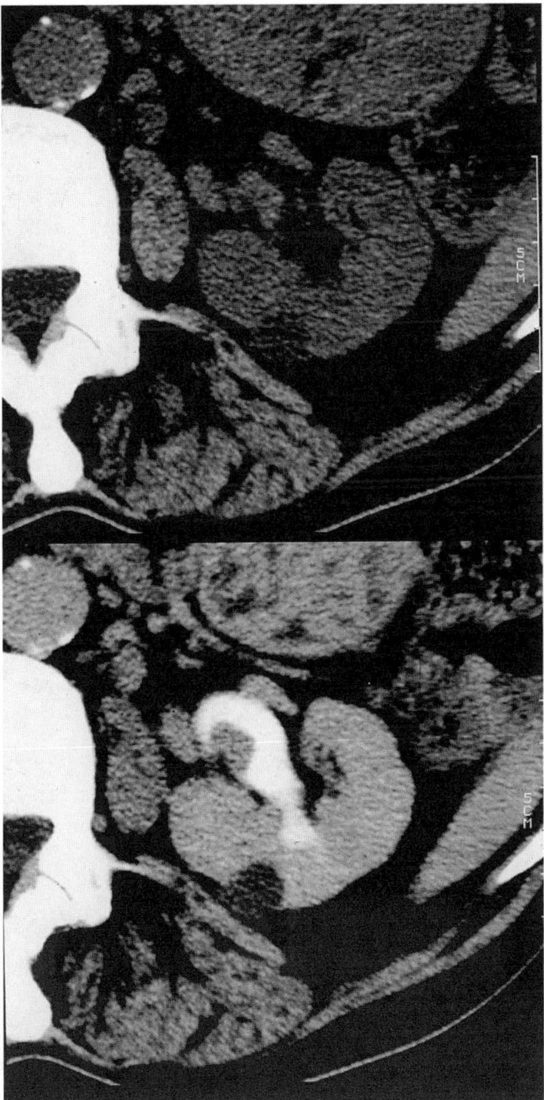

Figure 11.11 69-year-old male patient with proven TCC of the urinary bladder. CT-urography revealed an additional upper tract lesion presenting as a focal nodular lesion and filling defect in the left renal pelvis.

- Benign or inflammatory strictures may show similar findings.
- Irregular, nodular urothelial thickening that increases over time, particularly in the setting of positive urine cytology, raises the suspicion for urothelial cancer.
- **Magnetic Resonance Imaging (MRI)**
  - MRI has an intrinsic high soft tissue contrast and direct multiplanar imaging capabilities.

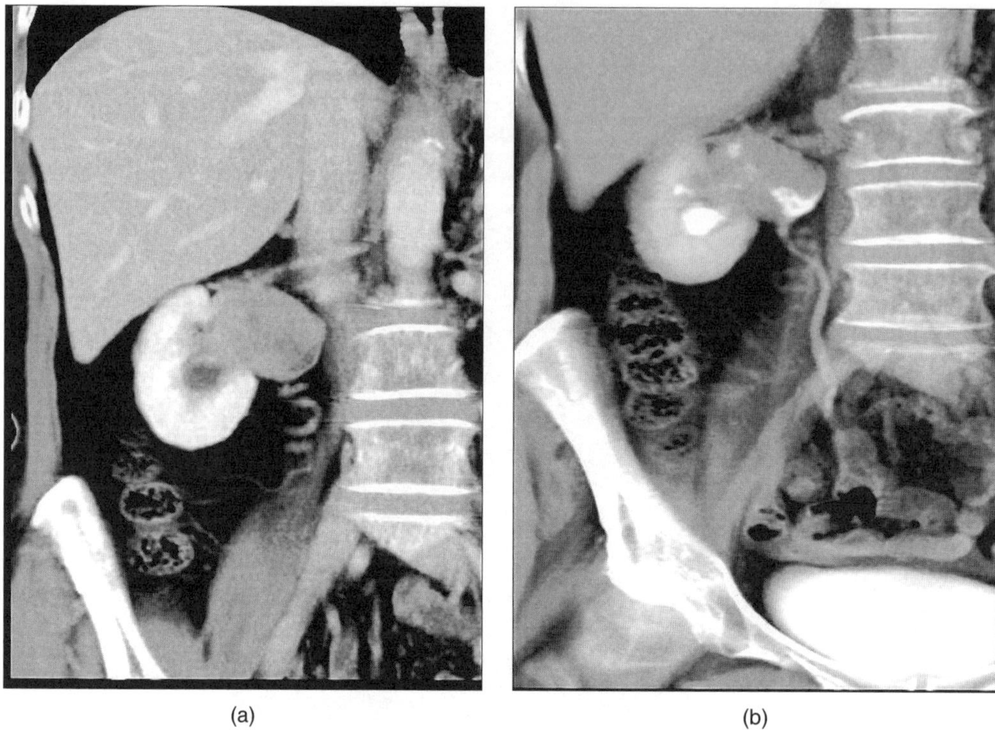

Figure 11.12 Venous phase renal CT in a 73-year-old female patient presenting with flank pain and hematuria shows a large solid mass in the right renal pelvis (a). On CT-Urography filling defects of the right renal pelvis and the pelvicalyceal system can be observed (b).

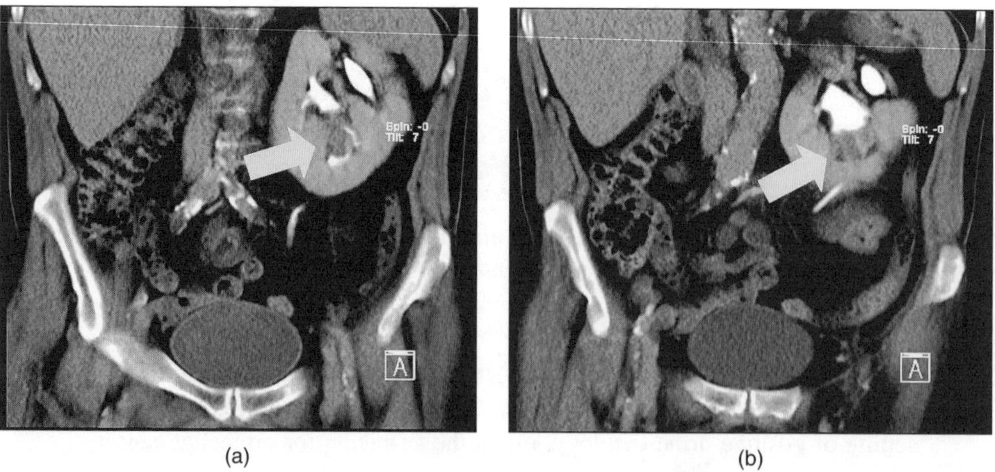

Figure 11.13 On CT-Urography in a 62-year-old male patient with one episode of hematuria minor filling defects of a left sided pancake kidney (a, b) are indicative for a small urothelial lesion. On histopathology a TCC was confirmed.

- Currently state-of-the art MR imaging of bladder masses includes T1-weighted spin echo images of the entire pelvis, T2-weighted fast spin echo images of the bladder in at least two different planes and dynamic contrast-enhanced T1-weighted images.

- Dynamic contrast-enhanced MR imaging yields higher accuracy than other imaging techniques in staging and tumor detection.

- Both overdistension and underdistension of the bladder may affect diagnostic accuracy.

- On MR imaging the normal bladder wall appears as a band of intermediate signal intensity on T1-weighted images and as bands of low (inner muscle layer) and intermediate (outer muscle layer) signal intensity on T2-weighted images.

- The band histologically representing the epithelium and lamina propria is obscured by water on T2-weighted images.

- The band is included on T1-weighted images, thus making the normal bladder wall appear thicker on T1-weighted images compared with T2-weighted images.

- Tumors of the urinary bladder can be detected with MR imaging if they exceed 7–8 mm in diameter.

- On T1-weighted images, the bladder tumor typically has a low-to-intermediate signal intensity (similar to that of the bladder wall and higher than the dark urine) (Fig. 11.14a).

- On T2-weighted images, the tumor tends to have intermediate signal intensity (brighter than the dark bladder wall muscle and lower than the high signal urine) (Fig. 11.14b).

- An intact, low-signal intensity muscle layer at the base of the tumor is indicative of non-muscle invasive bladder tumor of stage Ta or T1.

- Disruption of the muscle layer suggests deep tumor invasion.

- Immediately after intravenous administration of gadolinium contrast agent, tumor, mucosa, and lamina propria show earlier and greater enhancement compared with the muscle layer of the bladder wall (Fig. 11.15).

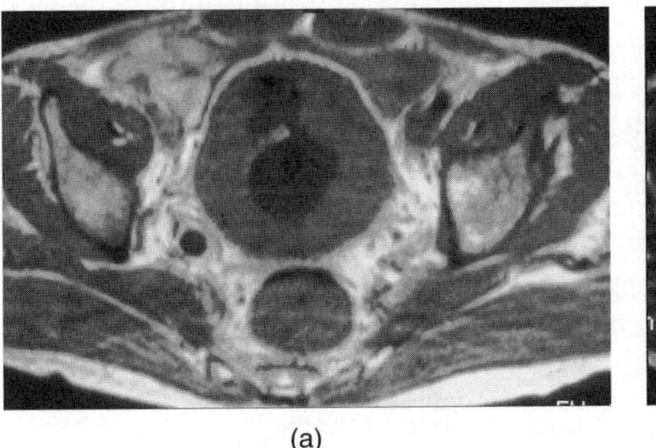

(a)

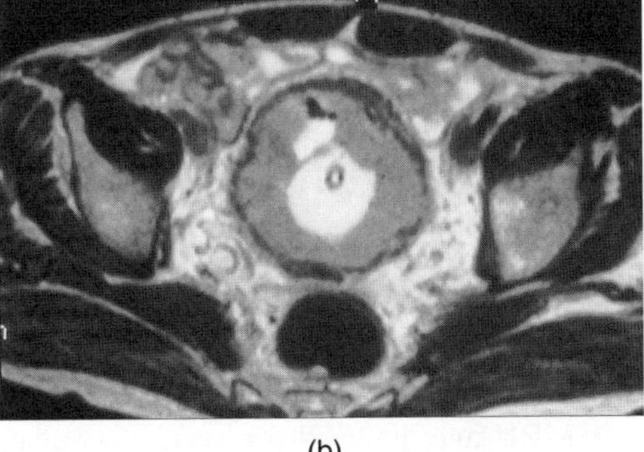

(b)

Figure 11.14 T1w (a) and T2w (b) MR images in a 84-year old male patient show an irregular circular wall thickening of the urinary bladder with disruption of the muscle layer on the left lateral aspect as depicted on the T2w image indicating a muscle invasive bladder cancer.

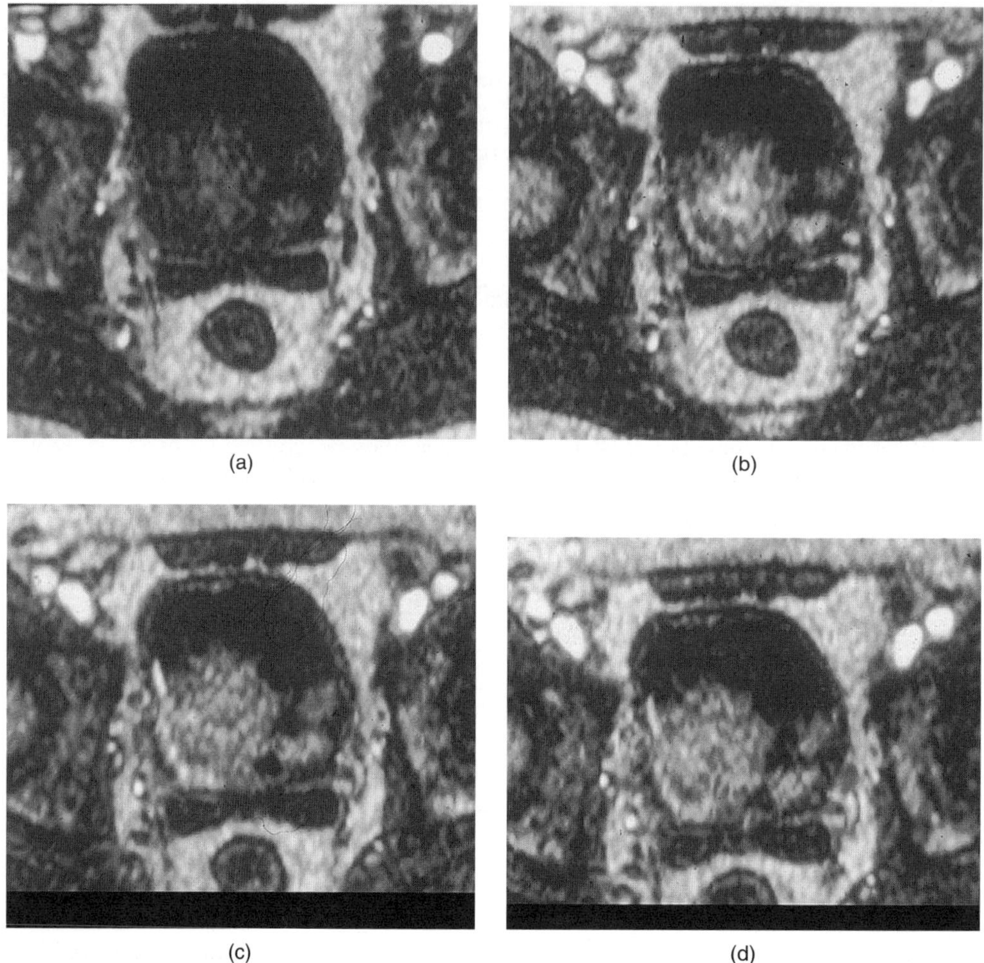

Figure 11.15 Dynamic MRU (a–d) in a patient with a large bladder cancer shows a hypervascularized, huge bladder lesion with infiltration of the muscle layer and infiltration of the perivesical fat on the right lateral aspect.

- A limitation of MR imaging is the differentiation between stages T2 and T3a.
- MRI allows evaluation of involvement of adjacent organs and structures.
- Multiplanar T2 weighted and contrast-enhanced images provide most information.
- Disadvantages of MRI in bladder imaging include poor detection of calcifications and air, and inferior spatial resolution compared with CT.

o **MR Urography**

o MRU may be used for evaluation of upper tract urothelial tumors.

o Can be performed in a static or a dynamic form.

o Static MRU is performed with heavily T2-weighted images.

o Dynamic MRU uses contrast enhanced T1-weighted images.

- A diuretic often is needed for optimal opacification of the collecting system on T1-weighted excretory MRU.

- TCC of the upper tract is lower in signal than water on T2-weighted sequences.

- TCC lesions demonstrate moderate early enhancement after intravenous contrast injection similar to the pattern on CT.

- **Excretory Urography (IVU)**

  - Most used imaging technique for evaluation of the upper urinary tract in the past.

  - Insensitive modality for diagnosis of TCC of the bladder.

  - Bladder cancers more than 1.5 cm in size can be seen on the bladder phase of an excretory urogram.

  - Can detect metachronous lesions in the upper urinary tract.

  - Can be used to detect other abnormalities such as stones or masses that could account for the patients' hematuria.

  - Negative findings cannot exclude urothelial cancer.

- **Ultrasonography**

  - Sonographic detection of bladder tumors depends on the size and location of the neoplasm.

  - Lesions <5 mm in size and tumors located in the bladder neck or dome areas are difficult to detect.

  - Bladder cancer appears as an intraluminal nonmobile mass or focal area of bladder wall thickening.

  - Doppler flow should be used to establish flow within the mass differentiating the mass from sludge and clot.

  - Urinary bladder should be fully distended.

  - The extent of invasion of the bladder wall and extravesicular extension cannot be assessed accurately by transabdominal ultrasound.

  - A few earlier studies reported efficacy of transurethral ultrasound in evaluation of bladder tumors.

- **Nuclear scintigraphy**

  - 18-fluorodeoxyglucose (FDG) is excreted into the collecting system and bladder.

  - Thus, evaluation of bladder cancer by 18-FDG positron emission tomography (PET) is limited.

  - Tracers not excreted in the urine such as 11 C methionine and 11 C choline may be useful for detecting the primary bladder tumor.

  - PET or PET-CT is used in the detection of metastases.

11.5 Treatment planning

- The treatment and prognosis of urinary bladder carcinoma is largely determined by the depth of tumor growth and the extent of tumor metastases.

  - Bladder saving treatment is used for superficial tumors (stages Ta–T1).

- o Radical cystectomy is performed for stage T2–T3b tumors.

- o Palliative radiation and chemotherapy is the treatment for stage T4a and T4b tumors and for metastatic disease.

- o CT plays an important role for patients selected for external beam irradiation
  - determining tumor extent
  - providing an accurate cross-sectional display of the tumor and related normal anatomy
  - superiority of CT integrated planning over conventional techniques in tumor localization,

11.6 Post-treatment Imaging

- Imaging of bladder cancer after recent treatment is challenging.

- Intravesical medication and transurethral resection or biopsy often cause inflammation and edema.

- Avid mucosal and submucosal enhancement after intravenous contrast administration can be observed.

- It is not possible on CT or MRI to distinguish edema, fibrosis, or recurrent or persistent tumor on the basis of CT attenuation values.

- CT may be required for restaging or to identify a recurrence in patients suspected or harboring progressive disease.

- Multiagent systemic chemotherapy using cisplatin/methotrexate-based regimens is currently employed in patients with inoperable advanced tumors.

- An objective response to treatment is achieved in up to 50% of patients.

- CT is an ideal method of follow-up.

- CT shows reduction in tumor volume.

- In some patients complete resolution of tumor is observed.

11.7 Summary

- Bladder cancer is the most common cause of painless hematuria.

- Evaluation of painless hematuria should include historical information, clinical evaluation, and laboratory testing with emphasis on urinalysis, urine culture, and urine cytology.

- Initial investigation includes lower urinary tract endoscopy followed by TUR in case of endoscopic visualization of a bladder tumor.

- TUR is a bladder-saving treatment for superficial tumors (stages Ta–T1).

- Imaging studies are required both in patients with negative cystoscopic findings and in patients with proven bladder cancer.

- CTU and contrast-enhanced dynamic MRU are most sensitive for evaluation of the upper urinary tract, contrast-enhanced MDCT and MRI tend to be equal in local staging of bladder cancer.

- Virtual endoscopic imaging proves to be a useful adjunct in imaging studies.

References

Sorahan, T, Lancashire RJ, Sole G (1994) Urothelial cancer and cigarette smoking: findings from a regional case controlled study. *Br. J. Urol.* **74**: 753–756.

Lamm DL, Griffith G, Pettit LL, 3 *et al.* (1992) Current perspectives on diagnosis and treatment of superficial bladder cancer. *Urology* **39**: 301–307.

Pode D, Fair W (1987) The development of bladder cancer. *AUA Update* **7**: 40.

Soloway MS (1985) Flexible cystourethroscopy: alternative to rigid instruments for evaluation of the lower urinary tract. *Urology* **25**: 472–474.

WongYou-Cheong JJ, Wagner BJ, Davis CJ (1998) Transitional cell carcinoma of the urinary tract: radiologic-pathologic correlation. *RadioGraphics* **18**: 123–142.

Song JH, Francis IR, Plat JF, Cohan RH, Mohsin J, Kielb SJ, Korobkin M, Montie JE (2001) Bladder tumor detection at virtual cystoscopy. *Radiology* **218**: 95–100.

Kim JK, Ahn JH, Park T, Ahn HJ, Kim CS, Cho KS (2002) Virtual cystoscopy of the contrast material-filled bladder in patients with gross hematuria. *Am. J. Roentgenol.* **179**: 763–768.

Stenzl A, Frank R, Eder R, Recheis W, Knapp R, Zur Nedden D, Bartsch G (1998) 3-dimensional computerized tomography and virtual reality endoscopy of the reconstructed lower urinary tract. *J. Urol.* **159**: 741–746.

Barentsz JO, Debruyne FMJ, Ruijs SHJ (1990) *Magnetic Resonance Imaging of Carcinoma of the Urinary Bladder*. Kluwer, Dordrecht, Boston, London.

Tachibana M, Baba S, Deguchi N *et al.* Efficacy of gadolinium-diethylene-triaminepentaacetic acid-enhanced magnetic resonance imaging for differentiation between superficial and muscle-invasive tumor of the bladder: a comparative study with computerized tomography and transurethral ultrasonography. *J. Urol.* **145**: 1169–1173.

Zhang J, Gerst S, Lefkowitz RA, Bach A (2007) Imaging of bladder cancer. *Radiol. Clin. N. Am.* **45**: 183–205.

12
Imaging of Urinary Diversion

Sameh Hanna[1] and Hesham Badawy[2]

[1] *Radiology Department, Cairo University*
[2] *Urology Departments, Cairo University*

12.1 Introduction

The term urinary diversion means diversion of the urinary stream away from the natural outlet. Famous forms of diversions include cutaneous vesicostomy, pyelostomy and loop ureterostomy. Nowadays, the term urinary diversion is most commonly used to describe the reconstruction of the lower urinary tract by the interposition of bowel segments and re-routing the constructed conduit or reservoir either to the skin or along natural orifices.

12.2 Indications for urinary diversion

- Post-cystectomy

- Neurogenic bladder dysfunction

- Congenital deformities as bladder or cloacal extrophy

- Traumatic injury of the bladder that may necessitate formation of a urinary diversion.

12.3 Types of urinary diversion

There are several types of urinary diversion procedures and description of all the techniques involved is beyond the scope of the chapter. Focus here is on presenting the concepts involved in the evolution and construction of important techniques of urinary diversions.

Urogenital Imaging: A Problem-oriented Approach   Edited by Sameh K. Morcos and Henrik S. Thomsen
© 2009 John Wiley & Sons, Ltd

The evolution of lower urinary tract reconstruction has developed along four distinct paths:

1. A non-continent cutaneous form of urinary diversion (ileal or colon conduit).

2. A continent cutaneous form of urinary diversion (continent catheterizing pouches).

3. Non-orthotopic continent diversion, relying on the anal sphincter for continence.

4. Orthotopic form of diversion to the native, intact urethra (neobladder).

12.4 Non-continent cutaneous form of diversion

- Diversion into a non-continent conduit is technically less difficult and associated with few postoperative complications.

- A 10–15 cm segment of the ileum or colon is commonly used.

- In the case of ileum, the segment should be at least 15 cm proximal to the ileocecal junction.

- The ureters are usually anastomosed to the proximal end while the distal end is anastomosed to the skin forming an abdominal wall stoma.

- The segment is placed in a properistaltic manner to promote urine drainage and minimize reflux.

- In the case of ileum, direct anastomosis of the ureters is carried out without any attempt at antireflux.

- In the case of colonic conduits, the tenia coli are used for antireflux reimplantation of the ureters.

12.5 Continent cutaneous urinary diversion (*Continent Catheterizing Pouches*)

In this type of diversion a continent reservoir (pouch) is constructed in which urine accumulates and is emptied at intervals by self-catheterization of the pouch through a continent skin stoma. The techniques include:

- **Mitrofanoff technique (Fig. 12.1)**

  o This is based on the implantation of a tubular structure as the appendix into a submucosal channel of a low-pressure reservoir.

  o The reservoir could be the native bladder or a pouch constructed from a bowel segment.

  o When the appendix is not available, a tube could be constructed from a short segment of ileum.

  o The Mitrofanoff technique has found wide application in pediatric urology in patients with neurogenic bladder dysfunction with:

    ▪ Difficulty in accessing urethral opening.
    ▪ Total incontinence that requires closure of the bladder neck.

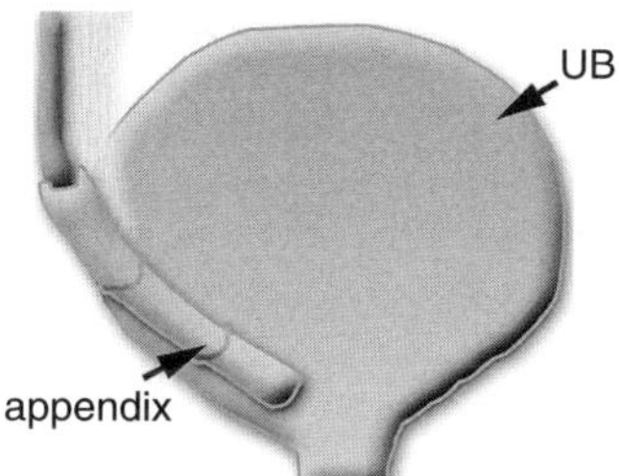

Figure 12.1   Mitrofanoff procedure. The urinary bladder (UB) is the reservoir with submucosal implantation of the appendix in the bladder wall. The appendix is used as the continent channel for self-catheterization.

- **Indiana Pouch**

  o The reservoir is constructed from the detubularized ascending colon with or without the incorporation of an ileal patch.

  o The catheterizable channel is constructed from the terminal ileum just proximal to the ileocecal valve.

  o The continence mechanism relies on tapering the ileal catheterizing channel and the reinforcement of the ileocecal valve.

- **Kock's Pouch (Fig. 12.2)**

  o The pouch is fashioned from a 40 cm segment of ileum 15–20 cm proximal to the ileo-cecal valve. Two one-way nipple valves, and their associated ileal limbs, are constructed in this procedure.

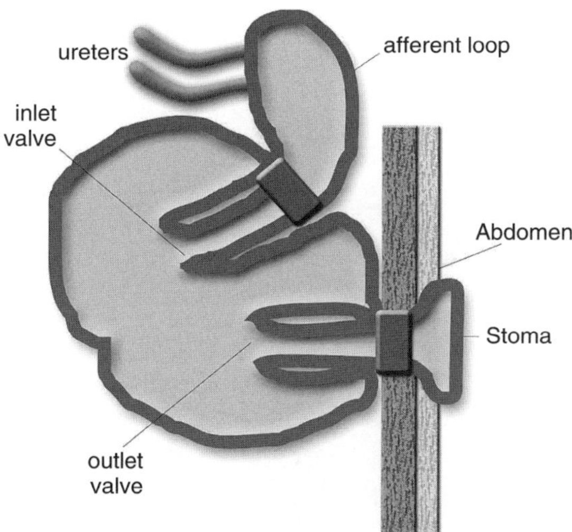

Figure 12.2   Kock's pouch. The pouch is fashioned from a 40 cm segment of ileum. The two ileal segments on either side of the reservoir are intussuscepted into the pouch and stapled into place, forming one-way nipple valves. The efferent limb is externalized via a flush abdominal wall stoma in the right lower part of the abdomen. The ureters are implanted at the proximal end of the afferent limb.

- o The two ileal segments on either side of the reservoir are intussuscepted into the pouch and stapled into place, forming one-way nipple valves.

- o The associated non-intussuscepted ileal portions are the afferent and efferent ileal loops. The efferent limb is externalized via a flush abdominal wall stoma in the right lower part of the abdomen.

- o The ureters are implanted at the proximal end of the afferent limb.

12.6 Non-orthotopic continent diversion, relying on the anal sphincter for continence

Ureterosigmoidostomy

- The ureters are anastomosed to the sigmoid colon using the tenia coli for creating an antireflux flap valve mechanism.

- The sigmoid acts as the reservoir, while continence relies on the anal sphincter.

Folded Rectosigmoid Bladder (Fig. 12.3)

- A folded rectosigmoid bladder is constructed with the ureters anastomosed into serosal troughs rather than into the taenia.

- It has the advantage of a larger sigmoid reservoir and the use of the serous lined tunnel or trough to prevent reflux.

- It appears to have a lower complication rate than that associated with direct taenial implantation.

  Ureterosigmoidostomy is associated with the following complications:

- Hyperchloremic acidosis

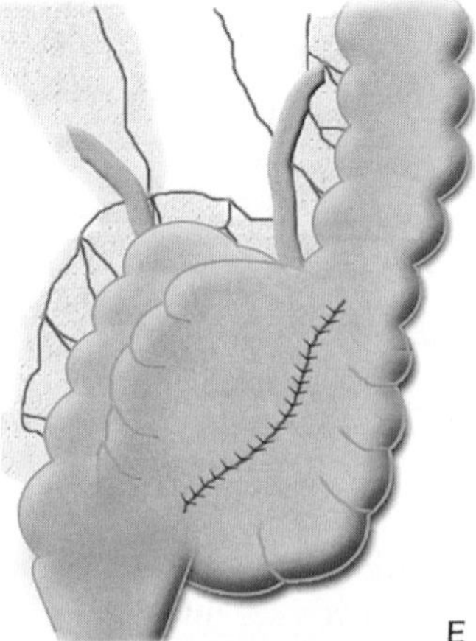

Figure 12.3   Folded rectosigmoid bladder. A folded rectosigmoid bladder is constructed with the ureters anastomosed into serosal troughs rather than into the taenia.

- Hypokalemia with nephropathy
- Pyelonephritis
- The development of colonic malignancy
- Kidneys tend to fail over time.

Careful selection of patients for continent diversion by ureterosigmoidostomy is crucial and this form of urinary diversion is not suitable for:

- Young patients because of the potentially long-term complications.
- Patients with neurogenic bladder because possible associated anal sphincter dysfunction.
- Individuals with dilated ureters owing to the increased risk for development of reflux and urinary infection.
- Patients with renal impairment.

12.7 Orthotopic form of diversion to the native, intact urethra (neobladder)

The success of any continent urinary diversion depends on construction of a large reservoir that can accommodate a large volume of urine under low pressure and not associated with ureteric reflux or absorption of urinary constituents. Continent urinary diversion includes the following operations:

Camey I

A segment of ileum 40 cm in length is detached from the intestinal tract and its midpoint sutured to the membranous urethra. One ureter is implanted into each end of the reservoir.

Camey II (Fig. 12.4)

It is a modification of the original Camey I and involves detubularization and folding to eliminate peristaltic activity. The Camey II has subsequently been modified to provide better functional results.

Ileal Neobladder (Hautmann) (Fig. 12.5)

A 40 cm segment of distal ileum is isolated and arranged in a W shaped pouch. A non-refluxing technique is used for the uretero-ileal anastomosis. This neobladder has a large-capacity which is important to reduce night-time incontinence.

Studer Ileal Bladder Substitute (Fig. 12.6)

The ileal bladder substitute has become a popular orthotopic form of diversion and is characterized by a long, afferent, isoperistaltic, tubular ileal segment.

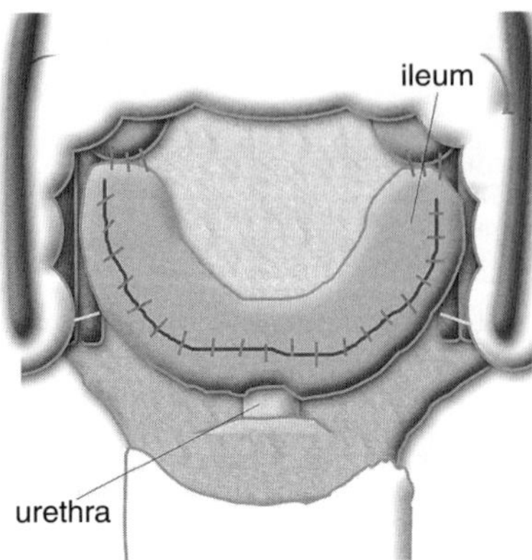

Figure 12.4 Camey II. A long ileal segment is necessary to construct the neobladder. The U-shaped neobladder properly fits into the pelvis and at its midpoint is anastomosed to the membranous urethra. One ureter is implanted into each end of the reservoir.

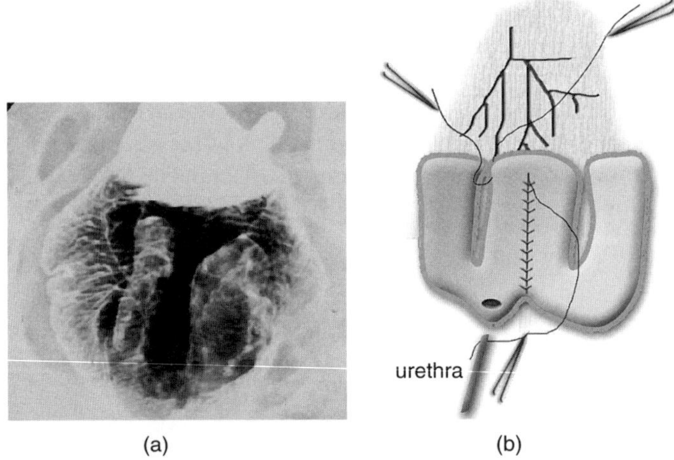

Figure 12.5 Ileal neobladder (Hautmann). The technique entails the creation of two serous-lined extramural tunnels in a detubularized ileal W-shaped bladder fashioned from 40 cm of the terminal ileum. Its advantage is to achieve a globular configuration of the neobladder and provides two serous-lined troughs for antireflux ureteral implantation (a). Double contrast pouchogram demonstrates two troughs within a globular shaped neobladder (b). (Courtesy of Prof. Tarek El Diasty, Nephrology and Urology Centre, Mansoura, Egypt.)

Orthotopic Kock's Ileal Reservoir (Fig. 12.7)

- The Kock ileal reservoir was first employed as a continent cutaneous ileal reservoir incorporating intussuscepted nipple valves for both the afferent (antireflux) and efferent (continence) limbs.

- This subsequently evolved into an orthotopic form of diversion in which the afferent intussuscepted limb was maintained to prevent urinary reflux.

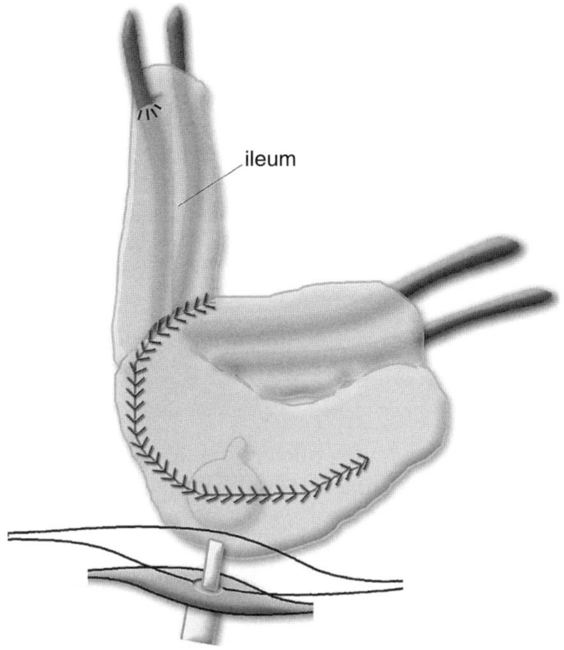

Figure 12.6   Studer bladder. The neobladder consists of two parts: a detubularized ileal spherical reservoir and an afferent antireflux ileal loop that receives both ureters.

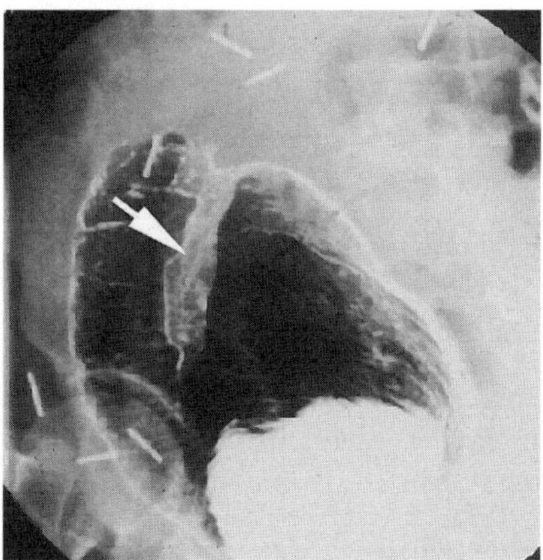

Figure 12.7   Orthotopic Kock's ileal reservoir. Double contrast pouchogram of urethral Kock's pouch showing ileal mucosal coating and the nipple valve (arrow) into which the ureters are implanted. (Courtesy of Prof. Tarek El Diasty, Nephrology and Urology Centre, Mansoura, Egypt.)

T-Pouch Ileal Neobladder (Fig. 12.8)

- The orthotopic T-pouch ileal neobladder maintains exactly the same geometric configuration as the Kock ileal neobladder, the only difference being the antireflux technique.

- The functional characteristics includes a large-capacity, low-pressure urinary reservoir.

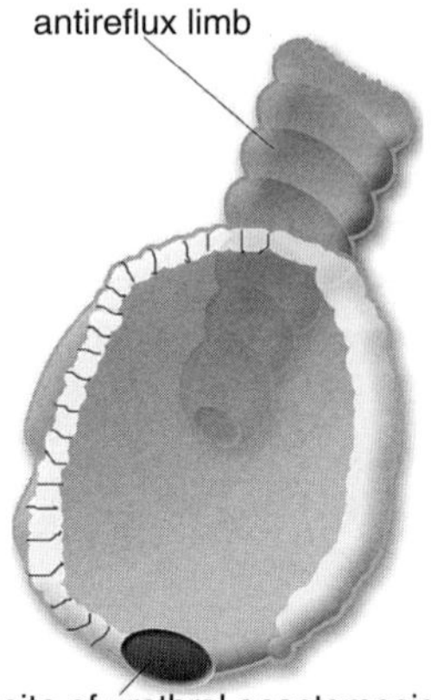

Figure 12.8   T-pouch. The T-pouch is constructed from a 44 cm ileal segment which forms the reservoir portion of the pouch, and a proximal 8–10 cm segment of ileum to form the antireflux limb.

- The unique aspect of the T-pouch surgical technique it allows permanent fixation of a segment of ileum within a serous-lined ileal trough creating an effective flap-valve technique without compromising the blood supply of the ileal segment.

12.8 Contraindications to urinary diversion

- Bowel-related contraindications
  - Refractory metabolic abnormalities, in these patients jejunal segments should be used only in the absence of another acceptable type of bowel segment.
  - Bowel abnormalities:
    - Post-radiation
    - Inflammatory bowel disease (Crohn disease, ulcerative colitis, severe irritable bowel syndrome)
    - Malabsorption.
- Poor hand coordination (e.g. elderly patients, cervical spinal cord damage) is an absolute contraindication for continent urinary diversion including neobladder.
- Patients with poor renal function (preoperative creatinine clearance less than 60 ml/min) or significant proteinuria.
- Patients with lack of motivation to catheterize their reservoirs as well as those who are not willing to accept some degree of incontinence that may be associated with orthotopic reservoirs are not good candidate for continent diversion.

12.9 Complications of urinary diversions

- Postoperative complications
  - Paralytic ileus

- ○ Anastomotic leak
- ○ Urinary tract infection
- ○ Pelvic or retroperitoneal infection
- ○ Postoperative fluid collections such as urinomas, hematomas, and lymphoceles
- ○ Ischemia and infarction of the constructed reservoir.

- Late complications

- ○ Deterioration of renal function
- ○ Ureteric reflux (Figs 12.9 and 12.10)

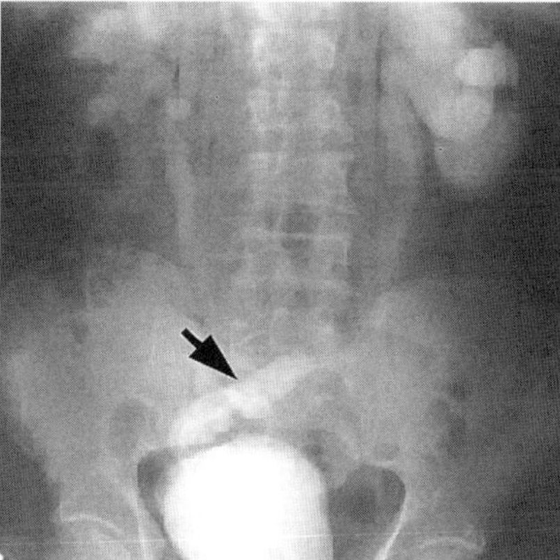

Figure 12.9 Retrograde pouchgram. Pouchgram showing bilateral ureteric reflux in a patient with orthotopic Kock's ileal reservoir. The afferent loop of the pouch which is anastomosed to the ureters is shown (arrow). Bilateral hydronephrotic changes are present.

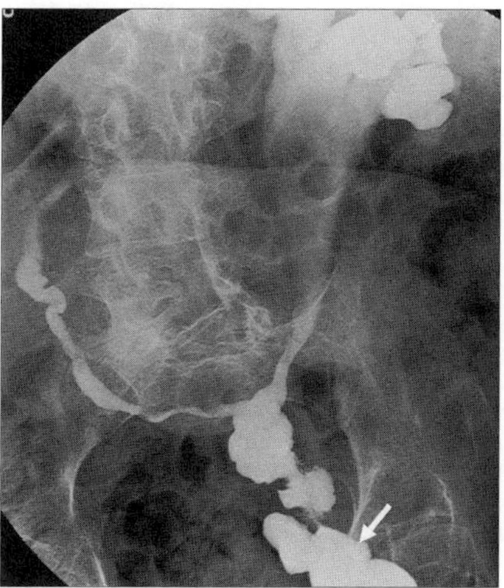

Figure 12.10 Loopgram. A retrograde loopgram showing the ileal loop (arrow) and bilateral ureteric reflux. The left kidney is grossly hydronephrotic. (Courtesy of Prof. S K Morcos, Sheffield, UK.)

- o Hydronephrosis
- o Stone formation
- o Strictures (Figs 12.11–12.13)
- o Pouch necrosis

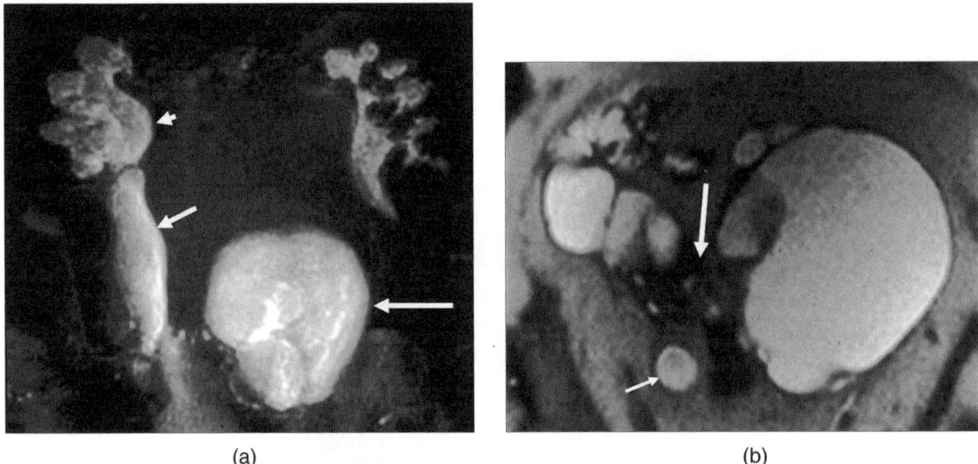

(a)   (b)

Figure 12.11 Stricture complicating colonic conduit urinary diversion. (a) T2 MRU (coronal image, MIP) of a patient the colonic conduit (long arrow) who developed stricture at the site of the anastomosis of the right ureter causing gross right hydroureter (short arrow) and hydronephrosis of the right kidney (arrow head). (b) T2 MRU axial image showing the site of the stricture of the colonic conduit (long arrow) and the dilated right ureter (short arrow). (Courtesy of Prof. S K Morcos, Sheffield, UK.)

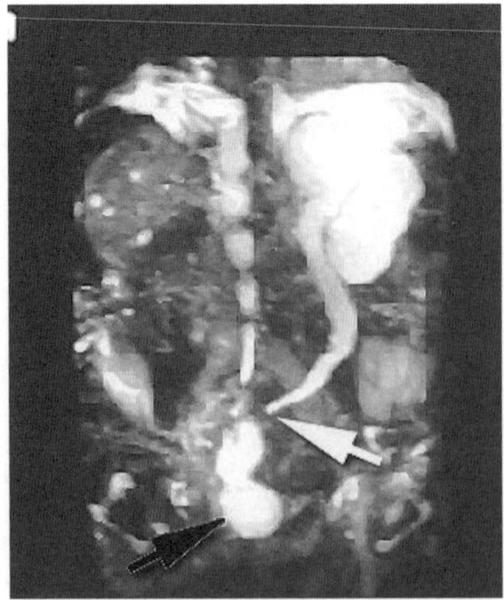

Figure 12.12 Uretric stricture posturinary diversion. T2 MRU (coronal image MIP) of a patient post cystectomy and orthotopic neobladder showing left ureteric stricture (arrow) associated with gross left hydronephrosis.

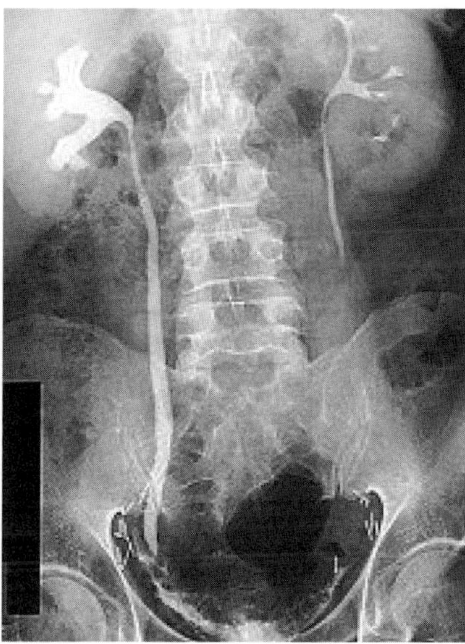

Figure 12.13 Intravenous urogram demonstrating a stricture at the lower end of the right ureter in a patient with ileal neobladder.

- ○ Retroperitoneal fibrosis
- ○ Tumor recurrence remains the most ominous late complication of cystectomy for bladder cancer and may present as an obstructing ureteral stricture, pelvic lymphadenopathy, and pelvic soft-tissue mass
- ○ Patients with a jejunal conduit may develop hyperkalemic, hypochloremic, hyponatremic metabolic acidosis
- ○ Patients with ileal conduits, colonic conduits, or continent reservoirs tend to present with hyperchloremic metabolic acidosis with normal or low potassium levels
- ○ Patients who have undergone ileal resection for diversion may present with megaloblastic anemia due to vitamin B12 deficiency
- ○ Patients with continent reservoirs are at risk of suffering from diarrhea, depending on the length of ileum used for the urinary diversion and whether or not the ileocecal valve was resected for construction of the urinary pouch.

12.10 The role of radiologist in urinary diversion includes:

- Pre-operative
  - ○ Evaluation of the urinary tract.
- Early postoperative
  - ○ Determine the integrity of the diversion.
  - ○ Detect any complications such as leaks from the pouch or at the sites of the anastomosis.

- Regular follow-up

  - Assess the capacity of the reservoirs.

  - The presence of ureteric reflux

  - Monitor upper tract changes.

  - Detect potential complications of the procedure.

12.11 Imaging studies

Pre-operative

- Having established the need for a urinary diversion it is important to have a baseline evaluation of the upper urinary tract. This would be helpful in monitoring changes that may develop in the future.

- Renal ultrasound and excretory urography whether with traditional intravenous urography (IVU) or CT urography (CTU) are very useful in this regard.

Postoperative

- *Intravenous urography (IVU)* and *retrograde loopogram* or *pouchography* are the two main imaging methods used for evaluating the urinary diversions.

  - The neobladder can have various shapes but is usually round or oval. The afferent segment is usually seen in the right lower quadrant and maintains a normal ileal mucosal fold pattern (Fig. 12.9). Minimal to mild dilatation of the upper urinary tract can be normal.

- *CTU* is a superior alternative to IVU allowing excellent evaluation of the urinary tract and the integrity of the urinary diversion with multiplanar and 3D imaging (Fig. 12.14).

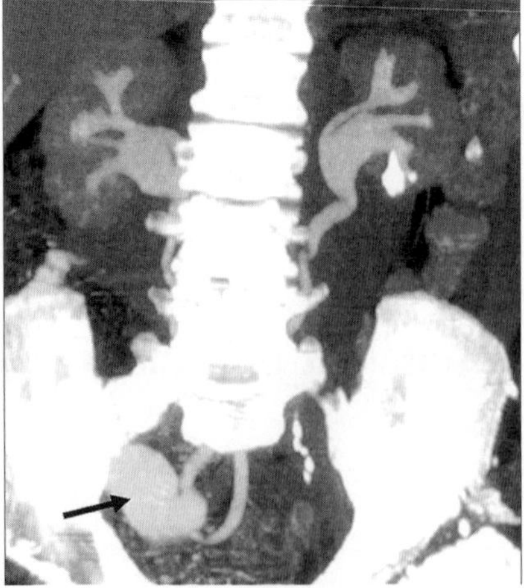

Figure 12.14   CT urography (thick coronal slab, MIP) demonstrating the anastomosis of the ureters to the blind end of the ileal loop (arrow). Normal kidneys and ureters are shown. (Courtesy of Prof. S K Morcos, Sheffield, UK.)

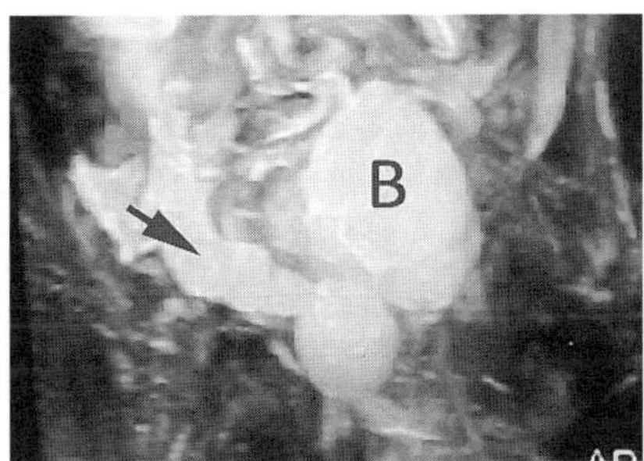

Figure 12.15   T2 MRU (coronal, MIP) showing the afferent segment (arrow) of Studer orthotopic neobladder (B). The neobladder capacity is usually small in the early postoperative period. The MRU was performed one week after the operation.

- *MRU* whether T2 weighted or excretory is an effective alternative to IVU or CTU in patients with contraindications to the use of ionizing radiation or use of iodinated contrast agents (Figs 12.11, 12.12 and 12.15).

- *^{99m}Tc-MAG 3* can offer important information about the function of the upper urinary tract and detect the presence of obstructive uropathy.

- *Ultrasound* is very useful in monitoring the kidneys and detecting hydronephrotic changes.

- *Urodynamic studies* of continent bowel segments can be helpful in the evaluation of patients with a continent urinary diversion and unrelenting incontinence.

12.12 Imaging of complications

Postoperative complications (extravasation, urinoma, haematoma)

CT is the modality of choice to assess extravasation and abnormal fluid collection such as urinomas or hematomas.

Hydronephrosis

- Minimal to mild dilatation of the upper tract can normally be seen postoperatively and remains stable on follow-up. Gross dilatation should raise the suspicion of obstruction usually caused by tumor recurrence or ureteral stricture.

- Hydronephrotic changes detected by ultrasound should be followed by an excretory urogram and or retrograde loopgram/pouchgram to determine the cause of dilatation of the upper urinary tract (Figs 12.9 and 12.10).

Complications of the urinary diversion system (rupture, dehiscence, reflux, stricture)

- *Retrograde pouchgram* can be carried out routinely after 2 weeks post-surgery to assess the presence of valve dysfunction, resulting in reflux (Fig. 12.9) or urinary incontinence.

- Distension of the continent reservoir with contrast is indicated when the patient is thought to have a ruptured segment. Assessing the reservoir in at least two views and ensuring that the conduit is adequately distended are imperative.

- Real-time imaging is important which allows the reservoir to be monitored throughout the entire distension phase.

- *Double contrast pouchgram* (Figs 12.5b and 12.7)

  - The pouch is filled with 50 ml of barium suspension (3 gm/ml) through a Foley catheter. Patient is asked to rotate several times to ensure mucosal coating with barium. The pouch is then inflated with air to achieve clear visualization of nipple valves.

- *Loopogram* (Fig. 12.10)

  - A Foley catheter of suitable size (10F) is inserted into the stoma, its balloon inflated and then retracted to the stomal site. Under fluoroscopic guidance, water-soluble iodinated contrast medium (200–300 mgI/ml) is injected into the Foley catheter to fill the loop until ureteric reflux is induced. Spot films are taken during the filling and a delayed radiograph of the whole abdomen is taken 20–30 min after removal of the catheter from the loop to assess the drainage of the upper tract and exclude the possibility of stricture at the uretero-ileal anastomosis. Oblique films are important for accurate assessment of the uretero-ileal anastomosis.

- *Micturating ileo-urethrography* is useful to assess the ileo-urethral anastomosis (Fig. 12.16).

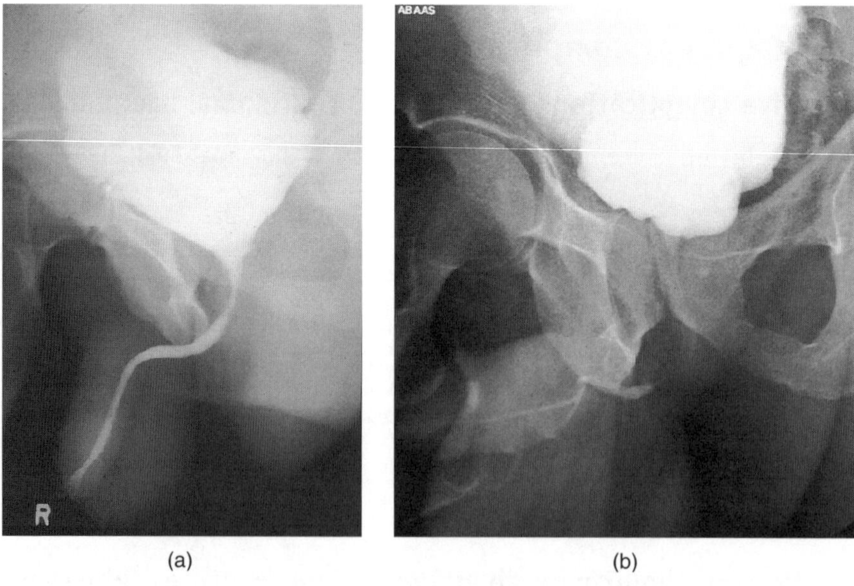

(a)   (b)

Figure 12.16   Micturating cystourethrogram showing different patterns of voiding in two patients with ileal neobladder. (a) Normal voiding pattern showing funneling at the ileo-urethral anastomosis and good urethral filling. (b) Ileo-urethral stricture showing poor urethral filling and difficulty in emptying the neobladder.

Urinary calculi

Imaging of stones of the urinary tract has been covered in details in Chapter 9 on urolithiasis.

12.13 Summary

- Several procedures are available for urinary diversion.

- The radiologists play an important role in the pre- and postoperative management of patients considered for urinary diversion.

- Excretory urography (IVU or CTU), retrograde loopgram/pouchgram and renal ultrasound are the main imaging techniques used for evaluating the urinary tract in patients with urinary diversion.

- Close cooperation between the urologist and radiologist is crucial for effective management of these patients.

Acknowledgement

We thank Drs. Nadine Barsoum and Mona Fouad of the Radiology Department of Cairo University, Egypt for their assistance with the medical illustrations.

References

Bissada NK (1995) Continent cutaneous diversion using the ileocecal segment. In Crawford ED and Das S (eds), *Current Genitourinary Cancer Surgery*, 2nd edn. Lea & Fabiger, Philadelphia, pp 414–425.

Elmajian DA, Stein JP, Esrig D *et al.* (1996) The Kock ileal neobladder: updated experience in 295 male patients. *J. Urol.* **156**: 920–925.

Ghoneim MA, el-Mekresh MM, el-Baz MA, el-Attar IA, Ashamallah A (1997) Radical cystectomy for carcinoma of the bladder: critical evaluation of the results in 1026 cases. *J. Urol.* **158**(2): 393–399.

Heaney MD, Francis IR, Cohan RH *et al.* (1999) Orthotopic neobladder reconstruction: findings on excretory urography and CT. *AJR* **172**: 1213–1220.

Stein JP, Skinner DG (2002) Orthotopic urinary diversion. In Retik AB, Vaughan ED, Wein AJ (eds) *Campbell's Urology,* 8th edn. Saunders, Philadelphia, PA, pp. 3835–3867.

Studer UE, Zingg EJ (1997) Ileal orthotopic bladder substitutes: what we have learned from 12 years experience with 200 patients. *Urol. Clin. N. Am.* **24**: 781–793.

Sudakoff G, Guralnick M, Langenstroer P, Foley D, Cihlar K, Shakespear J and See W (2005) CT urography of urinary diversions with enhanced CT digital radiography: preliminary experience. *AJR* **184**: 131–138.

13
Imaging of the Prostate Gland

Dr François Cornud

Consultant Radiologist, Service de Radiologie B (Pr Chevrot), Paris

13.1 Introduction

Imaging of the prostate gland improved considerably in the late 1980s when the transrectal approach started to be used for high resolution ultrasonography and Magnetic Resonance Imaging (MRI). Description of the zonal anatomy, according to the model of Mc Neal, became possible. Considerable synergy also came at the same period with the concomitant development of the PSA assay and the possibility to perform prostate biopsies under TRUS guidance with the biopty gun. The PSA era started which opened the way to the early diagnosis of prostate cancer (Pca) while MRI, in addition to its established ability to assess local extension, extended its capabilities to detect lymph node and bone extension of a newly diagnosed Pca.

13.2 Zonal anatomy and benign prostatic hypertrophy

It seems preferable to describe imaging of the normal prostate together with that of benign prostatic hypertrophy, because asymptomatic BPH can be considered as a physiological status in men over 40 years.

Zonal anatomy (Fig. 13.1)

- The prostate has three glandular zones located around two ductal structures (proximal urethra and ejaculatory ducts) (Fig. 13.1). In the absence of benign prostatic hyperplasia (BPH), the transion zone (TZ) only represents 5% of the glandular mass. The central zone (CZ) and the peripheral zone represent 25% and 75% of the glandular mass, respectively.

Urogenital Imaging: A Problem-oriented Approach Edited by Sameh K. Morcos and Henrik S. Thomsen
© 2009 John Wiley & Sons, Ltd

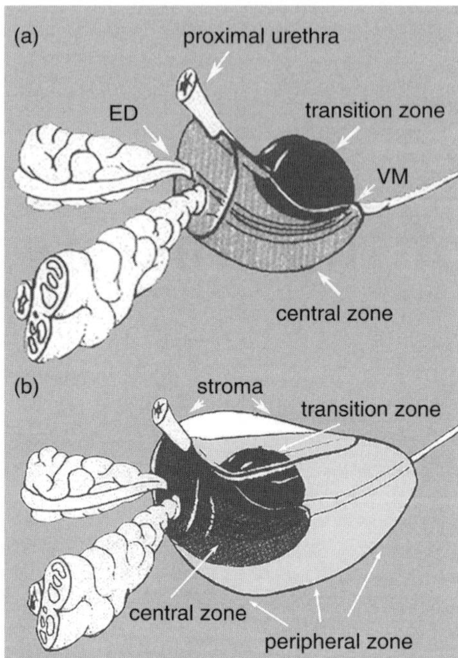

Figure 13.1   (a) The transition zone is around the proximal urethra. The central zone is around the ejaculatory ducts (ED). Its vertex is located at the level of the veru-montanum (VM). (b) The peripheral zone is posteriorly and laterally located covering the central zone at the prostate base and extends caudally to the apex. The anterior fibromuscular stroma covers the anterior aspect of the prostate.

- Zonal anatomy delineates two distinct areas (Fig. 13.2): the inner gland (TZ) and the outer gland (CZ + PZ). The most frequent affection of the inner gland is BPH whereas the most frequent affections of the outer gland are prostatitis and prostate cancer.

TRUS features of the normal prostate and BPH

- Normal prostate. The peripheral zone (Fig. 13.3) is posteriorly located and has a homogeneous pattern. Its echotexture is the reference to define hypo- or hyperechogenicity. At the prostate base (Fig. 13.4), the central is not detectable (same echostucture as that of the PZ). Above the prostate base are located the seminal vesicles and the ampullae of the vas deferens (Fig. 13.5).

- Benign prostatic hyperplasia

  - BPH has a heterogeneous pattern, commonly combined with a nodular pattern (Fig. 13.6a). Pure stromal nodules are very homogeneous and well marginated (Fig. 13.6b).

  - Other common findings in BPH are cystic glandular dilatation and corporea amylacea (Fig. 13.6c).

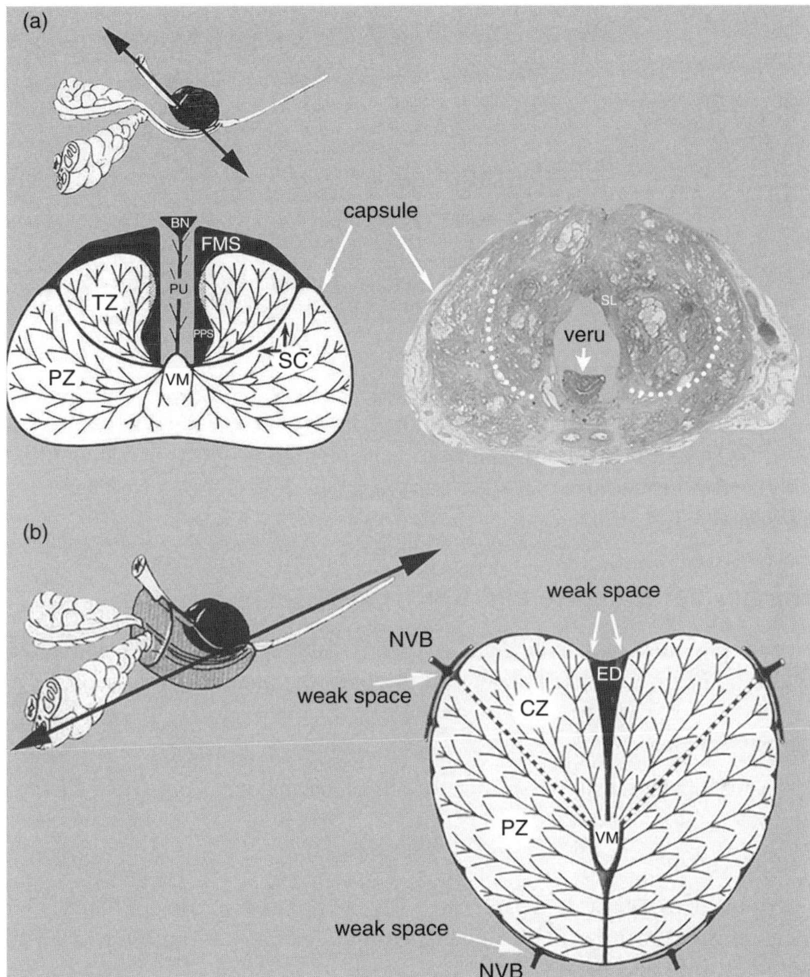

Figure 13.2 Relationships between the three zones. (a) Axial oblique section. The anatomical boundaries of the TZ are solid: the surgical capsule posteriorly (SC and white dots on the specimen), the prostatic capsule anterolaterally, the fibromuscular stroma anteriorly (FMS) and the preprostatic sphincter medially (PPS). Note the veru montanum (VM), key land mark of the zonal anatomy. (b) Coronal section, through the axis of the ejaculatory ducts. The CZ and PZ are contiguous without visible border (black dotted line). The weak spaces, pathways of extraprostatic spread of prostate cancer, are located along the neurovascular bundles (NVB) and ejaculatory ducts (ED).

Color and Power Doppler of the prostate (Fig. 13.7)

The peripheral zone has a hypovascular pattern. However, subcapsular and perforating vessels are commonly detected which can occasionally simulate prostate cancer due to their hypoechoic appearance. BPH is a hypervascular process.

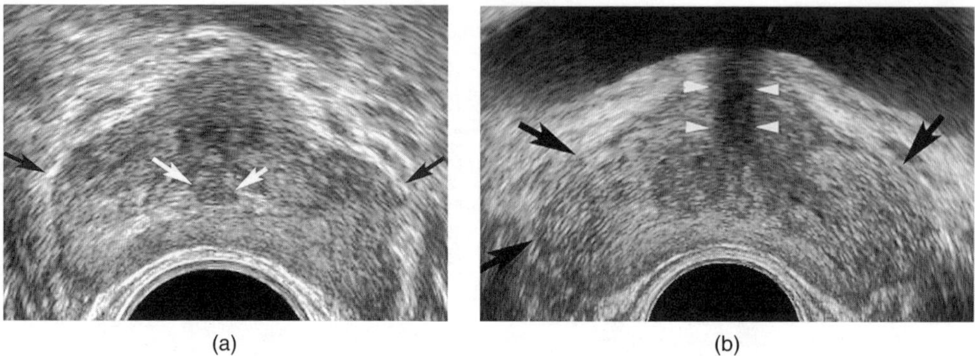

(a)   (b)

Figure 13.3 TRUS zonal anatomy. Mid portion. Transverse view. (a) the veru montanum has a hypoechoic appearance (white arrows). The bright boundary echo (black arrows) is an acoustic artefact. (b) with an 8–10 MHz probe, the moderately dilated PZ prostate glands (black arrows) are commonly visible in men over 50 YO. Note the hypoechoic appearance of the preprostatic sphincter (arrowheads).

MRI of the normal prostate and BPH (Fig. 13.8)

Endorectal coil provides exquisite details of the zonal anatomy. The endorectal coil is combined with an external phased array coil to cover the anterior portion of the gland.

- T1-weighted sequence

  o The prostate has an isosignal similar to that of the adjacent muscles. The sequence is used to detect biopsy artefacts.

- T2-weighted sequence

  o The peripheral zone is hyperintense. The hypointense capsule is visible at the mid-portion and the base of the gland, surrounded by periprostatic fat. The apex is devoid of capsule and periprostatic fat.

  o The transition zone has a heterogenous and nodular pattern. Glandular nodules are hyperintense. Stromal nodules are hypointense. Very often, nodules are mixed.

  o At the prostate base, the hypointense central zone is visible. The seminal vesicles and the ampullae (Fig. 13.9) join to become the ejaculatory ducts.

13.3 Diagnosis of prostate cancer: TRUS features

These depend on the findings of digital rectal examination.

Palpable prostate cancers

These correspond in most cases to tumors of the outer gland (PZ + CZ). PCa originates in the PZ and in the CZ in 70% and 5% of cases, respectively.

- The nodular hypoechoic appearance (Fig. 13.10) is due to the dense compact cellularity of the tumor (Fig. 13.11) and is not correlated to the Gleason grade.

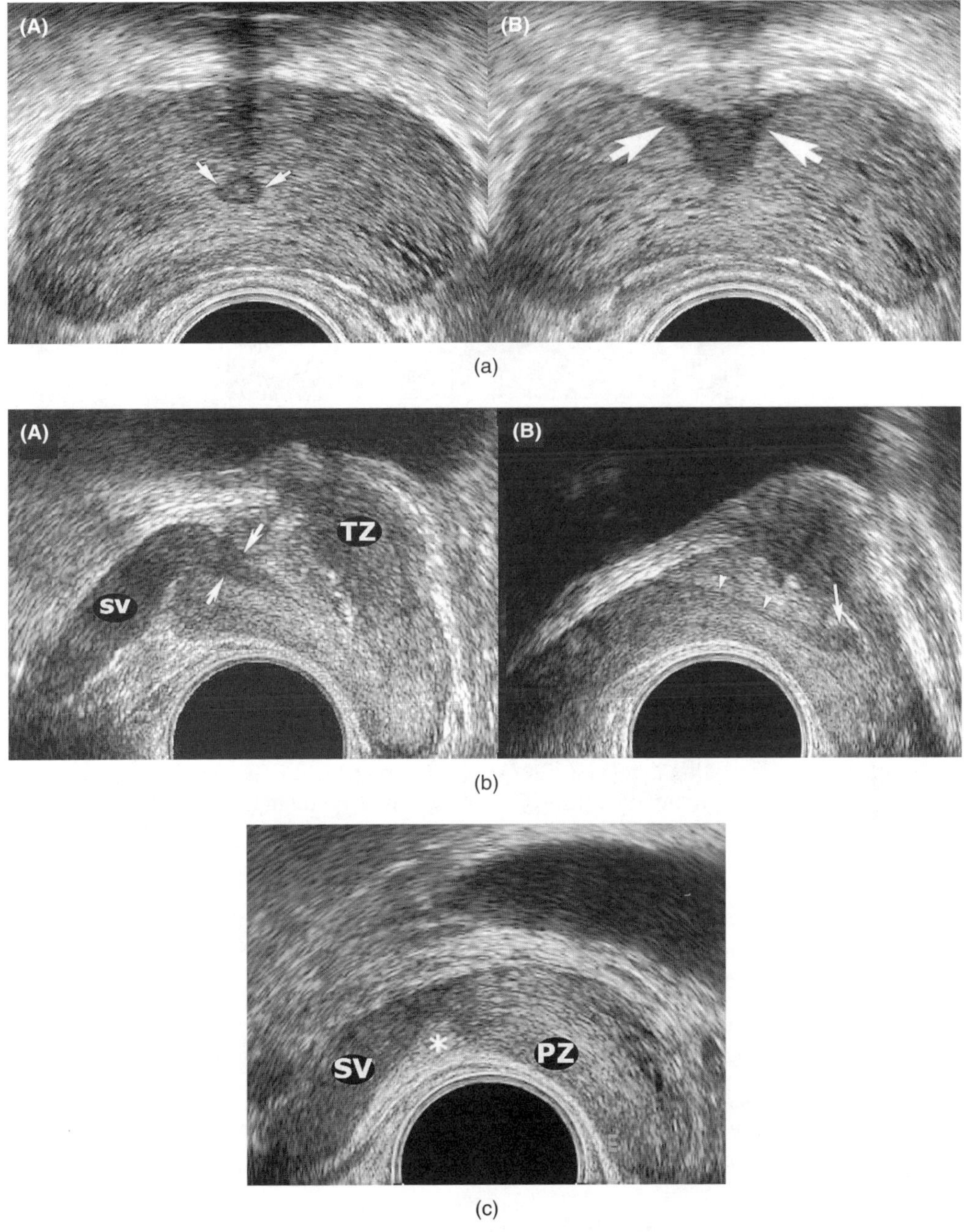

Figure 13.4 Prostate base. (a) transverse views. (A): Lower base: ejaculatory ducts visible within the CZ (white arrows). (B): Upper base: hypoechoic appearance of the caudal junction of the vas deferens (VD) and the seminal vesicles (SV) (white arrows, B). (b) sagittal views. (A): mid-sagittal. Hypoechoic appearance of the caudal junction of the vas deferens and the seminal vesicles (white arrows, A). The ejaculatory ducts (arrowheads, B) end at the veru montanum (white arrow, B). SV: seminal vesicles. TZ: transition zone. (c) parasagittal view. The fatty prostate-seminal angle (*) is located between the seminal vesicle (SV) and the PZ.

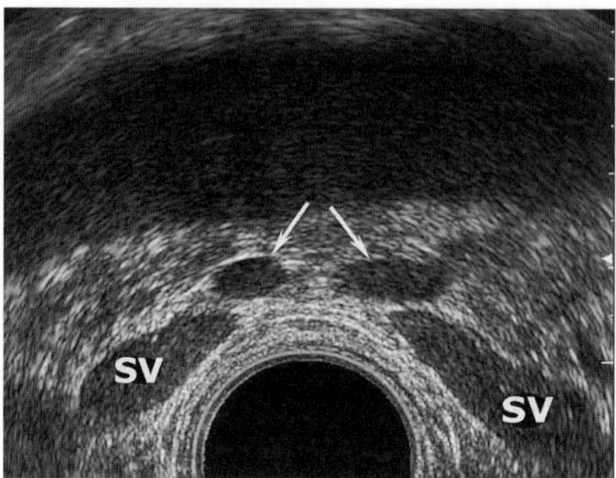

Figure 13.5   Transverse view above the prostate base. The ampullae of the vas deferens (white arrows) and the seminal vesicles (SV) are seen before they join to become the ejaculatory ducts.

- Cancer with intratumoral coarse hyperechoic foci (Fig. 13.12) are high grade tumors (grade 4–5), with comedonecrosis.

- Color Doppler (CD) shows a hypervascular pattern in 85–90% of cases (Fig. 13.1). The positive predictive value of CD is 95%. Hypovascular palpable cancers (10–15% of cases) correspond to large volume tumors, poorly differentiated, often T3 stage lesions.

Palpable abnormalities simulating prostate cancer

- Granulomatous prostatitis is related to tuberculosis or to local BCG instillation for superficial bladder tumor. It involves the PZ or TZ, has a nodular hypoechoic appearance, without vascularity (Fig. 13.13).

- Chronic prostatitis uncommonly simulates palpable PCa. The appearance is a palpable hypoechoic PZ nodule following an episode of acute prostatitis.

- Palpable calcifications without hypoechoic nodule (Fig. 13.14), corresponding to corpora amylacea (TZ calcifications) or to post-inflammatory changes (PZ calcifications).

- BPH nodules developing within the PZ (Fig. 13.15) are present in approximately 20% of cases at pathological examination of radical prostatectomy specimens and visible in approximately 6% of cases at TRUS.

- Whatever the cause, biopsy is mandatory to exclude malignancy. In case of a benign result, a repeat biopsy can be avoided if the TRUS features are typical.

TRUS features of non-palpable prostate cancer

Since the PSA era, most of detected prostate cancers are non-palpable. TRUS features of palpable cancer cannot be transposed to non-palpable tumors because many hypoechoic nodules are benign and non-palpable prostate cancer is commonly isoechoic.

- Visible cancer at TRUS (TNM-T2 stage) usually has a subtle hypoechoic appearance (fig. 13.16).

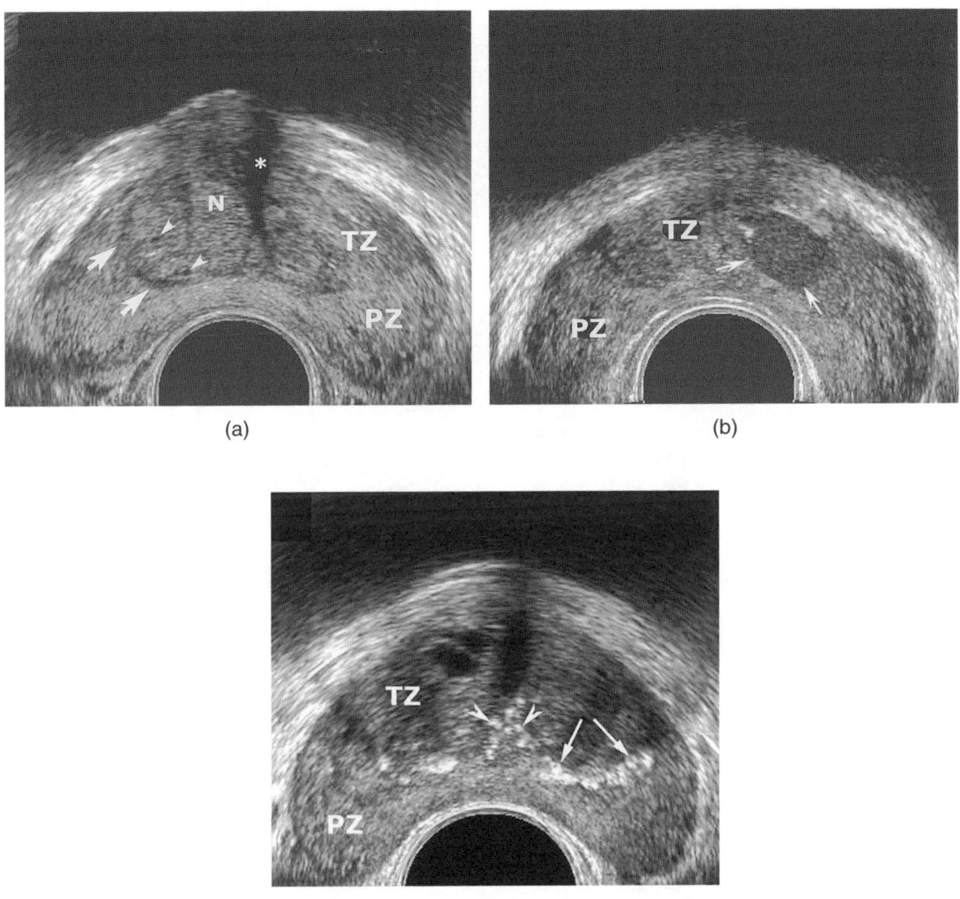

Figure 13.6 Benign prostatic hyperplasia. TRUS features. (a) Heterogeneous and nodular (N) pattern of the transition zone. The surgical capsule (white arrows) separates the PZ and the TZ. The preprostatic sphincter (*) has a hypoechoic appearance. Tiny cystic dilated glands are visible within the BPH nodule (arrowheads). (b) Pure TZ stromal nodule at TRUS guided biopsies (arrows). (c) Corporea amylacea visible along the surgical capsule (arrows) and within the prostatic ducts (arrowheads).

- The specificity of TRUS is low: benign hypoechoic non-palpable PZ nodules are visible on TRUS in approximately 30% of men over 50 years old and only 20% of them show cancer at biopsy.
- Factors influencing the specificity
  - Nodule size: cancer rate keeps increasing when tumor size is >10 mm.
  - Color Doppler sonography: the predictive value of a hypervascular nodule is approximately 60% and that of a hypovascular nodule 15%. The specificity is thus increased, but the sensitivity of CDS is lower than that of TRUS.
  - PSA level: above 4 ng/ml, the predictive value is at least 30–40%. It falls to 5% if the PSA level is <4 ng/ml.

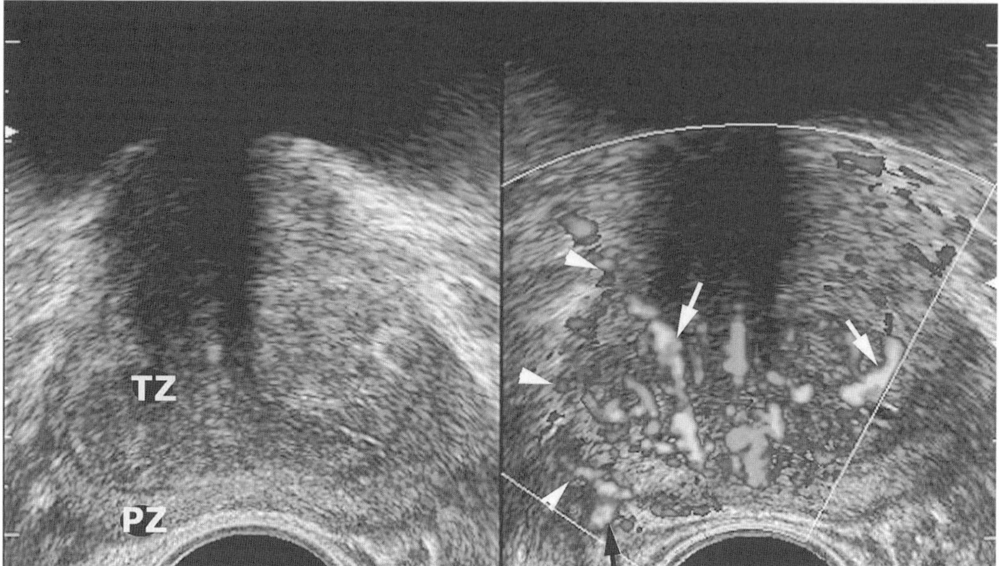

Figure 13.7 Color and Power Doppler of the prostate. Tranverse view. The TZ contains several macrovessels (white arrows). The posterolaterally located neurovascular bundle (black arrow) and the subcapsular vessels (arrowheads) are visible.

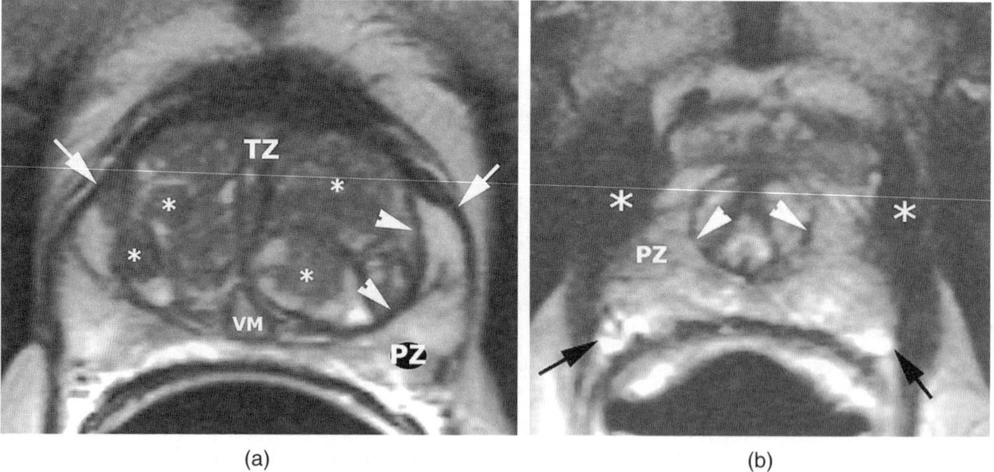

(a)   (b)

Figure 13.8 MR appearance of the normal prostate. (a) T2-weighted sequence. The capsule (white arrows) surrounds the PZ. The surgical capsule (arrowheads) separates the TZ and the PZ. Several BPH nodules (*) are visible in the TZ. VM: veru montanum. (b) Apex. The hypointense striated sphincter (arrowheads) represents the medial border of the PZ. The neurovascular bundles (arrows) are the posterolateral boundaries and laterally, the prostate abuts the levator ani muscles (*) without interposition of fat. (c) Prostate base. The CZ (arrows) is hypointense, located medially to the PZ. It is traversed by the ejaculatory ducts (arrowheads) running down to the veru montanum. SV: seminal vesicles.

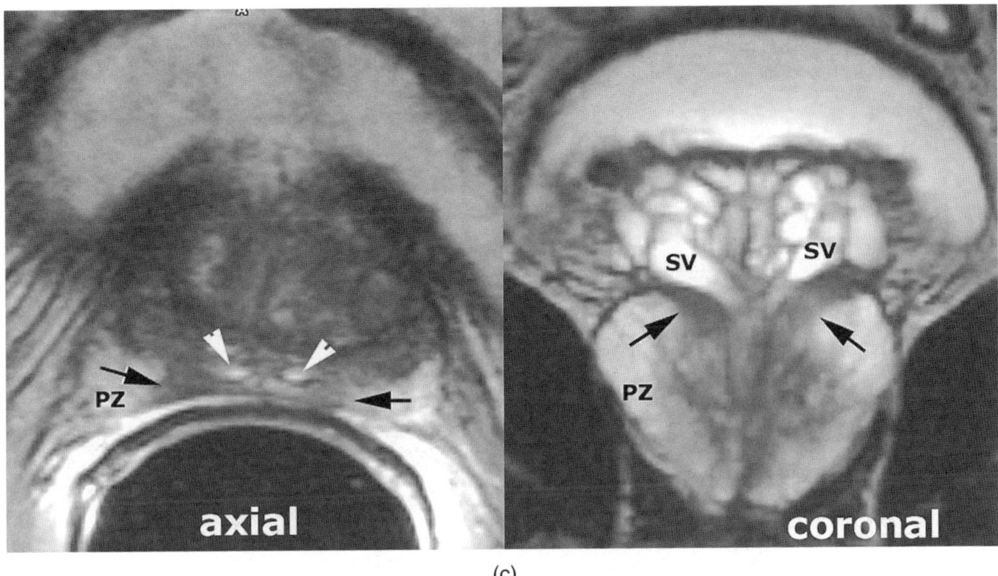

(c)

Figure 13.8   *(continued)*

- Non-visible non-palpable prostate cancer: T1c stage tumors (Fig. 13.17)

  o Are as frequent as non-palpable hypoechoic tumors

  o Factors contributing to their isoechoic appearance are

    - a histological infiltrative pattern (grade 3) with juxtaposition of tumoral and non-tumoral glands (Fig. 13.17a)

    - a non-significant volume (<0.5 cc) in up to 40% of cases

    - an origin in the TZ in up to 50% of cases.

  o Tumor conspicuity can be improved by contrast-enhanced TRUS (Fig. 13.17b), with an accuracy not >60%.

TRUS guided biopsies

A histological proof of malignancy is mandatory before treatment.

- The procedure is thoroughly explained to the patient to obtain an optimal cooperation, including the risk of complications (bleeding and sepsis). Contraindications are searched.

- Antibiotics (quinolone) are given orally prophylactically for 3 days (10 days in case of infectious risk factor), starting the day before biopsy. Rectal enema is recommended. Urinary infection or coagulation disorders are not routinely checked. In case of anticoagulation, the treatment must be temporarily interrupted.

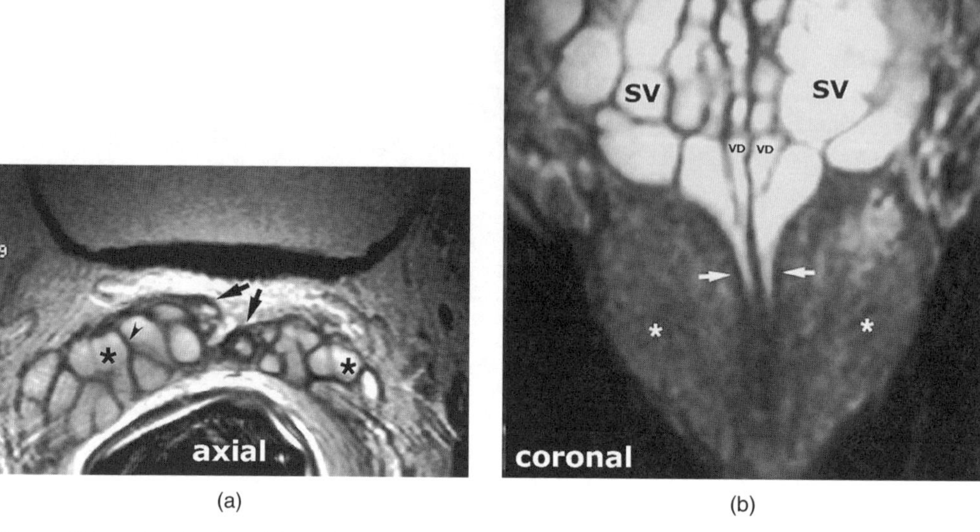

(a)   (b)

Figure 13.9 Seminal vesicles. (a) T2-weighted image. The ampullae of the vas deferens have a thick hypointense muscular wall (arrows). The seminal vesicles (*) are hyperintense and contain septa (arrowheads). (b) Coronal view. The ejaculatory ducts (white arrows) run within the prostatic tissue. The level of VD and SV junction occurs outside the prostatic tissue in most cases. Note the diffuse hyposignal of the peripheral zone due to post-inflammatory changes (*). The seminal vesicles (SV) are moderately dilated.

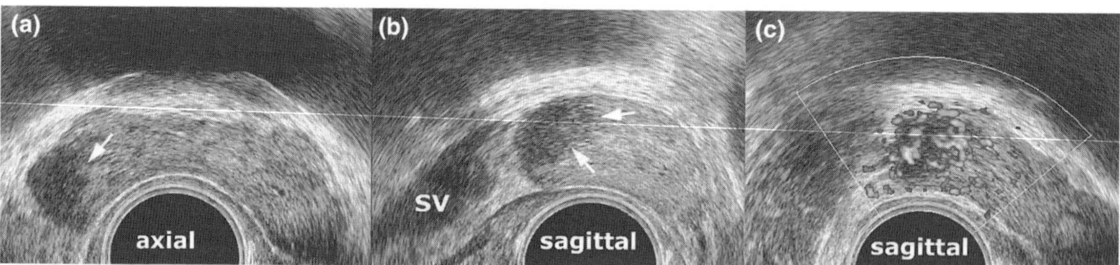

Figure 13.10 Typical palpable hypoechoic hypervascular prostate PZ cancer (arrows), originating in the prostate base (a–c). SV: seminal vesicle.

- Local anesthesia by transrectal TRUS-guided infiltration of the periprostatic spaces with lidocaine dramatically improves patient's comfort during the examination. General anesthesia is only required in a minority of cases, for local anatomical problems or at patient's request.

- Protocol (Fig. 13.18)

  - Palpable and visible lesion: a six sextant protocol is applied. In all other cases, a 12-sextant protocol is applied.

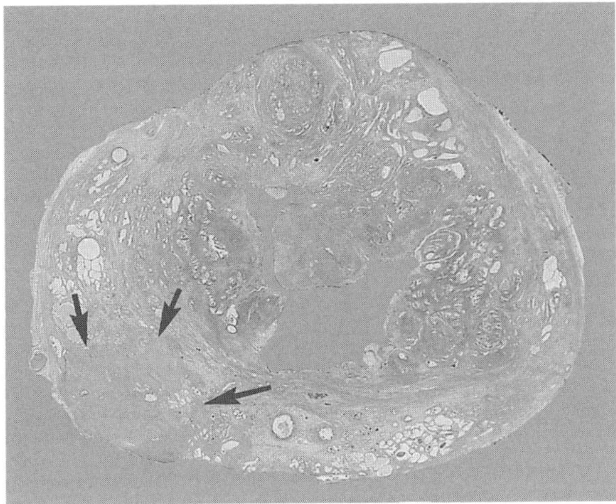

Figure 13.11 Prostatectomy specimen: the dense and compact cellularity (arrows) gives the hypoechoic appearance, whatever the Gleason grade.

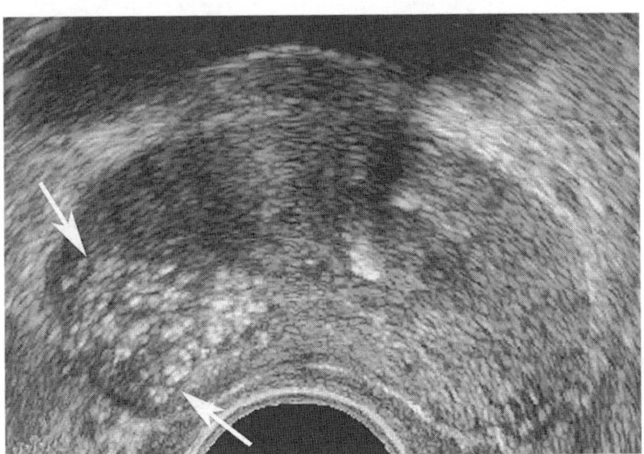

Figure 13.12 Grade 5 carcinoma with comedonecrosis: hyperechoic foci without little or no shadowing (arrows), corresponding to foci of comedonecrosis.

- o Repeat biopsies.
  - Twelve posterior and six deep anterior cores are taken to detect TZ cancers. Up to six sets of biopsies can be necessary to detect the tumor.
  - Saturation biopsies (≥ 30 cores) increase the cancer detection rate at the expense of a higher morbidity and of a higher detection rate of latent, insignificant tumors.
  - Functional MR Imaging guided biopsies (see below) permit targeted biopsies with fewer cores.

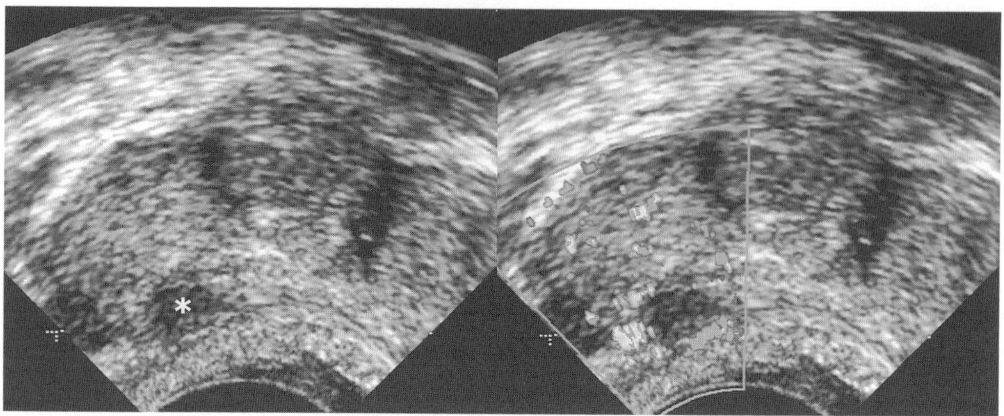

Figure 13.13 Granulomatous prostatitis. Palpable nodule detected 4 months after intravesical instillation of BCG. The nodule is hypoechoic and does not contain vessels (*). PSA level: 2 ng/ml. Granulomatous prostatitis at TRUS-guided biopsy.

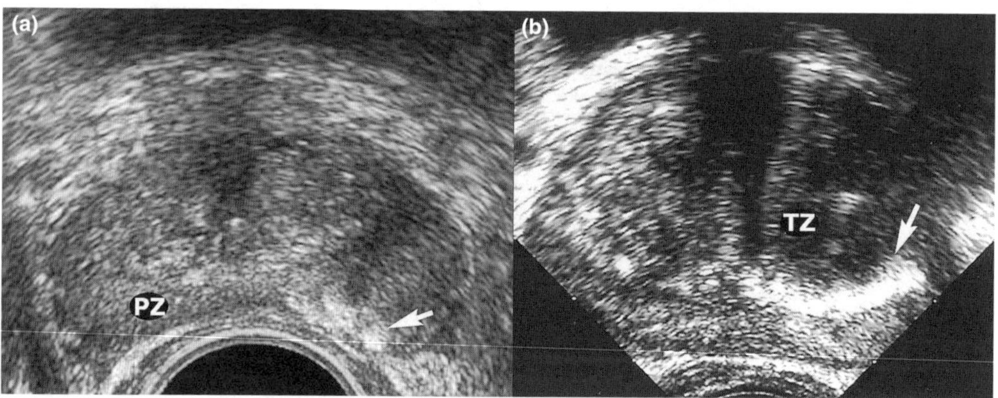

Figure 13.14   Palpable calcifications (arrow) within the PZ (a) and TZ (b).

13.4 Diagnostic of prostate cancer: MRI

PCa is hypointense on fast spin echo T2-weighted MR imaging. However, T2-W imaging lacks specificity to discriminate prostate cancer from benign tissue, due to the high rate of benign hyposignals simulating cancer. Functional MRI (contrast-enhanced MRI, spectroscopy and diffusion-weighted imaging) improve the accuracy of FSE-T2 imaging to localize PCa, and to estimate tumor volume of a newly diagnosed PCa.

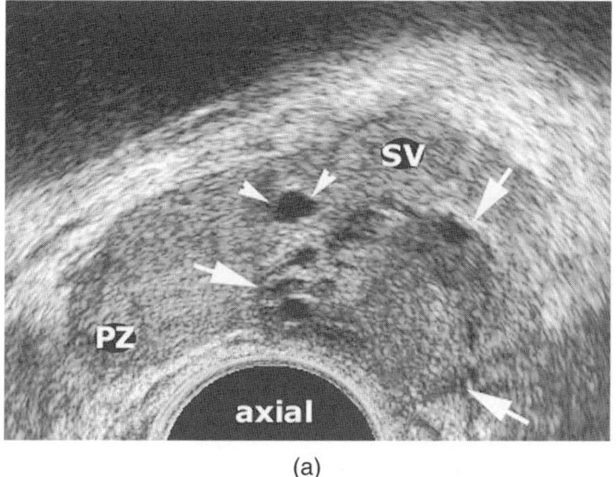

(a)

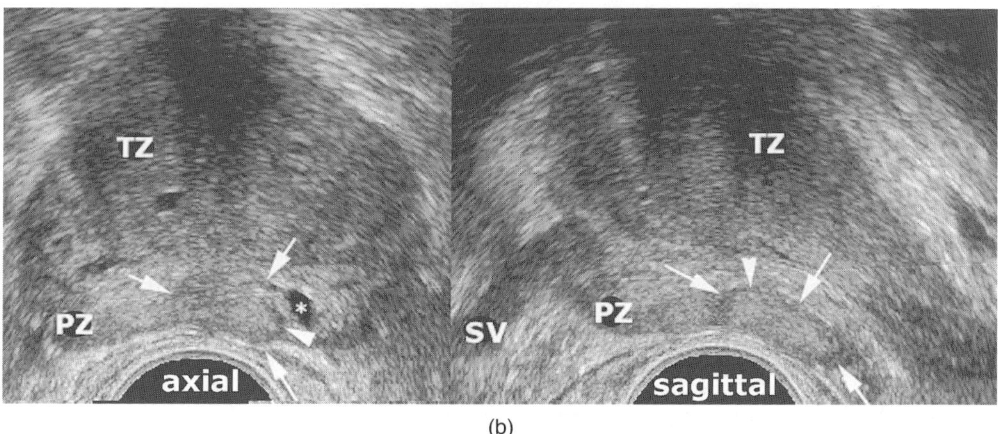

(b)

Figure 13.15   Palpable BPH nodules originating in the PZ. (a) Hypoechoic microcystic appearance (white arrows). A small utricular cyst is visible (arrowhead). SV: seminal vesicle. (b) Hypoechoic well marginated appearance (arrows) with a discrete perinodular halo and a few tiny microcysts (arrowheads). (*): dilated prostatic glands compressed by the nodule.

13.5 Contrast-enhanced (dynamic) MRI

Technique

- Eight weeks after the last series of biopsies to ensure no biopsy artefact.

- An endorectal coil is used is used in most series.

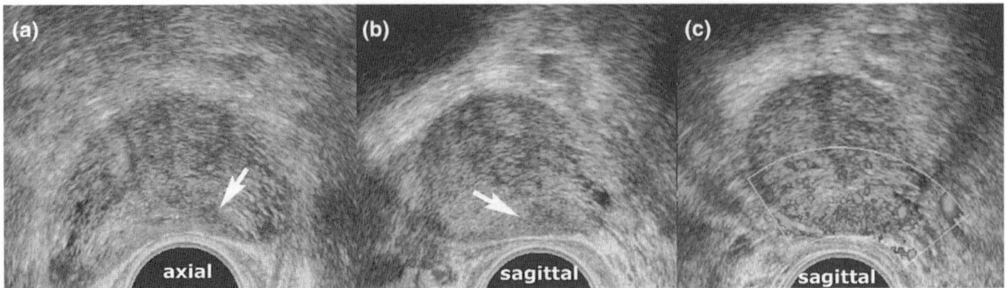

Figure 13.16 Non-palpable PZ cancer. Small left apical non-palpable cancer, barely visible (arrow, a–b). Hypervascularization is discrete (c).

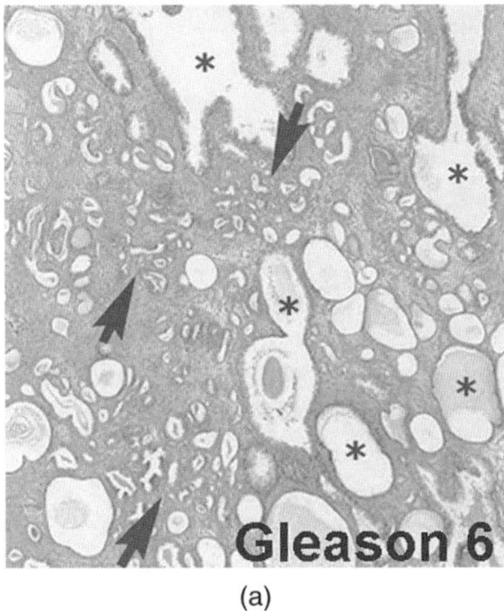

(a)

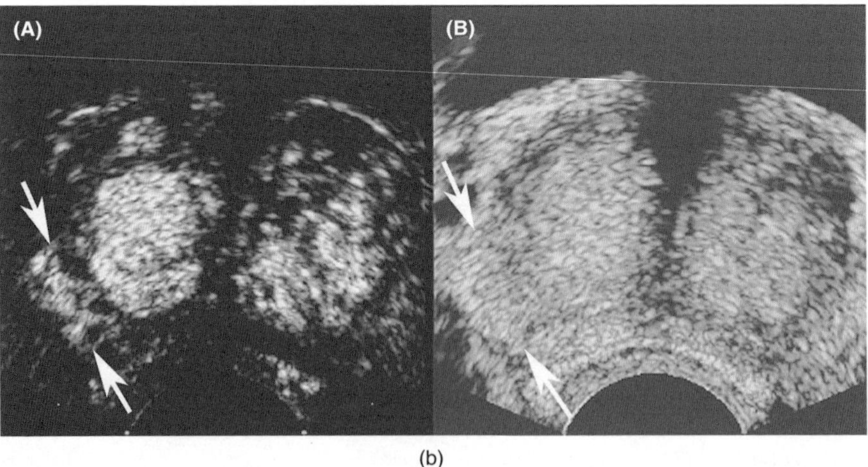

(b)

Figure 13.17 T1c stage (non-visible non-palpable) prostate cancer. (a) Histological view. Tumors cells (arrows) are blend with normal glands (*), without mass effect thus precluding TRUS visibility of this Gleason score 6 (3 + 3) tumor. (b) Contrast-enhanced TRUS: focal enhancement in the right PZ (arrow, a) in an isoechoic sextant (arrows, b) corresponding to a Gleason 6 score Ca (6 mm). PSA level 8, 7 ng/ml.

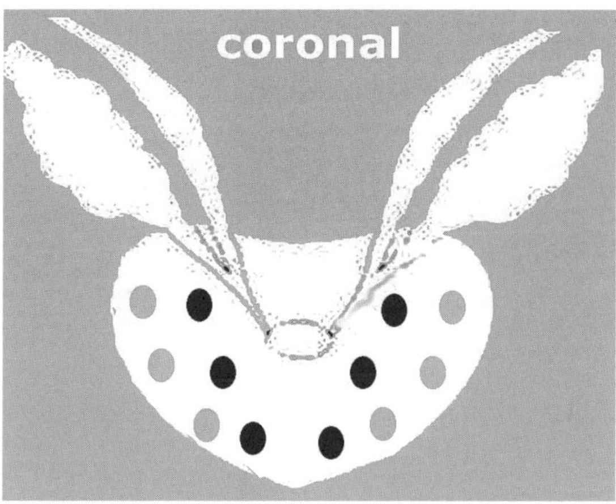

Figure 13.18 Six and 12 sextant biopsy protocol. In the 6 biopsy protocol (black dots), the cores are taken on the midline of each lobe, in the apex, mid-portion and base. In the 12 sextants protocol, six additional cores (gray dots) are taken laterally which increases the cancer detection rate by 15%.

- The sequence is a 3D gradient-echo T1-weighted gradient with bolus injection of 0.1 mmol/kg of gadolinium (power injector, rate: 3 ml/s), followed by a flush of saline (15 ml). Temporal resolution should not be >15 s and acquisitions are performed during five minutes.

Results

- Different approaches are used

  - Qualitative: visual assessment of the enhancement. Its value is under evaluation.

  - Semi-quantitative: after contrast injection, parameters calculate variations of *signal*: peak enhancement, time to peak and washout (Fig. 13.19). Persistent washout indicates benign tissue. Plateau-like is indeterminate and decreasing washout suggests PZ cancer.

  - Quantitative: parameters calculate variations of *concentration of gadolinium*: Ktrans (forward constant transfer) reflects the time to peak; maximum gadolinium concentration (AUC: area under the curve) reflects the peak enhancement and Kep (reverse flux rate) reflects the washout curve (Fig. 13.20). Carcinoma has high AUC, Ktrans and Kep values. Quantitative parameters are theoretically more reproducible from one patient to the other.

- Sensitivity of dynamic MR is higher (80–90%) than that of FSE-T2 imaging (50–60%) to detect PZ cancers with tumor volume >0.5 cc. The theoretical superiority of quantitative assessment has not yet been fully validated due to the lack of a standardized protocol.

- Whatever the approach, limitations of dynamic MRI come from PZ prostatitis and BPH.

  - Enhancement of PZ benign inflammatory sextants simulating carcinoma (Fig. 13.21) is a frequent pitfall. The specificity of dynamic MRI is thus not >70%.

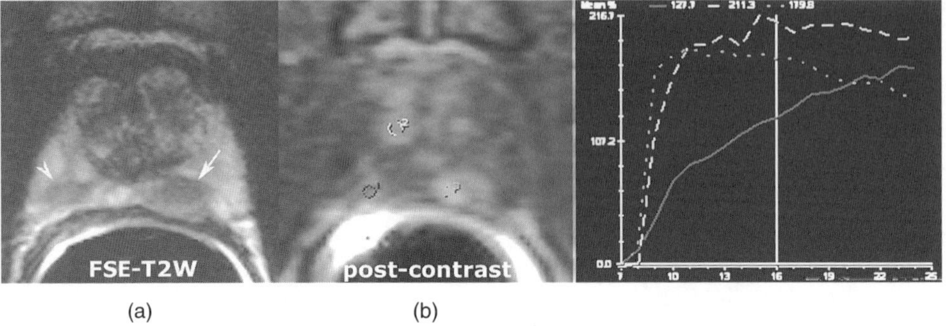

Figure 13.19 Left apical tumor (arrows, a) with a type 3 washout curve (green). Benign right hyposignal (arrowhead, a) with a type 1 washout curve (red). Note the type 2 washout curve in the TZ (yellow).

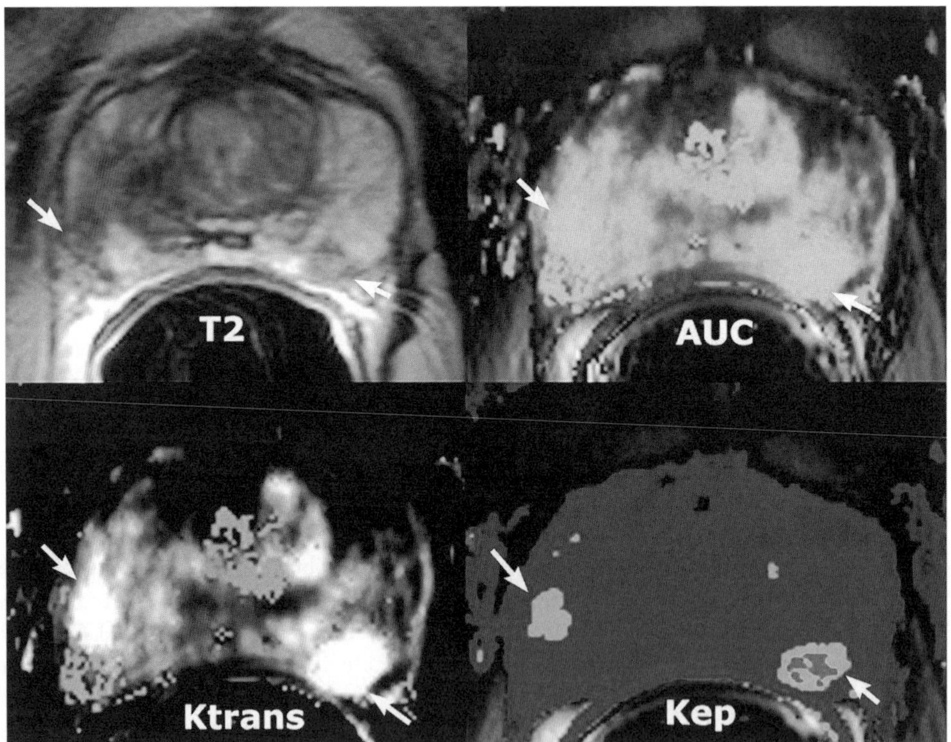

Figure 13.20 Quantitative dynamic MRI of a bilateral prostate cancer (arrows), Gleason score 6. PSA: 7 ng/ml. Color coded values of quantitative parameters show a bilateral high AUC, Ktrans and Kep.

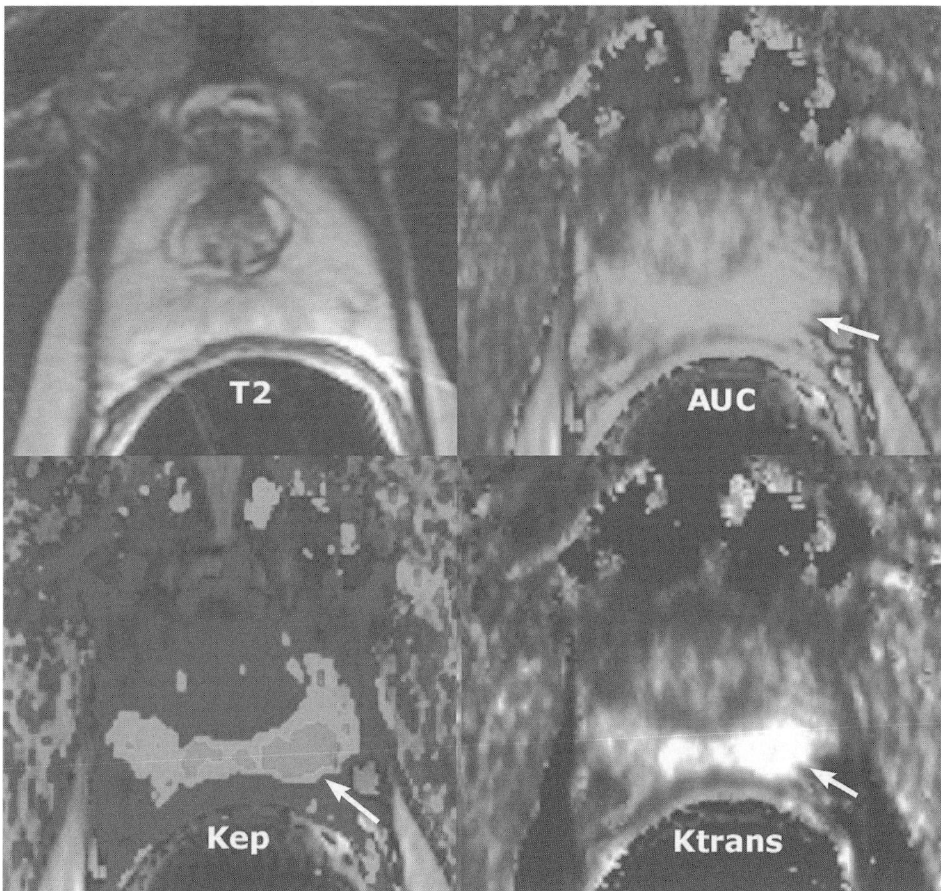

Figure 13.21 Prostatitis. 46 YO man. Raising PSA (2 to 4 ng/ml). Family history of PCa. MRI before biopsy. High AUC, Ktrans and Kep values in the left apex (arrow) with no hyposignal on the T2-W sequence. Saturation biopsies showed benign tissue and raising PSA was attributed to prostatitis.

- o Detection of TZ cancer remains difficult due to the high vascular permeability of BPH tissue which simulates Ca (Figs. 13.22 and 13.23).
- o FSE-T2W imaging remains an indispensable tool to interpret accurately a positive dynamic MR.
- Dynamic MRI significantly increases the accuracy of T2-W imaging to localize prostate cancer. Post-processing is dramatically facilitated by the quantitative approach, but its limited specificity suggests that it should be combined with a complementary functional MR modality.

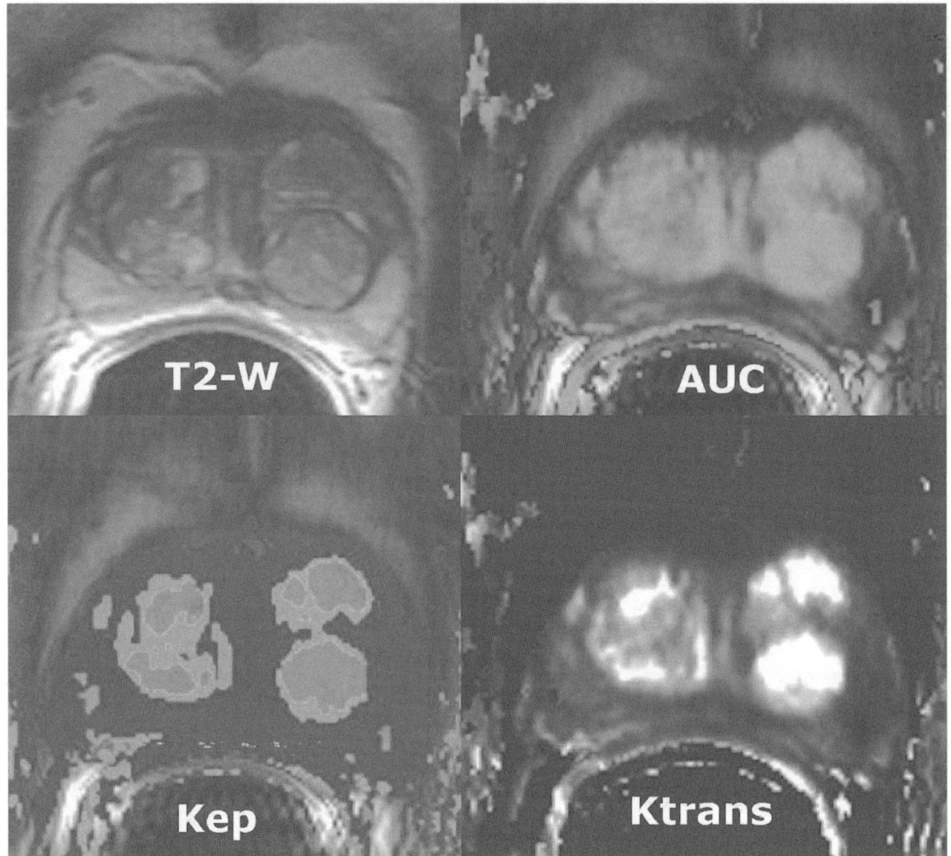

Figure 13.22 Dynamic quantitative MR and BPH nodules. Three typical BPH nodules (*) on the T2-W sequence with AUC, Ktrans and Kep values similar to those observed in cancer.

13.6 Magnetic Resonance Spectroscopic Imaging (MRSI)

Principle

- MRSI exploits the chemical shift (difference in resonance frequency) of hydrogen protons to produce a map of signal intensity versus frequency of different prostatic metabolites (choline, creatine and citrate) (Fig. 13.24).

Results

- Normal prostate tissue

  - The ratio of choline and creatine-to-citrate in sextants containing benign tissue is <0.75 in the PZ and <0.80 in the TZ (Fig. 13.24).

  - The periurethral glands and the area around the ejaculatory ducts contain a physiological high level of choline (Fig. 13.25)

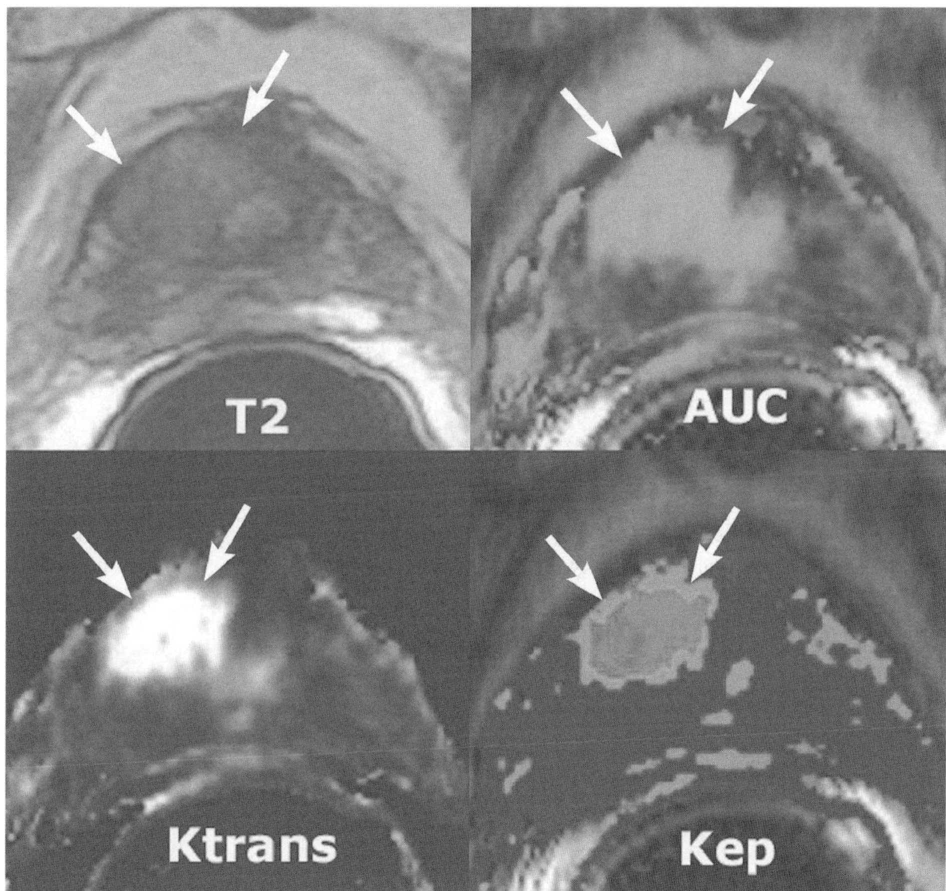

Figure 13.23 TZ carcinoma. 66 YO man, raising PSA (11 ng/ml). Two sets of posterior negative biopsies. Anterior ill-marginated hyposignal (arrow) with high AUC, Ktrans and Kep values. Combination of both sequences suggest cancer, which was confirmed by six directed right anterior biopsies (Gleason score 7, 13 mm of Ca).

- Prostate cancer originating in the peripheral zone

  - Is characterized by increased choline and reduced citrate (Fig. 13.26)
  - Results of MRI combined with those of MRSI have shown a wide range of sensitivity, specificity and accuracy for cancer localization, according to the findings of FSE-T2W imaging and the cut-off values of CC/Ci values (Fig. 13.27).

- Limitations of MR Spectroscopic Imaging

  - Artefacts or contamination by the periprostatic lipids occur in approximately 25–30% of cases.
  - Specificity of MRSI is limited by false-positive cases observed in case of PZ chronic prostatitis (Fig. 13.28) and in case of TZ stromal BPH (Fig. 13.29) which can simulate cancer.

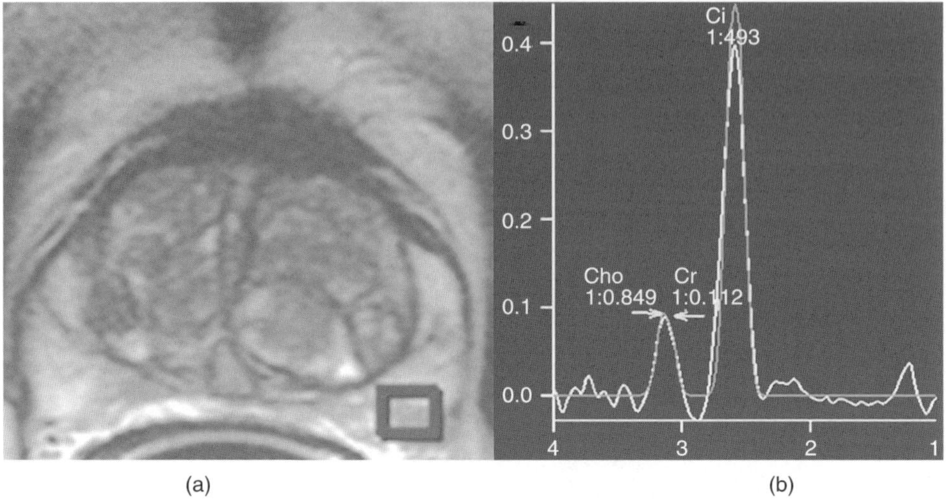

(a)   (b)

Figure 13.24   MRSI of normal PZ. (a): A voxel (blue box) is overlaid on a T2 image. (b): The x axis of the spectral trace from the voxel represents frequency. The y axis represents intensity which lacks absolute units. The ratio Cho + Cr/Ci is <0.6.

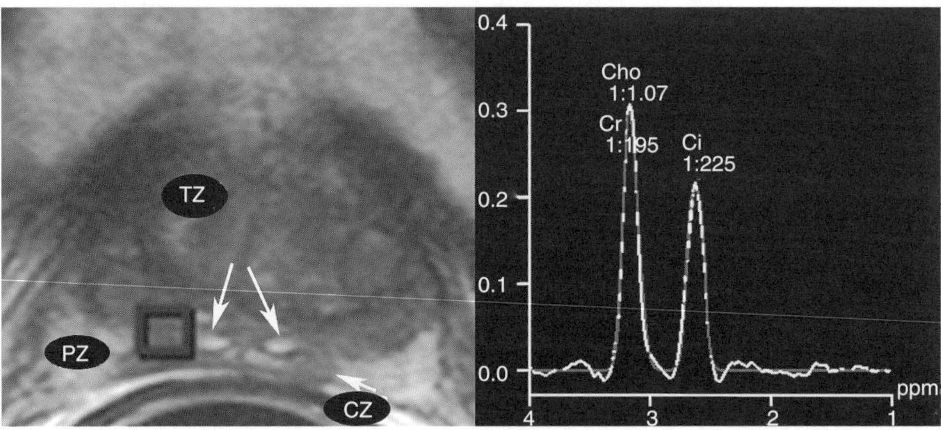

Figure 13.25   Physiological elevated CC/Ci ratio (>1) around the ejaculatory ducts (arrows). Note the hyposignal of the central zone (CZ).

- o MRSI has a low sensitivity (45%) for the detection of low grade carcinomas (Fig. 13.30), suggesting that MRSI at 1.5 Tesla should be used in conjunction with a complementary functional sequence (contrast-enhanced or diffusion).

13.7 Diffusion-weighted imaging

Principle

In a diffusion-weighted sequence, mobile protons of water molecules will be imperfectly rephased causing a decrease of signal in tumors proportionally to the cellular density. If

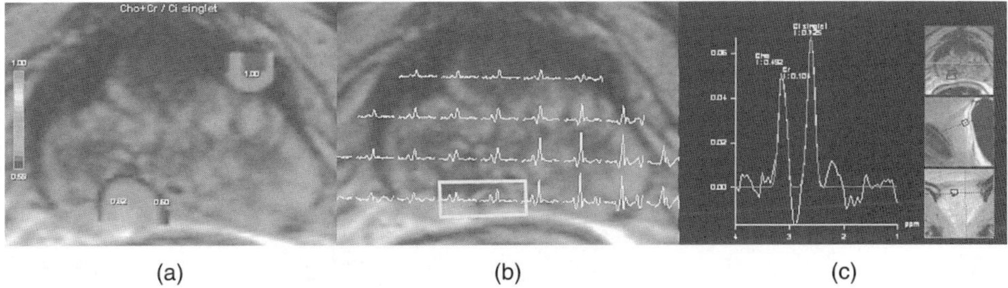

(a)   (b)   (c)

Figure 13.26 MRSI and detection of a PZ cancer. 69 YO man. PSA level: 7.6 ng/ml. One series of 12 negative biopsies. (a): Color-coded map of voxels with a CC/Ci ratio >0.6 in the right PZ. The upper left voxel is out of the prostate boundaries (b–c): spectral map with a detail (c) of one of the voxels in the yellow box with a CC/Ci ratio >0.6. Two directed biopsies were positive in the abnormal area (8 mm of Gleason score 7 cancer) on the repeat set of biopsies.

	Se	Sp	Acc
MRI+ *and* MRS+ (CC/Ci > 0.86)	50	90	65
MRI+ *or* MRS+ (CC/Ci > 0.86)	90	50	75
MRI+ *and* MRS+ (CC/Ci > 0.75)	70	75	85
MRI+ *or* MRS+ (CC/Ci > 0.75)	95	35	76

Figure 13.27 Sensitivity, specificity and accuracy of MRSI, according to the findings of FSE-T2 imaging and Choline + Creatine/Citrate ratio values (from Scheidler, Hricak *et al.* (1999)).

several gradients of diffusion are used (b0, b400, b800), it is possible to define a map of the apparent diffusion coefficient (ADC map).

Results

- The ADC is decreased in PZ PCa (<1). Values above 1.6 indicate benign tissue. Between 1 and 1.6, DW imaging lacks accuracy for a consistent localization of PCa (Fig. 13.31).

- The sequence is short (<5 mn) and robust. It represents a useful complement to dynamic MRI or spectroscopy to localize PCa, particularly when prostatitis is suspected (Fig. 13.32). Its accuracy in the detection of TZ cancer has not yet be evaluated.

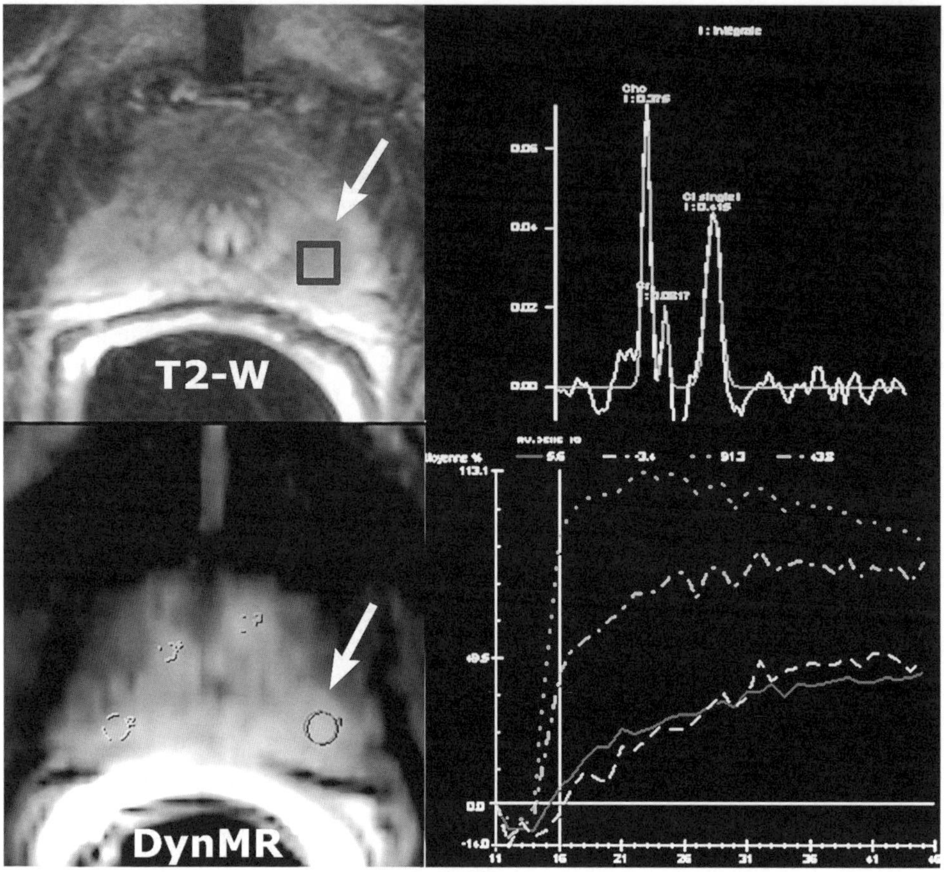

Figure 13.28 MRSI and chronic prostatitis. 63 YO man. Raising PSA (9 ng/ml). Two series of negative biopsies. Left apical hyposignal (arrow) on the T2-W image with a CC/Ci ratio >0.6 and a flat type 1 curve (red) on dynamic MR (DynMR). Saturation left apical biopsies (8 cores) showed interstitial prostatitis.

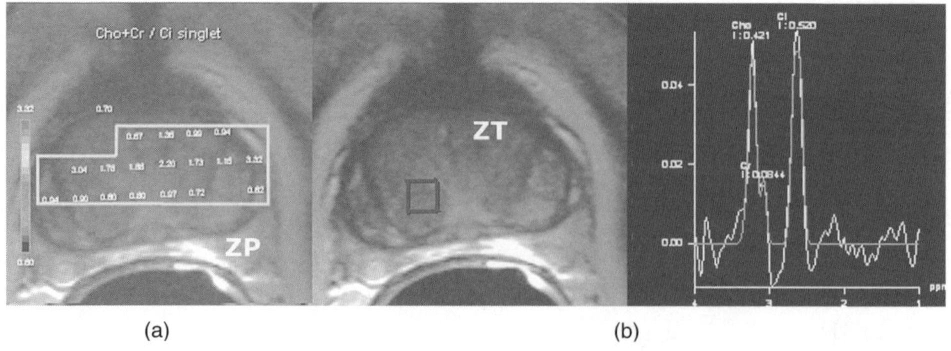

(a) (b)

Figure 13.29 MRSI and stromal BPH. Raising PSA (16 ng/ml) and three series of negative biopsies. (a): most of the voxels in the yellow box have a CC/Ci ratio >0.8 (b): detail of the spectrum of one of these voxels (CC/Ci: 1.21). Saturation biopsies (30 cores) showed benign tissue.

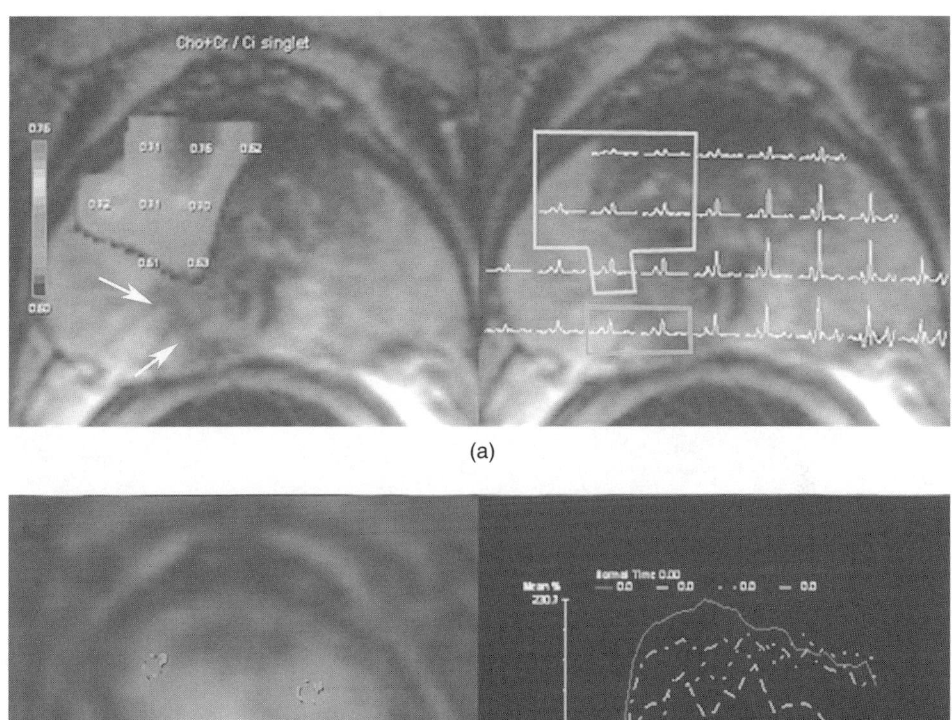

(a)

(b)

Figure 13.30 MRSI and low-grade cancers. Raising PSA (11 ng/ml). MRI before biopsy. (a): Hyposignal in the right PZ (arrow) with normal metabolic activity (green box). (b): dynamic MRI. Typical type 3 curve in the hyposignal (red). Targeted biopsies showed 6 mm of Gleason score 6 carcinoma.

13.8 Indications of functional MRI

Cancer localization after negative biopsies

- Although it has been reported a 30% detection rate by TRUS biopsies targeted on abnormalities detected on MRSI, it is not known yet after how many series of negative biopsies should functional be indicated.

- It should logically be indicated after a first negative series if the repeat series plans to perform anterior cores within the TZ.

- If MRI and biopsies are negative, the negative predictive value for the presence of a significant tumor remains to be defined.

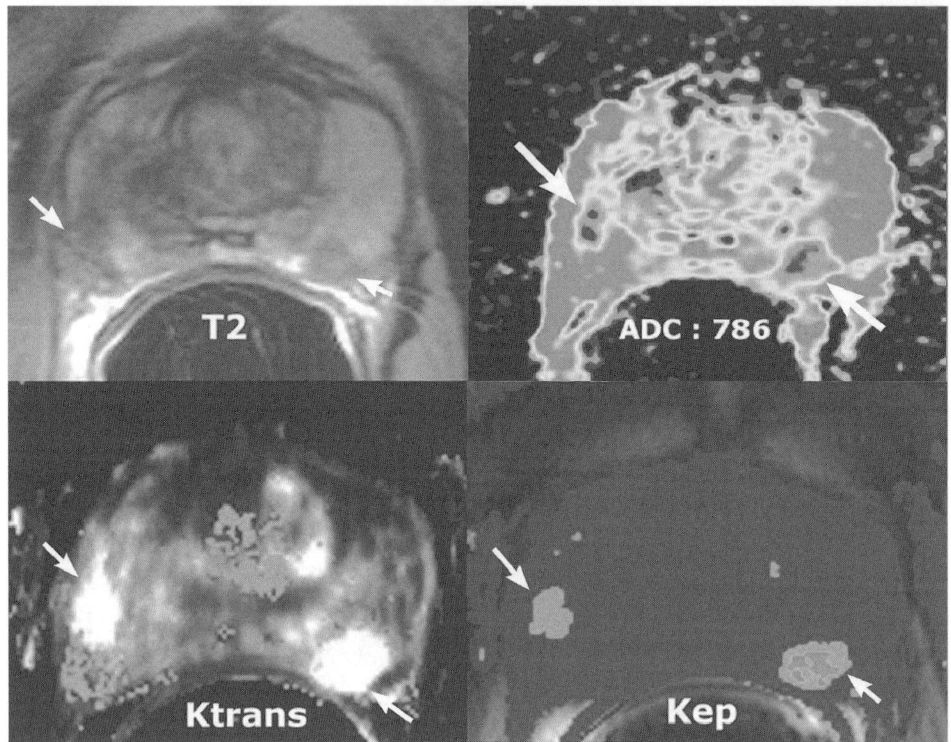

Figure 13.31 Combination of DWI and perfusion. Same patient as in Figure 13.20. bilateral Gleason 6 Ca with high AUC, Ktrans and Kep values. The ADC is low, suggesting cancer and increasing the specificity of dynamic MR. 57 YO patient.

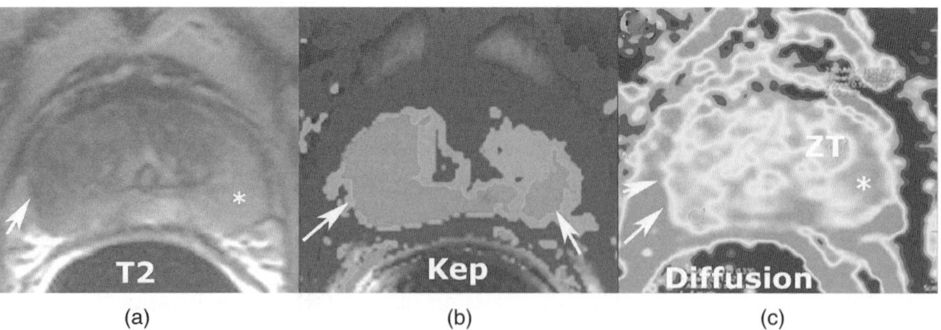

(a)   (b)   (c)

Figure 13.32 Combination of DWI and perfusion. Gleason score 7 (3 + 4).involving the three right sextants. (a): right PZ hyposignal (arrow) and heterogeneous signal of the left PZ (*). (b) Bilateral elevated Kep (arrows) suggesting a bilateral tumor (c): Low ADC (0.9, green area) in the right PZ (arrows). Normal ADC (1,9) on the left side (*, red and orange area). On the radical prostatectomy specimen, no tumor was present in the left lobe.

Estimation of tumor volume

- Biopsies often underestimate the number of sextants involved by the tumor. A single positive biopsy does not mean small volume tumor and a microfocus of less than 3 mm of carcinoma does not necessarily mean latent carcinoma.

- Functional MR can differentiate significant from latent tumors (fig. 13.33) and might play an important role in the selection of the most appropriate treatment option of clinically localised PCa.

13.9 Extension of prostate cancer

Precise local staging of prostate cancer is more necessary than ever, due to the rapid spread of non-surgical treatments such as brachytherapy which requires the selection of patients with a confined tumor. Endorectal MRI is the only imaging modality which can detect occult extraprostatic spread. However, TRUS and TRUS-guided biopsies can detect locally advanced lesions by biopsy of the periprostatic spaces or define a risk of pT3 stage disease by a combined use of PSA level and results of biopsies to establish a mathematical model (nomograms).

13.10 Local extension by TRUS and TRUS-guided biopsy

TRUS signs of locally advanced (T3 stage) tumors

Signs of macroscopic invasion of extraprostatic spread (Fig. 13.34) are very uncommonly observed since the PSA era which detects most cancers at an earlier stage. Specificity of TRUS in these advanced tumors is 100%.

Staging biopsies

- Should be performed to sample the periprostatic fat when TRUS findings are equivocal (Figs. 13.35 and 13.36). Seminal vesicles biopsy is recommended for tumors involving the prostate base (Fig. 13.37). When positive, these biopsies define a biopsy-T3 stage.

- Presumptive signs of stage T3 tumors are often subtle and more difficult to detect than the tumor itself.

- The specificity of staging biopsies is 100%.

Nomograms and extraprostatic spread

- PSA level and biopsy findings (Gleason score and % of positive biopsies) are integrated in a nomogram which defines three groups of patients according to the risk of pT3 disease (Fig. 13.38).

- In patients at intermediate risk, the nomogram has a poor accuracy and requires further evaluation (endorectal MRI).

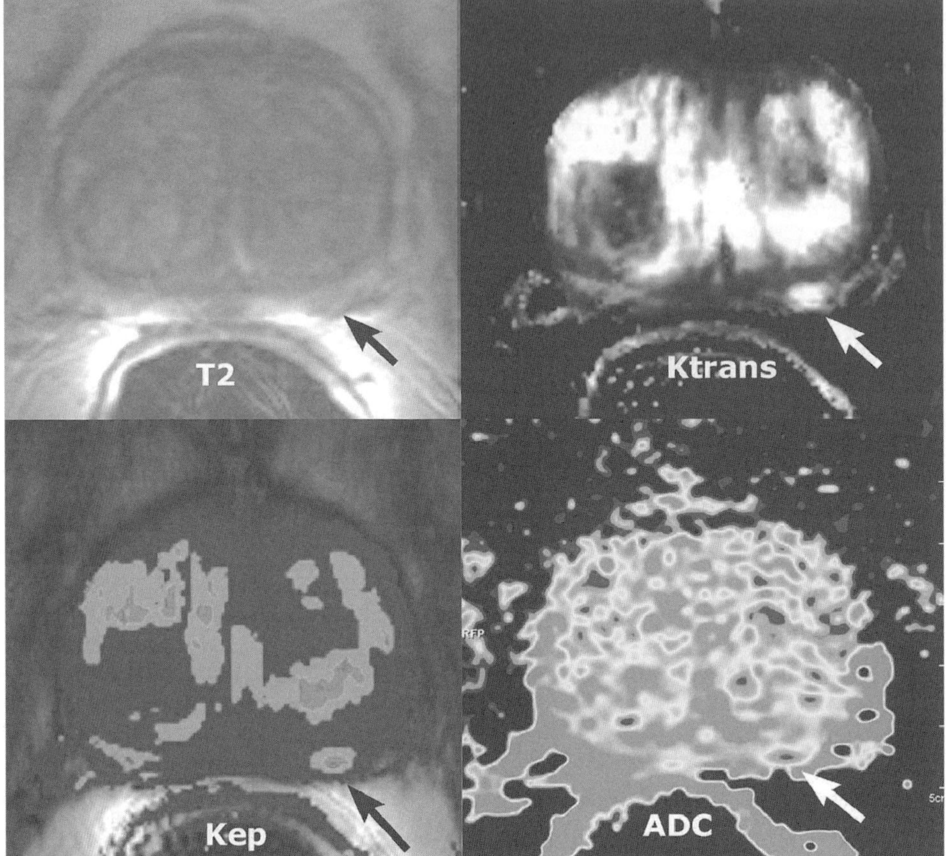

Figure 13.33   Functional MR and tumor volume. 68 Yo man. PSA: 6.5 ng/ml, 3 mm of Ca on a single left mid-sextant biopsy, Gleason score 6. Left non-specific 6 mm hyposignal (arrow) with high Ktrans and Kep values. Low ADC (blue area) increasing the specificity of dynamic MR: highly probable latent carcinoma (<0.5 cc) inviting to an active surveillance.

13.11 MRI and staging of prostate cancer F Cornud and D Portales

The role of endorectal MRI for local staging of PCa has been definitely established. Recently, lymph node staging has been considerably improved since iron particles have been developed and bone metastases staging, still under investigation, is now possible, with the development of whole marrow MRI. A whole in one MRI examination is now available and might replace in a short future all other examinations for staging a newly diagnosed prostate cancer. This assumption is reinforced by the continuing MR technical development, such as the use of three Tesla magnets or the increasing use of whole-body diffusion-weighted imaging in cancer patients.

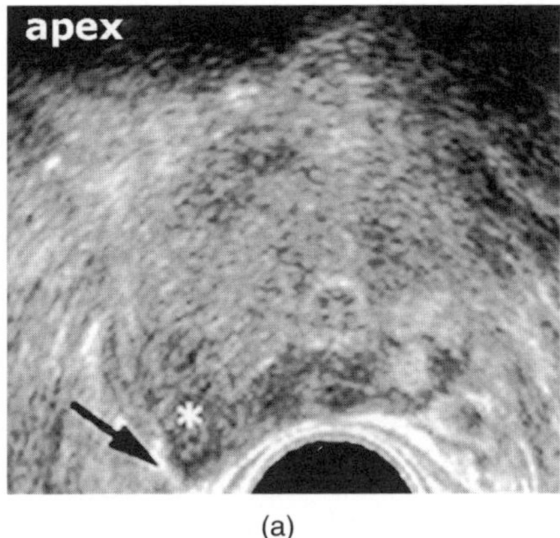

(a)

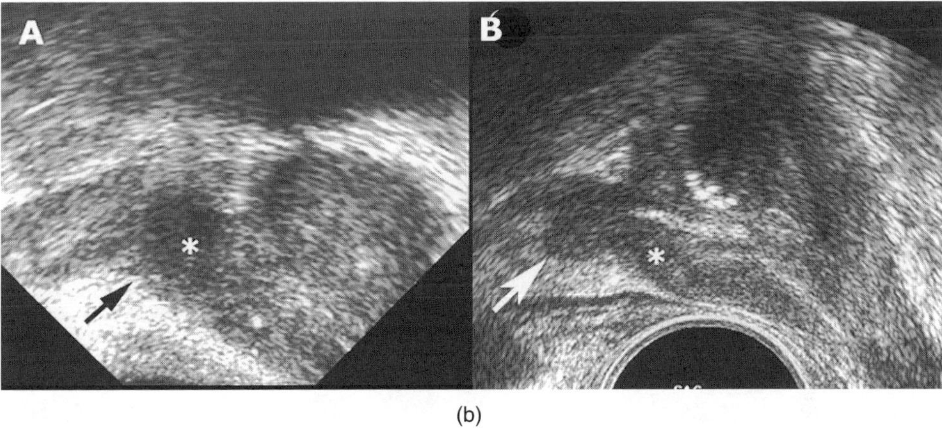

(b)

Figure 13.34 TRUS signs of extensive ECE. (a) Right apical PZ tumor (*). Extraprostatic extension is very conspicuous, with invasion of the neurovascular bundle (black arrows). (b) Extensive SVI in two different patients. (a) parasagittal view. Hypoechoic appearance of the root of the seminal vesicle (*) (arrow). (b) median sagittal view. Tumor (*) abuts the posterior aspect of the caudal junction of the vas deferens and the SV and extends above the prostate base within the periprostatic fat (arrow).

13.12 Local staging

Protocol

- A delay of at least 6 weeks should be respected between biopsies and MRI. It permits disappearance of parietal hematomas (which can simulate capsular effraction), and of biopsy artefacts which preclude tumor localisation (Fig. 13.39).

- To avoid motion artefacts, a careful recommendation to the patient not to contract the rectum during examination is a factor at least as important as the injection of glucacon.

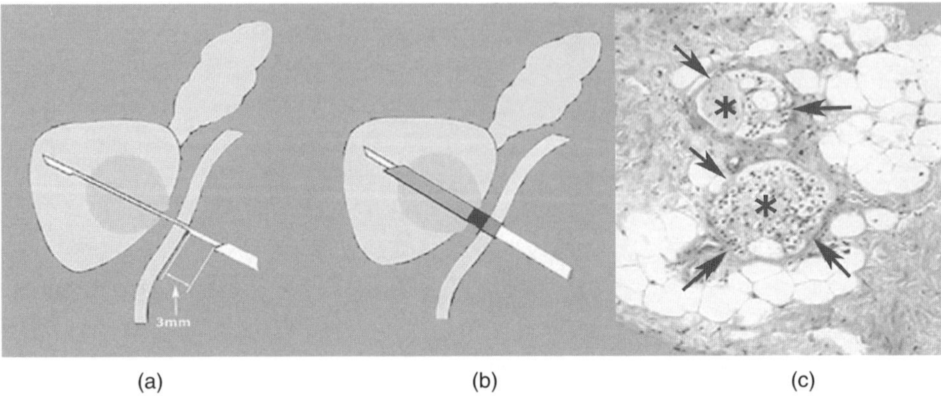

(a)   (b)   (c)

Figure 13.35 Periprostatic spaces biopsy. (a) the canula of the needle has been withdrawn to a few mm from the rectal wall (white arrow) before activation of the biopty. (b) when the canula is activated, an ideal sample contains a piece of the rectal wall (red), periprostatic fat (black) and primary tumor tissue (blue). (c) histology of biopsy-T3a stage: tumor cells (purple dots) are visible within the extraprostatic perineural spaces (arrows). (*): periprostatic nerves.

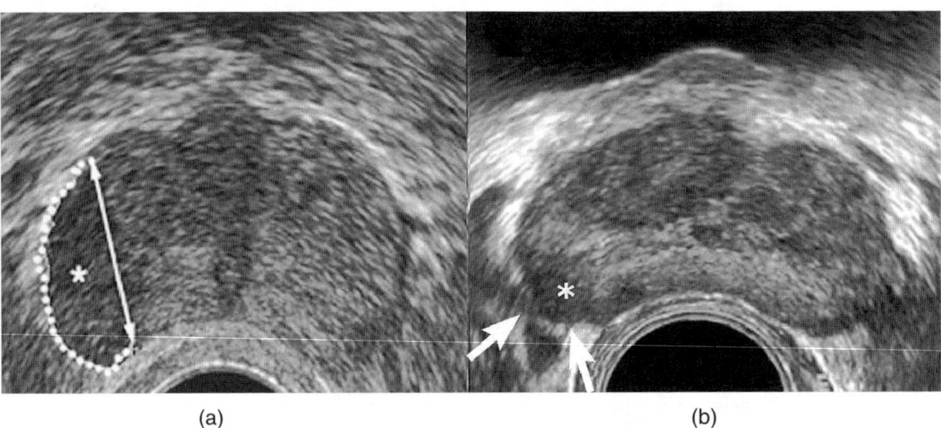

(a)   (b)

Figure 13.36 Presumptive signs of extracapsular extension (ECE). (a) broad contact (>23 mm, arrow) between the tumor (*) and the prostate contour (dotted line). (b) discrete tumor (*) bulging of the prostate contour at the mid-portion of the gland (arrows) in comparison to the normal appearance of the left side.

- The use of an endorectal coil is highly recommended for local staging of PCa. The incremental value of the endorectal coil has been demonstrated for 1.5T as well as 3T magnets.

Results

- Clinically confined tumors can be visible (MR-T2 stage), non-visible or obscured by biopsy artefacts (MR-T1 stage). The corresponding pathological stage (Fig. 13.40) is pT2. A MR-T2 stage tumor shows no sign of extension (Fig. 13.41). The margin status cannot be predicted by MRI and a pT2 stage tumor with a positive margin is the result of a surgical problem during dissection.

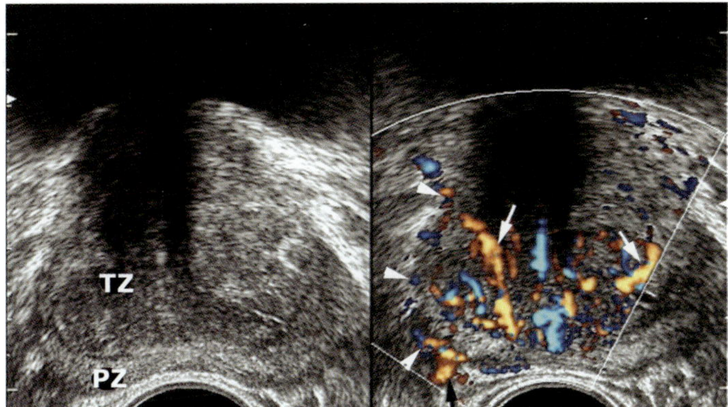

Figure 13.7 Color and Power Doppler of the prostate. Tranverse view. The TZ contains several macrovessels (white arrows). The posterolaterally located neurovascular bundle (black arrow) and the subcapsular vessels (arrowheads) are visible.

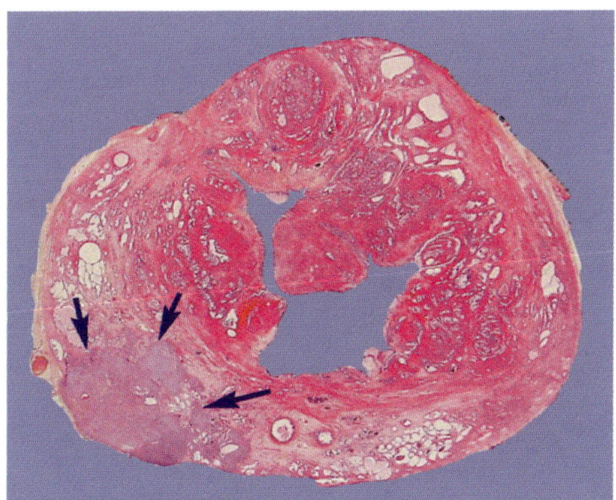

Figure 13.11 Prostatectomy specimen: the dense and compact cellularity (arrows) gives the hypoechoic appearance, whatever the Gleason grade.

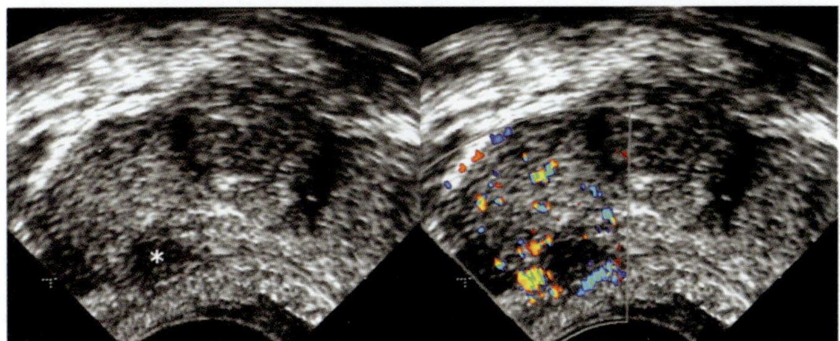

Figure 13.13 Granulomatous prostatitis. Palpable nodule detected 4 months after intravesical instillation of BCG. The nodule is hypoechoic and does not contain vessels (*). PSA level: 2 ng/ml. Granulomatous prostatitis at TRUS-guided biopsy.

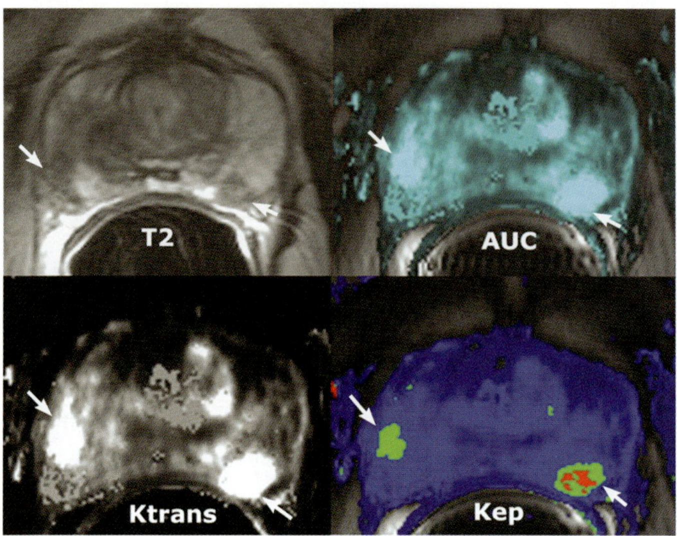

Figure 13.20   Quantitative dynamic MRI of a bilateral prostate cancer (arrows), Gleason score 6. PSA: 7 ng/ml. Color coded values of quantitative parameters show a bilateral high AUC, Ktrans and Kep.

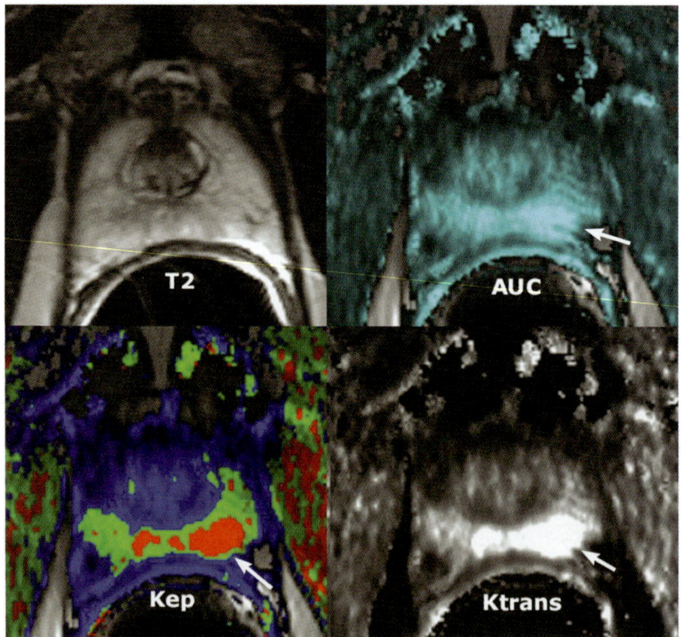

Figure 13.21   Prostatitis. 46 YO man. Raising PSA (2 to 4 ng/ml). Family history of PCa. MRI before biopsy. High AUC, Ktrans and Kep values in the left apex (arrow) with no hyposignal on the T2-W sequence. Saturation biopsies showed benign tissue and raising PSA was attributed to prostatitis.

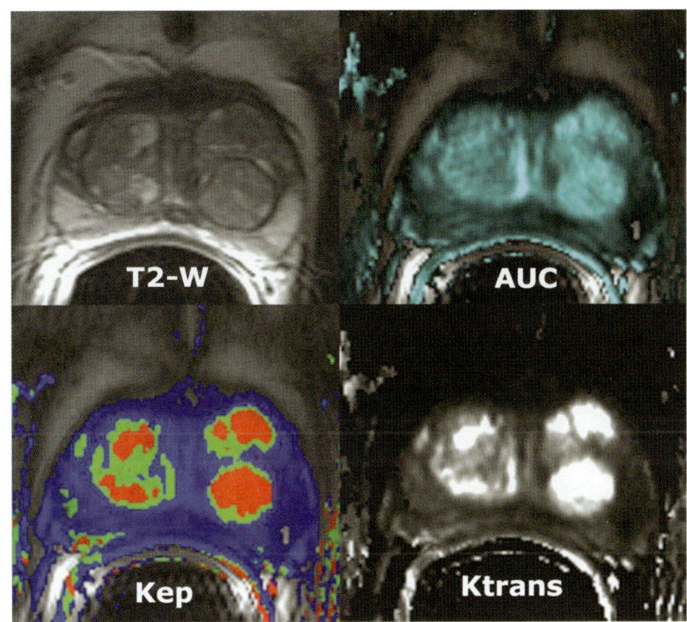

Figure 13.22 Dynamic quantitative MR and BPH nodules. Three typical BPH nodules (*) on the T2-W sequence with AUC, Ktrans and Kep values similar to those observed in cancer.

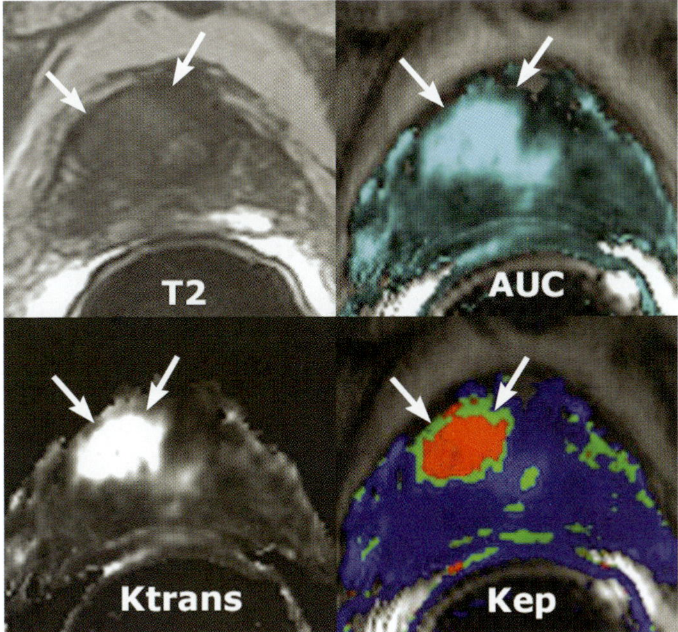

Figure 13.23 TZ carcinoma. 66 YO man, raising PSA (11 ng/ml). Two sets of posterior negative biopsies. Anterior ill-marginated hyposignal (arrow) with high AUC, Ktrans and Kep values. Combination of both sequences suggest cancer, which was confirmed by six directed right anterior biopsies (Gleason score 7, 13 mm of Ca).

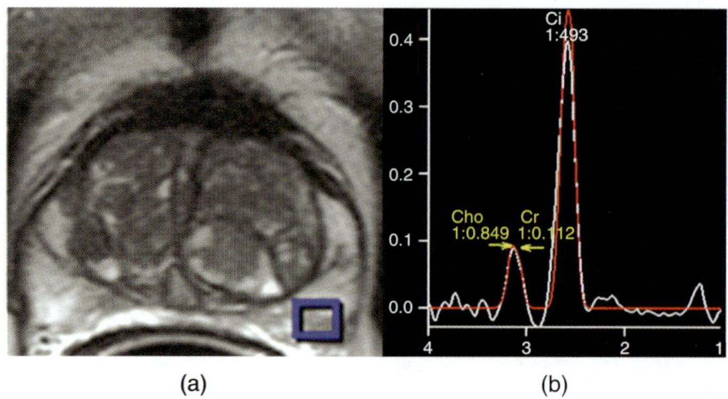

Figure 13.24 MRSI of normal PZ. (a): A voxel (blue box) is overlaid on a T2 image. (b): The x axis of the spectral trace from the voxel represents frequency. The y axis represents intensity which lacks absolute units. The ratio Cho + Cr/Ci is <0.6.

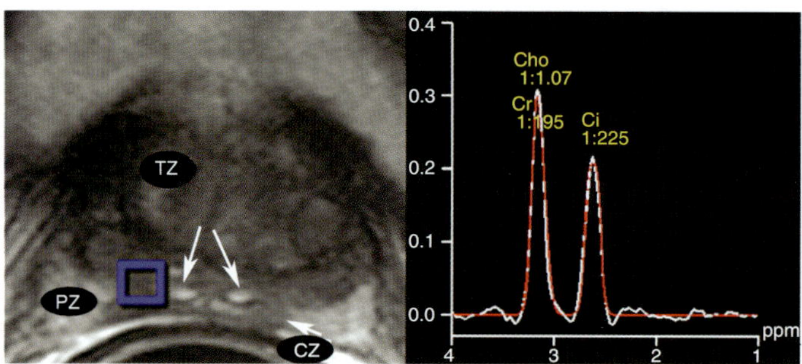

Figure 13.25 Physiological elevated CC/Ci ratio (>1) around the ejaculatory ducts (arrows). Note the hyposignal of the central zone (CZ).

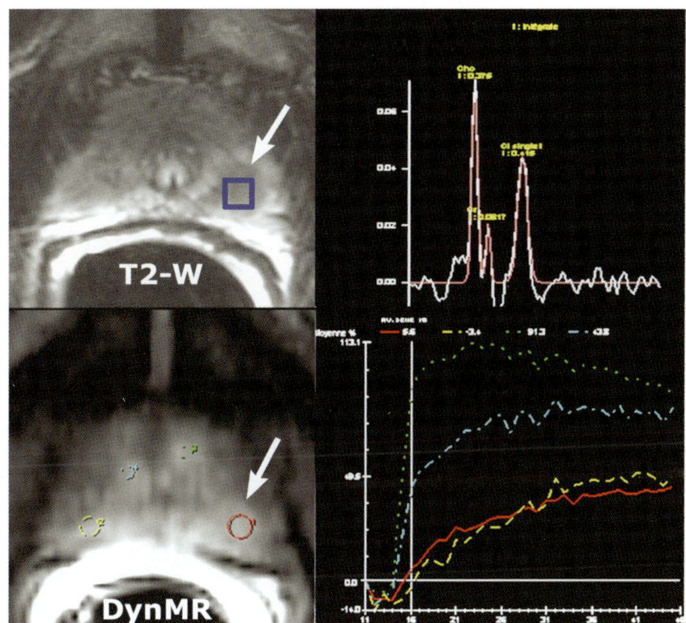

Figure 13.28 MRSI and chronic prostatitis. 63 YO man. Raising PSA (9 ng/ml). Two series of negative biopsies. Left apical hyposignal (arrow) on the T2-W image with a CC/Ci ratio >0.6 and a flat type 1 curve (red) on dynamic MR (DynMR). Saturation left apical biopsies (8 cores) showed interstitial prostatitis.

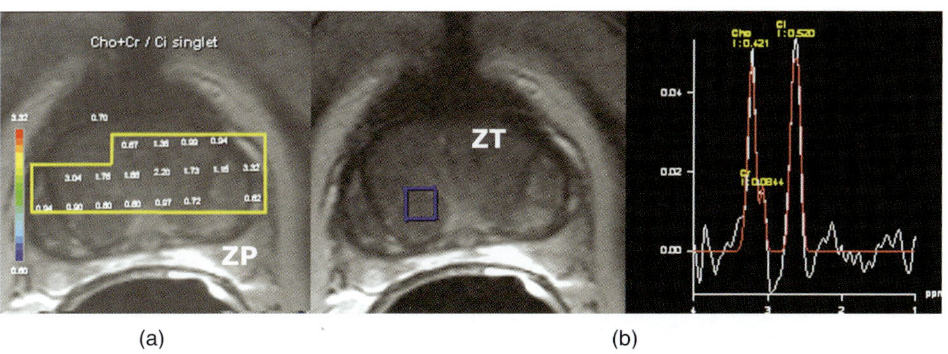

(a)   (b)

Figure 13.29 MRSI and stromal BPH. Raising PSA (16 ng/ml) and three series of negative biopsies. (a): most of the voxels in the yellow box have a CC/Ci ratio >0.8 (b): detail of the spectrum of one of these voxels (CC/Ci: 1.21). Saturation biopsies (30 cores) showed benign tissue.

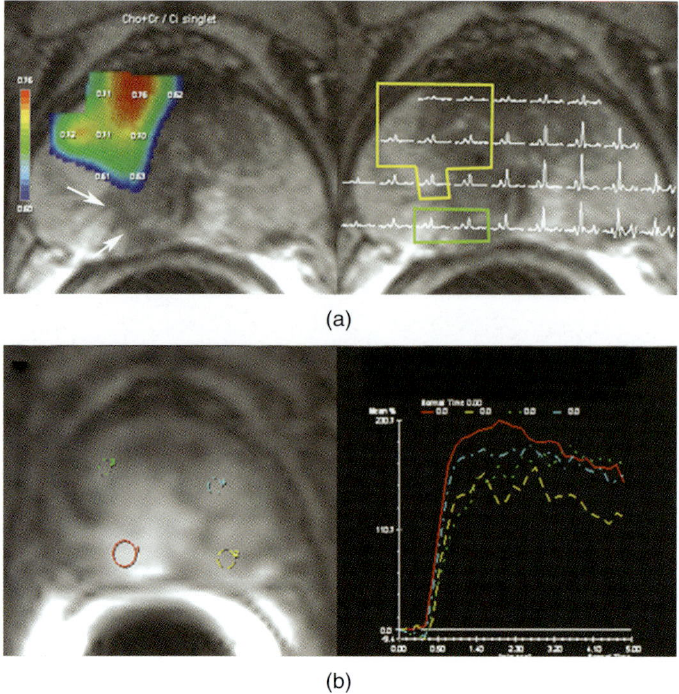

(a)

(b)

Figure 13.30 MRSI and low-grade cancers. Raising PSA (11 ng/ml). MRI before biopsy. (a): Hyposignal in the right PZ (arrow) with normal metabolic activity (green box). (b): dynamic MRI. Typical type 3 curve in the hyposignal (red). Targeted biopsies showed 6 mm of Gleason score 6 carcinoma.

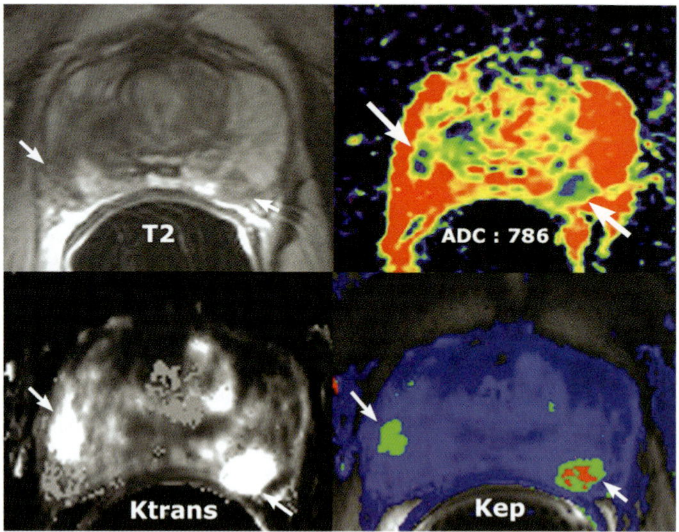

Figure 13.31 Combination of DWI and perfusion. Same patient as in Figure 20. bilateral Gleason 6 Ca with high AUC, Ktrans and Kep values. The ADC is low, suggesting cancer and increasing the specificity of dynamic MR. 57 YO patient.

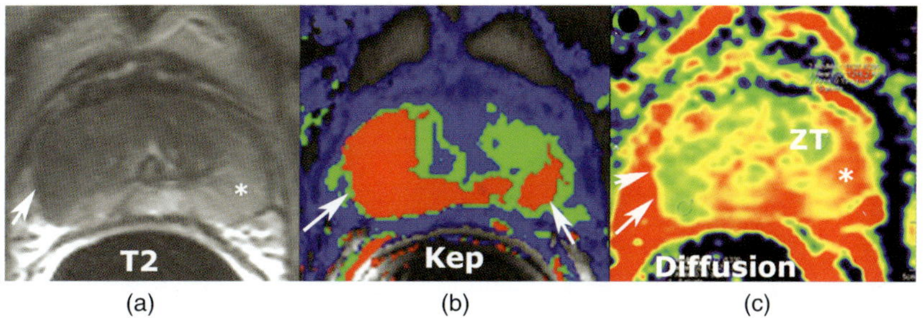

Figure 13.32 Combination of DWI and perfusion. Gleason score 7 (3 + 4).involving the three right sextants. (a): right PZ hyposignal (arrow) and heterogeneous signal of the left PZ (*). (b) Bilateral elevated Kep (arrows) suggesting a bilateral tumor (c): Low ADC (0.9, green area) in the right PZ (arrows). Normal ADC (1,9) on the left side (*, red and orange area). On the radical prostatectomy specimen, no tumor was present in the left lobe.

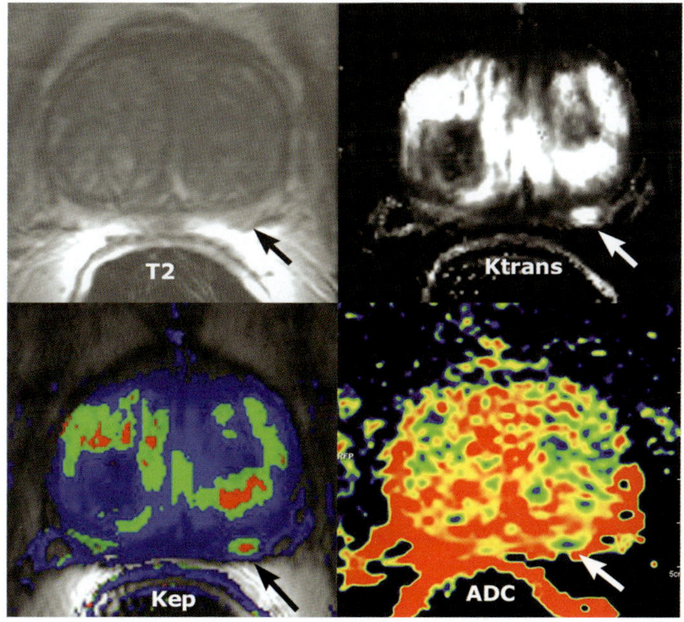

Figure 13.33 Functional MR and tumor volume. 68 Yo man. PSA: 6.5 ng/ml, 3 mm of Ca on a single left mid-sextant biopsy, Gleason score 6. Left non-specific 6 mm hyposignal (arrow) with high Ktrans and Kep values. Low ADC (blue area) increasing the specificity of dynamic MR: highly probable latent carcinoma (<0.5 cc) inviting to an active surveillance.

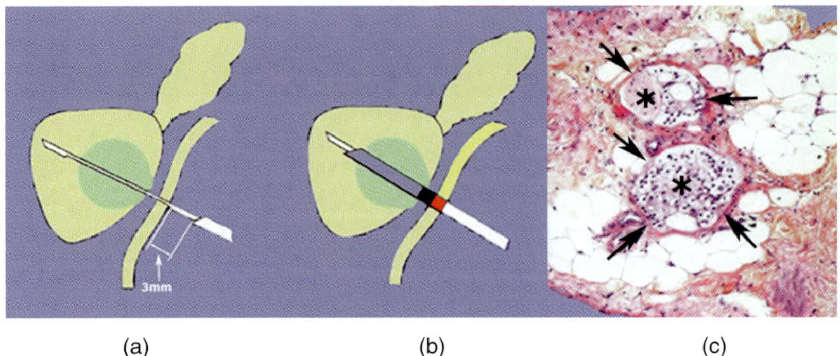

(a)   (b)   (c)

Figure 13.35 Periprostatic spaces biopsy. (a) the canula of the needle has been withdrawn to a few mm from the rectal wall (white arrow) before activation of the biopty. (b) when the canula is activated, an ideal sample contains a piece of the rectal wall (red), periprostatic fat (black) and primary tumor tissue (blue). (c) histology of biopsy-T3a stage: tumor cells (purple dots) are visible within the extraprostatic perineural spaces (arrows). (*): periprostatic nerves.

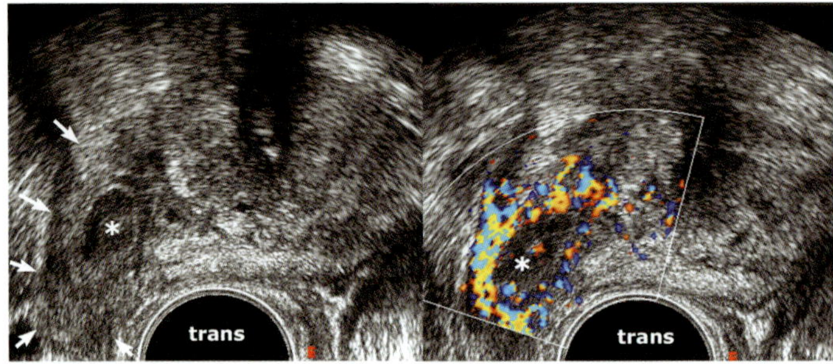

Figure 13.61 Prostatic abscess. Marked irregularity of the right prostate contour (arrows). Hypoechoic appearance of the right PZ with central cavitation (*). Intense vascularity around the abscess.

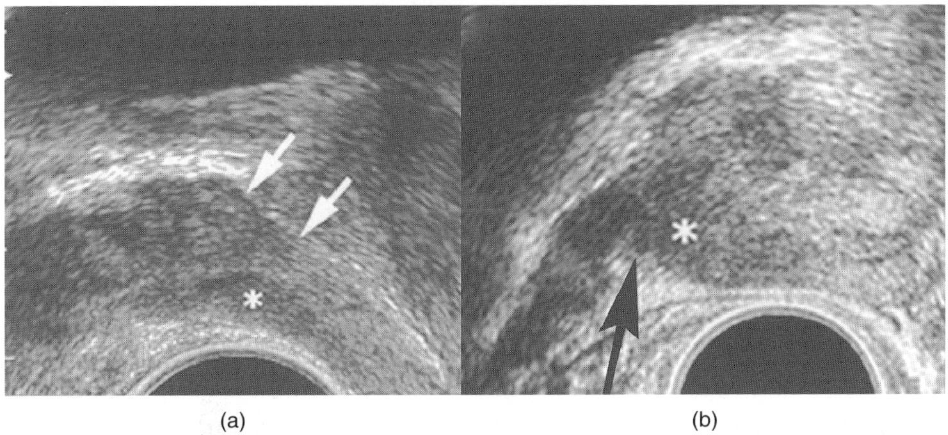

Figure 13.37   Presumptive signs of SVI. Sagittal views in two different patients. (a) The tumor (*) abuts the posterior aspect of the caudal junction of the vas deferens and the SV (arrows). Early SVI should be suspected. (b) Parasagittal view: the tumor (*) bulges within the periprostatic fat and partially obscurs the prostato-seminal angle (arrow). Transcapsular SVI should be suspected.

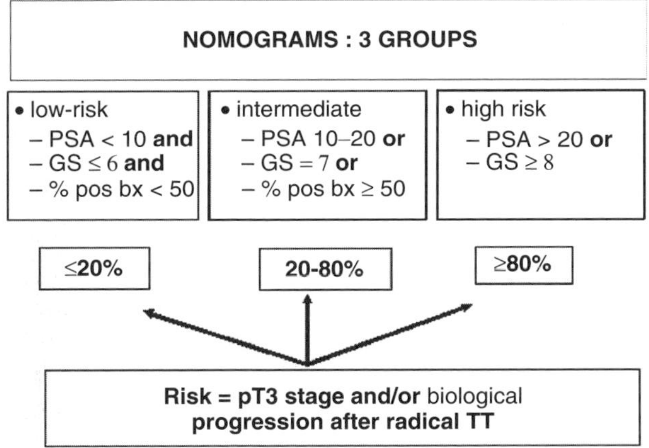

Figure 13.38   Classification of the risk at pT3 stage according to PSA level and biopsy findings.

- Extraprostatic capsular extension (ECE) can be detected by MRI if at least 1 mm of tumor extends within the prostatic fat (established pT3 stage).

  o Criteria are: tumor visible within the periprostatic (Fig. 13.42a), obliteration of the prostato-rectal angle (Fig. 13.42b), hyposignal of the neurovascular bundles (Fig. 13.42c) and invasion of the urethral sphincter for apical tumors (Fig. 13.42d).

  o They should be strictly applied to obtain a 90–95% specificity and avoid false-positive cases. Sensitivity is approximately 40% if focal (tumor extension <1 mm) and established pT3 stages are included and 70% if only established pT3 stage is taken into account.

- Seminal vesicle invasion is secondary to large volume tumors involving the prostate base.

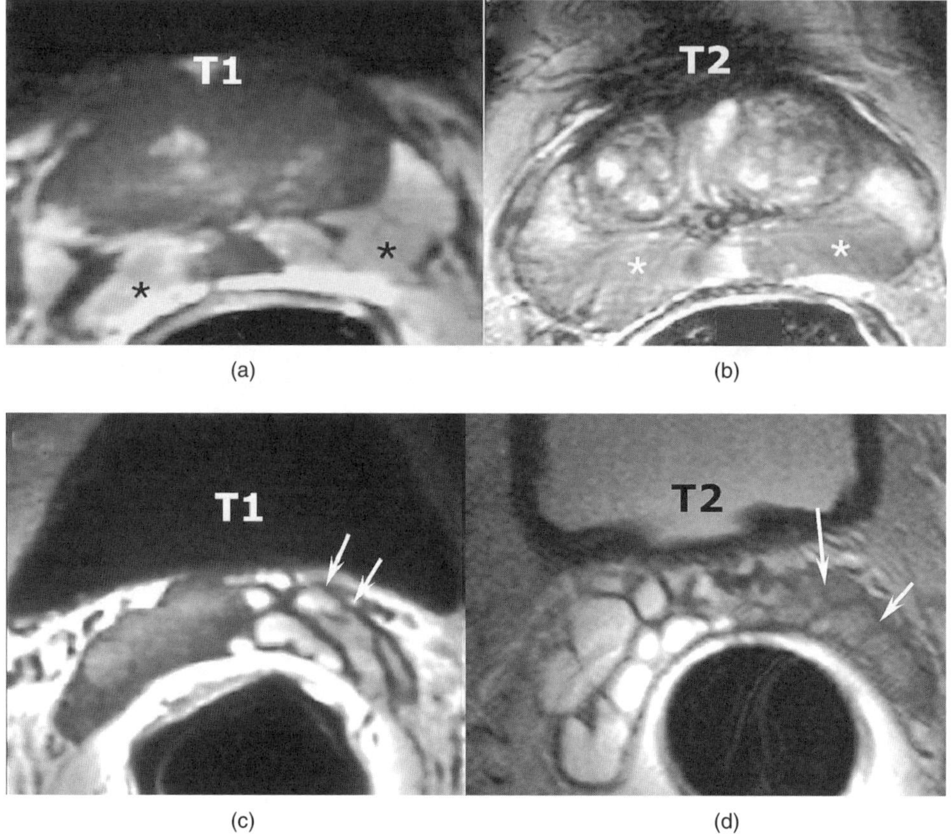

Figure 13.39 Biopsy artefacts. Bilateral hyperintense foci of hemorrhage on T1W images (black *, a) responsible for hypointense areas on T2W images (white *, b), precluding tumor localization. Seminal vesicles can be involved by the same artefacts (arrow, c-d).

- o Signs of gross SVI (Fig. 13.43) are consistently detected by MRI and have a specificity of virtually 100%.

- o Signs of early SVI are less conspicuous or less specific (Fig. 13.44) and may require TRUS-guided biopsies of the SV for confirmation.

- o Tumors originating in the central zone can cause extensive SVI (Fig. 13.45) without ECE.

- Extension to adjacent organs is a very uncommon finding since the PSA era.

  - o MRI remains the most accurate imaging modality to detect rectal invasion.

  - o Its accuracy is more limited for the detection of bladder neck invasion, considered as a pT4 stage by pathologists. Only advanced forms of bladder floor invasion can be detected (Fig. 13.46).

- False-positive cases. The direct signs can be misinterpreted and lead to an overdiagnosis of ECE.

- False-negative cases.

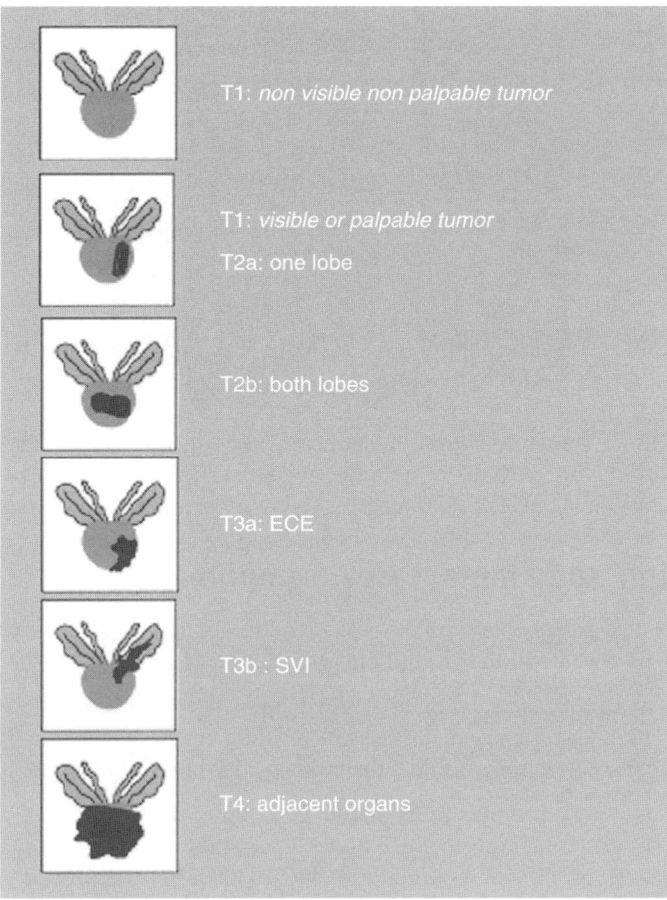

Figure 13.40 TNM clinical classification of PCa. T1 tumors are subclassified in T1a (<5% of positive chips of a TURP and Gleason score <7), T2b (>5% of positive chips of a TURP or Gleason score ≥7) and T1c (diagnosed on TRUS guided biopsies).

- Some of them can be avoided if ECE is thoroughly searched on the whole prostate contour and not only at the site of the broadest contact of the tumor (Fig. 13.47).
- In 30% of cases, established ECE cannot be detected on MRI, probably because slice thickness (3.5 mm) and the use of 1.5 Tesla magnets lack spatial resolution.

Indications of endorectal MRI for local staging

These are defined by the risk factors provided by the nomograms (Fig. 13.38).

- In low risk patients, endorectal MRI is only required when estimation of tumor volume is the objective.

- In intermediate and high risk patients, staging is indicated to convert a statistical risk provided by the nomogram to an almost certainty of pT3 stage if MRI is positive.

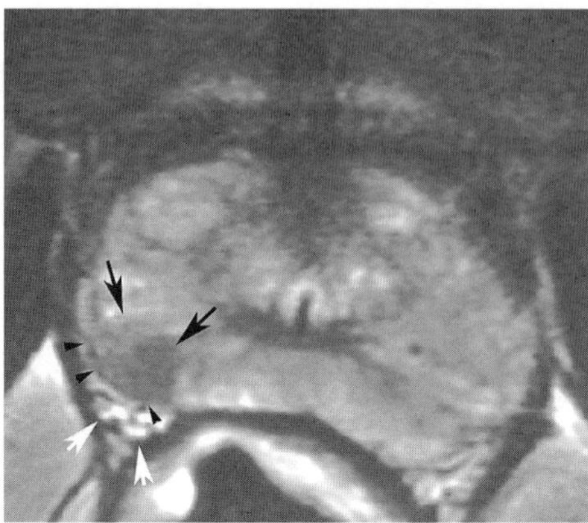

Figure 13.41 MR-T2 stage carcinoma. Hypointense well-marginated tumor (black arrows). Normal appearance of the prostate capsule (arrowheads). The neurovascular bundles (white arrows) are posterolaterally located. Pathological stage: pT2a stage, Gleason score 6.

13.13 Lymph node metastases: lympho-MRI

- They are suspected as soon as the PSA level reaches 10 ng/ml. When present, the cancer can no longer be cured and the overall survival rate decreases from 70% to 35%.

- Inflammatory and metastatic enlarged nodes cannot be differentiated with T1 or T2W imaging (Fig. 13.48) and many metastases of prostate cancer occur in normal size lymph nodes. Surgical dissection remains thus the gold standard to evaluate lymph node invasion.

- Lympho-MRI is a very promising technique. It exploits the property of macrophages to capture iron particles and store them in nodes when they are intravenously injected 24 h before MRI. However, the microparticules have not been FDA approved yet for a clinical routine use.

  - On a T2W or T2*W sequence, the signal of a normal lymph node (which stores the iron particles) dramatically decreases (Fig. 13.49).

  - The IV injection of particles does not modify the signal of a metastatic lymph node (which does not store the iron particles) (Fig. 13.50).

  - Diagnosis accuracy increases from 35% to 95% for lymph nodes with a long axis >5 mm and micrometastases can be detected within normal size lymph nodes.

13.14 Bone metastases: whole marrow MRI

- Bone metastases should only be searched in patients with a PSA level >15–20 ng/ml.

- Whole marrow MRI is performed by coupling several coils to cover the whole body. T1W, and diffusion sequences are used (Fig. 13.51). STIR sequences are optional.

- Imaging of the axial skeleton, pelvis and mid-femur has a 100% sensitivity to detect bone metastases of prostate cancer.

- This promising technique, in combination with lympho-MRI and local staging, provides a potential unique hole-in-one examination to evaluate a newly diagnosed prostate cancer.

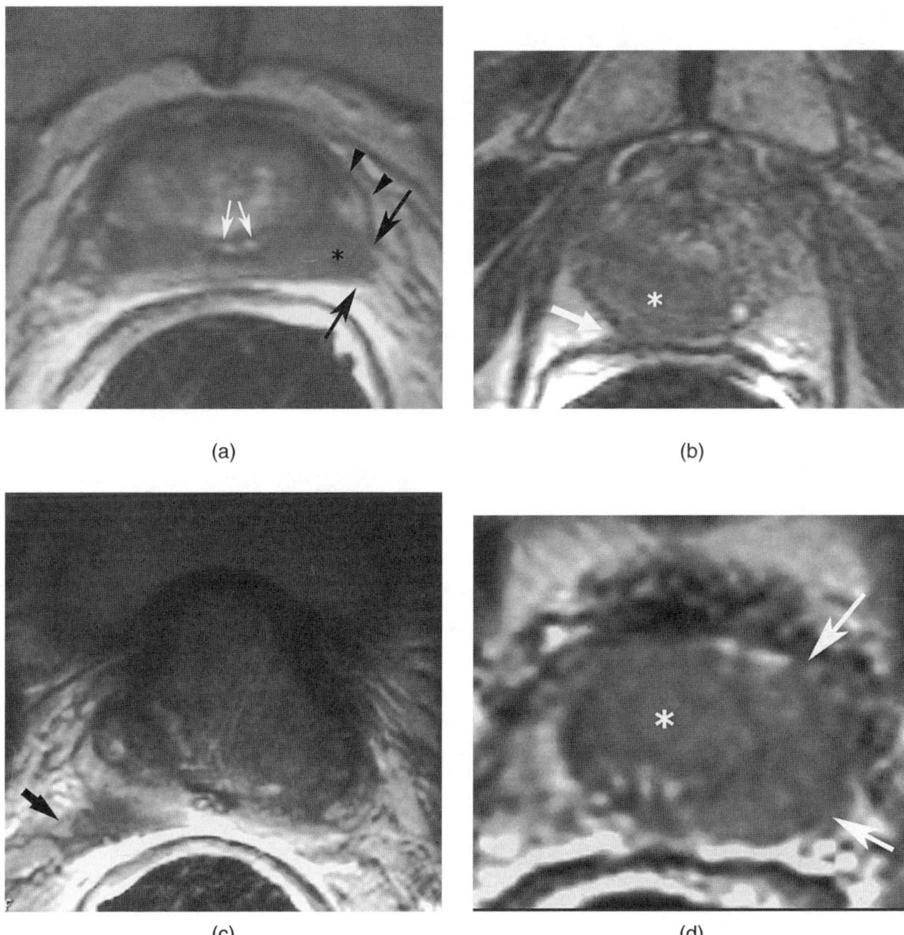

(a)　　(b)

(c)　　(d)

Figure 13.42　Established ECE. (a) Tumor within the periprostatic fat. Posterolateral extension of the tumor (*) within the periprostatic fat (arrows). More laterally, normal appearance of the capsule (arrowheads). Ejaculatory ducts are normal (white arrows). (b) Obliteration of the right apical prostate-rectal angle (arrow) by a pT3 stage tumor (*). (c) Invasion of the neurovascular bundle which is hypointense (arrow) when compared with the left side which has a normal appearance. (d) Invasion of the striated sphincter by an apical tumor. Apical tumor (white arrows) with invasion of the urethral sphincter (*) which is isointense to the carcinoma.

13.15　Benign disorders of the prostate (BPH excluded)

Besides prostate cancer and BPH, the prostate gland and the distal genital tract can be involved by embryological or inflammatory disorders.

Cystic disorders

Median cysts represent the most frequent abnormality.

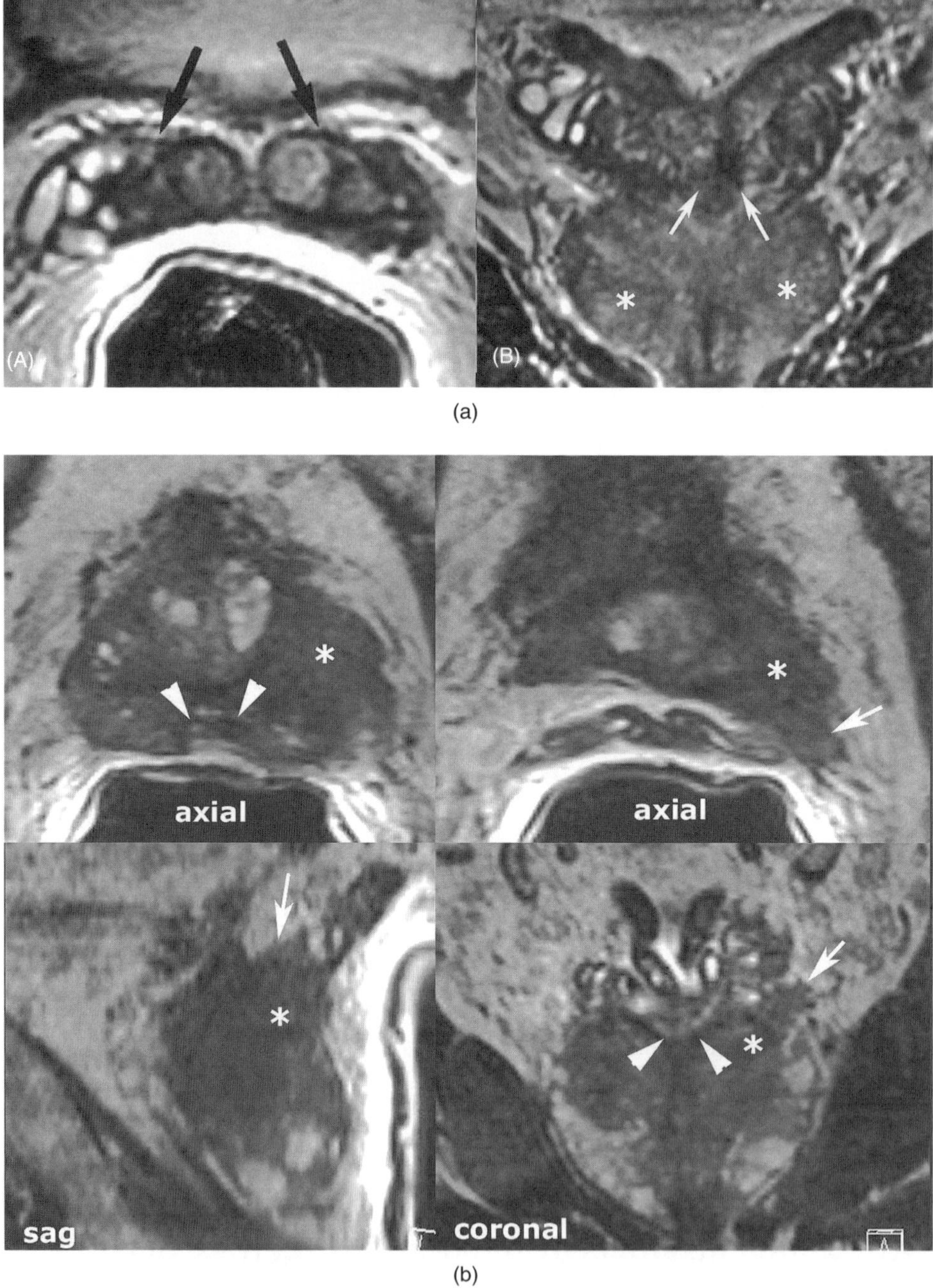

Figure 13.43 Extensive seminal vesicle invasion. (a) Bilateral massive invasion (arrows, A) through the two caudal junctions of the vas deferens and seminal vesicles (white arrows) by a bilateral tumor involving both bases (*, B), Gleason score 8. (b) SVI through the prostate capsule with invasion of the perivesicular fat. Basal tumor (*) with established ECE (white arrow) abutting the left SV. Pathological stage: massive pT3b. The ejaculatory ducts and the caudal junction of the vas deferens and SV (white arrowheads) are normal.

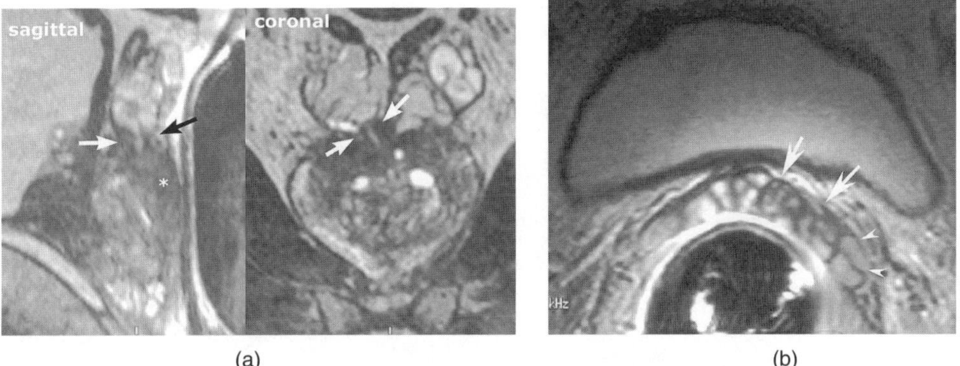

(a) (b)

Figure 13.44 Early SVI. (a) Invasion of the root of the left SV (arrows). (b) Focal thickening of the wall of the left seminal vesicle (white arrows) indicating possible early SVI. Pathological stage: pT3b.

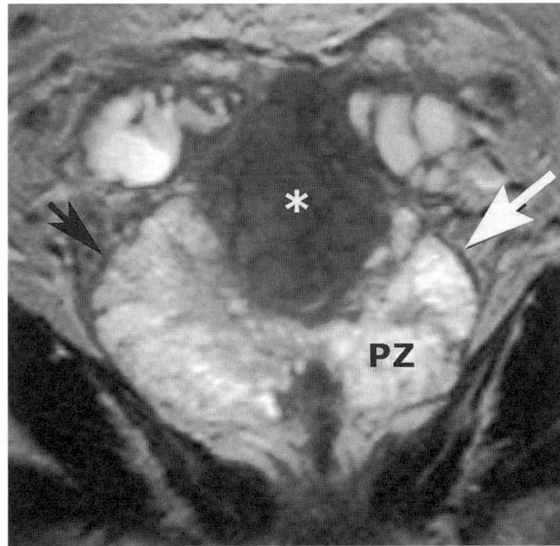

Figure 13.45 Massive SVI (*) by a carcinoma originating within the central zone (Gleason score 9). The PZ is isointense and surrounded by a normal capsule (arrow).

- Mullerian (utricular) cyst (Fig. 13.52)
  - Frequent in hypofertile men (11% of cases), versus 2% in the general population.
  - Complications include infection, bleeding (Fig. 13.53) and compression of the ejaculatory duct (complete or partial) responsible for hypofertility.
    - When the obstruction is complete, the volume of ejaculate is small (<1.5 ml), the semen pH is acid and the fructose level undetectable.

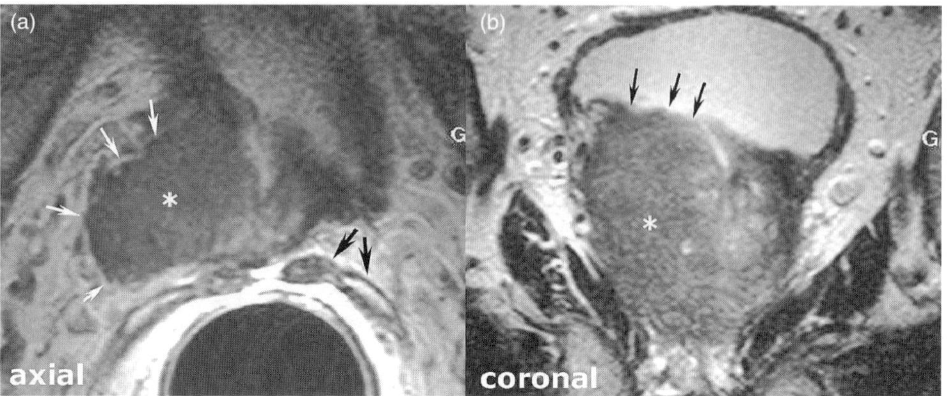

Figure 13.46   MR-T4 stage. Tumor involving both the PZ and TZ (*, a–b). Marked irregularity of the prostate contour (white arrows, a) and suspicion of invasion of the bladder floor (black arrows, b). The SV are normal (black arrows, a). Trigonal invasion confirmed at histology of endoscopic biopsies.

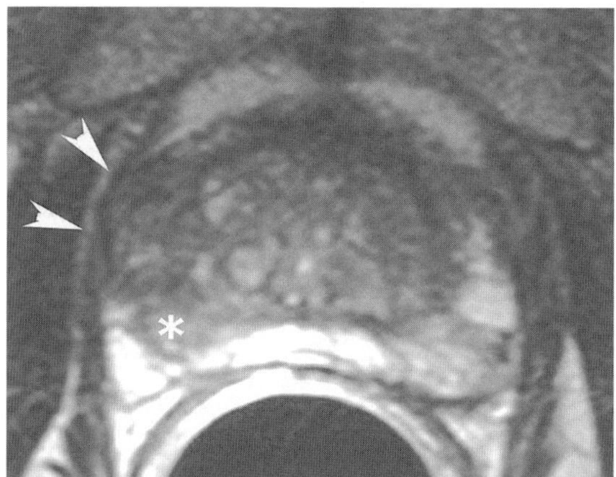

Figure 13.47   False-negative case. Tumor involving the three right sextants (*) with no posterolateral capsular abnormality. Tumor extension is only visible in the lateral horn of the PZ (arrowheads) and was not prospectively diagnosed.

- ■ Imaging confirms the dilatation of the seminal tract (Fig. 13.54) which can be masked by the presence of an inflammatory retraction of the seminal vesicles, only visible on MRI (Fig. 13.55).

- ● Median cyst of Wolffian origin

  - ○ They are much less common than the Mullerian cysts. They originate in the ejaculatory ducts, ampullae of the vas deferens or seminal vesicles and are well shown by TRUS (Fig. 13.56).

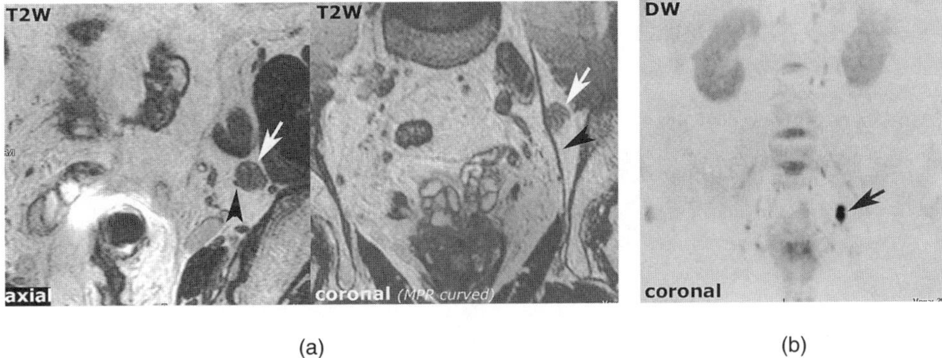

Figure 13.48   Lymph node metastasis. (a) Ilio-obturator enlarged lymph node (white arrow) located anterolaterally to the obturator nerve (black arrowhead), well displayed on the coronal curved MPR reconstruction. (b) Pelvic segment of a whole body DW-MRI. The enlarged lymph node is well visible, but lymph node dissection is necessary to confirm metastasis.

- Mega-seminal vesicles

  o Have been assimilated for years to SV cyst, because they are observed in patients presenting with an adult kidney polycystic disease. They are indeed due to an achalasia (unknown cause) of the seminal vesicles which are dilated and acontractile.

  o Can be detected during the work-up of hypofertile patients (Fig. 13.57) who typically present with high variability of the parameters of the ejaculate (volume, sperm count, motility) from one spermogram to the other, which reflects the intermittent functional stenosis.

Disorders of the vas deferens

- Congenital Bilateral Absence of the Vas Deferens (CBAVD)

  o Rare cause of male hypofertility (1–2% of all hypofertile patients).

  o Corresponds to a genital involvement by cystic fibrosis in more than 80% of cases. There is thus no associated renal agenesis. If one kidney is missing, CBAVD has an embryological origin and no mutation for the CFTR gene is found.

  o Clinical presentation includes no palpable vas deferens in the bursae, a very low volume of ejaculate with an acid pH and no detectable fructose. TRUS is helpful in when clinical findings are not obvious (Fig. 13.58).

- Congenital Unilateral Absence of the Vas Deferens (CUAVD).

  o Uncommon disorder (0.06–1%) which can be due to a mutation of the CFTR gene. The persistent vas deferens had a blind end in the pelvis. A genetic survey is thus recommended in case of CUAVD, particularly if no renal agenesis is present (Fig. 13.59).

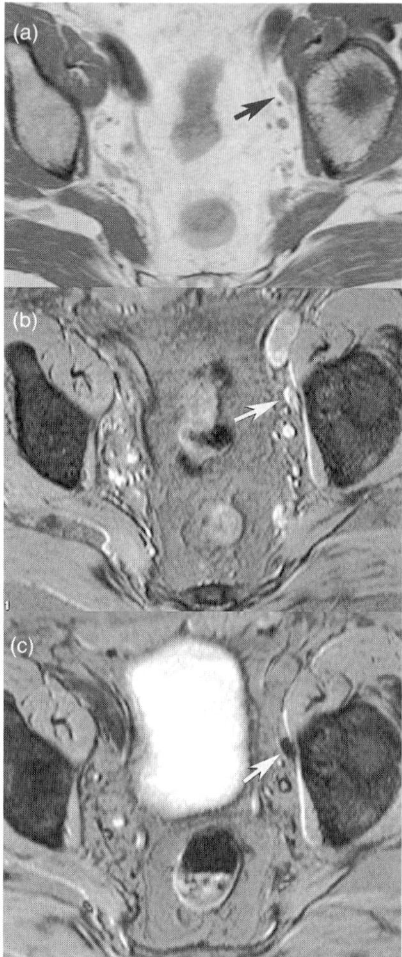

Figure 13.49   Normal lympho-MRI. (a): T1W image. Hyposignal of a normal size lymph node (arrow). (b): T2W image with fat saturation. Hypersignal of the lymph node (arrow). (c): T2W image with fat saturation, 24 h after IV injection of iron particles: marked signal decrease of the normal lymph node (arrow). Reproduced with courtesy of Professor Bellin, MD, Paul Brousse Hospital, 94804 Villejuif, France.

Ectopic joining of the ureter

This occurs above the level of the striated sphincter and do not cause incontinence. In most cases, the ectopic ureter comes from the upper half of a complete duplication of the collecting system (Fig. 13.60). It can be detected during the work-up of a hypofertile man or revealed by repeat attacks of urinary infection.

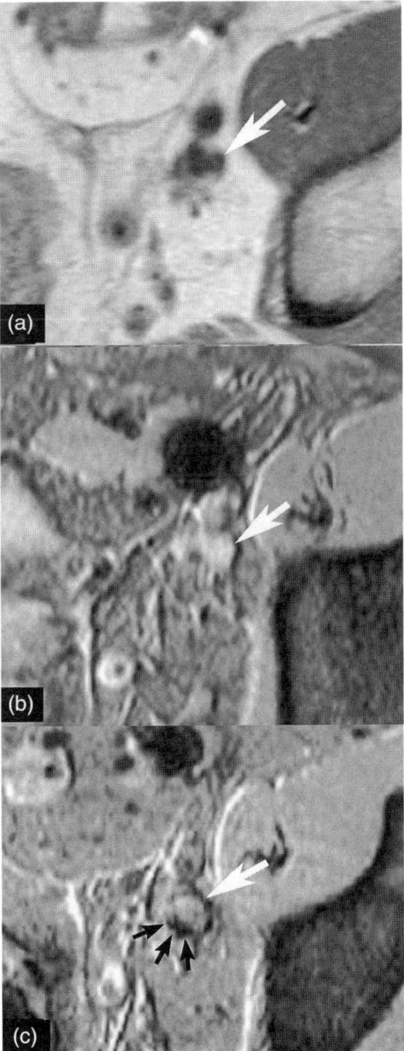

Figure 13.50 Metastasis in a normal size node (6 mm). (a): T1W image. Nodal hyposignal (white arrow). (b): T2W image with fat suppression. Hypersignal of the node (white arrow). (c): T2W image with fat suppression 24 h after IV injection of iron particles. Low signal of the posterior normal portion of the node (black arrows) and hypersignal of the anterior portion of the node (white arrow), invaded by tumor. Reproduced with courtesy of Professor Bellin, MD, Paul Brousse Hospital, 94804 Villejuif, France.

Inflammatory disorders

- Prostatitis

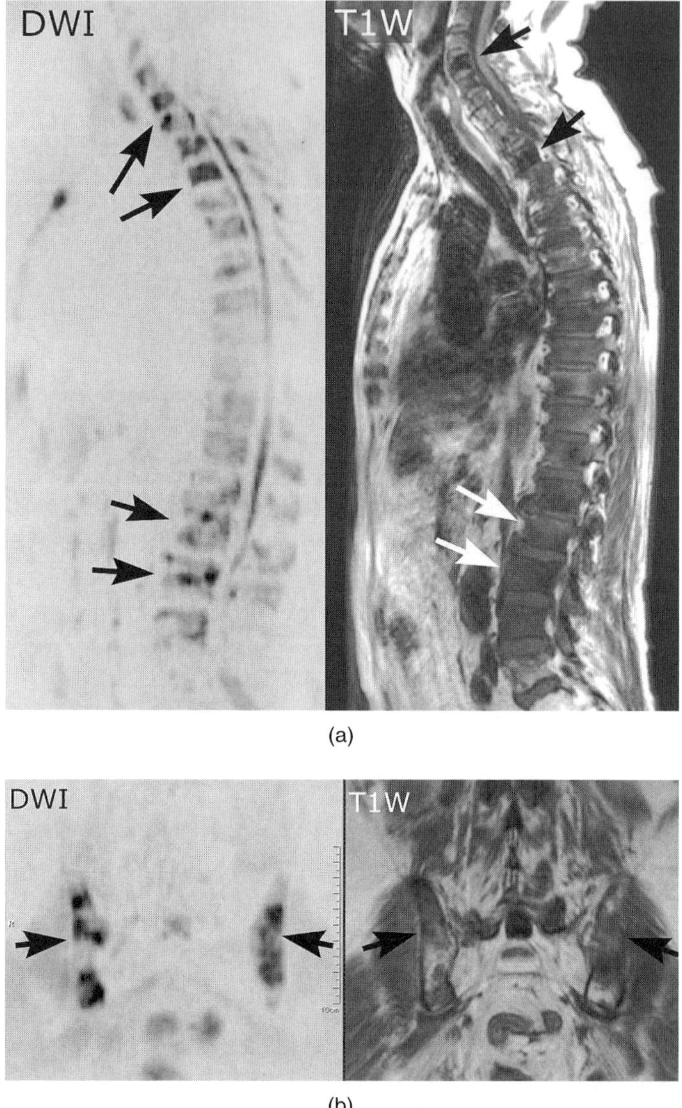

Figure 13.51 Bone metastases on DW and T1W images. (a) Several vertebras are involved by metastatic foci highly conspicuous on both sequences (arrows). (b) Coronal images, pelvic segment of the whole marrow MRI. On both DW and T1W sequences, several metastatic foci are visible in the pelvis bone (arrows).

- o The new classification includes acute prostatitis, chronic bacterial prostatitis and merges chronic non-bacterial prostatitis and prostadynia into a single new category called chronic non-bacterial prostatitis- pelvic pain syndrome (CNBP/CPPS), which is further divided into inflammatory and non-inflammatory subtypes based on the presence or absence of white blood cells in the prostatic secretions.

- o Acute prostatitis: imaging is not required in non-complicated cases.

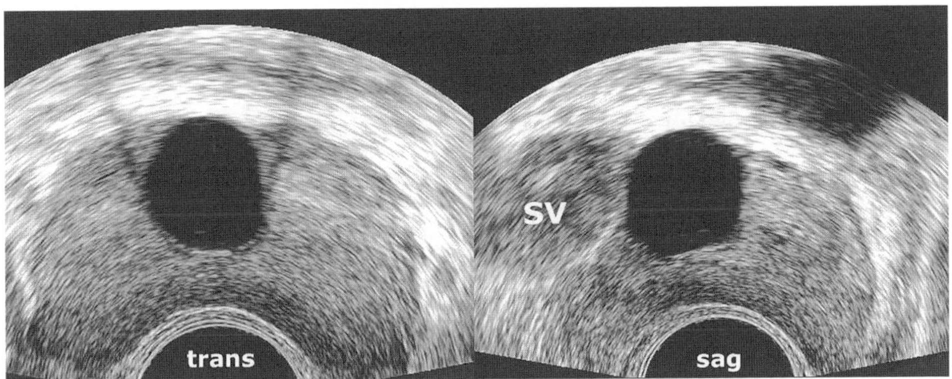

Figure 13.52   Mullerian median cyst. On the sagittal view (sag), the cyst slightly extends above the prostate base. SV: seminal vesicle.

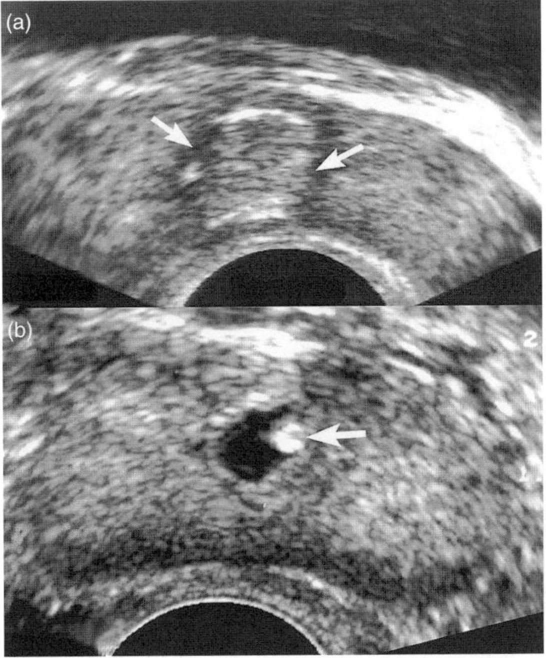

Figure 13.53   Complicated Mullerian cysts. (a): Echoic content of the cyst, which has a calcified wall (arrow). (b): intracystic stone (arrow).

- ○ Chronic bacterial prostatitis
  - ▪ Patients present with various symptoms (infectious and non-infectious) of the lower genito-urinary tract.
  - ▪ Over time, TRUS can detect PZ calcifications and hypoechoic areas of fibrosis (see below).
- • Prostate abscess

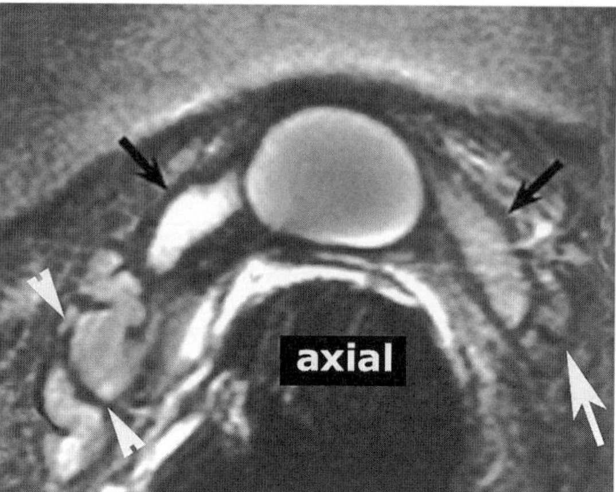

Figure 13.54 Mullerian cyst and ejaculatory duct obstruction. Endorectal MRI: both vas deferens (black arrows) and the right SV (arrowheads) are dilated. The left SV is barely seen (white arrow).

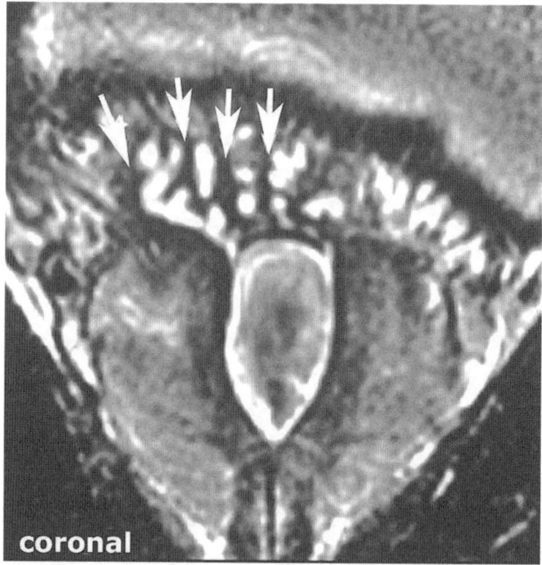

Figure 13.55 Seminal vesicle retraction. Azoospermic patient with a low volume of ejaculate (0.8 ml). Endorectal MRI, coronal view: diffuse thickening of the SV walls (white arrows).

- Uncommon since the introduction of broad-spectrum antibiotics to treat urinary tract infections.
- Risk factors include urethral manipulation and all causes of immunodeficiency.
- Fever and perineal pain are inconstant findings. DRE is painful in most patients, but fluctuation or induration are not commonly noted.
- TRUS confirms the diagnosis (Fig. 13.61) and is used for transrectal aspiration, when deemed necessary, which has a success rate of over 80% in curing the abscess, in combination with intravenous antibiotics.

trans
sag
28 cm

(a)

trans
sag (right)

(b)

sagittal
bladder
*
B
axial, T1W
*
A
C

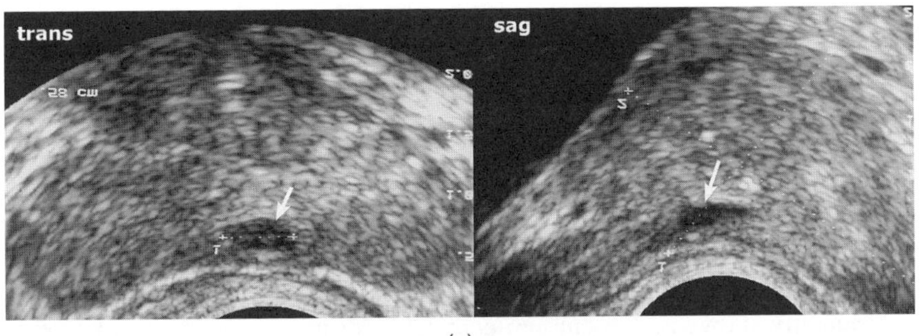

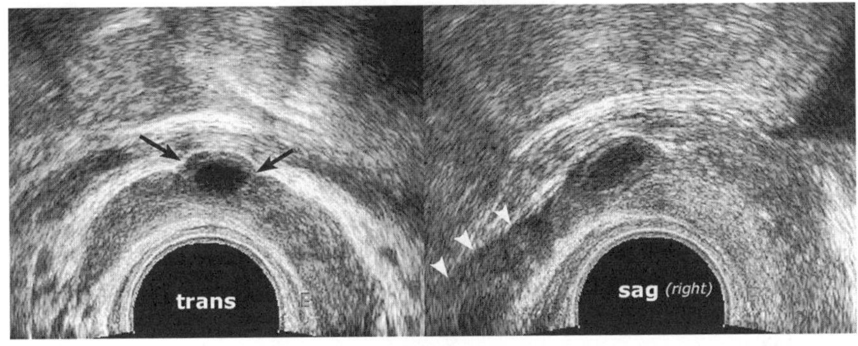

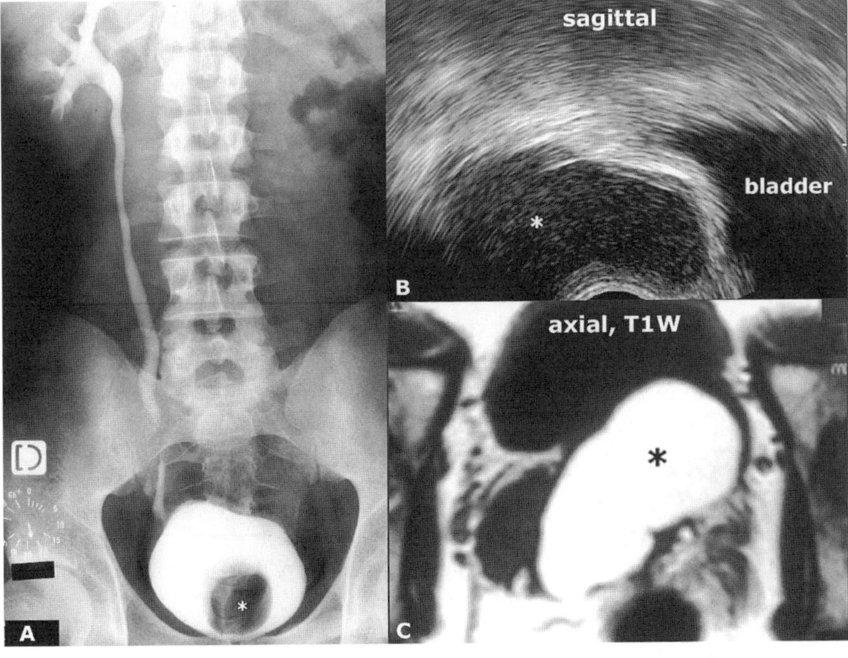

(c)

- Chronic Non-bacterial Prostatitis/Chronic Pelvic Pain Syndrome (CNP/CPPS)

  - Patients have lower genitourinary symptoms without evidence of a bacterial infection. In the inflammatory subtype, leukocytes are found in the post-prostatic massage urine or semen. The etiology of CNP/CPPS is not clearly understood.

  - TRUS findings include diffuse, focal or multifocal hypoechoic and hyperechoic areas in the peripheral zone (Fig. 13.62) and PZ calcifications (Fig. 13.63). TZ calcifications correspond in most cases to corporea amylacea and do not correspond to post-inflammatory changes (Fig. 13.63).

  - MRI most commonly shows multifocal non-contour deforming, triangular shape areas which have low signal on T2-weighted images. These lesions can simulate prostate cancer and functional MRI is helpful to differentiate the two entities (see above).

- Ejaculatory ducts obstruction (EDO)

  - The causes of EDO include midline or eccentric cysts, ejaculatory duct calcification or stones, and postoperative or post-infectious scar tissue. Several causes are often associated in the same patient. Patients may present with pelvic pain, hematospermia or infertility.

  - Complete EDO

    - is detected in 5% of hypofertile men. Semen abnormalities are those of CBAVD. Hemospermia or painful ejaculation may be present.

    - TRUS and MRI can detect signs of distal obstruction of the seminal tract (Fig. 13.64) and commonly shows signs of chronic prostatitis. MRI can be necessary to detect retraction of the seminal vesicles (see above).

    - EDO is associated with a more proximal obstruction in 20% of cases Diagnosis is made by TRUS-guided puncture aspiration of SV fluid which shows absence of motile sperm.

  - Partial ED stenosis

    - May be suspected in non-azoospermic patients with sperm motility <30%, a reduced or normal sperm count, and an ejaculate volume close to the lower limit of normal (2 ml).

    - Diagnosis is difficult to confirm by TRUS. MR imaging can detect, better than TRUS, early distension of the seminal vesicles (Fig. 13.65). More invasive and/or dynamic tests (TRUS-guided SV puncture, vesiculography, and chromotubation) are sometimes required to improve the accuracy of endorectal imaging. However, diagnosis of partial EDO still remains investigational.

  - Treatment of EDO.

Figure 13.56 Cysts of Wollfian origin. (a) Cyst of the left ejaculatory duct parasagitally located (arrow, trans) and extending along the tract of the left ED (arrow, sag). (b) Cyst of the vas deferens (arrows), located medially to the SV, originating in the right vas deferens (arrowheads, sag). (c) Seminal vesicle cyst. (a): IVU. Filling defect (*) corresponding to the cyst and renal agenesis (no excretion on the left side). (b–c): TRUS and pelvic MRI. The cyst (*) is posterior to the bladder wall and extends cranially.

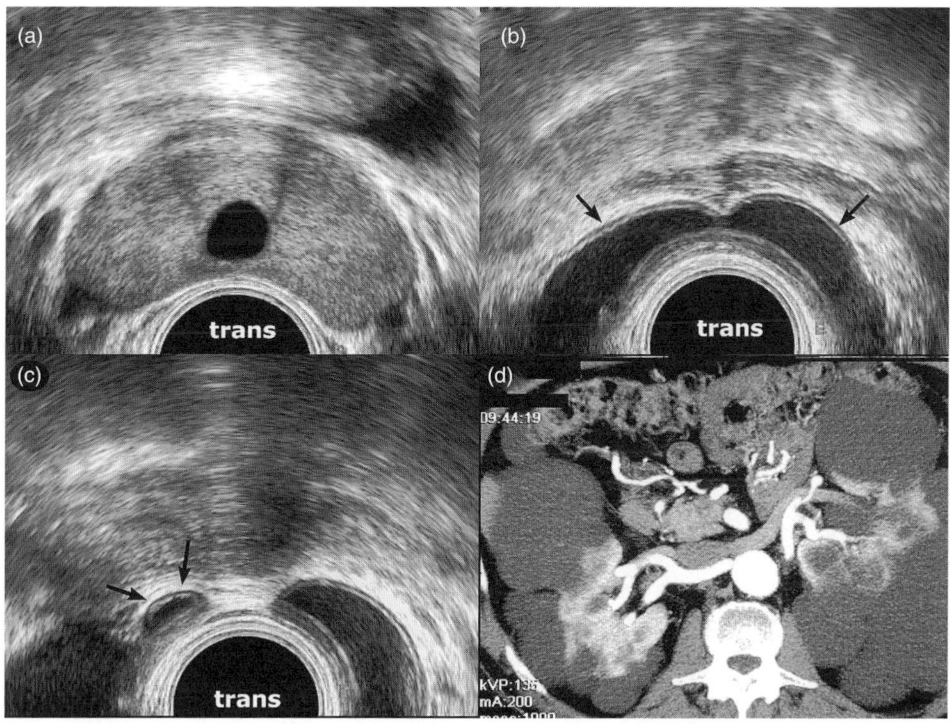

Figure 13.57 Megaseminal vesicles (megaVS) and PKRD. (a) Moderate size median cyst. (b) fully dilated seminal vesicles (arrows). (c) dilated right vas deferens (arrows). Similar appearance of the left VD (not shown). (d) CT scan showing the PKRD.

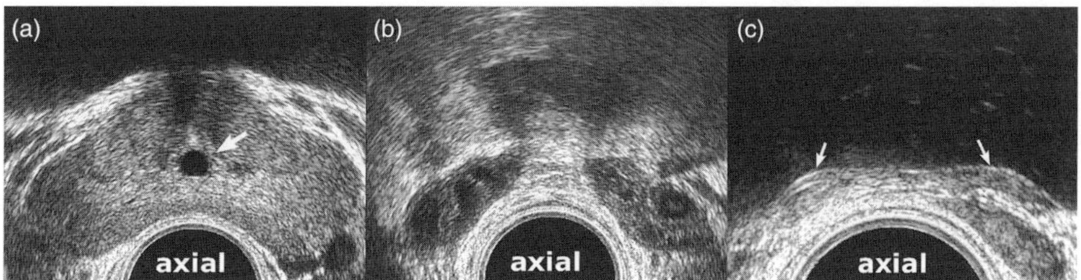

Figure 13.58 CBAVD. (a) Small median cyst and (b) absence of both vas deferens medially to the SV. The two SV are present, with a slightly dystrophic appearance. (c) The two ureteral meatus are present (white arrows), indicating the presence of both kidneys (not shown).

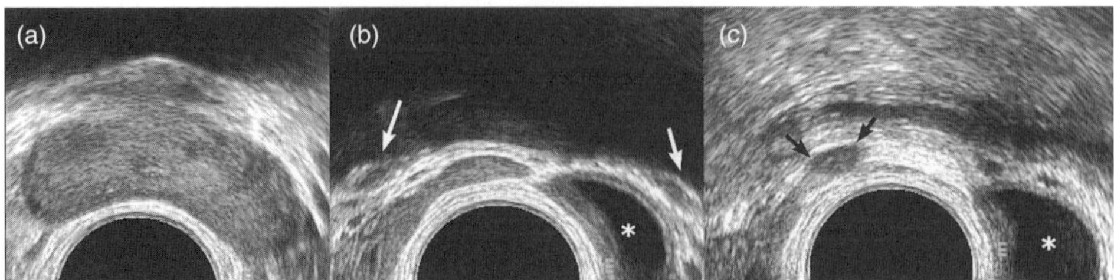

Figure 13.59 AUCD with genital cystic fibrosis. (a) Normal appearance of the prostate base. (b) Dystrophic and dilated appearance of the left SV and absence of ampullae. The two ureteral meatus are present (arrows), indicating two kidneys. (c) The right vas deferens is present (black arrows). No vas deferens on the left side.

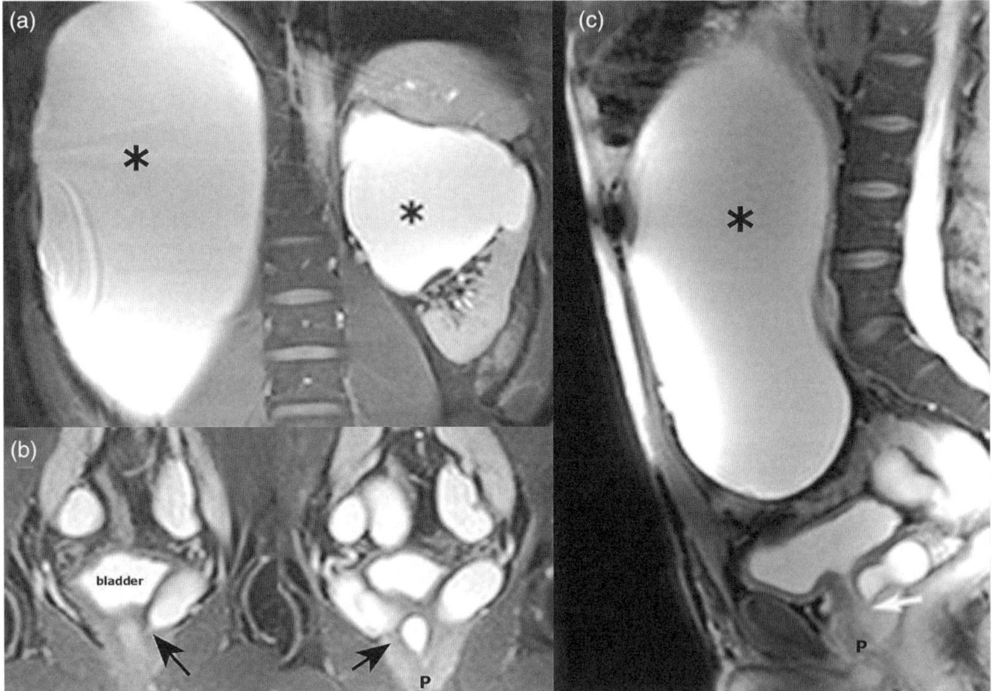

Figure 13.60 Bilateral ureteral ectopic joining. (a) T2-W MRI: hydronephrotic upper half of a bilateral duplication of the collecting system (*). (b) Pelvic MRI: bilateral ectopic joining of upper ureters, below the bladder level, within the prostatic urethra or the ED (black arrows) (c) Right sagittal view. The right upper ureter joins just above the veru montanum (arrow). (P) Prostate

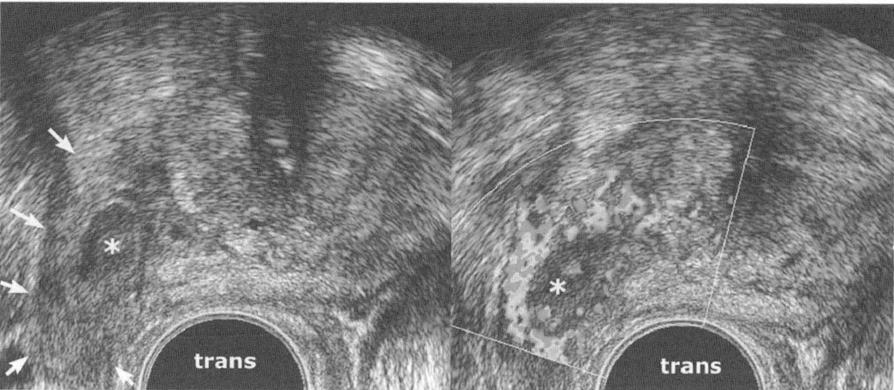

Figure 13.61   Prostatic abscess. Marked irregularity of the right prostate contour (arrows). Hypoechoic appearance of the right PZ with central cavitation (*). Intense vascularity around the abscess.

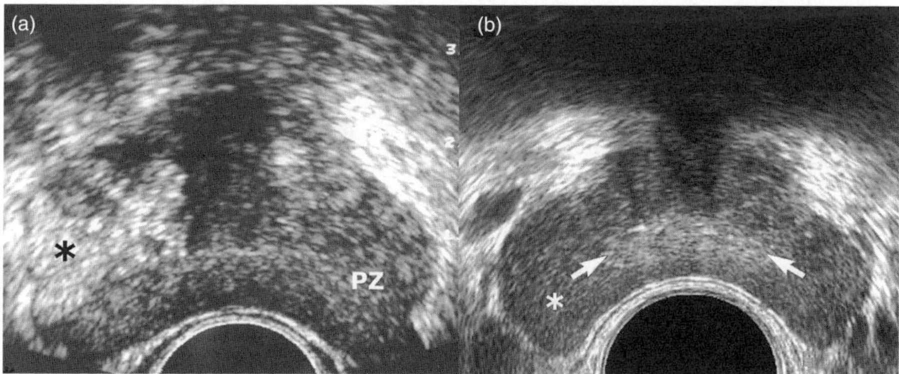

Figure 13.62   Chronic prostatitis. (a) Hypoechoic appearance of the left PZ and hyperechoic appearance of the right PZ (*) due to fibrotic changes. (b) Hypoechoic appearance of the whole PZ (*) outlining the normal isoechoic central zone (arrows).

- Endoscopic resection of the veru montanum or of the roof of a median cyst is the most common treatment for ED obstruction. The best outcomes are obtained in men with midline cysts. In patients with an inflammatory stenosis, short stenoses are more likely than longer stenoses to respond favorably to resection.

- Complications include chronic reflux of urine through the ED, giving a watery ejaculate, and also secondary fibrosis and reocclusion of the ED, which occurs in approximately 4% of cases. Candidates for TURED must therefore be selected with the utmost care.

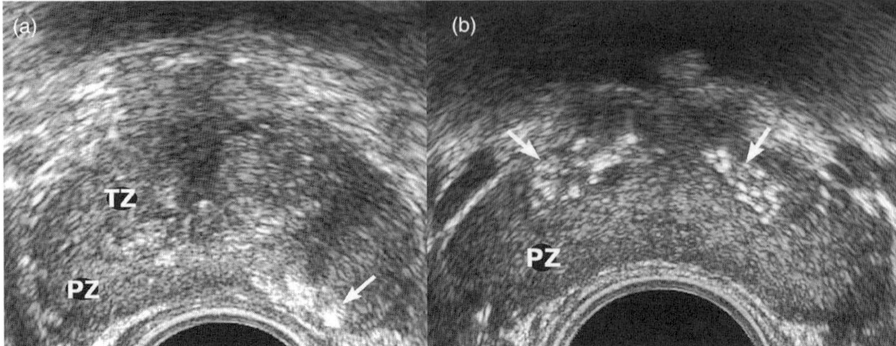

Figure 13.63 Prostatic calcifications. (a) Coarse calcifications within the PZ (arrow) corresponding to post-inflammatory changes. Hypoechoic appearance of the rest of the PZ. (b) Small calcifications (arrows) scattered within the TZ, suggesting corporea amylacea and not post-inflammatory calcifications.

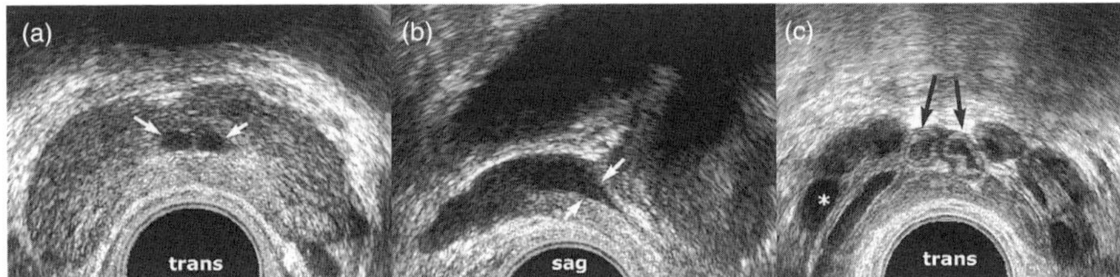

Figure 13.64 Complete distal inflammatory stenosis of the ED. Azoospermic patient with low volume of ejaculate (0.9 ml). (a–b) Dilatation of both ED (white arrows). (c) Dilatation of the vas deferens (black arrows) and the seminal vesicles (*).

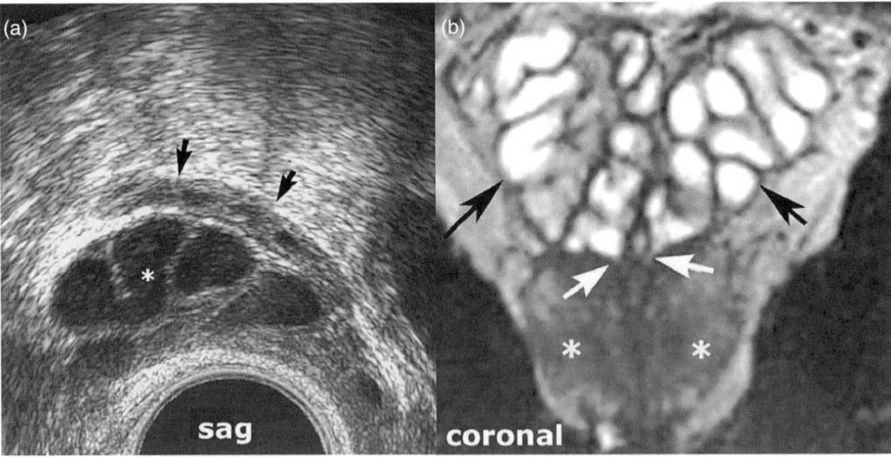

Figure 13.65 Partial stenosis of the ED in a non-azoospermic patient. Volume of ejaculate: 2.1 ml. (a) TRUS: moderately dilated SV (*). The vas deferens (black arrows) is normal. (b) endorectal MRI, coronal view: improved conspicuity of the early distension of both SV (black arrows). Normal appearance of the caudal junctions of the VD and the SV. (white arrows). Bilateral PZ inflammatory hyposignal (*).

References

Akin, O, Sala E *et al.* (2006) Transition zone prostate cancers: features, detection, localization, and staging at endorectal MR imaging. *Radiology* **239**(3): 784–792.

Boccon-Gibod LM, de Longchamps NB *et al.* (2006) Prostate saturation biopsy in the reevaluation of microfocal prostate cancer. *J. Urol.* **176**(3): 961–3; discussion 963-4.

Choi YJ, Kim JK *et al.* (2007) Functional MR imaging of prostate cancer. *Radiographics* **27**(1): 63–75; discussion 75–77.

Cornud F, Belin X *et al.* (1997) Imaging of obstructive azoospermia. *Eur. Radiol.* **7**(7): 1079–1085.

Cornud F, Belin X *et al.* (1995) [Zonal anatomy of the prostate using endorectal MRI]. *J. Radiol.* **76**(1): 11–20.

Cornud F, Belin X *et al.* (1997) Color Doppler-guided prostate biopsies in 591 patients with an elevated serum PSA level: impact on Gleason score for nonpalpable lesions. *Urology* **49**(5): 709–715.

Cornud F, Flam T *et al.* (2002) Extraprostatic spread of clinically localized prostate cancer: factors predictive of pT3 tumor and of positive endorectal MR imaging examination results. *Radiology* **224**(1): 203–210.

Cornud F, Hamida K *et al.* (2000) Endorectal color doppler sonography and endorectal MR imaging features of nonpalpable prostate cancer: correlation with radical prostatectomy findings. *AJR Am. J. Roentgenol.* **175**(4): 1161–1168.

Cornud F, Rocher L (2004) Benign conditions of the caudal junction of the vas deferens and the seminal vesicles. *Imaging of the Prostate.* F. Cornud. Paris, SAURAMPS.

D'Amico AV, Whittington R *et al.* (1996) Role of percent positive biopsies and endorectal coil MRI in predicting prognosis in intermediate-risk prostate cancer patients. *Cancer J. Sci. Am.* **2**(6): 343–350.

Elgamal AA, Van Poppel HP *et al.* (1997) Impalpable invisible stage T1c prostate cancer: characteristics and clinical relevance in 100 radical prostatectomy specimens – a different view [see comments]. *J. Urol.* **157**(1): 244–250.

Epstein JI, Pizov G *et al.* (1993) Correlation of pathologic findings with progression after radical retropubic prostatectomy. *Cancer* **71**(11): 3582–3593.

Girouin N, Mege-Lechevallier F *et al.* (2007) Prostate dynamic contrast-enhanced MRI with simple visual diagnostic criteria: is it reasonable? *Eur. Radiol.* **17**(6): 1498–1509.

Harisinghani MG, Barentsz J *et al.* (2003) Noninvasive detection of clinically occult lymph-node metastases in prostate cancer. *N Engl J Med* **348**(25): 2491–2499.

Heijmink SW, Futterer JJ *et al.* (2007) Prostate cancer: body-array versus endorectal coil MR imaging at 3 T – Comparison of image quality, localization, and staging performance. *Radiology* **244**(1): 184–195.

Langer JE, Cornud F (2006) Inflammatory disorders of the prostate and the distal genital tract. *Radiol. Clin. North. Am.* **44**(5): 665–677, vii.

Lecouvet FE, Geukens D *et al.* (2007) Magnetic resonance imaging of the axial skeleton for detecting bone metastases in patients with high-risk prostate cancer: diagnostic and cost-effectiveness and comparison with current detection strategies. *J. Clin. Oncol.* **25**(22): 3281–3287.

McNeal JE (1988) Normal histology of the prostate. *Am. J. Surg. Pathol.* **12**(8): 619–633.

Oyen RH, Van de Voorde WM *et al.* (1993) Benign hyperplastic nodules that originate in the peripheral zone of the prostate gland [see comments]. *Radiology* **189**(3): 707–711.

Qayyum A, Coakley FV *et al.* (2004) Organ-confined prostate cancer: effect of prior transrectal biopsy on endorectal MRI and MR spectroscopic imaging. *Am. J. Roentgenol.* **183**(4): 1079–1083.

Ravery V, Szabo J *et al.* (1996) A single positive prostate biopsy in six does not predict a low-volume prostate tumour. *Br. J. Urol.* **77**(5): 724–728.

Rifkin MD, Tessler FN *et al.* (1998) US case of the day. Granulomatous prostatitis resulting from BCG therapy *Radiographics* **18**(6): 1605–1607.

Scheidler J, Hricak H *et al.* (1999) Prostate cancer: localization with three-dimensional proton MR spectroscopic imaging–clinicopathologic study. *Radiology* **213**(2): 473–480.

Shukla-Dave A, Hricak H *et al.* (2004) Chronic prostatitis: MR imaging and 1H MR spectroscopic imaging findings – initial observations. *Radiology* **231**(3): 717–724.

Shukla-Dave A, Hricak H *et al.* (2007) The utility of magnetic resonance imaging and spectroscopy for predicting insignificant prostate cancer: an initial analysis. *BJU Int.* **99**(4): 786–793.

Villers A, Puech P *et al.* (2006) Dynamic contrast enhanced, pelvic phased array magnetic resonance imaging of localized prostate cancer for predicting tumor volume: correlation with radical prostatectomy findings. *J. Urol.* **176**(6 Pt 1): 2432–2437.

Villers A, Terris MK *et al.* (1990) Ultrasound anatomy of the prostate: the normal gland and anatomical variations. *J. Urol.* **143**(4): 732–738.

Zakian KL, Eberhardt S *et al.* (2003) Transition zone prostate cancer: metabolic characteristics at H MR spectroscopic imaging – initial results. *Radiology* **229**(1): 241–247.

Zakian KL, Sircar K *et al.* (2005) Correlation of Proton MR spectroscopic imaging with Gleason score based on step-section pathologic analysis after radical prostatectomy. *Radiology* **234**(3): 804–814.

14
Hemospermia

Drew A. Torigian[1], Keith N. Van Arsdalen[2] and Parvati Ramchandani[1]

[1]*Department of Radiology, University of Pennsylvania School of Medicine*
[2]*Department of Surgery, Division of Urology, University of Pennsylvania School of Medicine*

14.1 Introduction

Hemospermia (HS), or hematospermia, the presence of blood in the seminal fluid, has been recognized for centuries, was first reported in the USA in 1894 by Lydston, and was historically ascribed to sexual behavior such as 'unbridled license', excessive overindulgence, prolonged sexual abstinence, or interrupted coitus. Although HS is not uncommonly encountered in clinical practice, the exact prevalence and incidence are unknown. In this chapter, we present an overview of the clinical features, pathology, and imaging findings of HS.

14.2 Clinical features

- Typically a cause of great anxiety to men due to the imagined possibility of underlying malignancy.

- Most commonly idiopathic (in up to 79% of men under 40 years old).

- HS may either occur as a single episode or repeatedly over time.

- When a man $\geq$40 years old presents with HS, screening for prostate carcinoma may be prudent.

- Determination of origin of bleeding within the ejaculate is key, as post-coital hemorrhage from a sexual partner may be mistaken for HS.

- The 'condom test' can clarify this issue, where ejaculate from within a condom is collected and analyzed, and hemorrhage on the surface can be easily identified.

Urogenital Imaging: A Problem-oriented Approach   Edited by Sameh K. Morcos and Henrik S. Thomsen
© 2009 John Wiley & Sons, Ltd

- If hemospermia is associated with hematuria, evaluation of the urinary tract should be performed for renal and urothelial abnormality.

- Historical information acquired should include

  - amount and duration of HS
  - color of HS (red (acute) or brown (chronic))
  - presence of other coexistent symptoms
  - history of prior perineal, genital, or pelvic trauma
  - history of prior interventional procedures
  - medication history (in particular anticoagulant or antiplatelet therapy)
  - sexual history
  - travel history (with emphasis on travel to geographic regions endemic for mycobacterial or bilharzial infections)
  - history of severe systemic hypertension
  - history of bleeding diathesis.

- Physical examination should include evaluation of

  - vital signs
  - abdomen
  - pelvis including digital rectal examination
  - perineum
  - scrotum and spermatic cord structures
  - penis and meatus.

- Laboratory testing

  - urinalysis and urine culture (to exclude hematuria)
  - visual analysis of ejaculate for red discoloration
  - microbiological testing for infectious organisms
  - semen analysis
  - serum coagulation panel
  - serum chemistry panel
  - complete blood count.

- Serum prostate specific antigen (PSA) testing is also performed in men

  - ≥ 40 years old with family history of prostate cancer
  - ≥ 50 years old potentially at risk for prostate carcinoma.

- Watchful waiting, reassurance, and routine clinical evaluation may suffice in men <40 years old with transient HS as it is most often benign and self-limited.

- Non-invasive imaging techniques, predominantly transrectal ultrasonography (TRUS) and endorectal coil magnetic resonance imaging (MRI), may be used in men with

  - other associated symptoms or signs of disease

   ○ persistent HS (duration >1–2 months)

   ○ age ≥40 years old

   ○ to allay anxiety and provide reassurance that no significant pathology exists in patients with negative history and physical examination.

- When pathology is encountered in the setting of HS, treatment is tailored for the underlying pathology using current practice standards

   ○ antihypertensive therapy for severe hypertension

   ○ antimicrobial therapy for infectious disease or putative prostatitis

   ○ surgical, radiation therapy, and/or chemotherapy for neoplastic disease

   ○ aspiration, incision, or unroofing of prostatic, ejaculatory duct, or seminal vesicle cysts

   ○ transurethral resection of ejaculatory ducts for ejaculatory duct obstruction

   ○ transurethral resection or fulguration of prostatic urethral lesions

   ○ electrofulguration of prostate varices.

14.3 Pathology

- HS may be associated with abnormalities of the prostate gland, seminal tract, urethra, urinary bladder, epididymides, or testes.

- Table 14.1 provides a list of major pathologic entities associated with HS.

- The most common associated pathologies include

   ○ prostatic calcifications

   ○ chronic prostatitis

   ○ benign prostatic hypertrophy

   ○ prostate carcinoma

   ○ seminal vesicle or ejaculatory duct calculi

   ○ dilated seminal vesicles or ejaculatory ducts

   ○ prostate or seminal tract cysts

   ○ iatrogenic causes such as prostate or seminal vesicle biopsy.

14.4 Imaging findings

Table 14.2 provides a checklist of general cross-sectional imaging features that should be assessed in patients with HS.

Imaging techniques

- *Endorectal coil MRI (Fig. 14.1)*

   ○ a non-invasive radiation free imaging technique

   ○ provides multiplanar anatomic evaluation of prostate gland, seminal vesicles, ampullary portions of vasa deferentia, and ejaculatory ducts

Table 14.1 Major Entities Associated with Hemospermia (D.A. Torigian *et al.* (in press), Reproduced by permission of Springer)

Infection/inflammation
   Prostatitis
   Seminal vesiculitis
   Epididymo-orchitis
   Urethritis
   Urethral condyloma or stricture
Neoplasia
   Prostate adenocarcinoma or sarcoma
   Seminal vesicle carcinoma
   Urethral or bladder carcinoma
   Testicular carcinoma
   Secondary neoplastic involvement of seminal vesicles
      Melanoma
      Lymphoma
      Renal cell carcinoma
   Papillary adenoma or hemangioma of prostatic urethra
Vascular
   Prostate varices or telangiectasia
   Pelvic arteriovenous malformation
Traumatic
   Perineal, genital, or pelvic trauma
   Self-instrumentation
   Iatrogenic
      Prostate or seminal vesicle biopsy
      Prostate brachytherapy, cryotherapy, thermotherapy, or high-intensity focused ultrasound
         therapy
      Prostate or seminal vesicle injection of medication
      Local nerve block
      Lower ureteral extracorporeal shockwave lithotripsy
      Post-vasectomy or post-orchiectomy
      Post-hemorrhoidal sclerotherapy
Cysts
   Utricular cyst
   Müllerian duct cyst
   Seminal vesicle cyst
   Ejaculatory duct cyst
   Inclusion cysts in prostate in association with benign prostatic hypertrophy
Miscellaneous
   Benign prostatic hypertrophy
   Prostate calcification
   Seminal vesicle or ejaculatory duct calculi
   Seminal vesicle or ejaculatory duct dilation
   Seminal vesicle amyloidosis
   Severe hypertension
   Bleeding diathesis

Table 14.2 Checklist of general cross-sectional imaging features to assess in the man with HS (D.A. Torigian *et al.* (in press), Reproduced by permission of Springer)

Major organs or structures
    Prostate gland
    Seminal vesicles
    Ejaculatory ducts
    Ampullary portions of vasa deferentia
    Bladder/posterior urethra/Cowper's glands
Presence and symmetry of normal structures
Size, luminal caliber, and wall thickness of fluid-filled structures
Size and volume of prostate gland
Filling defects in fluid filled structures
    Calculi
    Inflammation/infection
    Neoplasia
Cystic lesions
    Size
    Site of origin
        Midline – utricular or müllerian duct cyst
        Paramedian – ejaculatory duct cyst
        Lateral – seminal vesicle cyst
    Relationship to adjacent structures
    Presence of associated findings of obstruction
    Presence of ipsilateral renal abnormality in case of seminal vesicle cyst
Solid lesions
    Size and extent
    Border deformation of involved organs/structures
    Alterations in echogenicity, color flow, signal intensity, attenuation or enhancement
        Hemorrhage
        Inflammation/infection
        Calcification
        Tumor
Vascular lesions
    Dilated or tortuous vessels
    High color or Doppler flow
    Signal voids
    Avid enhancement

- has excellent soft tissue contrast and is operator independent
- usually performed when TRUS is unsatisfactory or non-diagnostic
- may be slightly more sensitive than TRUS in detecting underlying abnormalities
- small field of view axial T1-weighted images and axial, sagittal, and coronal T2-weighted images provide high resolution evaluation of prostate gland and seminal tract
- large field of view axial T1-weighted and T2-weighted images allow for evaluation of pelvic lymphadenopathy and osseous metastatic disease.

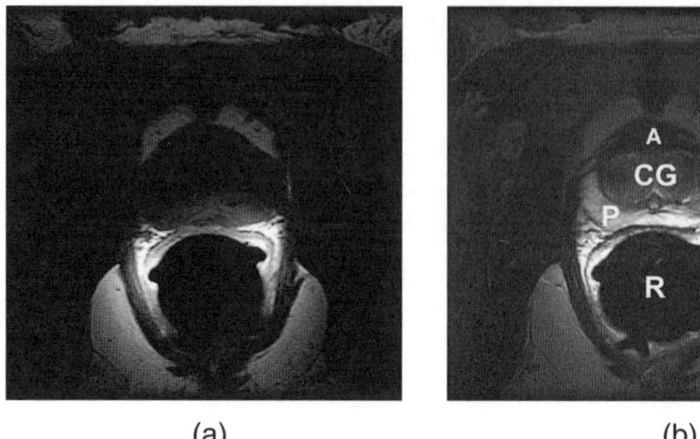

(a)   (b)

Figure 14.1 Normal MRI anatomy of prostate gland; focal chronic prostatitis. 50-year-old man with history of persistent hematospermia. (D.A. Torigian *et al.* (in press), Reproduced by permission of Springer.) (a) Axial T1-weighted endorectal MR image shows homogeneous low-intermediate signal intensity of prostate gland relative to skeletal muscle. (b) Axial T2-weighted endorectal MR image shows low signal intensity focus (*) in lateral peripheral zone of mid-gland of prostate relative to normal high signal intensity peripheral zone (P) in keeping with focal chronic prostatitis. Note that prostate carcinoma cannot be excluded based on this imaging appearance alone. Also note mildly enlarged low signal intensity central gland (CG) due to benign prostatic hypertrophy, normal thick low signal intensity anterior fibromuscular stroma (A), and very low signal intensity void in rectum (R) in location of endorectal coil placement.

- *Computed tomography (CT)*

  - a non-invasive operator independent imaging modality that uses ionizing radiation

  - can identify calcifications, gross soft tissue masses, or cystic lesions of prostate gland, seminal vesicles, or vasa deferentia

  - much less commonly used than TRUS or endorectal MRI in primary evaluation of HS due to limitations in

    - evaluation of small caliber structures such as the seminal tract

    - evaluation of internal architecture of prostate gland.

- *Vasoseminal vesiculography (or vasovesiculography) (VSV) or vasogram (Fig. 14.2)*

  - an invasive fluoroscopic imaging approach rarely performed for evaluation of HS

  - mainly reserved for men with azoospermia with normal spermatogenesis on testicular biopsy suspected to have aplasia or occlusion of vasa deferentia and ejaculatory ducts

  - after local anesthesia is applied, small scrotal incision is made, vas deferens is exposed, and 23G needle is inserted into its lumen

  - 3–5 cc of water-soluble iodinated contrast material is then injected, and frontal radiograph of pelvis is obtained

  - sequential opacification of vas deferens, ampulla of vas, seminal vesicle, and ejaculatory duct occurs, followed by opacification of the posterior urethra and urinary bladder

  - this verifies patency of ejaculatory duct and competence of external urethral sphincter.

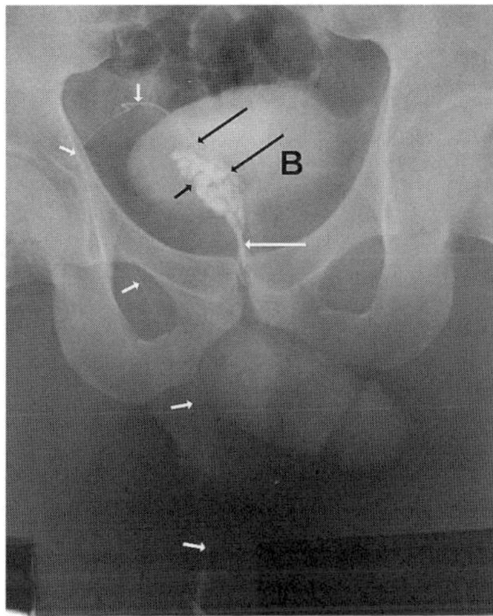

Figure 14.2 Normal seminal tract anatomy on vasovesical vesiculography. 31-year-old man with history of anorchia and right inguinal hernia repair with azoospermia and normal testicular biopsy. (D.A. Torigian *et al.* (in press), Reproduced by permission of Springer.) Frontal pelvic radiograph during vasovesical vesiculography demonstrates normal course and appearance of right vas deferens (white arrows), ampullary portion of right vas deferens (long black arrows), right seminal vesicle (black arrow), and right ejaculatory duct (long white arrow). Also note retrograde opacification of urinary bladder (B) with contrast material.

- *Retrograde urethrography (RUG), voiding cystourethrography (VCUG), or cystourethroscopy*

    o may be useful if HS is associated with hematuria, as urethra is then more likely to be the site of bleeding although retrograde ejaculation may also result in hematuria

    o upper and lower urinary tract imaging is recommended in patients with hematuria.

Normal imaging anatomy

- *Normal seminal tract*

    o *vas deferens*

        - 30–45 cm in length

        - uniform caliber, most often 1 mm in diameter

        - has thicker walls than seminal vesicle

        - low signal intensity walls and high signal intensity central fluid on T2-weighted MR images.

    o *ampullary portion of vas deferens*

        - 3–7 cm in length

        - 2.7–10.0 mm in diameter

        - symmetric length bilaterally

        - has thicker walls than seminal vesicle

- low signal intensity walls and high signal intensity central fluid on T2-weighted MR images.

  o *ejaculatory duct*

  - 16 ± 3.5 mm in length
  - 1.5 ± 0.6 mm in width in midportion with slight tapering distally
  - low signal intensity walls and high signal intensity central fluid on T2-weighted MR images.

  o *seminal vesicles*

  - symmetrically hypoechoic on TRUS
  - bow-tie configuration
  - few fine internal echoes or septations caused by saccular convolutions
  - less echogenic than prostate gland
  - homogeneous intermediate signal intensity on T1-weighted MR images relative to skeletal muscle on MRI
  - convolutions of tubules typically <5 mm in diameter, have low signal intensity walls, and have central high signal intensity fluid on T2-weighted MR images.

  o *verumontanum*

  - high signal intensity crescent in apical portion of prostate gland on T2-weighted MR images.

Imaging appearance of pathology

- *Hemorrhage (Figs 14.3–14.5)*

- *Müllerian duct cyst (Figs 14.3 and 14.6)*

  o congenital cystic remnant formed from caudal ends of fused müllerian ducts

  o mesodermal in origin

  o homologue of uterus and paranephric duct remnants

  o generally not associated with intersex problems, hypospadias, or other genital abnormalities

  o generally presents later in life than utricular cysts

  o does not contain spermatozoa or fructose at aspiration as it generally does not communicate with the seminal tract or urethra

  o typically occurs in midline of prostate gland

  o often has teardrop shape

  o may extend beyond the posterosuperior margin of prostate gland

  o lateral bowing of ejaculatory ducts or identification of ejaculatory ducts adjacent to the cyst walls may be visualized

  o does not become opacified with contrast material during RUG, VCUG, or VSV.

- *Ejaculatory duct cyst (Fig. 14.7)*

  o rare

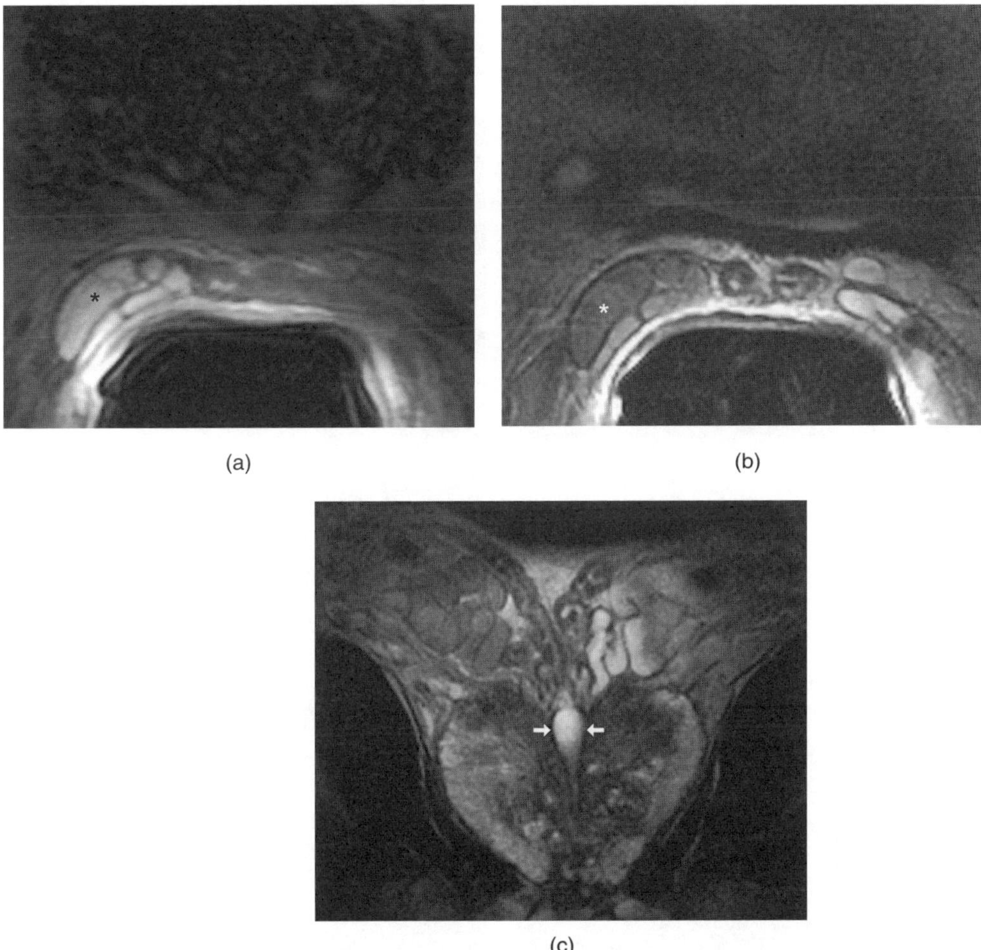

Figure 14.3 Seminal vesicle hemorrhage; müllerian duct cyst. 66-year-old man with history of hemospermia. (a) Axial T1-weighted endorectal MR image shows high signal intensity hemorrhage in right seminal vesicle (*) relative to normal low signal intensity fluid in left seminal vesicle. (b) Axial T2-weighted endorectal MR image shows low signal intensity hemorrhage in right seminal vesicle (*) relative to normal high signal intensity fluid in left seminal vesicle. (c) Coronal T2-weighted endorectal MR image reveals 13 mm midline prostate cyst (arrows) in keeping with müllerian duct cyst.

- o usually result of partial distal obstruction of ejaculatory duct
- o contains spermatozoa at aspiration
- o usually in paramedian location along course of ejaculatory duct
- o opacifies with contrast material at VSV.

- *Seminal vesicle cyst*
  - o uncommon congenital abnormality
  - o frequently associated with

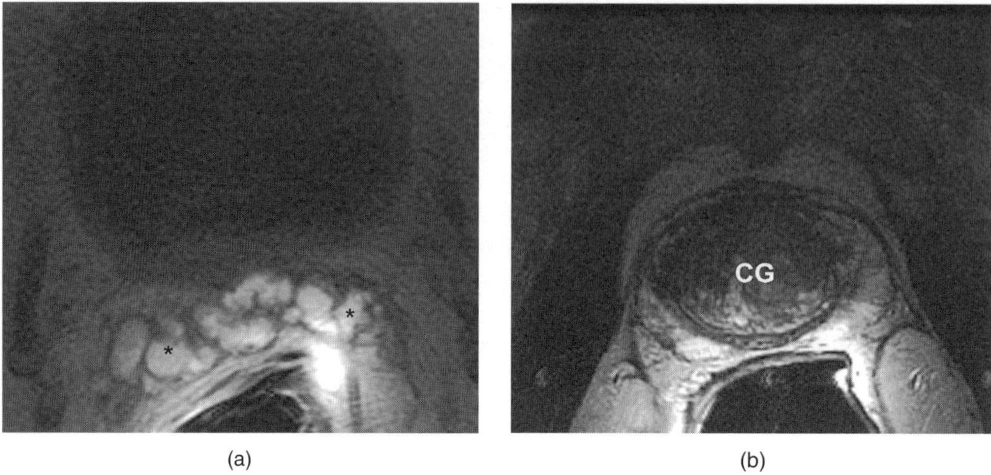

(a)   (b)

Figure 14.4 Seminal vesicle hemorrhage; benign prostatic hypertrophy. 70-year-old man with history of hemospermia. (a) Axial T1-weighted endorectal MR image demonstrates high signal intensity hemorrhage within seminal vesicles (*). (b) Axial T2-weighted endorectal MR image shows nodular enlargement of central gland (CG) due to benign prostatic hypertrophy.

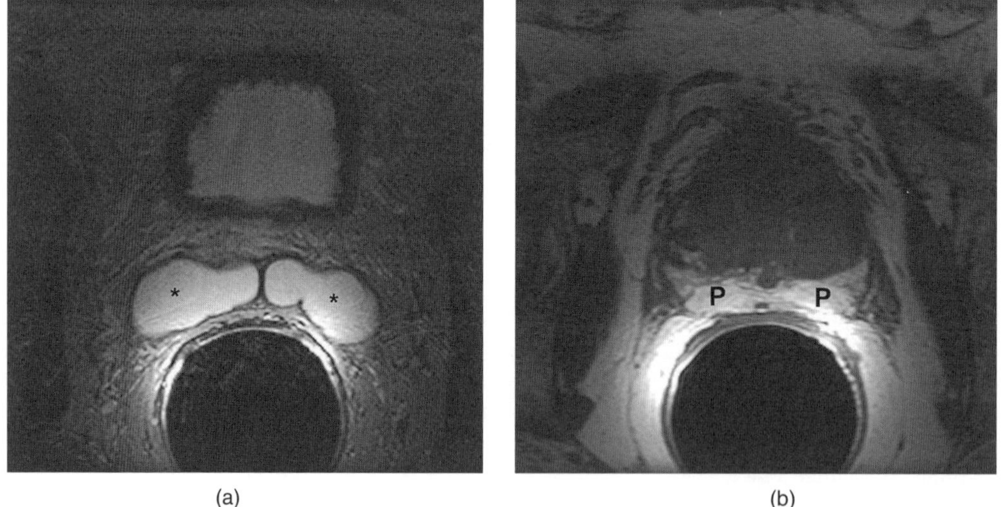

(a)   (b)

Figure 14.5 Dilated seminal vesicles; post-biopsy prostatic hemorrhage. 60-year-old man with history of prostate carcinoma status post-prostatic biopsy and hemospermia. (a) Axial T2-weighted endorectal MR image reveals markedly dilated seminal vesicles (*) and loss of normal convolutions due to chronic obstruction and inflammation. (b) Axial T1-weighted endorectal MR image shows diffuse high signal intensity in peripheral zone of prostate (P) in keeping with subacute post-biopsy hemorrhage.

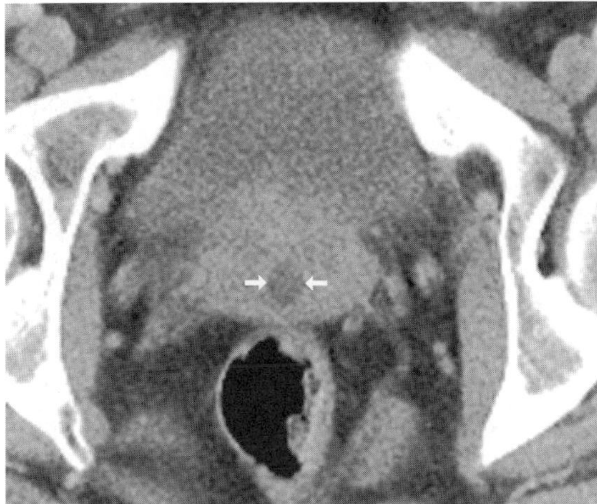

Figure 14.6 Midline prostatic cyst. 45-year-old man with history of low back pain and hemospermia. Axial contrast-enhanced pelvic CT image demonstrates fluid attenuation midline prostatic cyst (arrows) in keeping with either a utricular cyst or müllerian duct cyst.

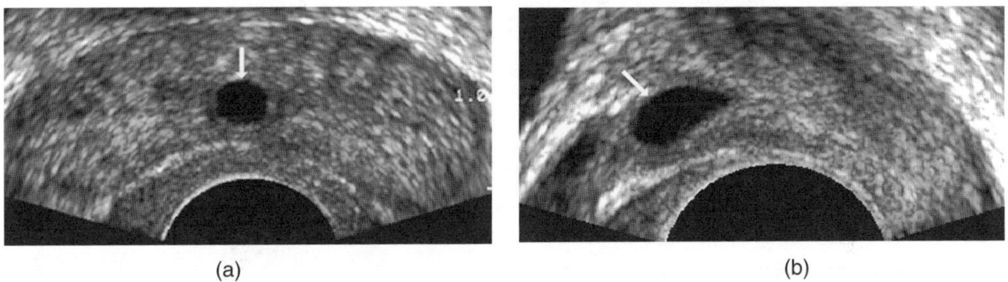

(a)   (b)

Figure 14.7 Ejaculatory duct cyst. 66-year-old man with history of microhematuria, pelvic discomfort, and hemospermia. A and B, Axial and sagittal TRUS grayscale images reveal 8 mm thin-walled well circumscribed anechoic teardrop shaped lesion (arrows) in right paramedian location in prostate in keeping with ejaculatory duct cyst. Note that it may be difficult at times to distinguish an ejaculatory duct cyst from a midline prostatic cyst.

- ■ autosomal dominant polycystic kidney disease
- ■ ipsilateral renal anomalies such as renal agenesis
- ■ ipsilateral congenital absence of vas deferens
- ■ ectopic ureteral insertion into mesonephric duct derivatives
- ○ contains fructose and spermatozoa at aspiration as communicates with seminal tract
- ○ typically occurs laterally within seminal vesicle
- ○ may be associated with ipsilateral ejaculatory duct dilation
- ○ may protrude into urinary bladder mimicking appearance of ectopic ureterocele
- ○ abnormality of ipsilateral kidney may be seen on imaging.

- *Calculi (Figs 14.8 and 14.9)*

  ○ may occur within prostate gland or seminal tract

  ○ well-circumscribed focal increased echogenicity with or without posterior acoustic shadowing on TRUS

  ○ very low in signal intensity on T1-weighted and T2-weighted MR images

  ○ very high attenuation on CT.

- *BPH (Figs 14.4 and 14.10)*

  ○ develops in nearly 80% of men with increasing age

  ○ increased overall size of prostate gland

  ○ arises from transitional zone of prostate gland with aging

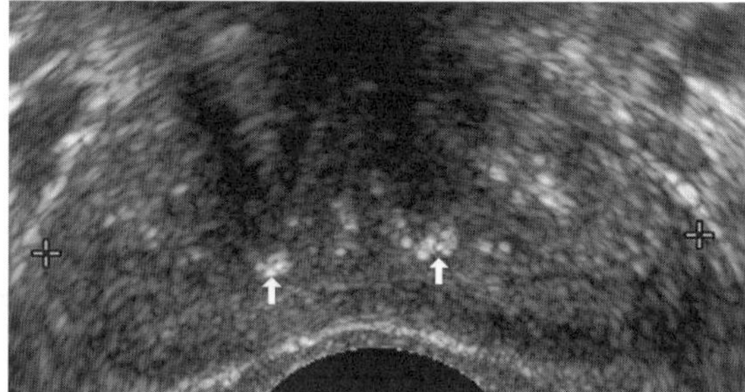

Figure 14.8 Ejaculatory duct calculi. 52-year-old man with history of chronic prostatitis and hemospermia. Axial TRUS grayscale image shows echogenic foci (arrows) with posterior acoustic shadowing in paramedian locations in prostate in keeping with ejaculatory duct calculi.

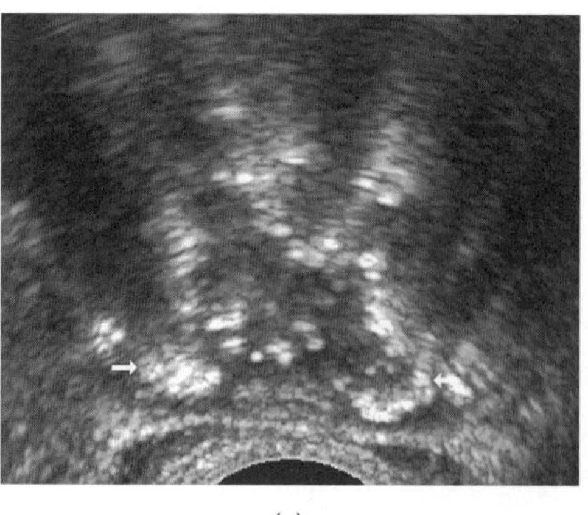

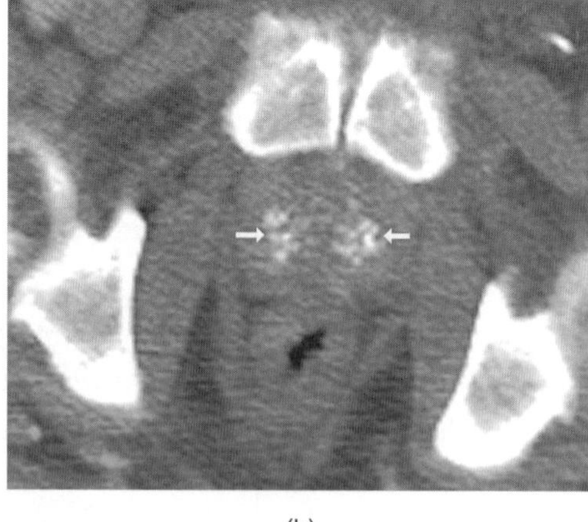

(a)   (b)

Figure 14.9 Prostate calcification. 72-year-old man with history of diabetes mellitus and hemospermia. (a) Axial TRUS grayscale image through prostate shows multiple echogenic foci (arrows) with posterior acoustic shadowing in keeping with prostate calcifications. (b) Axial contrast-enhanced CT image through pelvis demonstrates very high attenuation foci (arrows) within prostate gland in keeping with prostate calcifications.

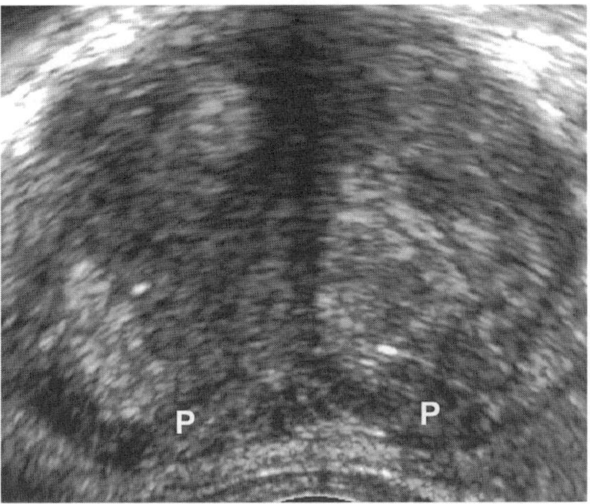

Figure 14.10 Benign prostatic hypertrophy. 77-year-old man with history of elevated serum PSA level and hemospermia. Axial TRUS grayscale image reveals marked enlargement of prostate gland and prostatic central gland with mild compression of peripheral zone (P) in keeping with benign prostatic hypertrophy.

  - o enlargement of central gland, which is often nodular and heterogeneous
  - o compression and distortion of peripheral zone
  - o cyst formation and calcification may be seen
  - o associated with bladder outlet obstruction, diffuse wall thickening, bladder trabeculation, or bladder diverticula.
- *Chronic prostatitis (Fig. 14.11)*
  - o chronic inflammation of prostate gland

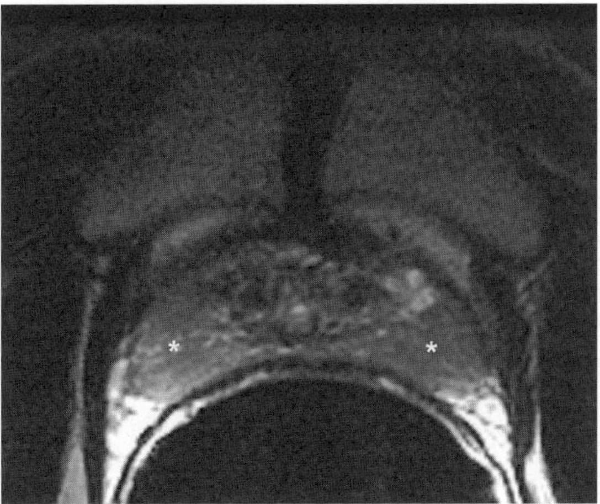

Figure 14.11 Chronic prostatitis. 42-year-old man with history of hemospermia. Axial T2-weighted endorectal MR image shows extensive low signal intensity (*) throughout peripheral zone in keeping with chronic prostatitis.

- o often associated with seminal vesiculitis (Fig. 14.5)

- o hyperechoic or hypoechoic foci, capsular irregularity or thickening, dystrophic calcification, and periurethral zone irregularity may be seen on TRUS

- o focal or diffuse low signal intensity in peripheral zone on T1-weighted and T2-weighted MR images, usually without contour deformation.

- *Seminal vesicle amyloidosis*

  - o common, particularly in the elderly

  - o rarely presents clinically, usually detected on MRI as an incidental finding

  - o nodular thickening of seminal vesicles

  - o focal or diffuse decreased signal intensity on T2-weighted MR images may be seen, potentially mimicking direct spread of prostate carcinoma

  - o definitive diagnosis via microscopy
    - positive staining with Congo red
    - typical green birefringence in polarized light.

- *Prostate carcinoma*

  - o the most commonly diagnosed malignancy in American men

  - o the second leading cause of cancer death in American men

  - o most commonly arises from peripheral zone of prostate gland

  - o most often hypoechoic relative to normal peripheral zone, but sometimes isoechoic or hyperechoic on TRUS

  - o may be hypervascular on color Doppler TRUS

  - o typically intermediate in signal intensity on T1-weighted MR images and low in signal intensity on T2-weighted MR images relative to normal peripheral zone

  - o other imaging findings best seen on MRI may include
    - asymmetry of prostate size particularly in peripheral zone
    - capsular distortion
    - loss of differentiation between central gland and peripheral zone
    - obliteration of rectoprostatic angle
    - asymmetry of neurovascular bundles
    - invasion of adjacent organs such as the seminal vesicles and urinary bladder by direct extracapsular spread of tumor
    - pelvic lymphadenopathy
    - osteoblastic metastases

  - o HS has been described in association with prostate carcinoma and also following prostate biopsy.

14.5 Summary

- HS is an anxiety provoking but otherwise generally benign and self-limited condition that is infrequently associated with significant underlying pathology.

- Most often idiopathic in nature.

- Management with routine clinical evaluation, watchful waiting, and reassurance generally suffice without further diagnostic work-up or treatment.

- Can be treated with short-course of broad spectrum antibiotics (quinolones, doxycycline, bactrim).

- Non-invasive imaging, most often with TRUS or endorectal MRI, may play an important role in the diagnostic work-up of men with HS, particularly in men

    o $\geq$40 years old, especially in association with hematuria

    o with other associated symptoms or signs of disease

    o with persistent HS.

- A wide variety of entities may be encountered in association with HS at imaging.

- Specific therapeutic interventions may be employed if certain treatable underlying pathologies are coincidentally detected.

References

Lencioni R, Ortori S, Cioni, D *et al.* (1999) Endorectal coil MR imaging findings in hemospermia. *MAGMA* **8**: 91–97.

Mulhall JP, Albertsen PC (1995) Hemospermia: diagnosis and management. *Urology* **46**: 463–467.

Munkelwitz R, Krasnokutsky S, Lie J *et al.* (1997) Current perspectives on hematospermia: a review. *J. Androl.* **18**: 6–14.

Papp GK, Kopa Z, Szabo F, Erdei E (2003) Aetiology of haemospermia. *Andrologia* **35**: 317–320.

Torigian DA, Ramchandani P (2007) Hematospermia: Imaging findings. *Abdominal Imaging* **32**: 29–49.

Yagci C, Kupeli S, Tok C *et al.* (2004) Efficacy of transrectal ultrasonography in the evaluation of hematospermia. *Clin. Imaging* **28**: 286–290.

15
Scrotal Masses

Lorenzo E. Derchi[1] and Alchiede Simonato[2]

[1]*DICMI-Radiologia, Università di Genova*
[2]*Clinica Urologica, Università di Genova*

15.1 Introduction

A scrotal mass is an important clinical problem and often a source of clinical anxiety to the patient. Radiologists play an important role in the management of these patients, since imaging is required to provide information about precise anatomical location of the lesion, size and, possibly, the nature of the disease process. Different mass lesions that can be seen in the scrotum are presented in this chapter.

15.2 Clinical features

- A scrotal mass is often identified by the patient as an abnormal lump in the testicle. Patients may also observe a change in the normal feeling of the testicle.

- Small, non-palpable, testicular nodules can be identified as an incidental finding during imaging studies performed for indications other than presence of a palpable mass.

- Testicular tumors are usually painless and present as a palpable mass. However, they may cause dull ache, or sense of fullness in the lower abdomen and scrotum. In some cases, a neoplasm can be associated with acute pain and be initially misinterpreted as epididymo-orchitis.

- Malignant tumors of the testis are relatively rare and account for 1% of all malignancies.

- Peak prevalence is at the age of 25 to 35 years.

Urogenital Imaging: A Problem-oriented Approach   Edited by Sameh K. Morcos and Henrik S. Thomsen
© 2009 John Wiley & Sons, Ltd

- They are more common in European and American men, and much less common in the African and African-American male population. The possibility of a benign nature of the disease process has to be considered when a testicular nodule is detected in this group of patients.

- Testicular masses in elderly patients over the age of 70 years are mostly lymphomas or metastases.

- Tumor markers (α-fetoprotein, human chorionic gonadotropin and lactate dehydrogenase) can be of great help in the diagnosis, staging and follow-up of testicular tumors.

- Increased α-fetoproteins are found in yolk-sac tumors and in mixed germ-cell tumors with yolk-sac elements; human chorionic gonadotropin is elevated in tumors containing syncytiotrophoblasts, such as seminomas and choriocarcinomas. Increase of one or both of these markers is found in more than 80% of cases with non-seminomatous germ cell tumors. Lactate hydrogenase is a less specific marker which correlates with the bulk of disease and can be used in staging.

15.3 Pathology

- The scrotum is a fibromuscular sac divided into two compartments by a median raphe. On each side, it contains the testis, epididymis, spermatic cord, and their fascial coverings.

- Masses can originate from any of the structures contained within the scrotum.

- Most solid lesions originating from the testes are malignant, while most lesions originating from extratesticular structures are benign.

- Testicular neoplasms can be classified into two categories: germ cell tumors and non-germ cell tumors. Also non-primary tumors, such as lymphomas, leukemia and metastases can be encountered.

  - Germ cell tumors arise from spermatogenic cells, and are almost invariably malignant.
  - Non-germ cells tumors derive from sex cords and stroma, and are malignant in only 10% of cases.

- The most common extratesticular neoplasms are benign lipomas, usually originating from the spermatic cord, and adenomatoid tumors, most often from the epididymis.

- Although rare, malignant extratesticular masses, such as rhabomyosarcomas, liposarcomas, malignant fibrous histiocytomas, and mesoteliomas, can develop.

15.4 Imaging

Ultrasonography

- The first imaging procedure to evaluate the scrotum.

- The study has to be performed with high frequency transducers ($>10\,\mathrm{MHz}$) with color Doppler facilities.

- The normal examination

  - The normal testis has homogeneous echotexture made of fine, medium level echoes, with the mediastinum testis presenting as an echogenic line that, on transverse images, has triangular shape.

  - The epididymis is seen as an elongated, generally isoechoic, structure adjacent to the testis. Intratesticular vessels are easily appreciated.

  - A small quantity of fluid around the testis is normal, and this allows, in many cases, to identify the testicular and the epididymal appendages.

  - Normal intratesticular vessels can be seen with color Doppler.

- Palpation during scanning helps to correlate physical findings with the results of US; this is particularly useful in cases with small, mobile extratesticular masses which may be easily missed if a focused examination is not performed.

Magnetic resonance imaging (MRI)

- MRI can be useful in the evaluation of scrotal masses as a problem-solving technique.

  - Discrepancies between US and clinical findings.

  - Diffuse, non-specific testicular involvement seen on US scanning.

  - Fibrous lesions, lipomas or hemorrhage are suspected.

- Surface coils should be used, and both T1- and T2-weighted sequences along axial, sagittal and coronal planes are routinely performed. Fat saturation sequences can be helpful.

- The normal examination

  - The normal testis has homogeneous intermediate signal on T1-weighted images and high signal intensity on T2-weighted ones.

  - The testis is surrounded by hypointense tunica albuginea. On T2 imaging the fluid around the testis has higher signal intensity.

  - The mediastinum testis appears as a hypointense structure of linear or triangular shape according to the scan plane used. On T2-weighted images, thin low signal intensity septa can be identified radiating toward the mediastinum testis.

  - The epididymis is isointense or slightly hypointense to the testis on T1-weighted images, and hypointense on T2.

15.5 Important principles in assessment of scrotal masses

- In patients with a scrotal mass, imaging is requested to answer the following five questions:

  - Is there a definite mass?

  - Is the mass intra- or extratesticular?

  - Is the mass bilateral?

- o Is the mass cystic or solid?
- o Is the nature of the lesion identifiable?

Is there a definite mass?

- US is almost 100% sensitive in the identification of presence of scrotal masses.

- Diagnostic difficulties leading to false-negative results are rarely encountered, and are mostly due to:
    - o presence of isoechogenic intratesticular lesions
    - o diffuse testicular involvement, especially in children with yolk-sac tumors
    - o extratesticular lipomas can be difficult to identify, being often isoechoic to surrounding subcutaneous tissue.

  In these cases, MRI can be helpful

- US imaging can also recognize the following abnormalities of the scrotum:
    - o Hydrocele: fluid collection within the tunica vaginalis.
    - o Varicocele: dilated pampiniform plexus, more frequent on the left side.
    - o Hematoma or edema of the scrotal wall.

Is the mass intra- or extratesticular?

- Differentiation can be made by US in almost all cases.
- Palpation during US examination can help to localize the mass.

Is the mass bilateral?

- Testicular tumors can be bilateral (38% of lymphomas, 2% of seminomas).
- A careful examination of both testes with US is essential, especially for identification of possible small, non-palpable lesions.

Is the lesion cystic or solid?

- US can easily differentiate a solid from a cystic lesion.
- Care should be taken before calling any intratesticular lesion as 'cystic' since hemorrhage or necrosis in a tumor may have a cystic-like appearance; however, a complex, multiloculated pattern is seen in most of these cases.
- A lesion may be defined as a 'cyst' only if it is completely anechoic, with increased through transmission and presence of thin walls, without any vegetations or irregularities.
- If any doubt exists, MRI examination may help further to characterize the mass. Contrast-enhanced MRI studies have been useful to show enhancement of solid portions of the tumor.

Is the nature of the lesion identifiable?

- Identification of the nature of scrotal masses cannot be based on imaging methods alone.

- Epidemiogical, clinical and laboratory findings, together with the results of imaging, are important in offering the differential diagnosis.

- Localization of the mass is important in predicting the nature of the lesion.

  - Most extratesticular lesions are benign

  - Most intratesticular masses are malignant.

- The structural pattern of the mass is the second important factor to consider.

  - Most cystic lesions are benign, while solid nodules are more often malignant.

- Combining location and structural pattern of the lesion is often helpful in narrowing the differential diagnosis

  - A cystic extratesticular mass is usually an epididymal cyst, a relatively common finding, which is almost certainly benign (Fig. 15.1).

  - A cystic intratesticular nodule can be encountered in up to 8% to 10% of patients; it can be classified as benign if it is purely cystic, without any mural irregularity, and if it is localized at the tunica albuginea or near the mediastinum testis.

  - A series of small, dilated, fluid-filled tubules with thin and regular walls, located at the mediastinum testis (Fig. 15.2) can be recognized as a dilated rete testis.

- Solid lesions, whether intra or extratesticular, cannot be classified with certainty, and most of them have no special US or MRI character to help identification of their nature.

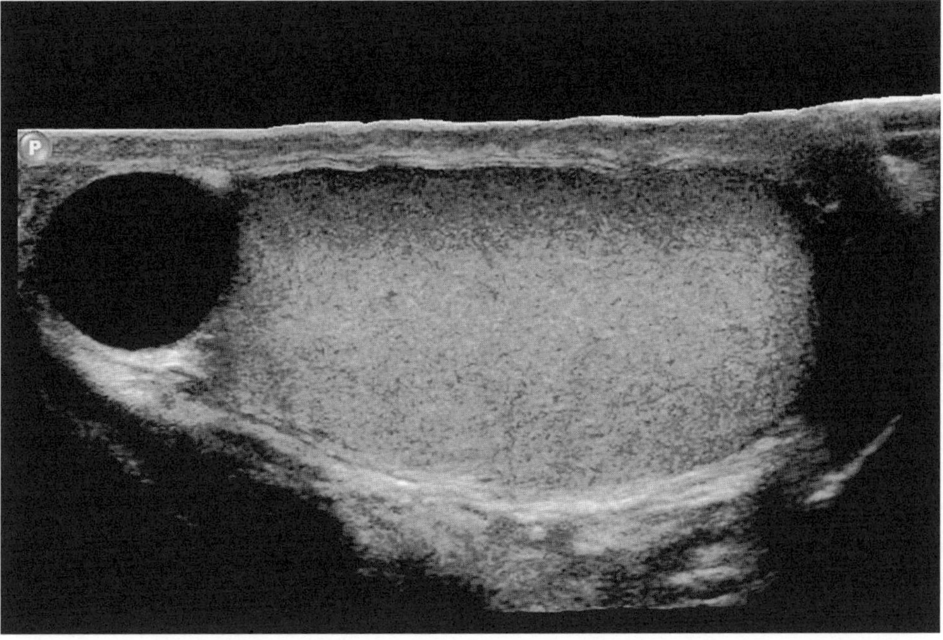

Figure 15.1 *Cyst of the head of the epididymis* (arrow) which has all the characteristics of a simple cyst (anechoic, regular borders, and increased through transmission).

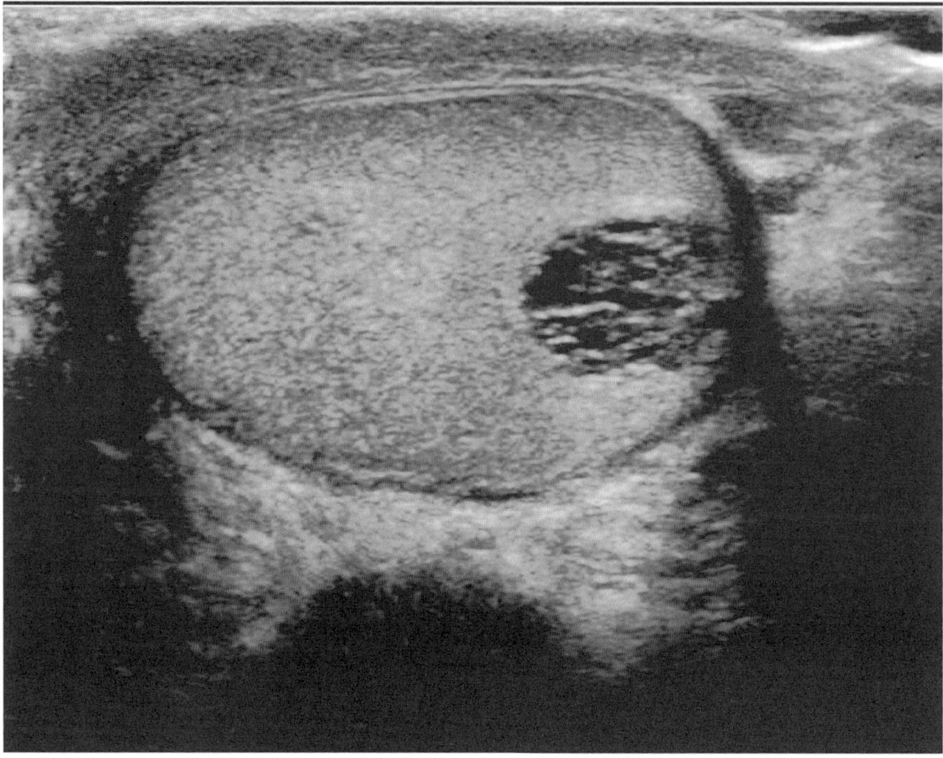

Figure 15.2 *Intratesticular dilatation of the rete testis* (arrow). This condition can be recognized both by its echotexture (many small tubular spaces divided by thin walls), and by its location at the mediastinum testis.

- Most seminomas seen at US are hypoechogenic homogeneous masses (Fig. 15.3).

- Presence of hemorrhage or necrosis may cause these tumors to appear heterogeneous, especially if large. This pattern can be seen with both germ cell and non-germ cell tumors (Fig. 15.4).

- Most malignant tumors larger than 1.6 mm are hypervascular at color Doppler.

- Color Doppler may help to identify isoechoic masses by demonstrating distortion of vasculature at the site of the lesion.

- At MRI:
  - Testicular tumors are generally isointense to normal testicular tissue on T1-weighted images and hypointense on T2-weighted images.
  - Heterogeneities are often encountered, and relate to presence of hemorrage, necrosis or calcification (Fig. 15.4).
  - These patterns are non-specific and cannot differentiate among the different types of tumors.

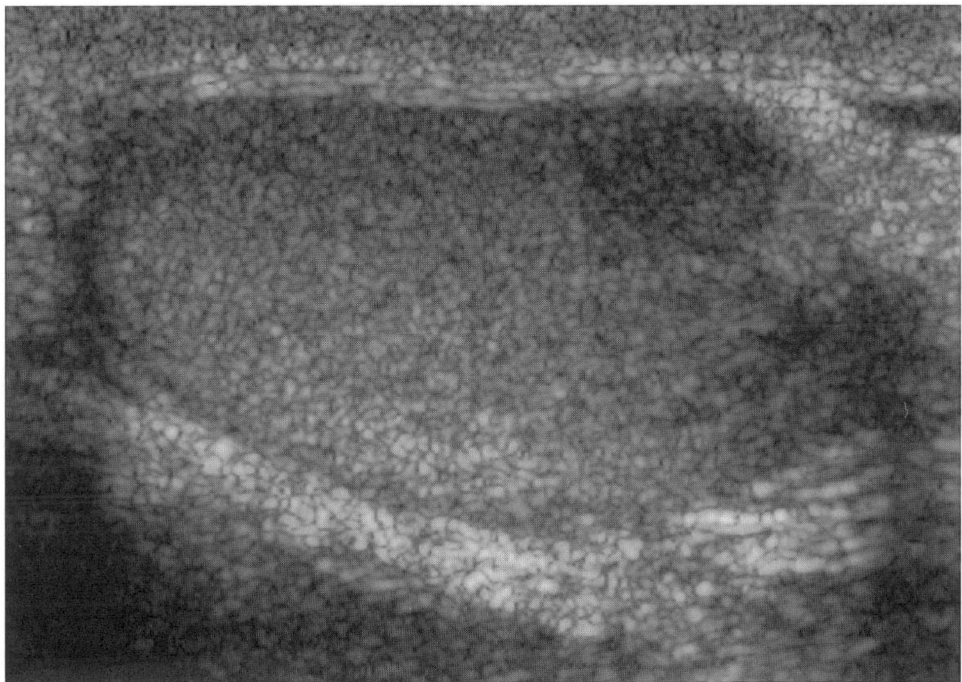

Figure 15.3 *Seminoma,* US shows a 1.5 cm hypoecoic lesion (arrow) with homogeneous echotexture.

15.6 Important problems in differentiating benign from malignant lesions

- A variety of non-neoplastic conditions may present as solid intra- or extratesticular masses. The most frequent include *epididymitis, orchitis, hemorrhage and focal intratesticular infarction.*

- The diagnosis of these lesions depends on combining the imaging features including disease location and Doppler US findings with the clinical history.

  ○ Acute inflammatory lesions such as *epididymo-orchitis* usually present as an acute scrotum with local clinical features of acute inflammation.

  ○ A solid nodule at the epididymis which is painful and tender at palpation with hypervascularity at Doppler US, can be safely diagnosed as an *epididymitis* (Fig. 15.5).

  ○ Lack of internal vascular signals at Doppler US can help in differentiating intratesticular *infarcts and hemorrhages* from epididymitis and focal orchitis.

- *Focal orchitis* presents as a solid intratesticular hypervascularized lesion which is impossible to differentiate, on imaging grounds alone, from a neoplasm. It is commonly associated with acute epididymitis. A follow-up study in a few weeks time is important since findings related to orchitis would evolve with time and adequate treatment.

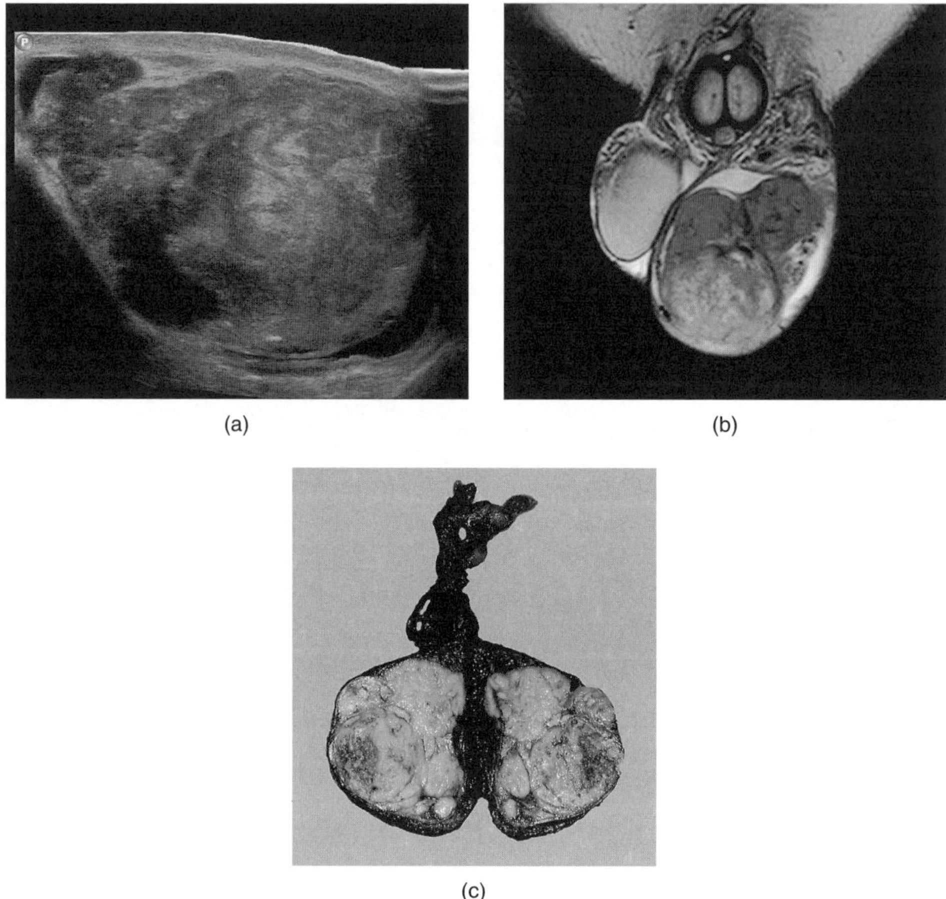

(a)

(b)

(c)

Figure 15.4 *Seminoma*, (a) US performed in a patient with diffuse testicular enlargement demonstrates involvement of the whole testis by a solid, heterogeneous mass. (b) Coronal T2 MRI confirms the US findings. (c) Macroscopic appearance of the lesion.

- *Chronic inflammatory lesions* associated with granulomatous reactions, such as tuberculosis, brucellosis, syphilis, parasitic and fungal infections are more difficult to identify. In these lesions:

  o Epididymal involvement is almost the rule.

  o Testicular lesions may also occur in addition to the epididymal involvement.

  o Clinical findings are crucial for proper diagnosis.

Solid lesions which can be properly identified as benign on imaging grounds.

- *Epidermoid cyst (Fig. 15.6)*

  o A rare benign tumor (approximately 1% of all testicular tumors).

  o It is a cyst filled with cheesy laminated material that appears solid on imaging.

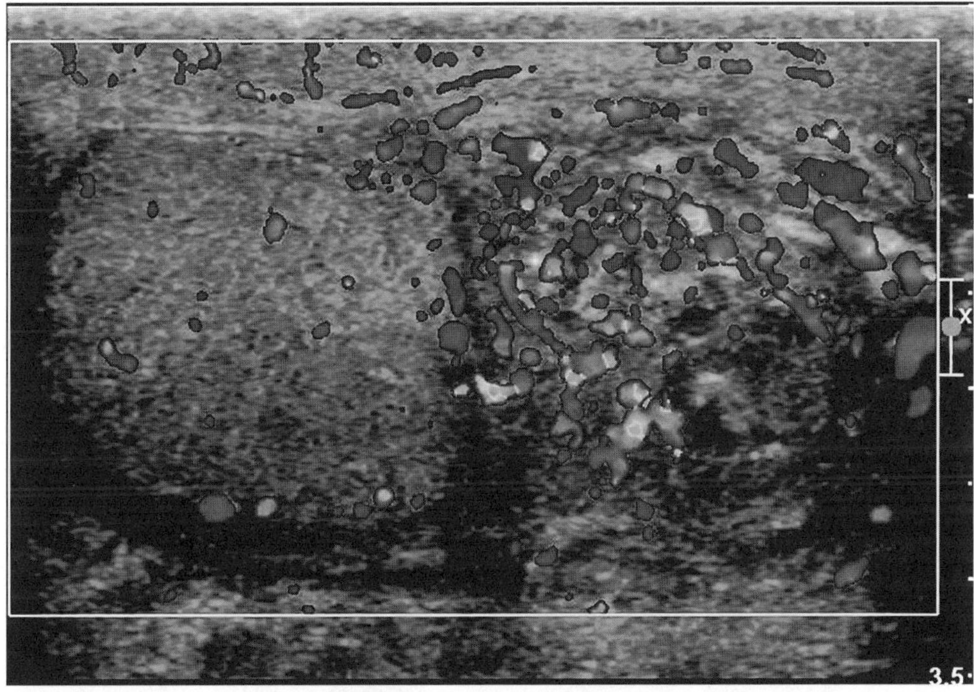

Figure 15.5 *Acute epididymitis.* Sagittal US scan of the testis (T) shows enlargement and heterogeneous texture of the tail of the epididymis (E). Color Doppler demonstrates marked hypervascularity.

- o At US, the lesion is seen as rounded or oval shaped nodule with regular outer margins. The lesion tends to be hyperechoic, sometimes calcific outer wall is seen, and an internal 'onion ring' structure is characteristic of an epidermoid cyst. No vascular signals are seen at Doppler evaluation.
- o At MRI, a laminated appearance, with alternate low-and high-signal intensity areas can be detected on T2-weighted images.
- o These findings, together with normal levels of tumor markers often allow a correct diagnosis to be made.
- o An epidermoid cyst is treated by testicular-sparing enucleation rather than orchidectomy.

- • *Uncommon benign testicular lesions*
  - o *Hyperplastic intratesticular adrenal rests (Fig. 15.7)*
    - ■ Aberrant adrenal rests may remain trapped within the developing testes during fetal development.
    - ■ They are usually very small (<5 mm) and can be found in the testis of 7.5% to 15% of newborns and 1.6% of adults.
    - ■ Their small size does not allow their identification at imaging.

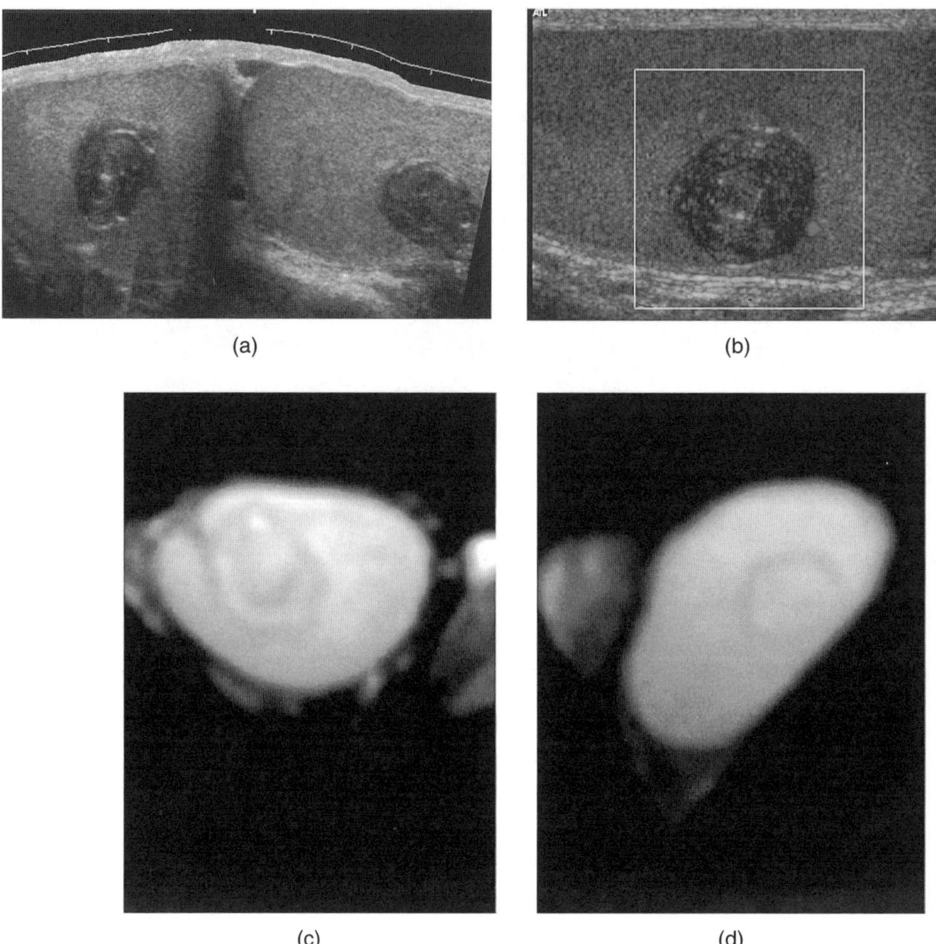

(a)

(b)

(c)

(d)

Figure 15.6 *Bilateral epidermoid cysts of the testis.* (a) Transverse extended-field-of-view sonogram demonstrates presence of a hypoecoic lesion (arrow), with sharp echogenic margins, in each testis. The lesion has an internal 'onion ring' appearance, suggesting an epidermoid cyst. (b) Color Doppler sonogram of the right testis showing absence of flow signals within the mass. (c) and (d) Fat-saturated T2-weighted axial MRI of the right (C) and left (D) testis shows a testicular nodule (arrow) with hypointense rim and alternating high-and low-signal intensity areas.

- In patients with congenital adrenal hyperplasia or, more rarely, with Cushing's syndrome, these cells are exposed to elevated levels of adrenocorticotropic hormone and may enlarge to form masses which are typically multiple, bilateral and eccentrically located.

- At US they have been described with variable appearances, from hypoechoic to heterogeneously hyperechogenic structure, with possible calcifications (Fig. 15.7).

- At MRI, these lesions have been reported to be hypointense on both T1- and T2-weighted images, and this can help in differentiating these lesions from tumors,

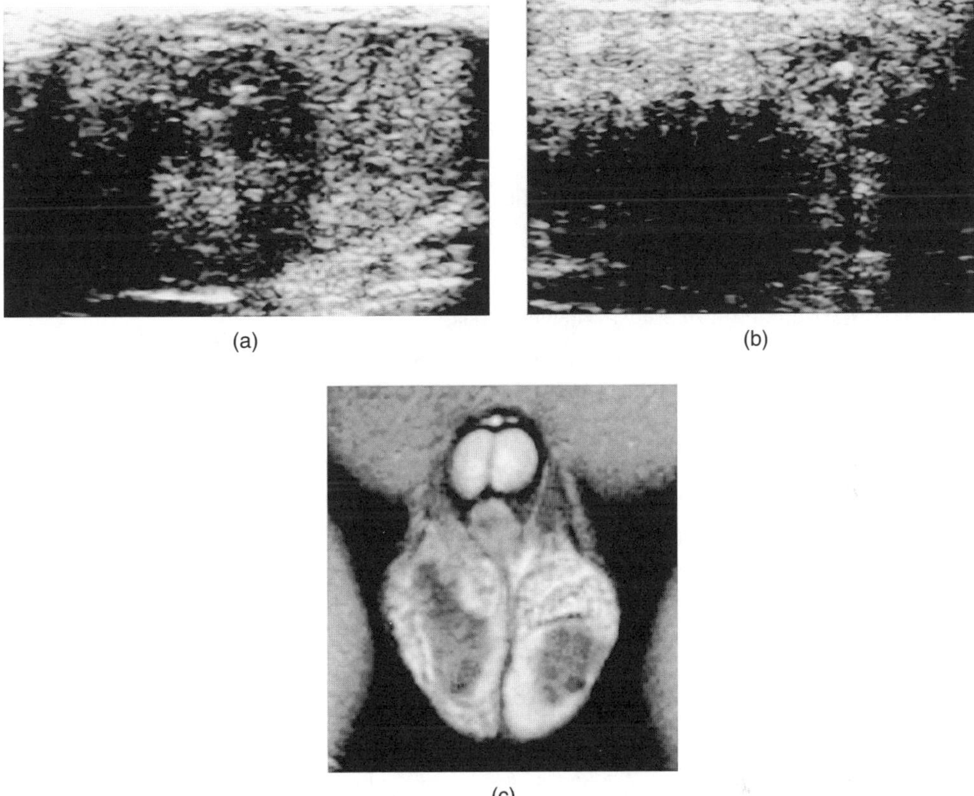

Figure 15.7 *Bilateral adrenal rests in a boy with congenital adrenal hyperplasia.* (a) A sagittal US view of the right testis demonstrates a heterogeneous mass (arrow). (b) A small calcification seen in the left testicle (arrow). (c) A coronal T2-MRI shows bilateral, low-signal-intensity lesions.

which are usually isointense to surrounding normal testicular tissue on T1-weighted images.

o *Sarcoidosis*

- This disease can involve the genital tract and produce solid nodules in the testis, often with associated epididymal enlargement.

- It is more frequent in the African and African-American male. In this group of patients testicular tumors are relatively rare, and this has to be taken into consideration in raising the possibility of benign disease.

o *Fibrous pseudotumors of the tunica vaginalis*

- Not a real tumor, but a benign fibroinflammatory reaction resulting in nodules (either single or multiple) at the tunica vaginalis or tunica albuginea.

- At US, they are seen as solid, hypoechogenic, non-specific lesions

- At MRI they have been reported with intermediate to low signal intensity on both T1- and T2-weighted images, addressing their fibrous nature.

- *Polyorchidism*

  - This is a rare condition thought to originate from abnormal division of the genital ridge, with up to five testes reported, mostly located within the scrotum.

  - At US, supernumerary testes have usually the same echogenicity as normal ones.

  - At MRI supernumerary testes have the same signal intensity of normal testes. The identification of the hypointense tunica albuginea. usually allows a correct diagnosis to be made.

- *Lipomas*

  - The most common extratesticular neoplasm.

  - Most often originating from the spermatic cord.

  - Most of these lesions have a hyperechogenic structure at US. However, this is not the case in many patients, and a specific diagnosis is not possible with this technique.

  - At MRI they have hyperintense signal on both T1-weighted and T2-weighted sequences, and can be differentiated from a hemorrhagic mass with the use of fat suppression sequences.

  - Differentiating a lipoma from a liposarcoma is not possible, and excision is needed to establish the diagnosis.

References

Akbar SA, Sayyed TA, Jafri SZH, Hasteh F, Neil JSA (2003) Multimodality imaging of paratesticular neoplasms and their rare mimics. *Radiographics* **23**: 1461–1476.

Baker LL, Hajek PC, Burkhard TK, Dicapua L, Leopold GR, Hesselink JR, Mattrey RF (1987) MR imaging of the scrotum: normal anatomy. *Radiology* **163**: 89–92.

Muglia V, Tucci S, Jr, Elias J, Jr, Trad CS, Bilbey J, Cooperberg PL (2002) Magnetic resonance imaging of scrotal diseases: when it makes the difference. *Urology* **59**: 419–423.

Woodward PJ, Sohaey R, O'Donoghues, Green DE (2002) Tumors and tumorlike lesions of the testis: radiologic-pathologic correlation. *Radiographics* **22**: 189–216.

Woodward PJ, Schwab CM, Sesterhenn IA (2003) Extratesticular scrotal masses: radiologic–pathologic correlation. *Radiographics* **23**: 215–240.

16
Gynecological Adnexal Masses

John A. Spencer and Michael J. Weston

Department of Clinical Radiology, St James's University Hospital, Leeds

16.1 Introduction

In this chapter we consider clinical investigation and management of the symptomatic and incidental adnexal mass.

16.2 Clinical features

- Women rarely present in clinical practice having felt a gynecological mass.
- Women with gynecological masses are often referred initially from primary care to non-gynecological specialists.
- Most presentations are with symptoms that result from pressure or displacement effects:
  - generalized abdominal distension from the mass or from ascites
  - intestinal symptoms from bowel compression
  - features of the urinary tract compromise affecting the bladder and later the ureters
  - lower limb swelling due to pelvic venous or lymphatic compromise.
- Symptoms are often vague or non-specific unless the mass causes vaginal bleeding or it prolapses into the vagina.
- Due to its insidious nature ovarian cancer, the 'silent killer', typically presents late with advanced abdomino-pelvic disease.
- A gynecological mass may be discovered incidentally during a cross-sectional imaging examination performed for a non-gynecological indication.

Urogenital Imaging: A Problem-oriented Approach   Edited by Sameh K. Morcos and Henrik S. Thomsen
© 2009 John Wiley & Sons, Ltd

- Tumor marker CA125

  - Serum level is raised in the presence of ovarian malignancy, particularly in advanced stages.

  - May be moderately raised in benign conditions such as endometriosis or pelvic inflammatory disease.

  - Raised only in 50% of patients with stage I (confined to the ovary) ovarian malignancy.

  - Therefore its interpretation needs care and a normal CA 125 should not prevent the diagnosis of a malignant ovarian lesion.

- Risk of Malignancy Index (RMI)

  - This is a calculation advocated by the Royal College of Obstetricians and Gynaecologists, UK in its web site (www.rcog.org.uk) based on a woman's menopausal status, her CA 125 level and the ultrasound appearances.

  - It can be a useful tool in predicting ovarian malignancy but as it uses CA125 measurement it has some of the problems described above.

  - It can be helpful to indicate which patients should be referred to specialist centers for further opinion and/or investigation.

Further relevant clinical features of different adnexal lesions are mentioned with the imaging findings.

16.3 Pathology

In this section the pathophysiology cystic of lesions that may affect the ovary is discussed and the pathology of solid and inflammatory adnexal masses is briefly presented with the imaging findings of these lesions.

Ovarian cyst

- The nature depends on the patient's age and the stage of her menstrual cycle.

  - *Neonatal*

    - Most pelvic cysts in female babies will be ovarian and secondary to the influence of maternal hormones that have crossed the placenta before birth.

    - They usually resolve spontaneously.

  - *Premenarchal*

    - Functional cysts may occur prior to the first menstruation.

  - *Menstrual*

    - The release of an egg with each cycle requires the maturation of follicles. One becomes dominant and egg release usually occurs once it reaches 2.5 cm in size; the follicle should then mature into a corpus luteum (Fig. 16.1) and, in the absence of pregnancy, regress.

    - Follicular or luteal cysts can develop if failure of regression occurs during the cycle.

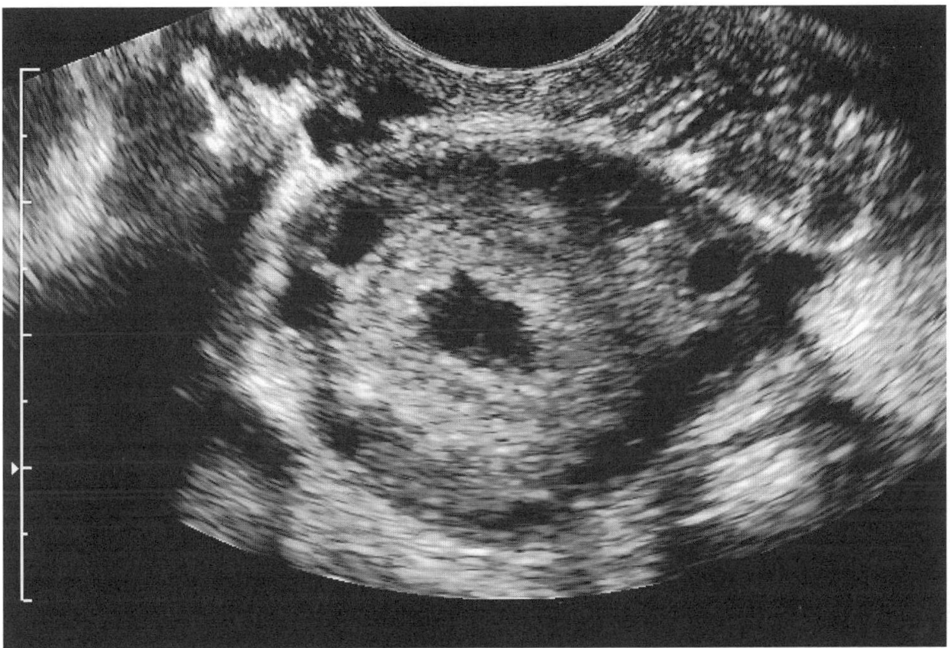

Figure 16.1   TVUS of a normal ovary showing a centrally placed thickwalled corpus luteum with surrounding stroma containing immature follicles.

- These functional cysts are
  - Usually 3 cm in diameter or less.
  - Have thin walls and contain clear fluid.
- The incidence of malignancy in this age group is low.
- *Pregnancy*
  - Persistent luteal cysts may occur.
  - Torsion is more common in pregnancy.
  - The likelihood of a cyst being malignant during pregnancy is higher than in age matched non-pregnant women.
- *Post-menopausal*
  - Simple cysts are surprisingly common in post-menopausal women but incidence of malignancy in this age group is relatively high.
  - Benign cysts have thin walls, clear fluid and usually less than 5 cm in diameter. Thin septae may also be found.
  - A true simple cyst 'never' transforms to a malignant lesion.
  - Malignant ovarian cyst have the following features
    - Thick wall and septa
    - Nodular growth from the wall
    - Partial solid and partially cystic
    - May have areas of calcification.

16.4 Imaging

The cross-sectional imaging modalities ultrasound (US), magnetic resonance imaging (MRI) and computed tomography (CT) are the main diagnostic tools that are used in modern imaging departments for the evaluation of the adnexal mass. The goals of imaging (Table 16.2) are to determine the nature, origin, extent of the adnexal mass and to guide therapy with the intention that:

- benign lesions do not undergo inappropriate cancer surgery

- ovarian cancers do not undergo surgery limited to simple resection

- ovarian cancers do not undergo non-therapeutic surgery because of unrecognized non-resectable features

- cancer metastatic to the ovary is not mistaken for primary ovarian cancer.

Table 16.1   Common adnexal lesions and their histological classification

Functional
Follicular cyst
Luteal cyst

Inflammatory
Hydropyosalpinx
Tubo-ovarian abscess

Hemorrhagic
Within pre-existing mass – 'cyst accident'
Endometriotic cyst

Vascular
Ovarian torsion/massive edema
Ovarian vein thrombosis

Epithelial neoplasm
Cystadenoma/adenofibroma
Borderline neoplasm
Invasive carcinoma
Malignant mixed Mullerian tumor

Stromal neoplasm
Fibroma/Thecoma
Granulosa cell tumor
Sex cord stromal tumor

Germ cell neoplasm
Mature teratoma
Dysgerminoma
Malignant teratoma

Other neoplasms
Metastasis
Lymphoma
Sarcoma

Table 16.2 Imaging algorithm for suspected newly diagnosed ovarian cancer

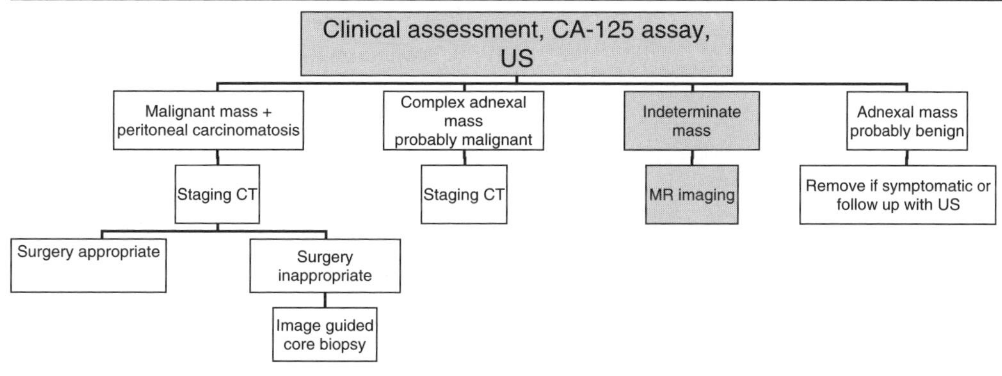

16.5 Standard radiographic techniques

- Plain chest radiograph is obtained as a baseline investigation in women with ovarian cancer and may be required as part of the anesthetic assessment.

- Plain abdominal radiography has no role in the assessment of an adnexal mass but can be useful when women present with an acute abdomen.

- There is no role for intravenous urography as CT provides relevant information in cancer patients.

16.6 Ultrasound (US)

US is the first-line investigation of the suspected gynecological mass (Table 16.2).

US technique (Table 16.3)

- Essential information

  o The patient's age and menstrual status – adnexal masses in premenarchal or older post-menopausal women are more likely to be malignant.
  o The date of the first day of last menstrual period (LMP) and the normal length of cycle.
  o Medications, such as hormone replacement, contraceptives or tamoxifen.
  o Her history of gynecological procedures and any other co-morbidity.

Table 16.3 Relative merits of US techniques

Transabdominal US	Transvaginal US
Full bladder	Empty bladder
Large field of view	Restricted field of view
Lower frequency/poorer resolution	Higher frequency/better resolution
Good for large masses	Good for detailed views of pelvic structures
Useful for checking upper abdomen.	Can provide information on 'visceral slide'

- Ideally, an ultrasound examination of the pelvis should comprise both transabdominal and transvaginal approaches.

- If an abnormality is found in the pelvis, then the scan should be extended to include the upper abdomen.

US imaging features

Adnexal cysts and their differential diagnosis (Table 16.4)

- A simple cyst is a well-defined, anechoic structure with an imperceptible wall and posterior acoustic enhancement (Fig. 16.2).

- It is important to identify normal ovarian tissue related to the cyst in order to confirm its ovarian origin. This may not always be possible, particularly in the post-menopausal age group.

- Finding a simple (follicular) ovarian cyst of 3 cm diameter or less on ultrasound in a woman of child-bearing age is essentially normal and follow-up is not required unless there are some symptoms attributable to the cyst.

Table 16.4 Differential diagnosis of an ovarian cyst

Diagnosis	US features
Fimbrial cyst	ipsilateral ovary should be seen separately
Hydrosalpinx	tubular in shape 'cysts' interconnect plicae do not completely traverse the lesion may show a 'waist' (Fig.16.3)
The bladder	a classic pitfall for the unwary
Bladder diverticulum	look for the communication with the bladder.
Ureterocele	dilated distal ureter communicates with an expansion that protrudes into the bladder
Peritoneal inclusion cyst	usually occurs following previous pelvic surgery or infection the classic feature is angular extensions of the cyst interleaving between adjacent structures
Lymphocele	relevant surgical history
Aneurysm	obvious if color Doppler is used
Abscess	clinical history and signs are paramount here
Mucocoele of appendix	bowel related lesions typically show a multilayered wall and may be traced back to join a recognizable loop of bowel. However, this connection may be obscured by bowel gas.
Necrotic/cystic fibroid	fibroids can present diagnostic difficulties try to join the lesion to the uterus look at previous scans to see if there was a fibroid at that site

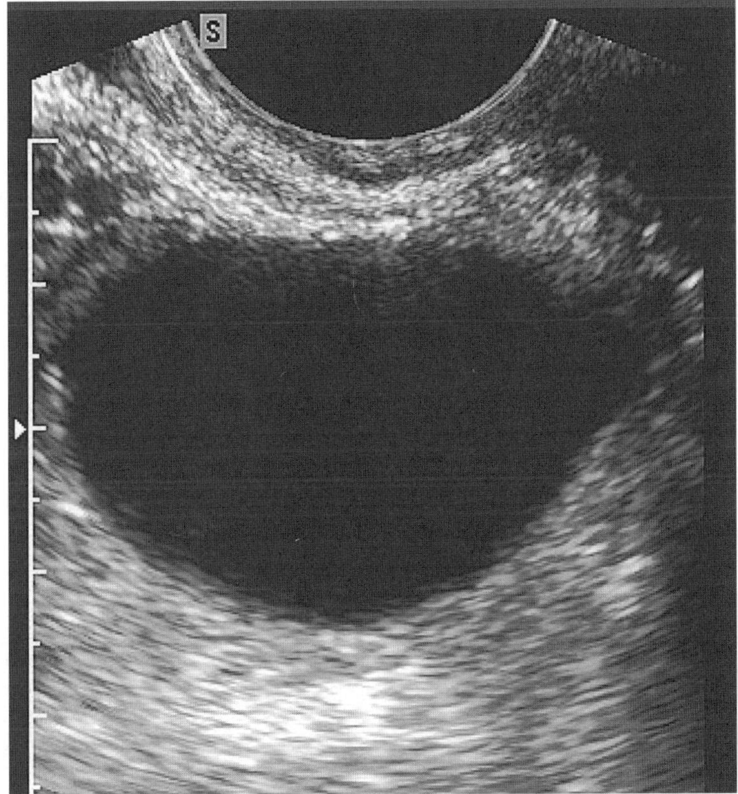

Figure 16.2 TVUS of a simple unilocular ovarian cyst showing a thin regular wall, purely anechoic contents and through transmission of sound with posterior acoustic enhancement.

- Larger cysts in women of child-bearing age are worth a follow-up scan after an interval (at least one menstrual cycle) to check they are not continuing to enlarge.

- Truly simple cysts that are stable over time and less than 5 cm in diameter can be ignored in a post-menopausal patient.

- Persistent, simple cysts of over 5 cm in size in a post-menopausal patient should be considered for removal notably if believed to be symptomatic. MR imaging may be useful to confirm benignity in larger cysts left *in situ*.

US signs used to distinguish benign from malignant cysts
Size

- Large lesions >5 cm in diameter are more likely to be malignant.

- However, very large cysts of 20 cm or more in size (without any signs of disease outside the cyst) are more likely to be benign, usually mucinous cystadenomas.

Calcifications

- The presence of calcification in otherwise normal ovaries is a feature of no concern.

- Calcification in abnormal ovaries is a feature of concern.

- Benign calcifications as seen in teratomas or endometriomas should be differentiated from calcifications seen in some malignant tumors.

Septa

- A single smooth thin (less than 3 mm thick) septum may be present in simple bilocular cysts.

- Even multiple smooth thin septae are unlikely to indicate malignancy (Fig. 16.4).

- Septae of over 3 mm thickness, particularly those with an irregular 'lumpy bumpy' profile, are pointers towards malignancy (Fig. 16.5).

Wall thickness

- Thick walls (greater than 3 mm) and irregular walls are pointers towards malignancy.

- Care has to be taken not to mistake remaining normal ovarian tissue around the margin of the cyst for an area of wall thickening.

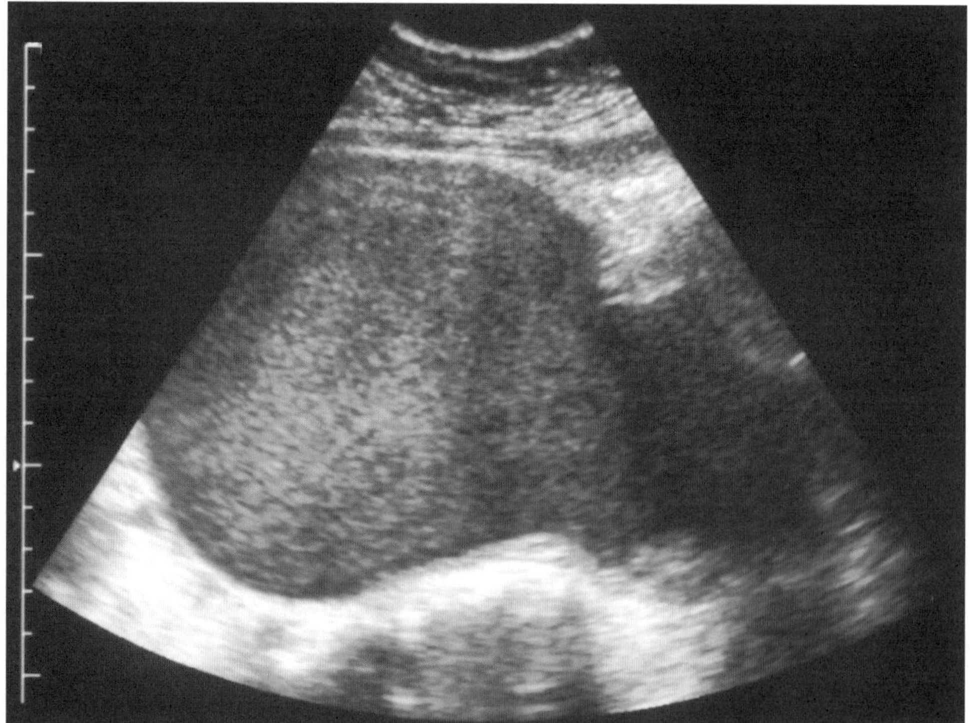

Figure 16.3 TVUS of a hematosalpinx in a woman with endometriosis. Notice the tubular shape of the structure and the prominent 'waist'. It contains uniform low-level echoes and still shows enhanced through-transmission of sound (indicating fluid).

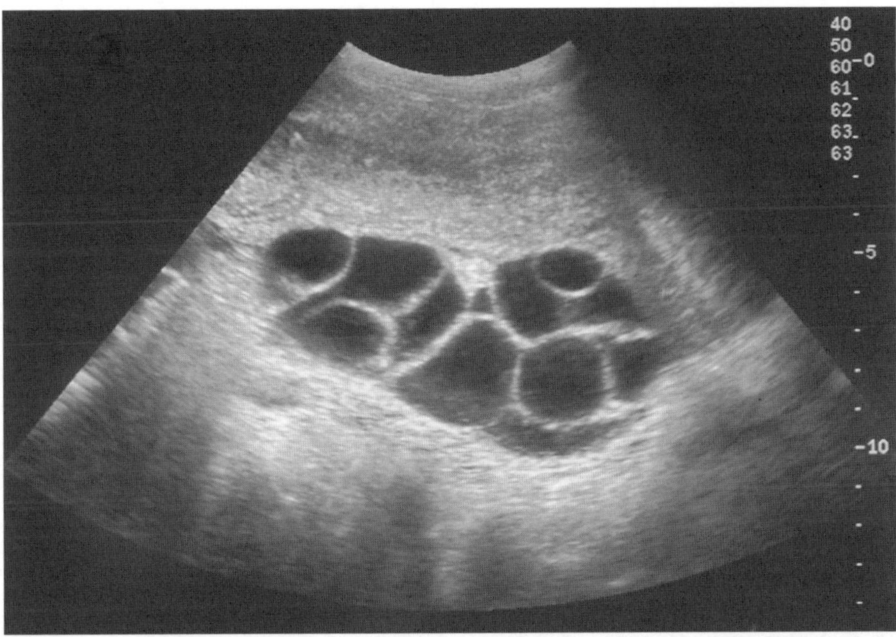

Figure 16.4 TVUS of a multilocular cystic ovary in a woman undergoing stimulation for assisted conception. It is the patient's history that allows the diagnosis of a stimulated ovary rather than any other lesion.

Papillarities

- Nodules or papillary excrescences or vegetations of over 3 mm in size protruding from the wall or septa into the lumen of a cyst are a very strong marker for malignancy.

- Transabdominal examination may miss these if the lesion is deep and the spatial resolution is poor.

- Transvaginal scans may miss them if the cyst is large and the far wall extends out of the range.

Mixed cystic and solid mass

- A truly mixed cystic (i.e. septated) and solid mass is pathognomic of malignancy (Fig. 16.5) though note that some solid benign masses may outgrow their blood supply and undergo cystic necrosis.

Blood flow

- Color and spectral Doppler ultrasound is an adjunct but not the dominant determinant of the nature of the lesion. The main determinant of lesion classification in the authors' view is its grayscale appearance.

Contrast enhancement

- Lesions with solid areas which show enhancement are more likely to be malignant.

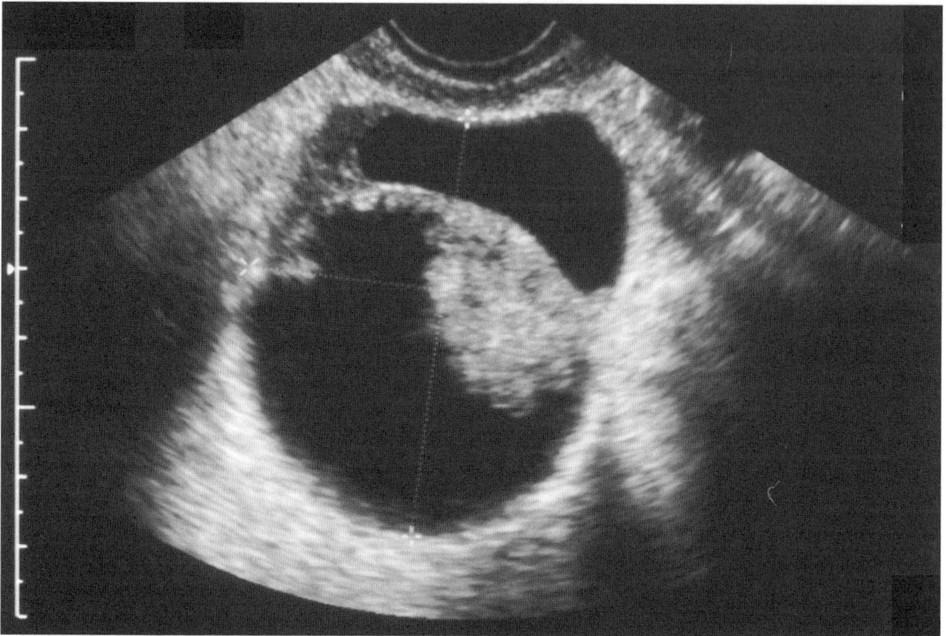

Figure 16.5   Small ovarian cancer shown by TVUS with irregular 'lumpy-bumpy' septa and solid mural nodule/papillarity.

- Washin and washout times for contrast agents may also help. Ovarian malignancies have prolonged washout times.

Abnormalities outside the adnexal lesion

- Ascites is a very strong pointer to peritoneal dissemination of malignant tumor.

- Small amounts of free fluid may be observed in the pelvic recesses of women of menstrual years.

- Ascites is also seen in women with acute presentations due to infection, torsion, cyst accidents and ectopic pregnancy.

- Rarely ovarian fibroma is associated with ascites and/or pleural effusion.

- Omental cake or peritoneal thickening/serosal deposits and lymphadenopathy are highly indicative of advanced malignancy.

US features of other ovarian and adnexal lesions

Hemorrhagic ovarian cyst

- Hemorrhage into a physiological follicle or luteum is common in women of menstrual age.

- Some women form complex hemorrhagic cysts with each menstrual cycle.

- When associated with pain it is termed a 'cyst accident'.

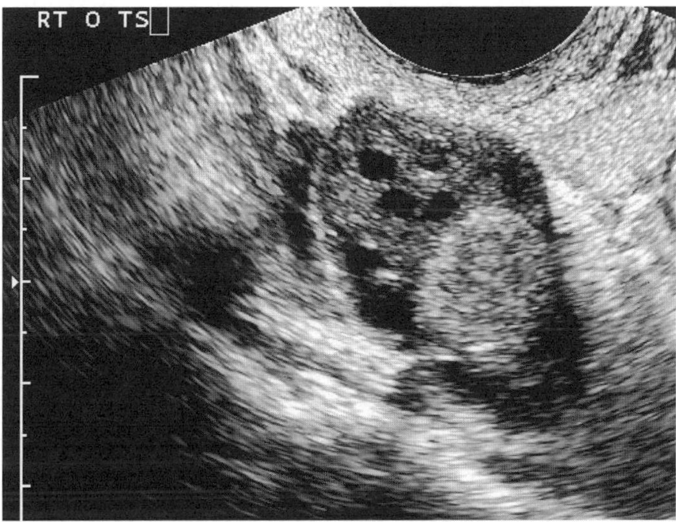

Figure 16.6 TVUS of a small echogenic fatty dermoid within an otherwise normal ovary. Only time allows the diagnosis to be made as an acute bleed into a follicle looks similar. Follow-up scans show that a dermoid persists unchanged whereas a bleed resolves.

- Blood shows a variety of appearances on US depending on its age.
  - Fresh blood, particularly in a small lesion, can be echogenic.
    - This can be confused with the bright echoes seen from fat in small dermoid tumors (Fig. 16.6).
    - Repeating the scan after an interval of a few weeks will show that fat still looks the same whereas blood will have matured and become less echoic.
    - Blood may also show layering out of its components.
    - Blood may mimic the cystic/solid appearances of malignancy.
    - An absence of detectable blood flow in the lesion is reassuring but repeat examination after an interval is vital to show clot maturation.
  - Classic appearance of mature clot
    - The clot retracts in upon itself to form a smaller nodule or cast of the lesion.
    - Showing an acute angle between the clot retraction (Fig. 16.7) and the cyst wall is a good sign to distinguish it from a tumor nodule, which will have an obtuse angle.

Endometrioma (Endometriosis)

- Defined as the presence of endometrial glandular tissue outside of the uterus.
- The most frequent site of endometriosis is the ovary leading to the formation of a hemorrhagic 'chocolate cyst'.
- On US a chocolate cyst has a uniform grayscale level of echoes across the whole cyst (Figs. 16.3 and 16.8). A malignant ovarian lesion may show a similar appearance.
- Endometriomas persist over time and may become larger.

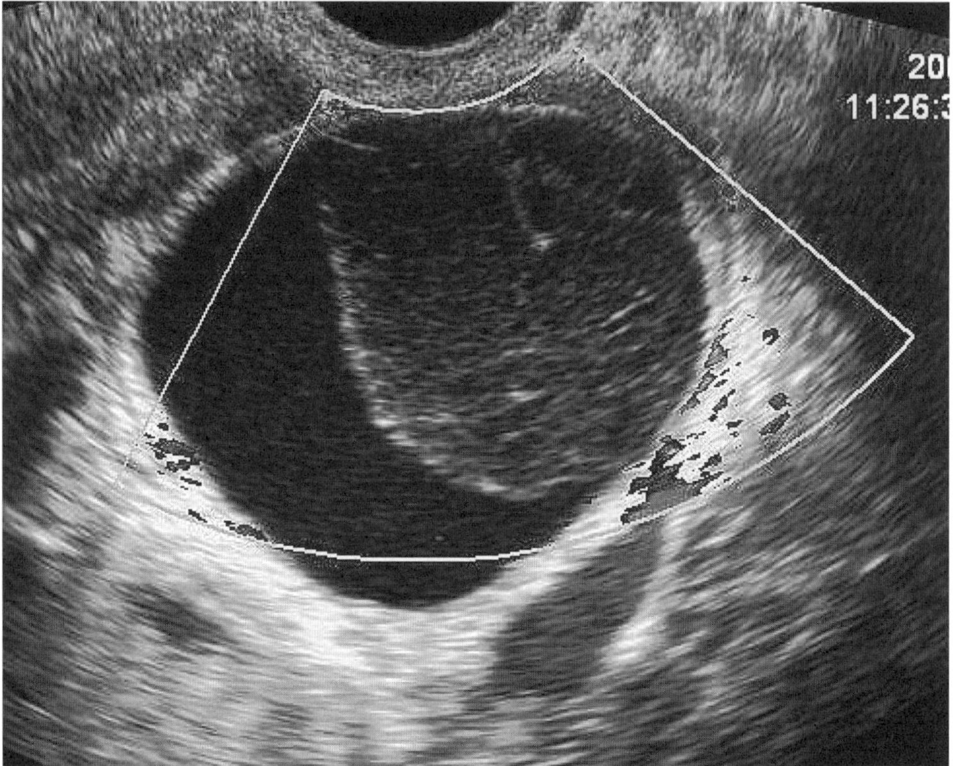

Figure 16.7 TVUS of clot retraction within a hemorrhagic cyst using color Doppler imaging to show absence of blood flow. Note the typical feature of the acute angle made between the clot retraction and the cyst wall.

- Small calcifications may occur in their walls.

- The size, wall thickness and internal complexity are variable and may be indistinguishable from other complex benign and malignant pelvic pathology.

- MR imaging is an extremely useful tool in this setting as it can define the signal characteristics of blood of differing ages.

- Rarely malignancy can arise in pre-existing endometriosis. Finding a new area of soft tissue should alert to this complication.

Dermoid (mature cystic teratoma)

- This lesion commonly presents in younger women of reproductive age but can be seen in any age group.

- Small fatty dermoid lesions are relatively common findings and manifest as echogenic 'bright' nodules within ovarian stroma (Fig. 16.6).

- Larger lesions may present with very complex ultrasound features (Figs 16.9 and 16.10).

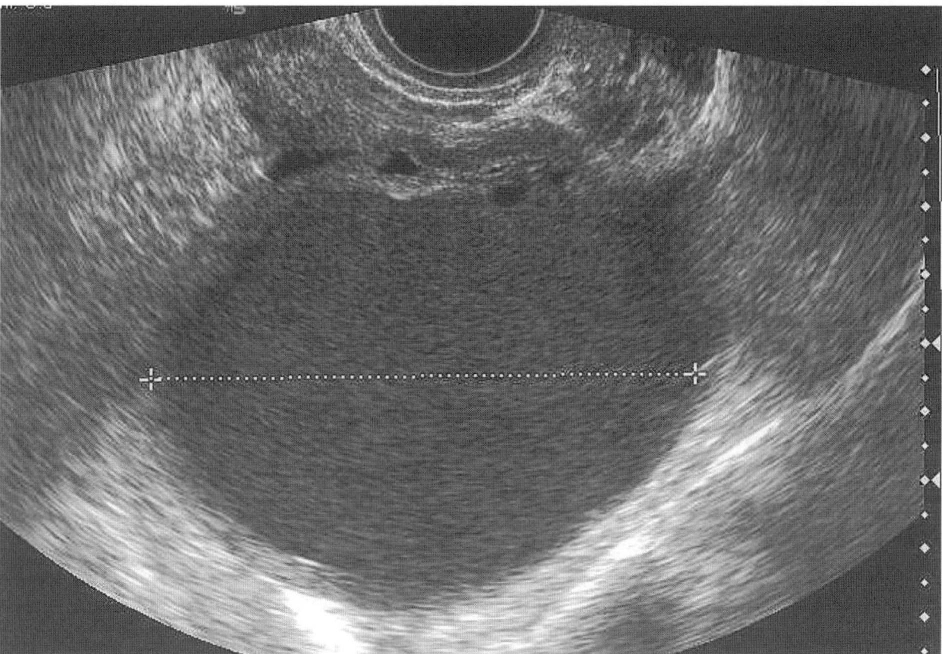

Figure 16.8 Typical features of an Endometriotic cyst containing uniform low-level echoes. However, this is not specific.

- ○ *Fat/fluid level* might be observed. The uppermost layer is the fat or oil. If there is oil this will show as anechoic fluid on US rather than the echogenicity usually associated with fat.

- ○ A *dermoid plug* is a hyperechoic nodule in a cyst (Fig. 16.9) which contains hair or teeth. A dense acoustic shadow might be observed.

- ○ *Dermoid mesh* (Fig. 16.10): small echogenic particles or lines are seen suspended in a hypoechoic medium.

- ○ These complex internal features need to distinguished from the complex solid and cystic internal features of a large epithelial ovarian neoplasm (Fig. 16.11).

Solid adnexal lesions

- Solid ovarian masses are uncommon amounting to only 5% of all ovarian tumors.

- A pedunculated uterine fibroid has to be considered (Fig. 16.12) and then ovarian stromal tumors such as fibromas, thecomas and granulosa cell tumors.

- They usually show a uniform isoechoic or hyperechoic mass. The degree of acoustic shadowing or enhancement is very variable.

- Areas of cystic degeneration (necrosis) may occur.

- Fibromas may have foci of calcification.

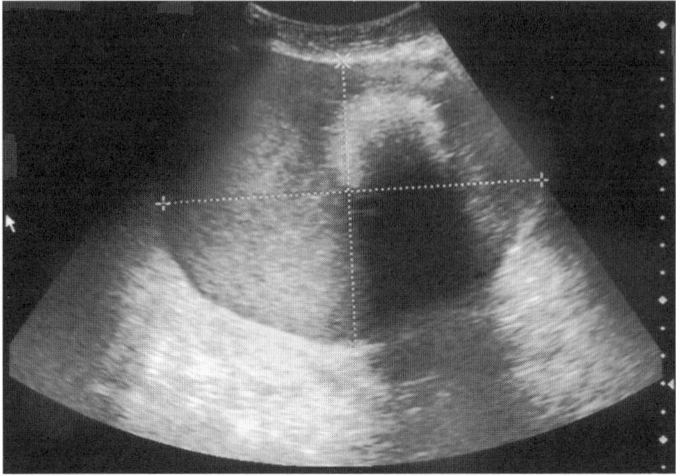

Figure 16.9 Characteristic appearances of an echogenic plug casting a posterior acoustic shadow in this dermoid cyst.

- A uniformly solid mass on ultrasound carries a lower risk of malignancy than a mixed cystic and solid lesion.

- US cannot provide a confident diagnosis for many solid lesions which are therefore US indeterminate masses (Table 16.2).

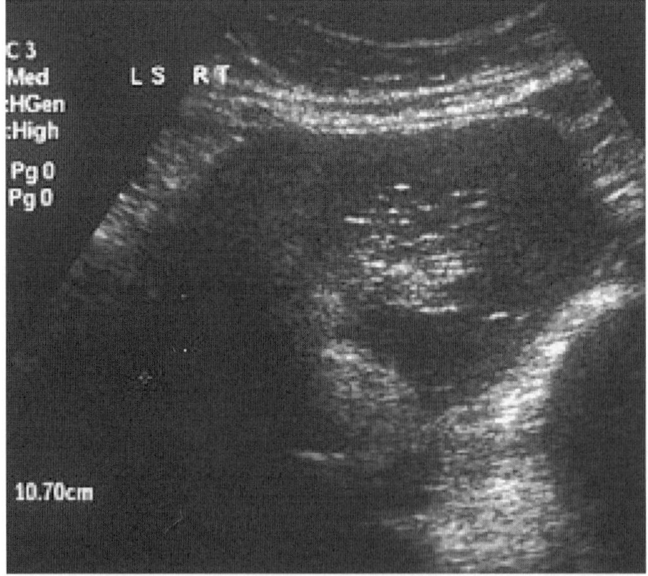

Figure 16.10 US showing a right-sided dermoid with a typical dermoid matrix of reflectors. This pattern of incomplete, thin, almost parallel lines of reflection is almost pathognomonic of a dermoid.

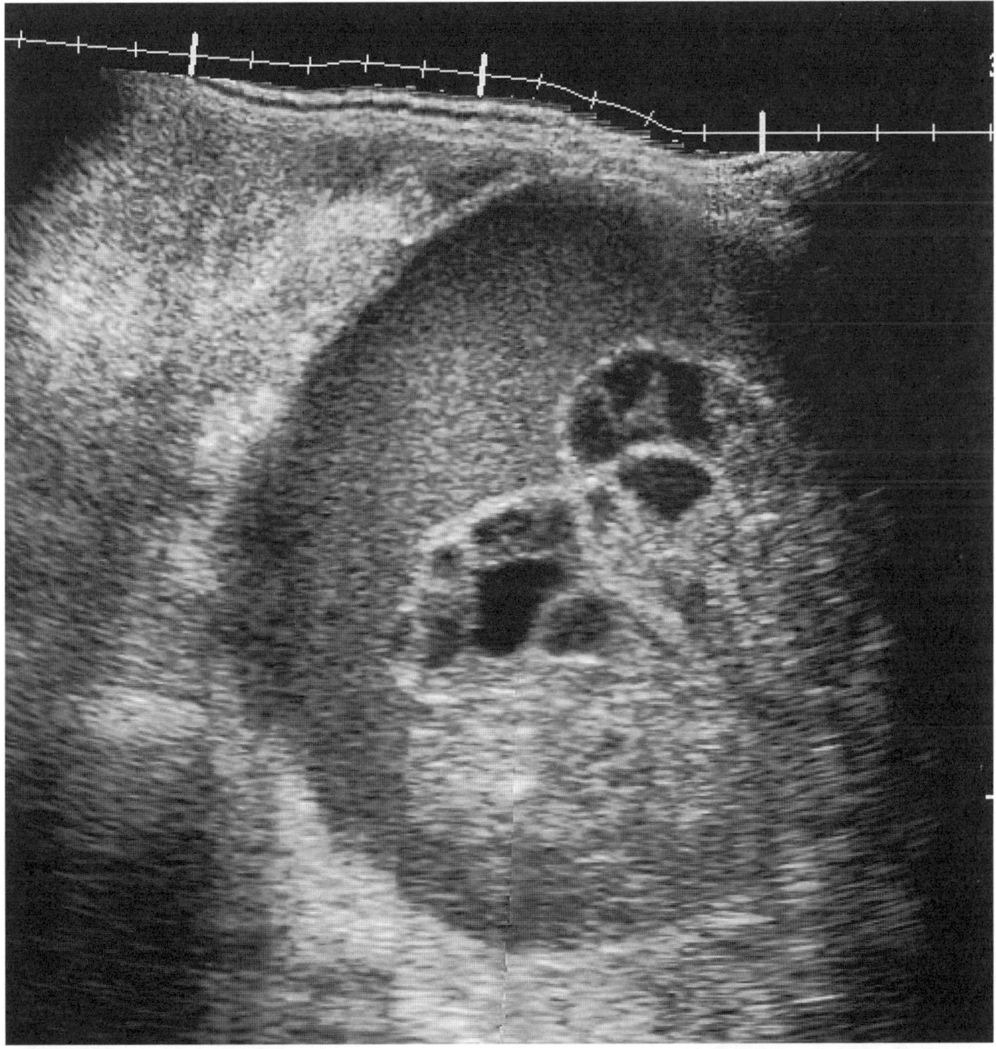

Figure 16.11 US of classical cystic solid ovarian cancer. The fluid component shows low-level echoes illustrating that this sign is non-specific and does not always correspond to blood.

- MR imaging is a valuable adjunct as fibroma has characteristic appearances which distinguish it from pedunculated fibroids and solid malignant masses.

Pelvic inflammatory disease

- This is an infective condition caused by ascending lower genital tract infection.

- Risk factors include previous episodes of sexually transmitted disease, multiple partners, intrauterine contraceptive devices and septic abortion.

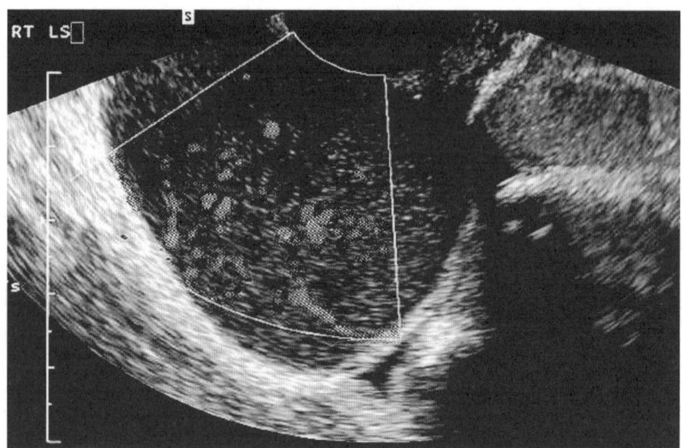

Figure 16.12 The colour Doppler shows flow within this lesion confirming that is a solid mass with a uniform echogenicity.

- An appropriate clinical picture with acute pain, fever, vaginal discharge, tenderness and cervical 'excitation' on internal examination and raised inflammatory markers is most useful in suggesting that a complex adnexal mass represents a tubo-ovarian abscess.

- Endocavity (transvaginal) ultrasound may indicate the site of pain by direct 'palpation'.

- Transvaginal US has a key role in guiding drainage of abscesses and may enable surgery to be avoided.

The outcome of the US assessment of an adnexal mass (Table 16.2)

- Benign lesion, no follow-up is needed.

- Benign, but needs removal or other treatment for symptoms.

- Most likely benign but follow-up with ultrasound is required after an interval. *(NB. Repeated scans every few months to see what is happening to a cyst without any decision being made are wasteful and unhelpful. Once an adnexal cyst is shown to be benign and there is no intention to intervene there is no need for further scans).*

- Indeterminate lesion, proceed to MR imaging for further characterization

- Malignant lesion, proceed to CT for staging which allows prediction of complete surgical resection. If surgery is not felt appropriate CT allows planning of image-guided biopsy (IGB). Imaging algorithm for suspected newly diagnosed ovarian cancer is presented in Table 16.2.

16.7 MR Imaging (MRI)

MRI is the investigation of choice for the US indeterminate adnexal or pelvic mass (Table 16.2).

Technique

- Should use a high field system of 1T to 3T strength.

- There is no patient preparation necessary and the patient may empty her bladder beforehand so she is not uncomfortable during the 30 minute examination.

- IV injection of a smooth muscle relaxant is advisable to reduce bowel peristalsis.

- A pelvic phased array coil system should be used.

- The protocol is divided into two stages: identification of the mass and then its characterization. Identification should include a minimum of these basic sequences:

    o Sagittal T2-weighted sequence through the uterus from pelvic sidewall to sidewall.

    o Axial T2-weighted sequence of the uterus along the long axis of the uterus.

    o A pair of axial or coronal T1- and T2-weighted sequences of the whole pelvis to show best the mass and its relationship to other pelvic organs.

- After these basic sequences it is possible to divide the mass into one of three categories and to decide if it arises from the ovary, uterus or another pelvic organ (Table 16.5):

    o a T1 'bright' mass (high T1 signal intensity) (Fig. 16.13)

    o a complex cystic or cystic-solid mass (Fig. 16.14)

    o a T2 solid mass, either T2 'dark' (low signal intensity) or intermediate/inhomogeneous intensity (Fig. 16.15).

- The purpose of this algorithm is to place a mass into a category which defines its management. Detailed description of the MR features of every adnexal tumor is beyond the scope of this chapter.

Table 16.5   Algorithm for assessment of the US indeterminate mass using MR imaging

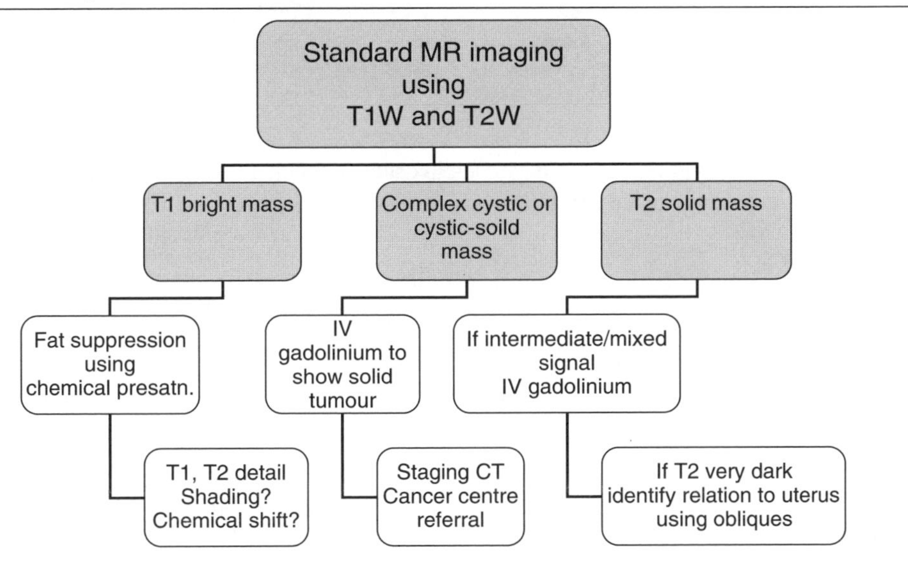

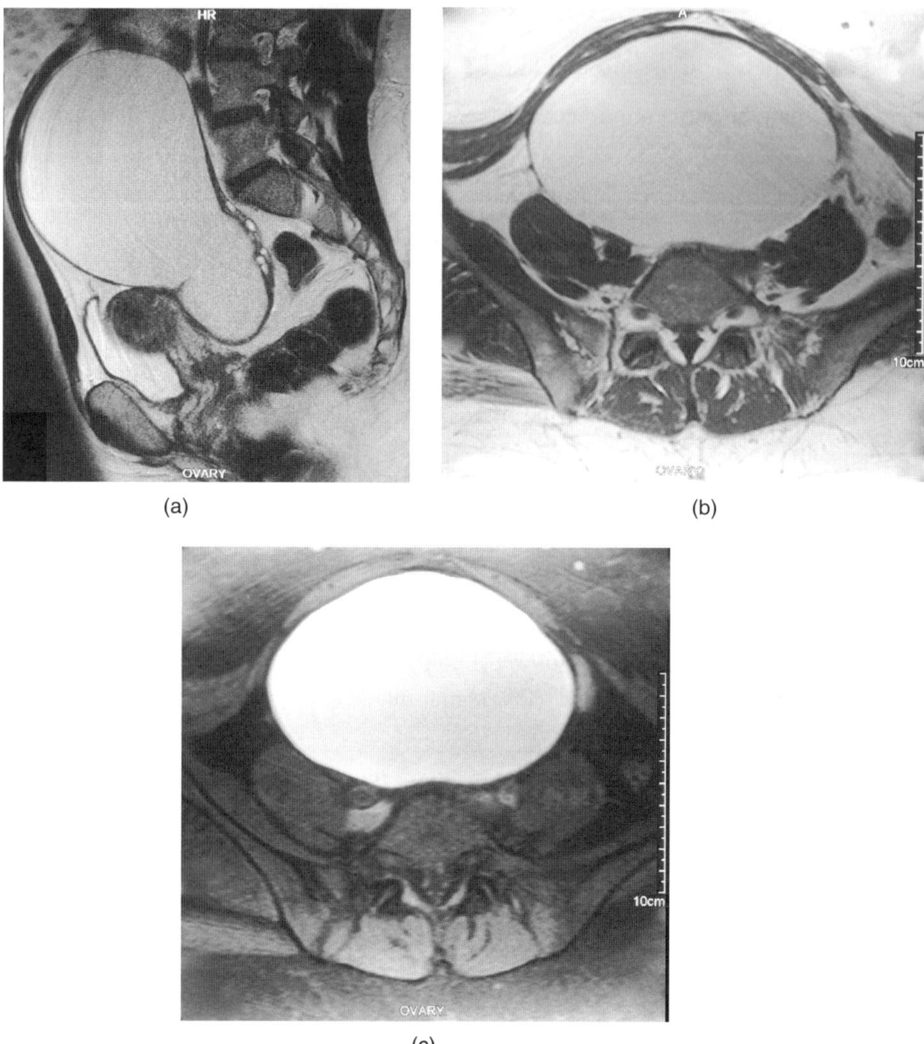

Figure 16.13   MR imaging of the hematosalpinx shown in Fig. 16.3 with (a) sagittal T2W image showing the tubular, waisted structure with a mural linear structure which unlike a septum incompletely crosses the lesion and (b), (c) axial T1W and fat suppressed T1W images showing 'bright' blood which does not undergo fat suppression.

- Some masses will have more than one of these features, e.g. an endometrioma may contain blood products that are both T1 bright and T2 dark, a mature cystic teratoma may contain T1 bright fat and other mature cutaneous elements which have cystic-solid appearances.

- T1 'bright' masses require a fat suppressed T1-weighted (FST1W) sequence using chemical presaturation to distinguish fat from blood, mucin or other proteinaceous material (Figs 16.13 and 16.16).

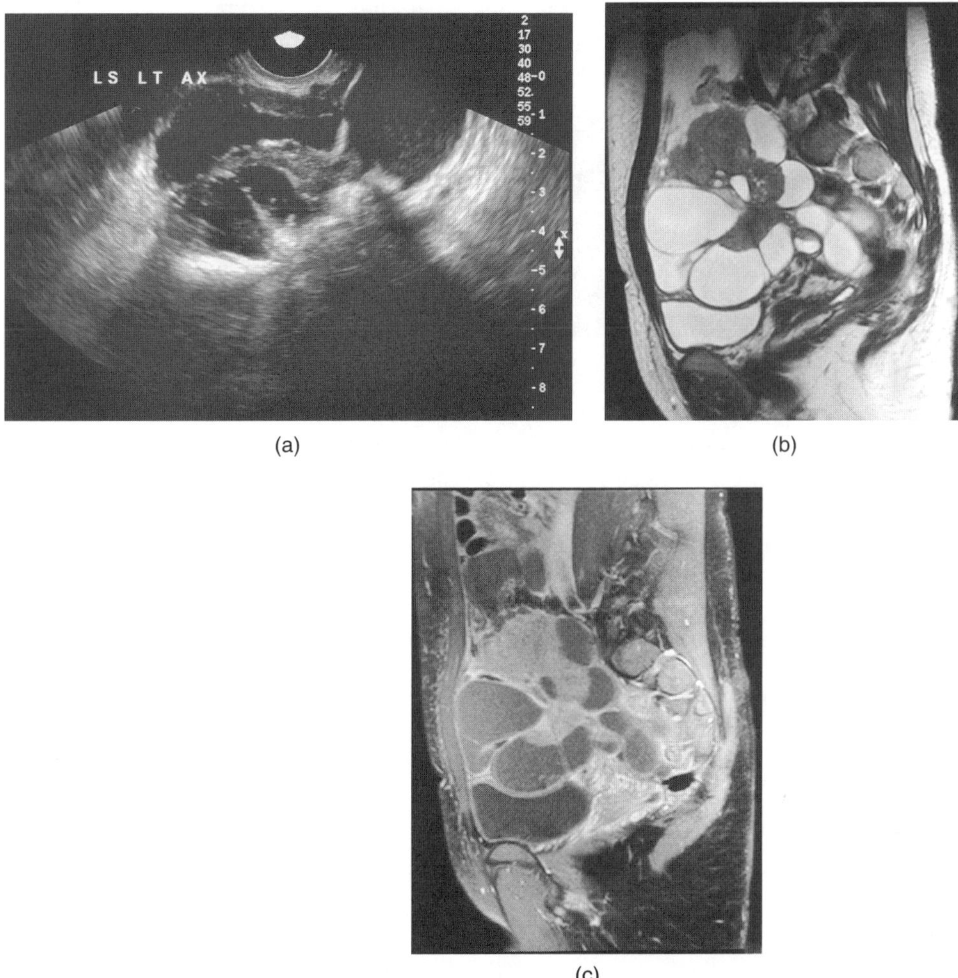

(a)

(b)

(c)

Figure 16.14   Classical ovarian cancer shown (a) by US and (b) (c) by T2W and fat suppressed contrast-enhanced T1W MR imaging with irregular solid enhancing elements.

- T2 'dark' masses require additional T2-weighted oblique sequences to identify the relationship with the uterus (is the lesion connected to the uterus as with a pedunculated fibroid or separate as in an ovarian fibroma) (Fig. 16.15).

- Fibroid masses may be shown to have bridging vessels arising from the uterus but ovarian masses are supplied by the gonadal vascular pedicle.

- Cystic-solid or solid masses with soft tissue components require gadolinium enhanced T1-weighted (CET1W) sequences to confirm the presence of neoplastic tissue (Fig. 16.14) and overview sequences of the abdomen and pelvis to look for evidence of metastases.

- In some cases T2 dark masses require CET1W imaging as this further helps distinguish a fibroma by virtue of its non-enhancement from a solid malignancy which does enhance.

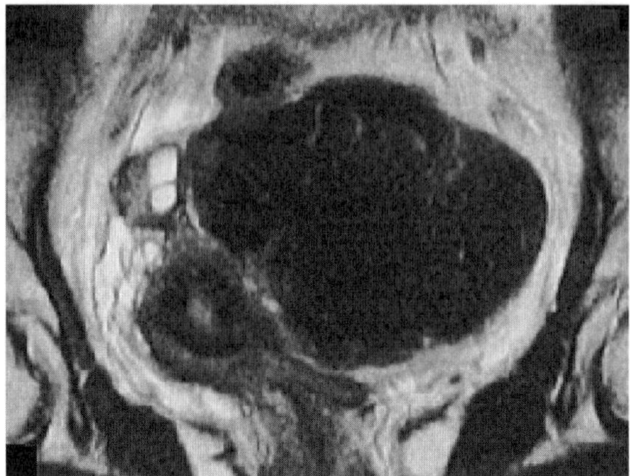

Figure 16.15 Oblique T2W image of a normal uterus and right tube and ovary with a left ovarian fibroma clearly shown to be separate from the uterus.

MRI signs of adnexal masses (Table 16.5)

T1 bright masses

- A variety of adnexal masses have T1 bright characteristics.

  - Mature cystic teratoma (dermoid tumor)
  - Endometrioma
  - Hemorrhagic cyst
  - Mucinous tumors
  - Melanoma metastasis.

- The only T1 bright mass to undergo fat suppression is a mature cystic teratoma (dermoid tumor).

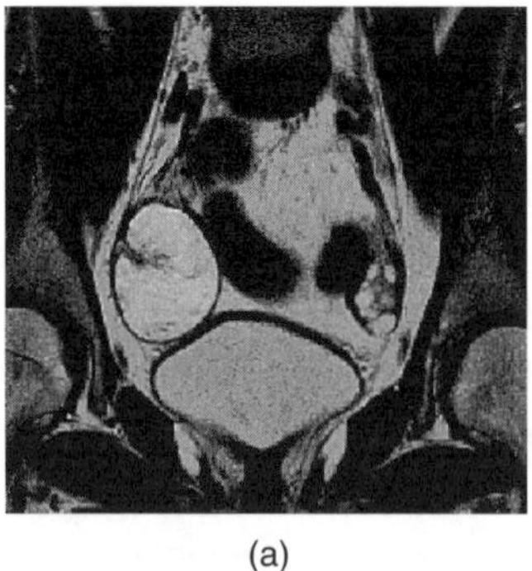

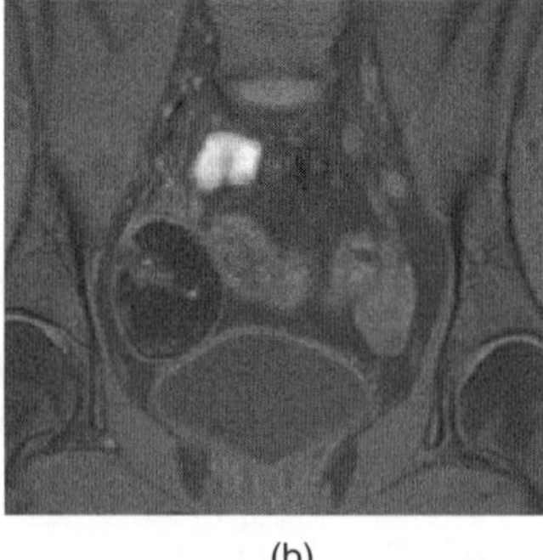

(a) (b)

Figure 16.16 Classical MR appearances of a dermoid with (a) coronal T2W image showing really quite complex internal elements which represent skin appendages but also the presence of chemical shift artefact with small bright-dark nodules and then (b) virtually complete fat suppression of the major content.

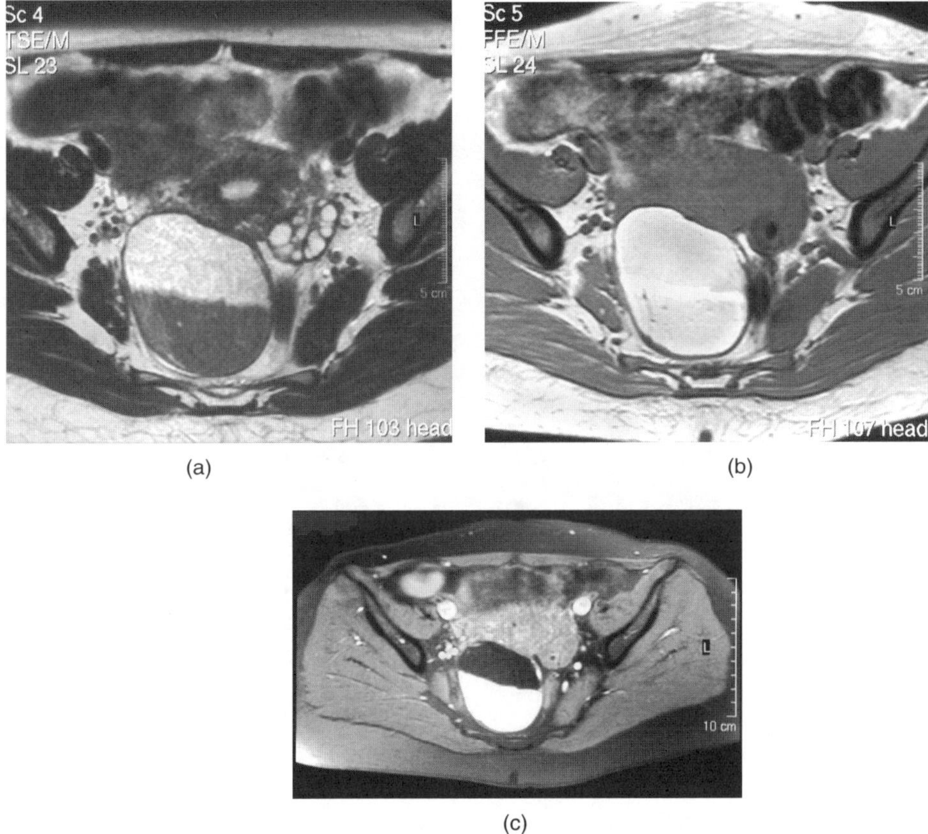

(a)   (b)

(c)

Figure 16.17   MR imaging of the dermoid mass shown by US in Figure 16.10 with complex and potentially confusing appearances (a) axial T2W image showing a fluid level with bright material above (fat) and dark material below (blood) and some tiny bright fatty elements within this which (b) show prominent chemical shift artefact on the axial T1W image on which both fat and blood are bright, their nature revealed by (c) the axial fat suppressed T1W image.

- Dermoid tumors can have protean appearances but the presence of even very small amounts of fat indicates the diagnosis.

- The presence of fat also results in the chemical shift artefact (Figs 16.16 and 16.17) and this can be helpful to identify very small fatty elements.

- Some dermoids contain no fat and there may be enhancing elements as skin appendages are very vascular. Such lesions can be misclassified as malignant.

- Malignant change within a dermoid tumor is very rare but should be suspected when there is a dominant solid component with wall thickening, breach or invasion of adjacent fat or other pelvic organs.

- The presence of non-suppressing T1 bright components in a dermoid cyst could be due to blood from prior torsion or proteinaceous fluid from glandular components (Fig. 16.17). However, the presence of fatty elements indicates that the lesion is a dermoid.

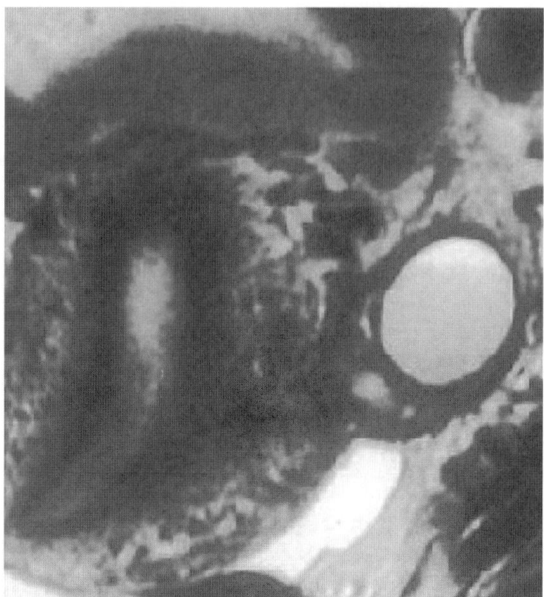

Figure 16.18 Axial T2W MR imaging showing 'shading' and faint fluid level due to sedimentation of chronic blood products in an endometrioma with adenomyosis evident in the uterus as widening of the junctional zone.

- A hemorrhagic cyst may present as T1 bright mass due to the presence of methemaglobin and as a dark lesion in T2 due to the presence of deoxyhemoglobin or hemosiderin.

  o Blood products of different ages are diagnostic of repeated bleeding, a feature of endometriosis and the uterus may show signs of adenomyosis (a junctional zone >12 mm) (Fig. 16.18).

  o Shading, a graded darkening in dependent portions, on T2W sequences results from sedimentation of blood products (Fig. 16.18).

  o In some cases there are frank fluid-fluid levels.

Complex cystic and cystic-solid or inhomogeneous solid masses

- These masses include:

  o Cystadenoma

  o Adenofibroma

  o Primary cancer

  o Metastasis

  o Lymphoma.

- The majority of these lesions are correctly defined by US.

- MRI should be performed when the US examination is not conclusive.

- Gadolinium enhanced T1-weighted imaging allows confident delineation of even very small vascularized mural and septal elements (Figs 16.14 and 16.19) which define the neoplastic nature of the mass.

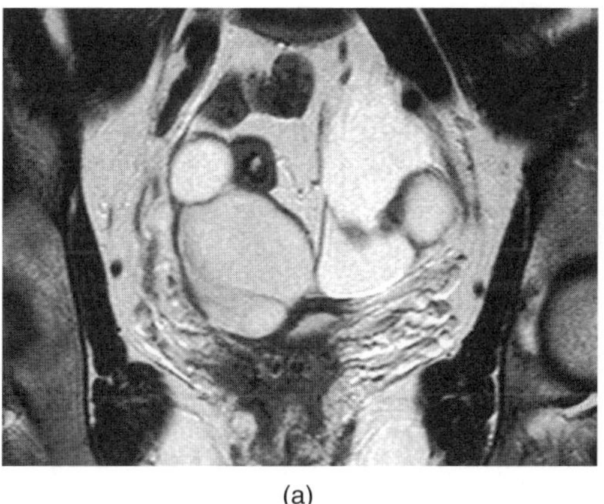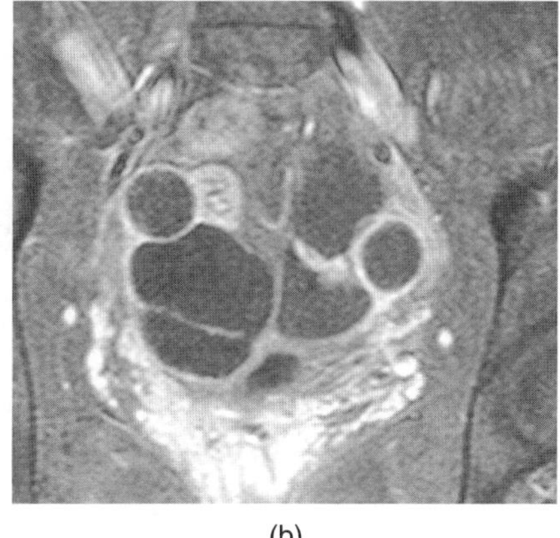

(a)   (b)

Figure 16.19   Coronal MR imaging of bilateral ovarian cystic lesions the right benign and the left a borderline malignancy of the ovary showing within it a single irregular septum on (a) T2W and (b) fat suppressed contrast-enhanced T1W images.

T2 dark adnexal masses

- These lesions include:

  - Fibroma/thecoma
  - Brenner tumor
  - Uterine fibroid
  - Metastasis.

- Oblique T2W sections help to determine if a lesion is attached to the uterus as in a pedunculated fibroid or separate as in an ovarian fibroma (Fig. 16.15).

- Most T2 dark solid adnexal masses have such low signal intensity as to be diagnostic of a fibroma or other benign stromal tumors such as Brenner tumor.

- Usually solid malignant masses which have intermediate or inhomogenous soft tissue signal intensity.

- A feature of larger solid lesions of all types is necrosis as they outgrow their blood supply. This feature should not be confused with a cystic nature.

- These T2 bright components are irregular and not bounded by septa as found in cysts.

- When there is uncertainty CET1W is able distinguish the nature of the mass by showing bright enhancement in malignant lesions.

- A mass with solid soft tissue elements which is enhancing and not attached to the uterus should be managed as a cancer, referred to a Cancer Centre for further management.

Key points

- Most T1 'bright' and non-enhancing T2 'dark' masses are benign and can be managed on the basis of symptoms.

- Most enhancing non-fatty cystic-solid or solid masses are malignant and need referral to a Cancer Centre.

- The presented MR imaging algorithm will characterize the vast majority of lesions and define their pattern of referral.

- For the few lesions which remain 'indeterminate', referral for specialist imaging or an opinion from a specialized oncology center should be considered.

16.8 Computed Tomography

Indications

- staging of suspected ovarian cancer (Tables 16.2 and 16.6)

- planning surgical options or image guided biopsy (Table 16.2)

- staging of metastatic gynecological cancer to monitor chemotherapy response

- imaging the acute abdomen in women with ovarian cancer

- CT is not indicated for assessment of the indeterminate adnexal mass as it is inferior to MRI and given that most masses prove to be benign imparts unnecessary ionizing radiation

- CT is also inferior to US in assessment of the nature of adnexal masses

- therefore incidental and indeterminate adnexal masses may be found on CT studies performed for other reasons require US assessment to enter the imaging algorithm (Table 16.2)

Technique

- The standard CT technique includes the abdomen and pelvis.

- Patient preparation requires the patient to drink oral contrast for bowel preparation

- 5 ml of Gastrografin in 200 ml of water 6 to 8 hr prior to examination to improve colonic opacification.

- The patient fasts for 4 h prior to the CT examination. On arrival in the CT department the patient is asked to drink slowly and steadily a further 1000 ml of 3% Gastrografin over the hour prior to examination with the final 200 ml of this taken immediately prior to the examination in order to distend and opacify the stomach and duodenum.

- A vaginal tampon may be used, when tolerated to define the vaginal vault.

- Intravenous contrast is routinely administered, typically 100 ml of a 300 mg iodine strength non-ionic agent at 3 ml/s using a pump injector.

- A helical examination technique using a maximum of 5 mm collimation is recommended.

- The image acquisition is timed to coincide with maximal portal venous enhancement beginning at 65 s and covers from the domes of the diaphragm to the lower border of the pubic symphysis.

Table 16.6 FIGO (International Federation of Gynecological Oncology) staging classification for ovarian cancer

Stage	Characteristics
I	Growth limited to the ovaries
Ia	Growth limited to one ovary; no malignant ascites; negative peritoneal cytology finding; no tumor on the external surface, capsule intact
Ib	Growth limited to both ovaries; no ascites; negative peritoneal cytology finding; no tumor on the external surface; capsule intact
Ic	Tumor either stage Ia or Ib, but with tumor on the surface of one or both ovaries; or with capsule ruptured; or with ascites present containing malignant cells; or with positive peritoneal washings
II	Growth involving one or both ovaries with pelvic extension
IIa	Extension or metastasis to the uterus, tubes or both
IIb	Extension to the pelvic tissues
IIc	Tumor either stage IIa or IIb, but with tumor on surface of one or both ovaries; or with capsule(s) ruptured; or with ascites present containing malignant cells; or with positive peritoneal washings
III	Tumor involving one or both ovaries with peritoneal implants outside the pelvis or a positive finding in retroperitoneal or inguinal glands; superficial liver metastases; tumor limited to the true pelvis but with histologically proven malignant extension to small bowel or omentum
IIIa	Tumor limited to the true pelvis, unaffected nodes but histologically confirmed microscopic seeding of abdominal peritoneal surfaces
IIIb	Tumor involving one or both ovaries with histologically confirmed implants on abdominal peritoneal surfaces, none exceeding 2 cm in diameter, nodes unaffected
IIIc	Abdominal implants greater than 2 cm in diameter or unaffected retroperitoneal or inguinal nodes
IV	Distant metastases; if pleural effusion is present there must be a positive cytology finding; parenchymal liver disease

- With the advent of multidetector CT it is possible to reconstruct high quality reformatted images in the coronal and sagittal plane and imaging parameters should be chosen to allow this.

- Additional scanning might be required following a delay of 30 min after further oral contrast or in decubitus positions in selected cases to allow distinction of unopacified bowel from pelvic, peritoneal or omental masses.

- The chest is only examined if:
  - pleural effusion, lung metastasis or mediastinal lymphadenopathy are evident on baseline chest radiography
  - suspected relapse when the abdomen and pelvis show no evidence of this.

- It is important to be aware of patients with renal impairment and to take measures to minimize contrast medium-induced nephrotoxicity (CIN). Patients at risk should receive a small dose of either non-ionic iso-osmolar dimeric or non-ionic low osmolar monomeric contrast medium and intravenous fluid. Intravenous infusion (1 ml/kg body weight/h) of 0.9% saline starting 4 h before contrast injection and continuing for at least 12 h afterwards is effective in reducing the incidence of CIN.

- For examination of the acute abdomen the technique may be modified.

  - Patients with established small bowel obstruction do not require oral contrast.

  - For patients with suspected subacute obstruction oral contrast is encouraged as passage into the large bowel may indicate the degree of obstruction (three aliquots of 5 ml of Gastrografin in 200 ml of water taken over a 24 h period prior to CT examination).

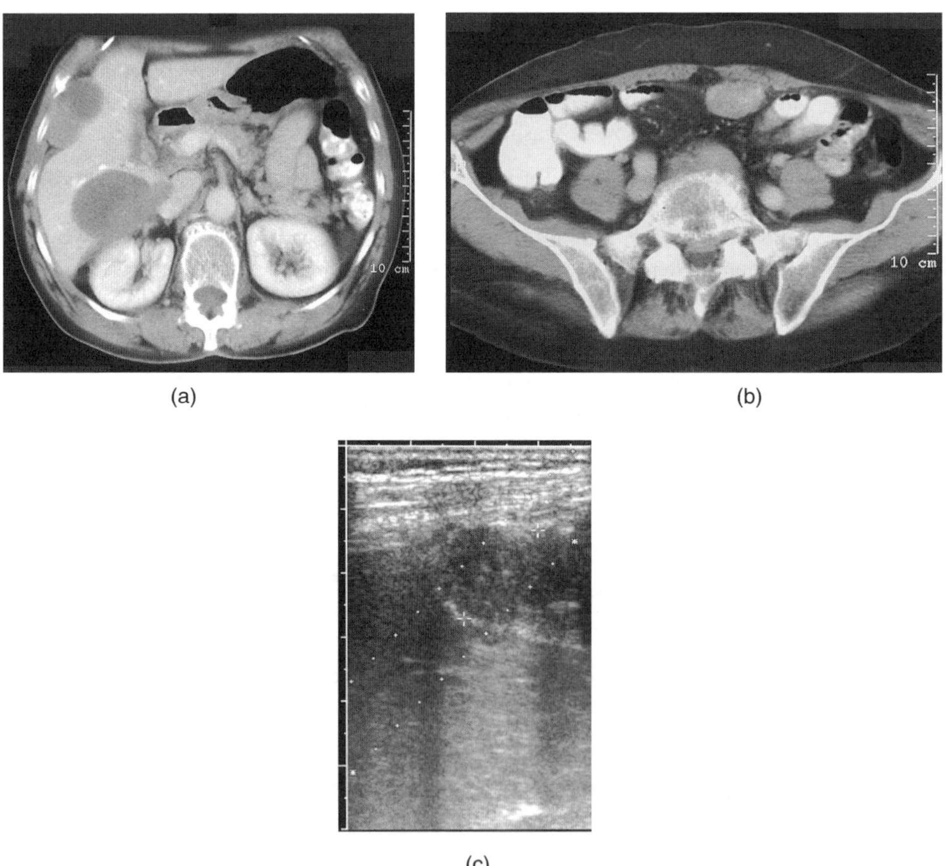

(a) (b)

(c)

Figure 16.20 (a) Staging CT of newly diagnosed ovarian mass showing surface metastases scalloping the surface of the liver, (b) CT of the mid-abdomen showing one of several omental masses and (c) localizing US image prior to cutting needle biopsy. Biopsy showed granulosa cell cancer of the ovary.

The goals of CT at diagnosis are:

- detection of the sites and extent of metastatic spread

- indication of when disease bulk and spread is beyond effective cytoreductive surgery (Fig. 16.20)

- indication of when ovarian disease may result of metastasis from another primary tumor

- planning image guided biopsy to achieve a histological diagnosis (Fig. 16.20).

The goals of CT in the treated patient are:

- recognition of disease complications

- monitoring treatment response

- evaluation of the residual mass

- confirmation of remission/assessment of suspected relapse.

CT features of ovarian cancer

- The primary malignant ovarian tumor/s

  - a cystic mass with a solid mural nodule
  - circumferential mural thickening and irregularity
  - multilocularity with differing cyst contents
  - multiple irregular internal solid elements
  - a predominantly solid mass with areas of necrosis
  - calcifications and contrast enhancement may be present in the cyst wall or within solid tumor components
  - apart from detection of calcifications and fat CT is inferior to both US and MRI in determining internal structure of the ovarian lesion.

Metastases to the ovaries

- May be indistinguishable from that of primary ovarian cancer. Both may produce bilateral masses.

- The stomach, colon, appendix and pancreas should be inspected as potential primary cancer sites within the abdomen.

The metastatic spread (Table 16.6)

- Metastatic spread via:

  - The peritoneal cavity
    - Usually leads to the development of ascites.

- Detection of peritoneal seedlings is easier in the presence of ascites.
- CT can detect the calcified tumor implants containing psammoma bodies from serous cystadenocarcinoma of the ovary even in the absence of ascites. Conversely densely calcified tumor implants from serous tumors may be mistaken for bowel containing oral contrast.
- CT can detect 50% of implants that are 5 mm or more in size.

  - Lymphatics, affecting the pelvic and para-aortic lymph nodes.
  - Hematogenous spread to the liver (stage IV).
  - Spread to the pleura with effusion (stage IV).

- Direct invasion of adjacent structures (stage II).

  - small and large bowel
  - the pelvic sidewall
  - the iliac veins leading to thrombosis
  - the pelvic ureter leading to hydronephrosis. Hydronephrosis is, however, more commonly due to simple mass effect upon the pelvic ureter.

- Metastatic spread to the abdomen (stage III) may manifest as

  - Peritoneal and mesenteric masses and omental cakes (Fig. 16.20).
  - Pelvic or retroperitoneal lymphadenopathy.
  - Involvement of the surface of the liver (Fig. 16.20) and spleen (parenchymal deposits within the liver upstage the patient to stage IV).
  - Spread to the pleura or mediastinal/neck nodes is also stage IV disease.

CT features of other adnexal masses

- CT is not indicated for assessment of the indeterminate adnexal mass as it is inferior to MRI and given that most masses prove to be benign imparts unnecessary ionizing radiation.

- Incidental complex adnexal masses may be found on CT studies performed for other reasons and may require US/MRI assessment.

- Benign incidental lesions which can be confidently diagnosed by CT include a simple cyst and a mature teratoma by virtue of its fat content and mature calcifications, classically representing dental elements.

- acute tubo-ovarian sepsis may mimic appendicitis and diverticulitis and thus be discovered on emergency CT examinations.

Image-guided biopsy (IGB)

IGB using CT or US guidance is a valuable and useful alternative to laparoscopy or exploratory surgery in the following circumstances:

- In women believed to have ovarian cancer but with poor performance status or with advanced disease believed beyond the scope of primary cytoreductive surgery (Fig. 16.19).

- In women with a history of cancer whose metastases may mimic ovarian cancer (e.g. breast, GI tract, melanoma).

- When there is diagnostic uncertainty, e.g. unusual imaging patterns of disease such as peritoneal carcinomatosis with bilateral solid ovarian masses or non-enlarged ovaries or with an unusual tumor marker profile.

- In a woman with undiagnosed peritoneal carcinomatosis biopsy findings can focus the search for the primary tumor when appropriate, e.g. to the bowel when mucinous carcinoma is found.

- IGB may have a role in determining if pelvic masses represent recurrence of gynecological cancer, e.g. a long interval since the primary diagnosis.

CT of gynecological emergencies

Gynecological masses may present as an acute abdomen with no specific gynecological symptoms. The symptoms could be due to torsion or hemorrhage of an ovarian mass, spread of infection from an inflammatory tubo-ovarian mass or to a secondary effect such as bowel obstruction. The principal differential diagnoses include acute appendicitis, diverticulitis or bowel obstruction/ischemia from other causes. With pelvic inflammatory disease (PID) and other complex gynecological infections CT may show

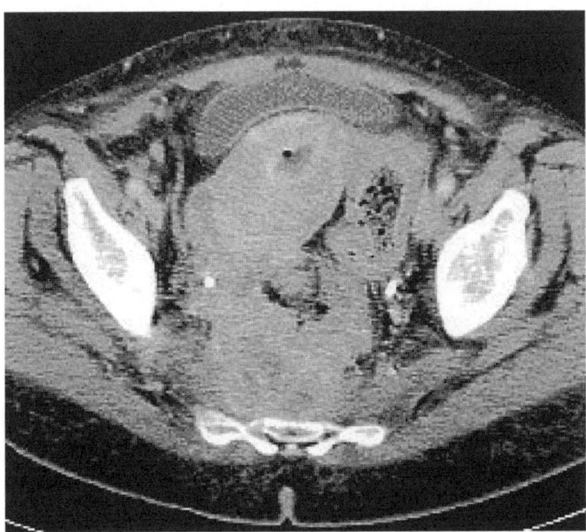

Figure 16.21 Complicated pelvic inflammatory disease in a woman with acute pelvic pain and lower gastrointestinal symptoms. CT shows a diffuse pelvic process infiltrating most of the visible organs but with gas and fluid in the gynecological apparatus, notably the left adnexa. The diagnosis was actinomycosis in a woman with recent removal of an intrauterine contraceptive device.

- complex adnexal masses

- fluid collections

- gonadal vein thrombosis

- hydronephrosis

- features of peritonitis (Fig. 16.21).

References

Hricak H, Chen M, Coakley FV *et al.* (2000) Complex adnexal masses: detection and characterization with MR imaging – multivariate analysis. *Radiology* **214**: 39–46.

Kurtz AB, Tsimikas JV, Tempany CMC *et al.* Diagnosis and staging of ovarian cancer: comparative values of Doppler and conventional US, CT, and MR imaging correlated with surgery and histopathologic analysis – report of the Radiology Diagnostic Oncology Group. *Radiology* 1999; **212**: 19–27.

Meyer JI, Kennedy AW, Friedman R, Ayoub A, Zepp RC (1995) Ovarian carcinoma: value of CT in predicting success of debulking surgery. *AJR* **165**: 875–878.

Sohaib SA, Mills TD, Sahdev A *et al.* (2005) The role of magnetic resonance imaging and ultrasound in women with adnexal masses. *Clin. Radiol.* **60**: 340–348.

Spencer JA, Swift SE, Wilkinson N *et al.* (2001) Peritoneal carcinomatosis: image guided peritoneal core biopsy for tumor type and patient management. *Radiology* **221**: 173–177.

Tempany CMC, Zou KH, Silverman SG *et al.* (2000) Staging of advanced ovarian cancer: comparison of imaging modalities – report from the radiological diagnostic oncology group. *Radiology* **215**: 761–767.

17
Imaging of Abnormal Uterine Bleeding

Patricia Noël[1], Evis Sala[2] and Caroline Reinhold[3]

[1]Department of Radiology, Université Laval, Québec, Canada
[2]University Department of Radiology, Addenbrooke's Hospital, Cambridge
[3]Department of Radiology, McGill University Health Center, Montreal and Medical Director, Oncology, Synarc Inc., San Francisco, CA

17.1 Abnormal uterine bleeding

Abnormal uterine bleeding (AUB) is a frequent clinical complaint, accounting for 20% of gynecologic visits and two-thirds of hysterectomies. It can affect pre-, peri- and post-menopausal women. In pre-menopausal women, AUB is defined as substantial change in frequency, duration or amount of bleeding during or between menstruations. The most likely cause in this group is dysfunctional anovulatory bleeding (40%). Other causes are pregnancy-related events, disorders of coagulation, and uterine masses, including endometrial polyps, fibroids, adenomyosis and rarely, endometrial hyperplasia and carcinoma. In post-menopausal women, any vaginal bleeding occurring at least 6 months after complete cessation of menses is abnormal unless they are receiving hormone replacement therapy (HRT). Non-cyclic vaginal bleeding in women who are receiving HRT is also abnormal. Endometrial atrophy accounts for most cases (60–80%) of post-menopausal bleeding (PMB), whereas endometrial carcinoma occurs in 10% of patients presenting with PMB. The role of the physician in this group is to exclude endometrial carcinoma and to identify a source of bleeding that can be treated.

Transvaginal ultrasound (TVS) is the imaging modality of choice for the evaluation of endometrial pathology in women presenting with PMB. Endometrial thickness at TVS should be evaluated in mid-sagittal plane measuring the thickest portion of the endometrium,

Urogenital Imaging: A Problem-oriented Approach   Edited by Sameh K. Morcos and Henrik S. Thomsen
© 2009 John Wiley & Sons, Ltd

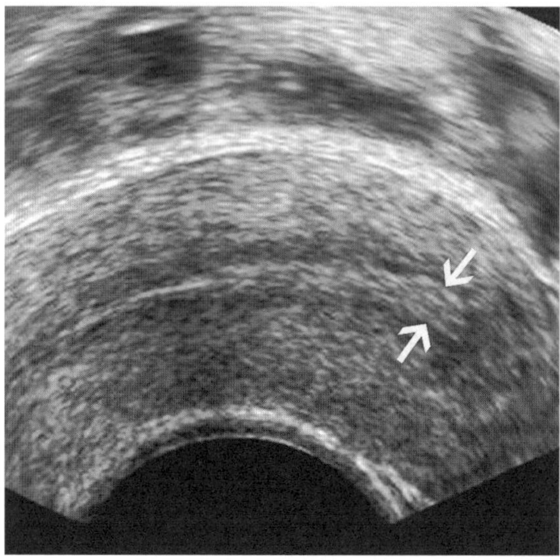

Figure 17.1   TVS demonstrating normal appearances to the endometrium. Endometrial thickness (arrows) on endovaginal ultrasound is measured on the mid-sagittal plane, on the thickest portion of the hyperechoic endometrium, excluding the hypoechoic inner myometrium. Both endometrial leaflets are measured (basalis to basalis layer) excluding endometrial fluid.

excluding fluid within the endometrial cavity and the hypoechoic inner myometrium (Figure 17.1). TVS has a sensitivity of 96% for detecting endometrial cancer using a threshold value of greater than 5 mm in non-HRT users and 8 mm in HRT users. Women who meet these thresholds should be referred for endometrial biopsy. Pre-menopausal women presenting with AUB are referred for endometrial biopsy if endometrial thickness is more than 16 mm during secretory phase, or more than 8 mm during proliferative phase. TVS, sonohysterography and MRI are also used in evaluation of other causes of AUB such as adenomyosis, leiomyomas, endometrial polyps and endometrial hyperplasia.

17.2 Adenomyosis

Clinical features

- Common gynecological disorder.

- Affects women during reproductive and perimenopausal years (in 5th and 6th decades).

- Menorrhagia is the most frequently encountered symptom (50% of patients).

- May present with pelvic pain, metrorrhagia and dysmenorrhea of increasing severity.

- On physical examination the uterus is enlarged, soft and tender.

- Uterine sparing treatment: GnRH analog therapy, endometrial ablation, myometrial excision, uterine artery embolization.

- Definitive treatment: Hysterectomy.

Pathology

- Defined as presence of ectopic endometrial glands and stroma embedded within the myometrium with adjacent myometrial hyperplasia.

- Predominance of endometrial zona basalis (refractive to cyclical hormonal milieu, no cyclical bleeding).

- Can be diffuse or focal, superficial (inner myometrium) or deep (mid and outer myometrium).

- Present in 20–60% of hysterectomy specimen.

Imaging

TVS

- Initial imaging modality

- Real-time examination

- Poorly marginated, heterogeneous, hypoechoic areas in myometrium, with or without myometrial cysts (Figure 17.2)

- Fine, linear areas of attenuation producing "rain shower" appearances

- Widening and poor definition of endometrial-myometrial junction

- Echogenic finger-like projections or linear striations extending from endometrium to myometrium

- Lack of contour abnormalities or mass effect, ill-defined margins between normal and abnormal myometrium, elliptical shape of myometrial abnormality

- Color Doppler: increased vascularity, no large peripheral vessels

- Accuracy of TVS diagnosis: 68–86%

MRI

- T1WI

  o High signal intensity (SI) foci (hemorrhage or endometrial tissue)

- T2WI

  o Thickening of low SI junctional zone (JZ), symmetric or asymmetric

    ▪ JZ $\geq$ 12 mm: Highly predictive

    ▪ JZ $\leq$ 8 mm: Diagnosis essentially excluded

    ▪ JZ between 8 and 12 mm: Indeterminate, look for ancillary findings

  o Ancillary criteria

    ▪ Ill-defined JZ

    ▪ Poorly defined low SI myometrial mass

    ▪ High SI foci within JZ

    ▪ Linear high SI striations (finger-like) radiating out from endometrium

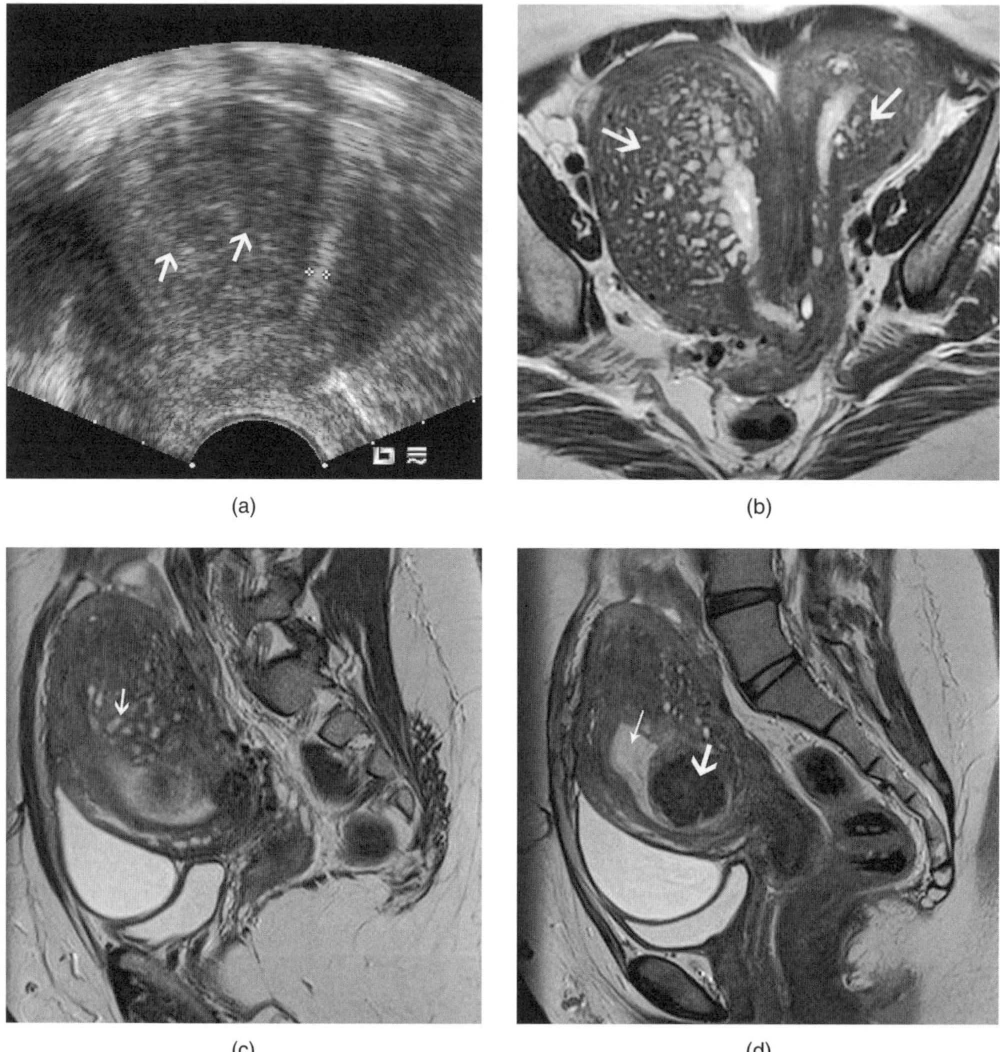

Figure 17.2 Adenomyosis. Longitudinal TVS (a) shows an enlarged uterus, with heterogeneous myometrium and fine, linear areas of attenuation (arrows) in a patient with adenomyosis. Endometrium is noted between calipers. Axial T2W MRI (b) shows a dydelphis uterus with ill defined asymmetric thickening of junctional zone (arrows). There are high signal intensity striations radiating out from endometrium into myometrium and multiple foci of high SI in keeping with endometrial glands. These findings are consistent with diffuse adenomyosis. Sagittal T2W MRI (c) in another patient shows focal adenomyosis with focal thickening of junctional zone involving dorsal aspect of uterus with multiple foci of high SI (arrow). Sagittal T2WI MRI (d) of the same patient as previous also shows a hypointense submucosal leiomyoma (thick arrow) as well as thickening of endometrium (thin arrow) which was due to endometrial hyperplasia at surgery.

- T1WI C+

  - Early-phase perfusion anomalies

  - Swiss-cheese appearance: Signal void of dilated glands

- Accuracy of MRI diagnosis: 85–90%

- Sagittal T2WI images to best depict uterine junctional zone

- During menstrual/periovulatory phases, uterine peristalsis may cause pseudothickening of JZ: Cine MRI may be used to assess peristalsis.

17.3 Leiomyomas

Clinical features

- Most common tumor of female genital tract: 20–30% of women >30 y.o.

- Most commonly asymptomatic.

- If symptoms occur, AUB is most common symptom, in pre- and post-menopausal women.

- Other signs and symptoms: pressure-effect, pain, infertility, palpable mass.

- Torsion or infection are rare occurrences, presenting with acute abdominal pain.

- Treatment: depends on location

  - Hysteroscopic resection in submucosal

  - Uterine artery embolization

  - Myomectomy

  - Thermo-ablative techniques

  - Hysterectomy.

Pathology

- Well-defined, pseudoencapsulated mass.

- Composed of smooth muscle cells arranged in a whorl-like pattern with variable amount of collagen, extracellular matrix and fibrous tissue.

- Classified according to location within uterine corpus:

  - Intramural (most common)

  - Submucosal (most likely to bleed)

  - Subserosal (most likely to cause pressure effect).

- Submucosal leiomyomas are the most likely to bleed, followed by intramural ones.

- May involve uterine cervix, broad ligament or detach from genital tract and parasitize.

- Estrogen stimulated: increase in size during pregnancy.

- Progesterone inhibited: decrease in size after menopause.

- Types of degeneration: calcific, hemorrhagic, hyaline, cystic, myxoid, sarcomatous.

Imaging

TVS

- Initial modality of choice.
- Homogeneous attenuating hypoechoic mass.
- When submucosal, continuous with myometrium, covered by thin echogenic endometrial line, often broad based (Figure 17.3).
- May show calcification or be hyper- or anechoic if degeneration present.
- Color Doppler: marked peripheral flow, decreased central flow
  - When submucosal, usually multiple vascular pedicles.
- Limitations of TVS: Limited field-of-view, patient's body habitus, distorted anatomy.
- Transabdominal scanning is necessary with multiple large leiomyomas.

Sonohysterography

- Submucosal leiomyoma presents as a mass indenting endometrial cavity.
- Intraluminal extension.
- Better visualization of covering hyperechoic endometrial stripe (Figure 17.4).
- Shows continuity with myometrium.
- Diffuse or peripheral vascularity.
- Multiple vascular pedicles.
- Useful for surgical planning: >50% of mass must be intraluminal to beneficiate from hysteroscopic removal.

MRI

- T1WI
  - Intermediate signal intensity (SI) mass
  - May be low to high SI if degenerated.
- T2WI
  - Sharply marginated low SI mass (relative to adjacent myometrium)
  - Frequently surrounded by high SI rim
  - Orthogonal views allow precise evaluation of leiomyoma location.
- T1WI C+
  - Variable enhancement
  - Non-enhancing areas if degeneration is present.
- Imaging characteristics vary with types of degeneration
  - Hemorrhagic: High SI T1WI with fat saturation, no enhancement

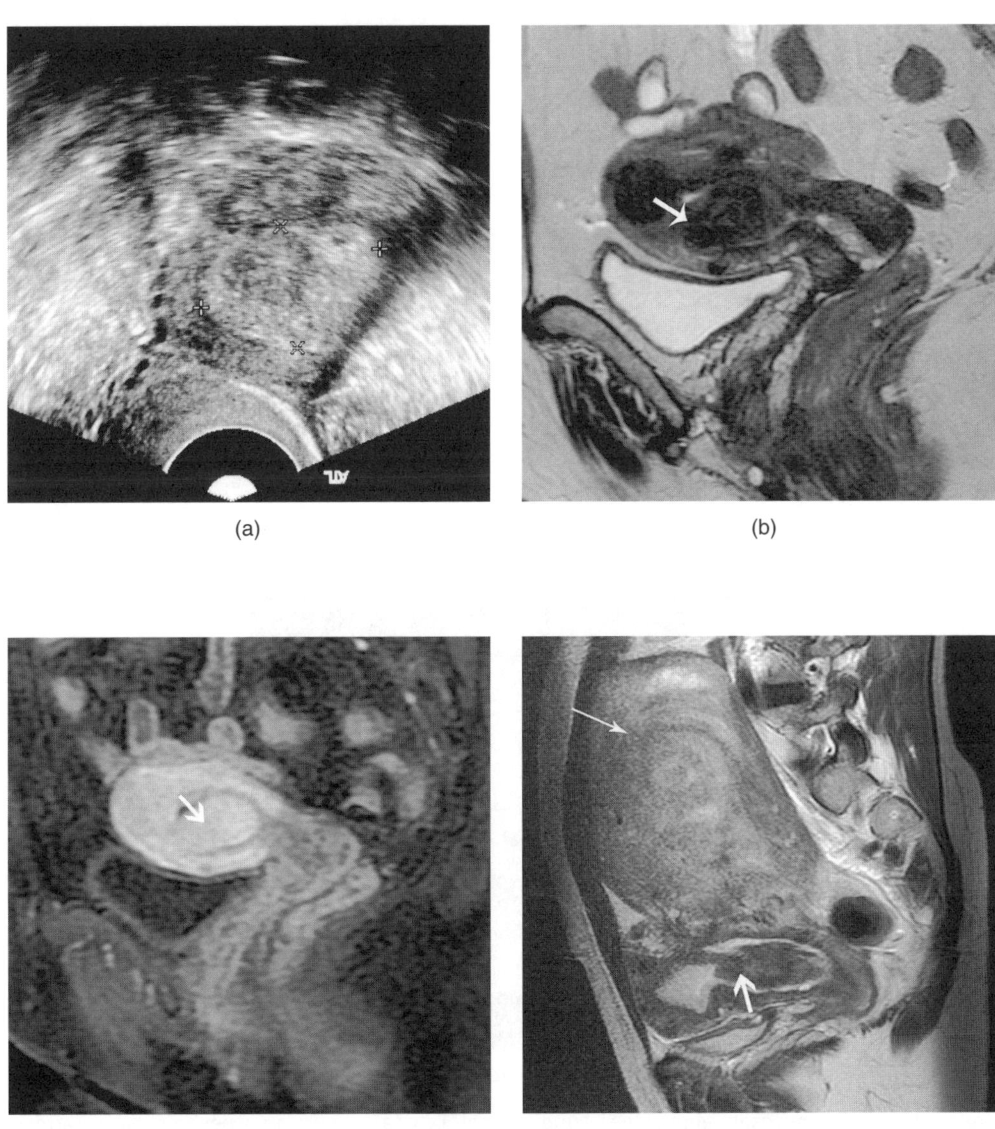

Figure 17.3 Submucosal leiomyoma. Longitudinal TVS (a) shows a hyperechoic mass (calipers) distending the endometrial cavity. Sagittal T2W MRI (b) in the same patient shows multiple leiomyomas. The mass noted at TVS shows low SI and it is continuous with the myometrium (arrows). More then 50% of the surface of the mass is in contact with the endometrium indicative of a submucosal leiomyoma. Sagittal T1W FS C+ MRI (c) confirms avid enhancement of the mass (arrows) similar to the adjacent myometrium. Sagittal T2W MRI (d) in a different patient demonstrates a submucosal leiomyoma as a pedunculated low SI intra-cavitary mass (thick arrow). Also note the presence of another large subserosal leiomyoma arising from the dorsal myometrium (thin arrow).

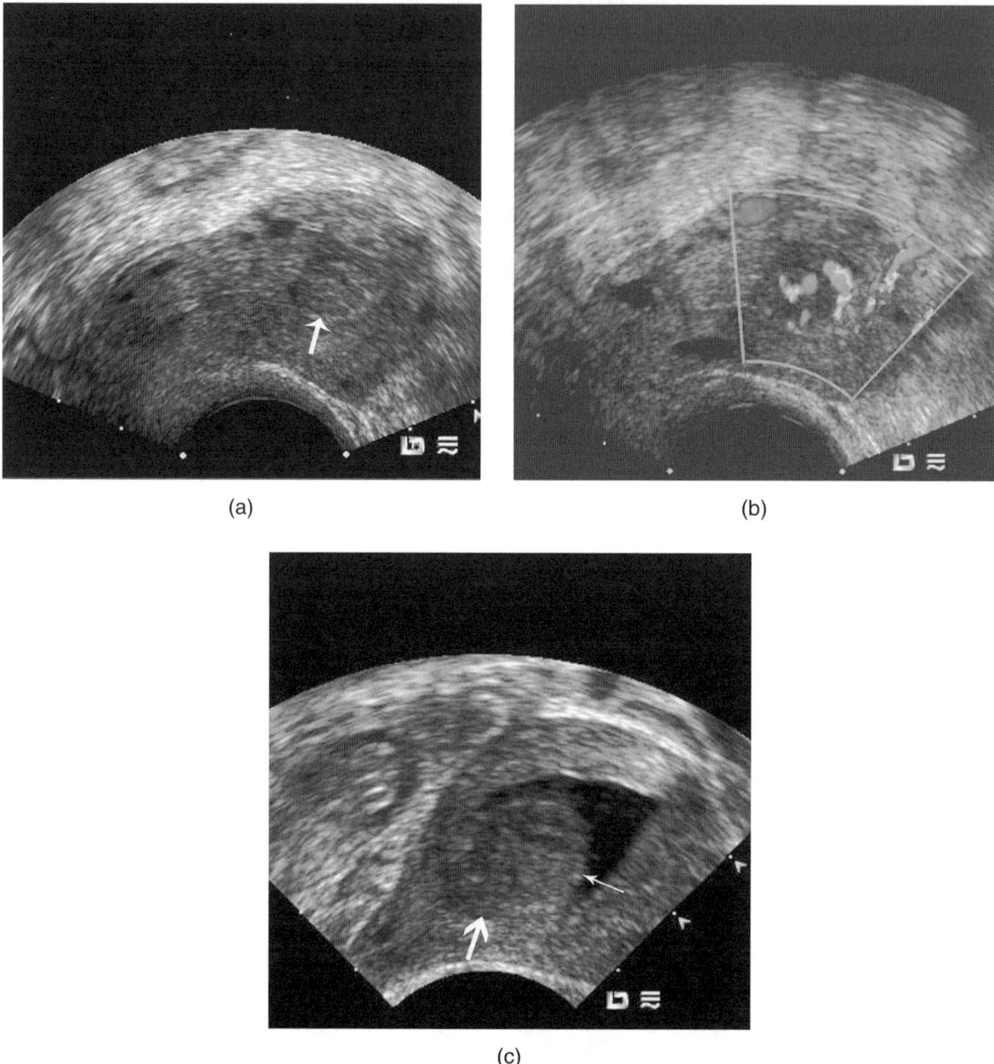

Figure 17.4   Submucosal leiomyoma. Longitudinal TVS (a) shows an isoechoic mass (arrow) distending the endometrial cavity. Longitudinal TVS (b) with color Doppler shows diffuse vascularity with several vascular pedicles connecting it to the myometrium. Longitudinal sonohysterography (c) shows continuity of the mass with myometrium (thick arrow) and thin covering hyperechoic endometrium (thin arrow).

    ○ Hyaline: Low SI T1WI and T2WI

    ○ Cystic: Low SI T1WI, high SI T2WI.

- MRI is the most accurate modality to diagnose leiomyomas: Precise delineation of size, number and location.

- MRI may confirm uterine origin of an indeterminate adnexal mass: look for splaying of uterine serosa or myometrium, bridging vessels originating from myometrium.

17.4 Endometrial polyp

Clinical features

- Most common cause of endometrial thickening, more frequent than endometrial hyperplasia and carcinoma.

- Incidence higher in post-menopausal women treated with tamoxifen.

- Usually asymptomatic.

- When symptomatic: AUB is the most frequent symptom, secondary to ulceration and necrosis.

- Polyps should be removed in post-menopausal women because of risk of malignancy.

Pathology

- Broad-based or pedunculated endometrial mass with thin or thick stalk.

- Composed of focal glandular and stromal hyperplasia covered by endometrium.

- May occur in isolation or with endometrial hyperplasia or carcinoma.

- Multiple in 20% of cases.

- May also involve cervix.

Imaging

TVS

- May present as non-specific focal endometrial thickening.

- Pedunculated intraluminal echogenic endometrial mass (Figure 17.5).

- Separate, intact overlying endometrial stripe.

- Subendometrial hypoechoic halo intact.

- May contain small, anechoic cysts.

- Color Doppler shows single feeding vessel in stalk.

- Sensitivity 56–96%, specificity 82%.

Sonohysterography

- More precise than TVS.

- Same imaging criteria as TVS, but polyp is better outlined with fluid distension of endometrial cavity.

MRI

- T1WI

  - Intermediate SI, isointense to endometrium.

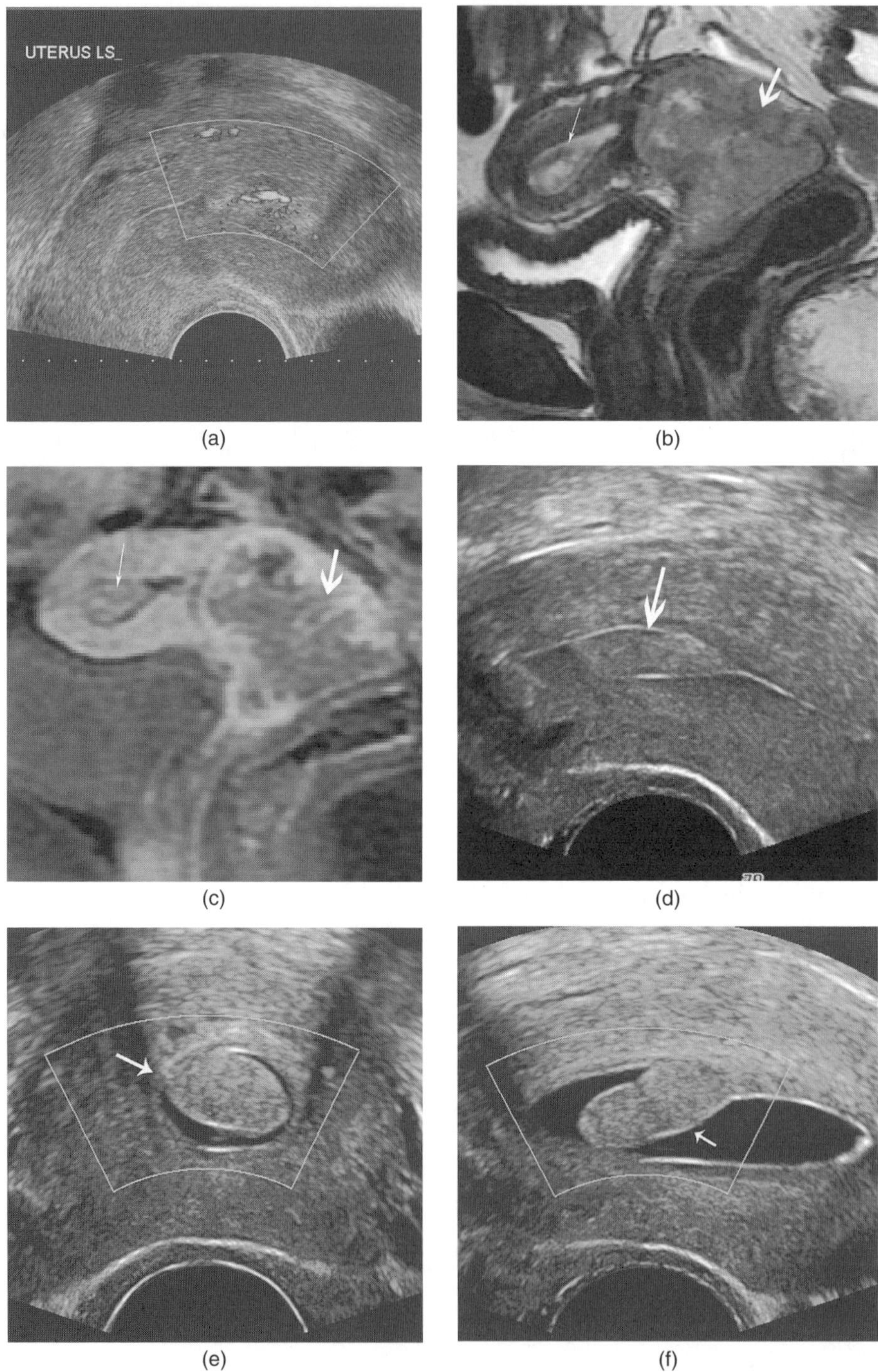

(a)   (b)

(c)   (d)

(e)   (f)

- T2WI

  - Slightly hypo- to isointense to normal endometrium
  - May show heterogeneous signal if high SI cystic changes
  - Low SI central fibrous core or stalk.

- T1WI C+

  - Variable enhancement
  - Early enhancement of small lesions: higher than the adjacent endometrium
  - Delayed hypointensity relative to endometrium.

17.5 Endometrial hyperplasia

Clinical features

- Typically presents with abnormal uterine bleeding.

- Common sequela of unopposed estrogen or sequential estrogen-progesteron hormone replacement therapy in post-menopausal women.

- Less commonly seen in pre-menopausal women, in association with polycystic ovary disease, obesity and persistent anovulatory cycles.

- May be encountered with estrogen producing tumors (granulosa cell tumors, thecomas).

- Simple and complex hyperplasia is treated with progesterone therapy with follow-up endovaginal sonogram and/or endometrial sampling. Continuous combined hormone replacement therapy may reverse hyperplasia.

- Atypical hyperplasia is treated with curettage or simple hysterectomy.

Pathology

- Local hyperestradiolemia considered main factor of development of hyperplastic lesions in the endometrium.

Figure 17.5 Endometrial polyp. Longitudinal Doppler TVS (a) demonstrating a hyperechoic endometrial lesion. Note the presence of a vascular pedicle highly suggestive of a polyp. Hysteroscopy confirmed the presence of an endometrial polyp. Sagittal T2W MRI (b) in a different patient referred for staging of cervical carcinoma (thick arrow). Note presence of a second lesion (thin arrow) in the endometrial cavity which shows heterogeneous SI with a low SI fibrous core. Sagittal T1W FS C+ MRI (c) shows homogeneous enhancement of the endometrial lesion (thin arrow) and heterogeneous enhancement of the cervical mass (thick arrow). Histopathology confirmed the presence of an endometrial polyp and cervical carcinoma. Longitudinal TVS (d) shows a slightly hyperechoic endometrial lesion (arrow). Transverse sonohysterography (e) with color Doppler shows a single vascular pedicle connecting the lesion to the myometrium (arrow). Longitudinal sonohysterography (f) in the same patient as previous shows a pedunculated intraluminal echogenic endometrial mass covered by endometrial stripe (arrow). Histology confirmed an endometrial polyp. (Figures 5d, e and f are courtesy of Dr Deborah Levine, md).

- Excessive proliferation of endometrial glands with increased ratio of glands to stroma.
- Three categories
  - Simple hyperplasia without atypia: cystically dilated glands with increased interglandular stroma
  - Complex hyperplasia: crowded and irregularly branched glands with minimal stroma
  - Atypical hyperplasia (intraendometrial neoplasia): atypical epithelial cells with high malignancy risk: 25–33% malignant degeneration.

Imaging

Non specific imaging appearance, overlaps with other endometrial disorders.

TVS

- Diffusely thickened, echogenic, homogeneous endometrium, although focal endometrial thickening has been reported (Figure 17.6).
- Anechoic cystic foci may be present.
- Heterogeneity may be seen with atypical hyperplasia.
- Color Doppler: several feeding vessels, diffuse vascularity.

Sonohysterography

- Same imaging appearance as on TVS.
- May direct biopsy by clearly delineating focal areas of thickening.

MRI

- T1WI
  - Isointense to myometrium.
- T2WI
  - Diffuse or focal thickening of endometrial complex
  - Iso- to slightly hypointense to normal endometrium
  - Endometrial-myometrial interface is well defined
  - Small hyperintense foci when cystic changes present.
- T1WI C+
  - Hypoenhancing compared with myometrium on early post-contrast images
  - Iso- to hyperenhancing on delayed contrast images
  - No enhancement in small cystic foci.
- Limited usage: should be used when TVS indeterminate and hysteroscopy and endometrial sampling are not possible.

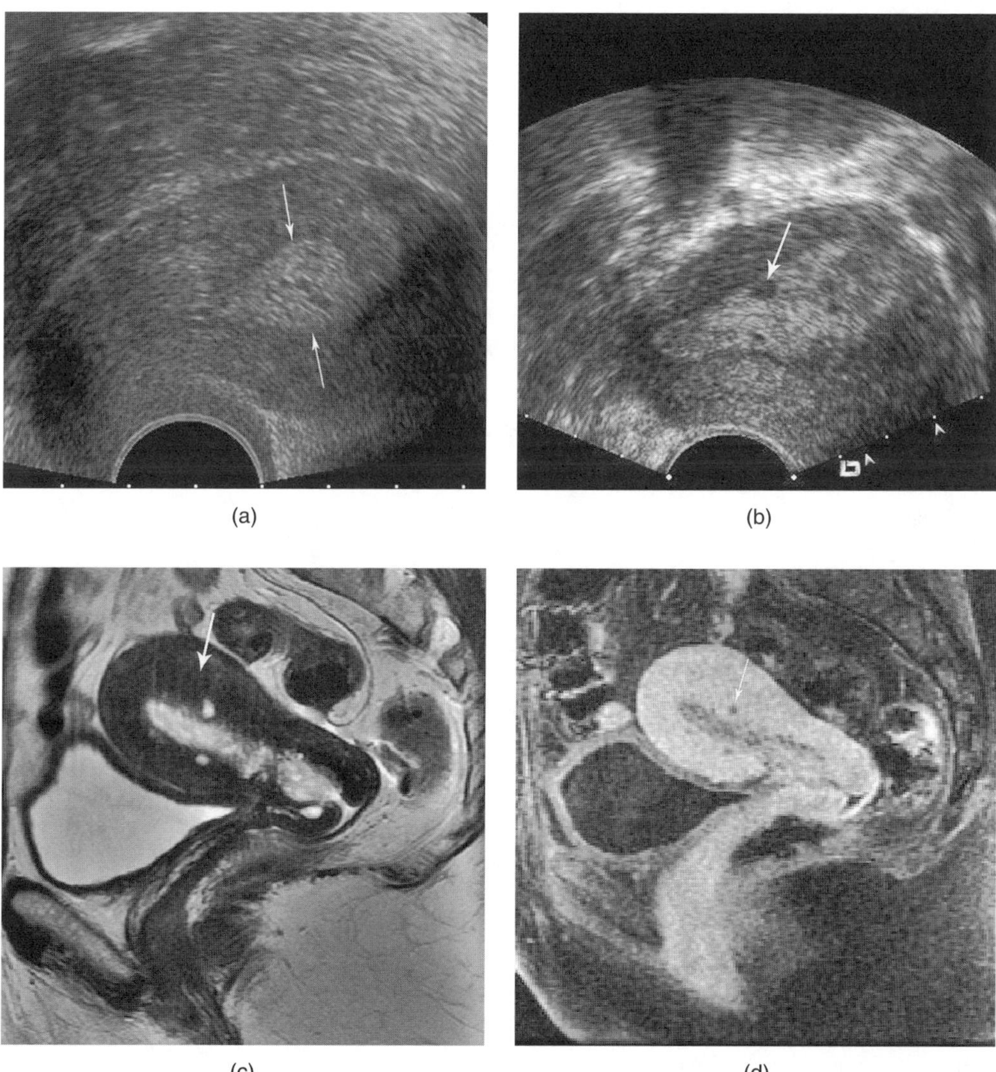

Figure 17.6 Endometrial hyperplasia. Longitudinal TVS image (a) demonstrating non specific thickening of endometrium (thin arrows). Histology confirmed endometrial hyperplasia. Longitudinal TVS image (b) demonstrates heterogeneous thickening of endometrium with hypoechoic foci (arrow) in a patient with atypical endometrial hyperplasia. Sagittal T2W MR image (c) shows a thickened heterogeneous endometrium with hyperintense cystic foci. Cystic glandular hyperplasia was found at biopsy. Also note the presence of a diffusely thickened low SI junctional zone (arrows) consistent with diffuse adenomyosis. Subendometrial hyperintense foci are also present in keeping with adenomyosis. Sagittal T1W FS C+ MRI (d) shows heterogeneous hypoenhancement of the endometrium compared with myometrium, with absence of enhancement of the subendometrial cysts (arrow).

17.6 Endometrial carcinoma

Clinical features

- Most common malignancy of the female genital tract.

- Peak age at diagnosis is 55–65 years.

- Most commonly (>75%) presents with post-menopausal or intermenstrual bleeding.

- 10% of patients presenting with post-menopausal abnormal uterine bleeding will have endometrial carcinoma.

- 2% of pre-menopausal patients presenting with AUB will have endometrial carcinoma, with increasing incidence after the age of 40 years old.

- Risk factors: nulliparity, unopposed estrogen therapy, adenomatous endometrial hyperplasia, PCOS, diabetes mellitus, hypertension, obesity, tamoxifen.

Pathology

- 90% are adenocarcinomas.

- Other subtypes include squamous, papillary and clear cell carcinomas.

- Histological subtype is a strong prognostic indicator, as well as FIGO staging.

Imaging

TVS

- May mimic benign endometrial lesions.

- Focal or diffuse endometrial thickening, homogeneous or heterogeneous.

- Heterogeneous mass-like lesion (Figure 17.7).

- Irregular borders, or disruption of subendometrial halo suggests malignancy.

- Irregular endometrium myometrium interface.

- Color Doppler: several feeding vessels, moderate vascularity.

Sonohysterography

- Irregular broad-based mass.

- Poor distensibility of uterine cavity.

MRI

- Focal or diffuse thickening of endometrial complex.

- T1WI

  o Hypo- to isointense to endometrium.

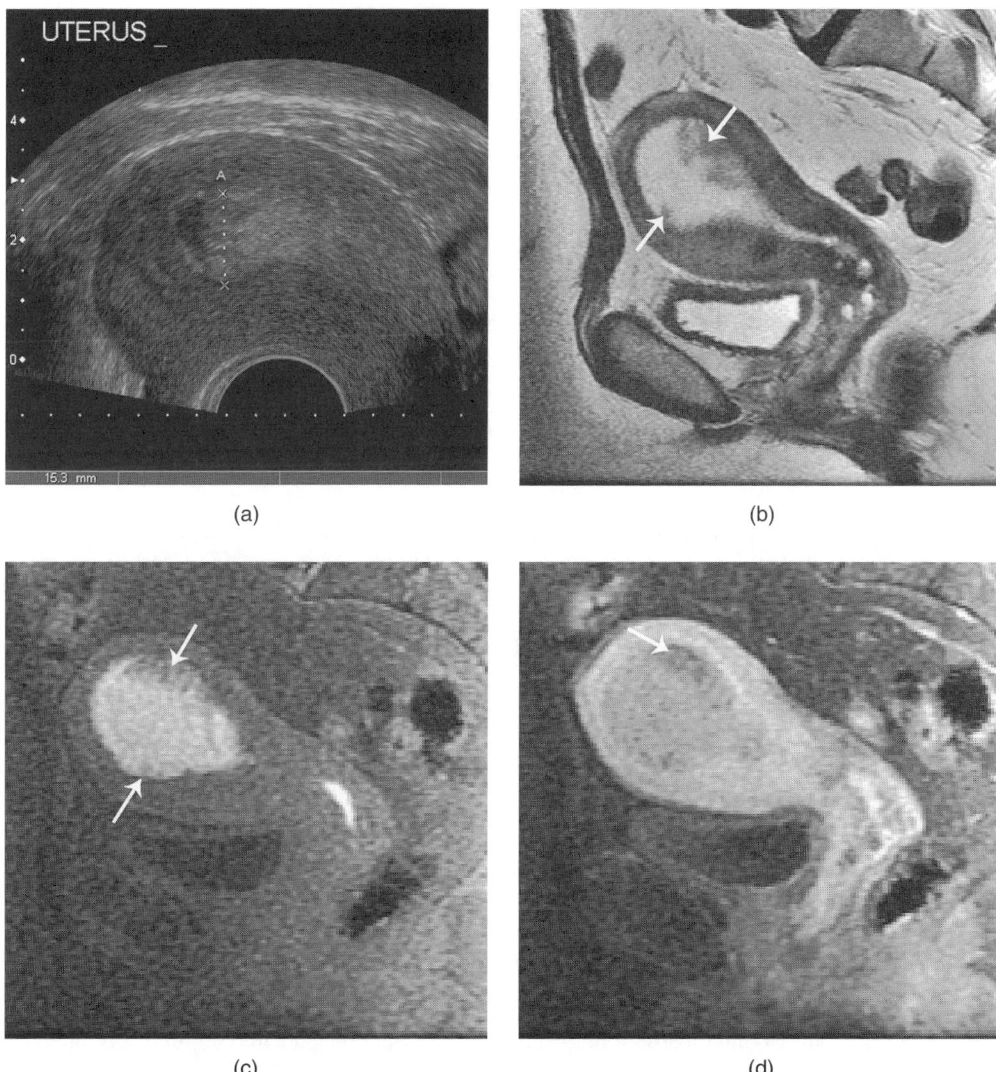

Figure 17.7 Endometrial carcinoma. Longitudinal TVS (a) in a patient presenting with PMB shows a thickened, heterogeneous endometrium (calipers) proved to be endometrial carcinoma at histopathology. Sagittal T2W MRI (b) in a different patient shows a fluid distended endometrial cavity with intermediate SI polypoid multifocal endometrial-based masses (arrows). Sagittal T1W MRI FS (c) shows high signal intensity fluid within endometrial cavity consistent with blood and multiple endometrial lesions isointense to myometrium (arrows). On sagittal T1W FS C+ MRI (d) the endometrial masses enhance less (arrow) than the adjacent myometrium. Clear cell endometrial carcinoma was found at histopathology.

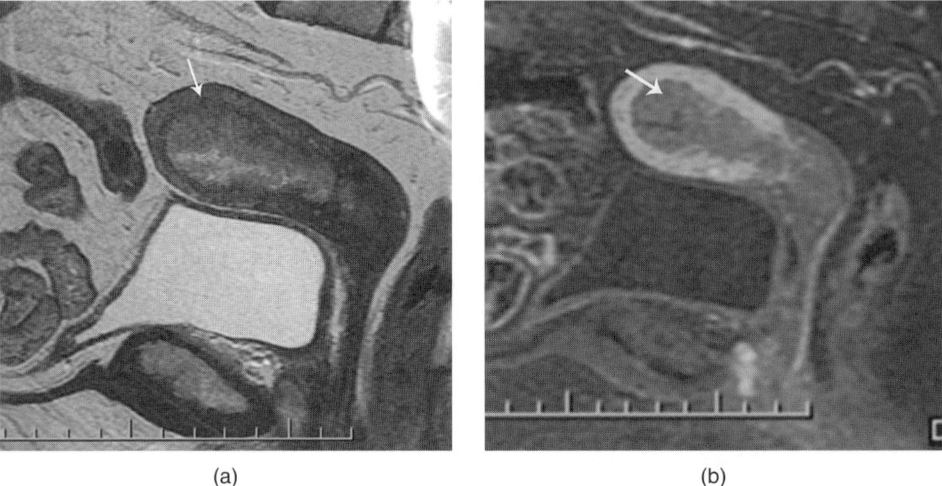

(a)   (b)

Figure 17.8   Endometrial carcinoma, endometrioid adenocarcinoma type. Sagittal T2W MRI (a) shows an intermediate SI endometrial mass with ill-defined endometrial/myometrial interface (arrow), in keeping with superficial myometrial invasion (stage 1B). Sagittal T1W MRI FS C+ (b) demonstrates the endometrial mass is hypoenhancing (arrow) compared with myometrium. The endometrium–myometrium interface is ill-defined, due to superficial myometrial invasion.

- T2WI

    - Heterogeneous iso- to hypointense to endometrium (Figure 17.8)
    - No myometrial invasion if JZ intact
    - Irregular endometrial/myometrial interface suspicious for myometrial invasion.

- T1WI C+

    - Hypoenhancing compared with myometrium
    - Differential enhancement less marked on delayed scans
    - Dynamic contrast enhancement helps determining the presence and depth of myometrial invasion
    - Useful for differentiating tumor from fluid or blood in endometrial cavity.

- If no myometrial invasion, may look identical to endometrial hyperplasia or polyp.

- MRI is only indicated to stage known endometrial carcinoma.

17.7 Summary

- Imaging has a significant role in the evaluation of abnormal uterine bleeding in both pre- and post-menopausal women.

- TVS can confidently exclude endometrial carcinoma in post-menopausal women when endometrial thickness is ≤5 mm.

- Endometrial hyperplasia and stage 1 endometrial carcinoma are indistinguishable on both TVS and MRI.

- TVS and MRI can accurately diagnose other causes of AUB such as adenomyosis, submucosal leiomyomas and endometrial polyps, as well as identify patients who need an endometrial biopsy or hysteroscopy.

References

Williams SC *et al.* (2007) Developing a robust and efficient pathway for the referral and investigation of women with post-menopausal bleeding using a cut-off of ≤ 4 mm for normal thickness. *Br. J. Radiol.* **80**: 719–723.

Goldstein SR (2006) Abnormal uterine bleeding: The role of ultrasound. *Radiol Clin North Am.* **44**: 901–910.

Dubinsky TJ (2004) Value of sonography in the diagnosis of abnormal vaginal bleeding. *J. Clin, Ultrasound* **32** (7): 348–353.

Ascher S *et al.* (2003) Benign myometrial conditions: leiomyomas and adenomyosis. *Top Magn. Reson. Imaging* **14** (4): 281–304.

Reinhold C *et al.* (2002) Postmenopausal bleeding: value of imaging. *Radiol Clin North Am.* **40** (3): 527–562.

18
Female Pelvic Floor Dysfunction

Rania Farouk EL Sayed, MD

Radiology Department, Cairo University Hospitals, Cairo, Egypt

18.1 Introduction

Pelvic floor dysfunction (PFD) is a term applied to a wide variety of clinical conditions including urinary incontinence (UI), pelvic organ prolapse (POP), defecatory dysfunction, sensory and emptying abnormalities of the lower urinary tract, sexual dysfunction and several chronic pain syndromes.

This chapter briefly reviews the definitions, pathophysiology, clinical features and the traditional imaging modalities of UI and POP. The chapter is structured to be problem oriented: examples of cases with PFD will be presented together with a newly developed MR imaging analytic approach.

18.2 Anatomical considerations

Pelvic floor

- 'Pelvic Floor' is used broadly to include all the structures supporting the abdominal and pelvic cavity (Fig. 18.1)

- Conceptually, it is useful to divide the pelvic floor anatomy artificially into passive and active structures.

  ○ Passive structures

    ■ The pelvic bones

    ■ Supportive connective tissue of the pelvis which consist of ligaments and endopelvic fascia.

Urogenital Imaging: A Problem-oriented Approach   Edited by Sameh K. Morcos and Henrik S. Thomsen
© 2009 John Wiley & Sons, Ltd

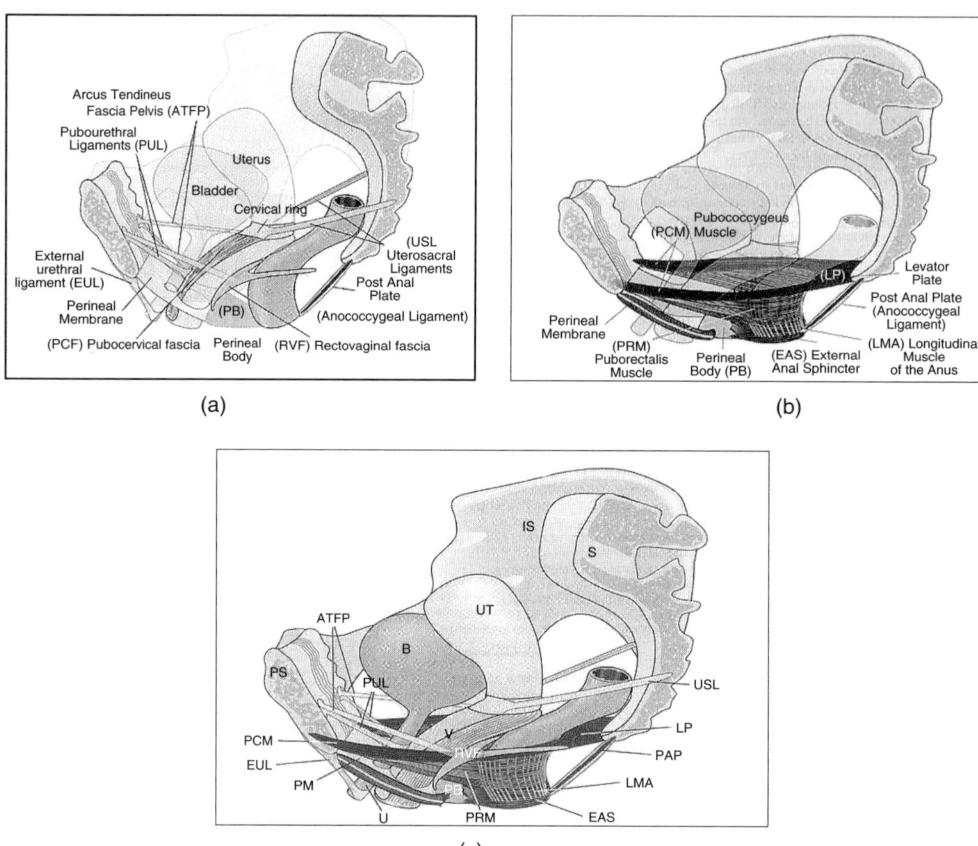

Figure 18.1 Diagram of the pelvis. (a) Pelvic organs, the ligamentous and membranous structures are indicated by gray color. (b) Muscles are marked with striation. (c) The relationship of the pelvic muscles to organs, ligaments and fascia is shown (Reproduced by permission of Springer).

- ○ Active support structures
  - ■ Pelvic floor muscles with its neurologic 'wiring' that result in sustained (tonic) and intermittent voluntary muscle contractions during activity.

- These passive and active components of the pelvic floor function as integrated multilayer system from superior to inferior consist of four principle layers:

  - ○ The endopelvic fascia; include the parametrium and paracolpium giving support to the uterus and upper vagina. The paracolpium that attach the upper vagina to the pelvic walls has two portions.
    - ■ Level I (the upper portion) consists of relatively long sheet of tissue that suspends the vagina to the pelvic wall.
    - ■ Level II attaches the mid portion of the vagina more directly to arcus tendineus fascia pelvis (ATFP) at the lateral pelvic wall.

- o The pelvic diaphragm including the levator ani and the coccygeus muscles, both acts as a shelf supporting the pelvic organs.
- o The perineal membrane (urogenital diaphragm),is triangular in shape and spans the anterior pelvic outlet. Trilaminar structure with the deep transverse perineal muscle sandwiched between the superior and inferior fascia.
- o The superficial layer, (External Genital Muscles) comprising the superficial transverse perineal muscle, bulbospongiosus and ischiocavernous muscles.

- From a functional point of view it is useful to divide the pelvic organ support system into the urethral supporting system, the vaginal supporting system and the anal sphincter complex. The later will not be described as defecatory dysfunction is beyond the scope of this chapter.

  - o Urethral supporting structures consist of:
    - The ventral and dorsal urethral supporting ligaments
    - The endopelvic fascia that support the middle and proximal urethra known as (level III fascial support)
    - The puborectalis muscle.
  - o Vaginal supporting structures include:
    - Level I and II endopelvic vaginal fascia
    - The iliococcygeus muscle.

18.3 Pathophysiology of pelvic floor dysfunction

- Stress urinary incontinence (SUI) can be due to:
  - o Structural defects in the urethral supporting structures.
  - o A poorly functioning urethral sphincter muscle, termed 'intrinsic sphincter deficiency' (ISD).

- Pelvic organs prolapse (POP):
  - o Weakness of the levator ani may cause widening of the levator hiatus, and descent of the central portion of the pelvic diaphragm. The resultant loss of support to the pelvic organs places tension on the pelvic fascial support system.
  - o Excessive tension results in breaks, separations, and attenuation of the pelvic fascial support system. Cystocele, rectocele, and uterine prolapse are caused by specific defect in one of the vaginal support levels.

18.4 Clinical features

Urinary incontinence (UI)

Subtypes include stress (SUI) which is the most common, urge (UUI) and mixed (MUI).

- The main symptom of SUI is the involuntary leakage of urine on effort, sneezing or coughing.
- A urinary diary for pad use, UI episodes and urinary frequency is important in patient's assessment.

- A cotton swab test to identify bladder neck hypermobility.

- Full bladder cough stress test to elicit the sign of SUI.

- Testing for urinary tract infection.

Urodynamic studies

- Correlation between urodynamic findings and symptoms of UI is generally poor particularly in patients with symptoms of mixed UI.

- Medium-fill cystometry

  - It differentiate SUI from urge incontinence.

  - A rise in the intravesical pressure is consistent with a bladder detrusor muscle contraction, which implies detrusor instability or urge incontinence.

- Abdominal leak point pressure

  - It can identify SUI owing to intrinsic urethral sphincter deficiency.

  - At different volume intervals during filing cystometry, the patient is asked to strain until leakage is observed and the pressure within the bladder is measured.

  - Valsalva leak point pressure (VLPP) of less than $60\,cm\ H_2O$ at a volume of 150 filling correlates with intrinsic sphincter deficiency (ISD).

Pelvic organ prolapse (POP)

POP includes anterior vaginal prolapse (cystocele), apical or uterine prolapse, posterior vaginal prolapse which include (enterocele, rectocele, and perineal descent but does not include rectal prolapse). Refer to Table 18.1 for POP quantitation.

Cystocele

- Mild cystocele is asymptomatic but can be associated with SUI.

- Marked cystocele is commonly symptomatic and can be associated with:

  - Vaginal bulging

Table 18.1　Pelvic Organ Prolapse Quantification (POPQ)

Stage 0	No prolapse is demonstrated.
Stage I	The most distal portion of the prolapse is more than 1 cm above the level of the hymen.
Stage II	The most distal portion of the prolapse is 1 cm or less proximal to or distal to the plane of the hymen
Stage III	The most distal portion of the prolapse is more than 1 cm below the plane of the hymen but protrudes no further than 2 cm less than the total vaginal length in centimeters.
Stage IV	Essentially complete eversion of the total length of the lower genital tract is demonstrated.

- o Dyspareunia
- o Urinary tract infection
- o Obstructive voiding symptoms
- o Urinary retention

Uterine prolapse

- Mild uterine prolapse is usually asymptomatic but higher grades can present with:

  - o A vaginal mass
  - o Dyspareunia
  - o Urinary retention
  - o Stretching of the uterosacral ligaments may lead to low back pain
  - o Obstructive uropathy due to ureteral obstruction
  - o Difficult defecation is experienced by one-third of patients.

Enterocele

- *Simple enterocele* exists when there is no associated vault prolapse and the cuff of the vagina is well supported.

- *Complex enterocele* is associated with vault prolapse and tend to coexist with other forms of the anterior or posterior vaginal wall.

- Symptomatic enterocele may cause

  - o Vaginal pressure
  - o Dyspareunia
  - o Dragging sensation in the pelvis as well as pelvic pressure
  - o Stretching of the mesentery with straining can cause pain in the lower abdomen or back
  - o Patients may complain of severe constipation, feeling of incomplete evacuation or symptoms of bowel obstruction.

Rectocele

- A rectocele may be present in up to 80% of asymptomatic patients.

- Symptoms include vaginal pressure, vaginal mass and dyspareunia.

- Difficult emptying of the rectum, tenesmus, and rectal splinting.

Difficulties in clinical assessment and management of patients with POP

- It is frequently difficult to different a high grade cystocele from an enterocele, a vaginal vault prolapse or a high rectocele by physical examination.

- A high grade cystocele may mask SUI; results of anti-incontinence procedure are usually improved by restoring the normal pelvic floor anatomy.

- Repair of cystocele without attention to the rest of the pelvic floor may predispose the patient to an increased incidence of enterocele, rectocele or uterine prolapse after the operation.

- Due to vaginal overcrowding, an enterocele is often missed on physical examination. In addition, physical examination cannot reliably distinguish the content of an enterocele.

- The size of the uterus and the presence of concomitant uterine or ovarian pathology determine if a vaginal or abdominal hysterectomy is performed at time of the prolapse repair.

- Clinical findings may not correlate with symptoms. These patients may have a degree of descent sufficient to cause symptoms but because they have a deep pelvis, the extent of the prolapse is not appreciated by clinical examination.

Recommendations

- It is essential that concomitant vaginal wall prolapse to be diagnosed prior to repairing cystocele or prior to incontinence surgery.

- It is sometimes necessary to reduce the enterocele to examine adequately the rest of the vaginal canal and rule out any associated cystocele or rectocele.

- Imaging, particularly MRI, is crucial in assessment of POP.

18.5 Imaging of pelvic floor dysfunction

Urinary incontinence (UI)

Cystourethrogram (CUG)

- The diagnostic criteria for SUI include:

  - The bladder neck and proximal urethra open and descend more than 2 cm in relation to symphysis pubis during straining (Fig. 18.2).
  - Posterior vericourethral angle (PVUA) beyond $100°$ during straining.
  - Angle of urethral inclination more than $30°$ from the longitudinal axis of the body.
  - Limitations

    - It provides only a silhouette view of the contrast agent-filled organ with little, if any information about the organ composition, surrounding soft tissue, or associated PFD.
    - There are controversies about the value of the PVUA as an indicator of SUI being of extremely variable value among continent and incontinent women.

Transvaginal ultrasound (TVUS)
Change in bladder position in relation to the symphysis pubis during stress maneuvers in patients with SUI include:

- Postero-inferior rotation of the urethrovesical junction.

- Opening of the bladder neck, urethra leading to urinary leakage.

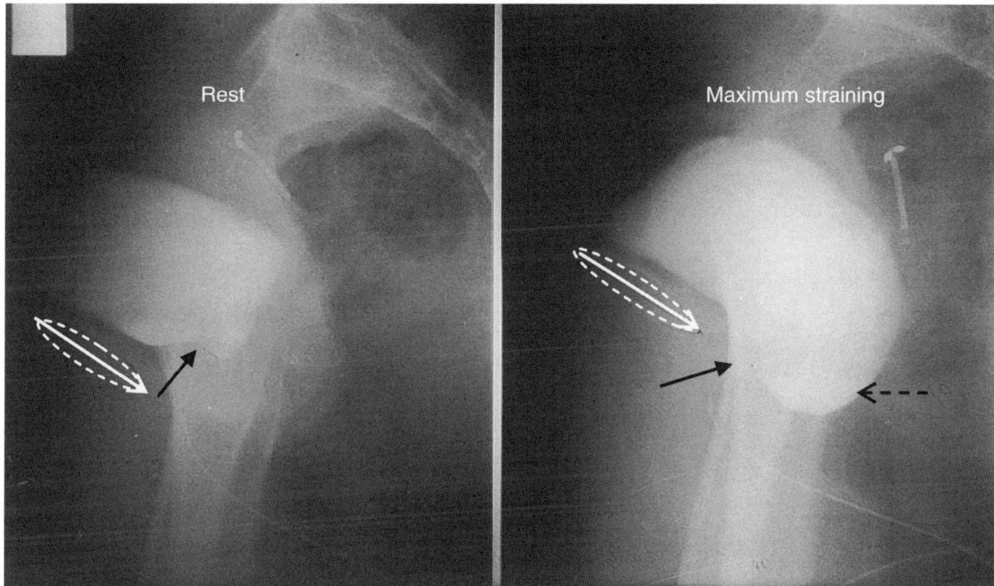

Figure 18.2 Cystourethrogram (CUG) of a 35-year-old patient with stress urinary incontinence (SUI). The bladder neck (BN) (solid arrow) is labeled by a soft guide wire placed inside the Foley's catheter; the symphysis pubis, outlined by the dotted line. At rest, the BN is seen above the level of the symphysis pubis. During straining, the BN is below the level of the pubococcygeal line (PCL) with an associated moderate cystocele (dashed arrow).

- Limitations
  - During endocavitary scanning, there is always the problem that the probe is stenting the vagina and limiting the movement of the bladder neck.
  - The examination is operator-dependent.
  - It does not provide adequate visualization of soft tissue planes.

MR imaging

- Provides detailed anatomic information on the status of the urethral supporting elements due to the high inherent soft tissue contrast. Details are provided with MRI of POP.

Pelvic organ prolapse (POP)

Dynamic contrast cystocolpoproctography

- Requires opacification of the pelvic organs (bladder, vagina, small bowel and rectum).

- The study can be done with all organs opacified or in phases with each organ opacified individually prior to each straining phase (Fig. 18.3).

- The diagnostic criteria include:
  - Prolapse of pelvic organs is defined radiologically by reference to the pubococcygeal line (PCL), which extends from the inferior margin of the pubic symphysis to the sacrococcygeal junction.

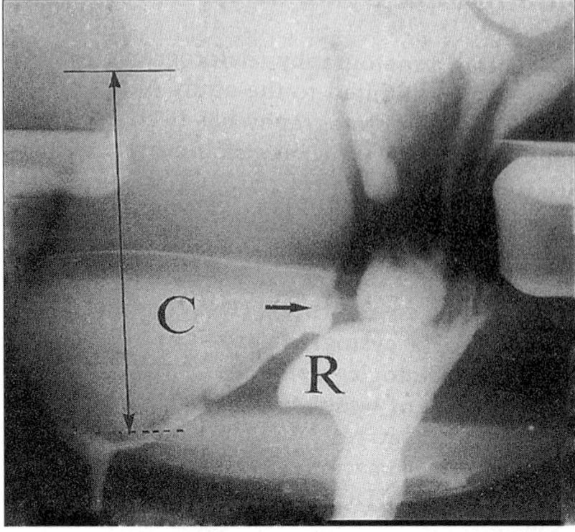

Figure 18.3 Cystoproctogram image taken during evacuation shows a very large cystocele (C). The uninterrupted line represents the pubococcygeal line (PCL), the dotted line indicates the bladder base and the arrowed line indicates the depth of the cystocele below the PCL. There is a rectocele (R) but its size is minimized by the pressure from the large cystocele. The arrow indicate the uppermost point of the vagina.

- A cystocele, enterocele or sigmoidocele, and vaginal vault prolapse are defined by extension of the bladder base, small bowel or sigmoid colon, and vaginal apex respectively below this reference line.
- Prolapse of any of these organs is graded as small if there is organ descent up to 3 cm below the PCL, moderate if this extension measures between 3–6 cm, and large if descent is greater than 6 cm.
- Anterior rectocele is defined as anterior rectal wall bulge, the depth of bulge is measured from line extended upward from the anterior wall of anal canal. Lateral and posterior rectocele may also occur.
- Rectocele is graded as small if its depth is less than 2 cm, moderate between 2–4 cm and large if it measures more than 4 cm.
- Limitations
  - Time consuming
  - Exposes the patient to a significant amount of ionizing radiation
  - It may fail to detect enterocele in 20% of patients with this condition.

Perineal ultrasound

- In dynamic transperineal ultrasound the probe is placed on the perineum, scanning is performed in the sagittal and coronal planes with the movement of the pelvic floor observed during straining and squeezing.
- This study has a considerable potential as simple, cheap and non-invasive technique.
- Its relationship to other imaging methods and reliability await further assessment.
- During straining cystocele, enteroceles and rectocele may become apparent.

18.6 Magnetic resonance (MR) imaging

- MRI has been effectively used to evaluate pelvic floor disorders, with very good reported sensitivity, specificity and positive predictive value.

- An MRI analytic approach that defines the most predominant pelvic supporting system defects to which the treatment can be directed is described below.

- This analytic approach gives new insight into the diagnosis of these complex pathologies. Based on this insight, a defect-specific approach for management could be applied and thus can allow an individually tailored surgical technique to be employed.

- All data obtained from MRI are presented in a schematic form (Table 18.2) for easier comprehension by the clinicians.

- A diagnostic algorithm is suggested in Figure 18.4.

Table 18.2 A proposed form for magnetic resonance (MR) reporting. Data reproduced from Radiology, August 2008: Volume 248: Number 2, 528–530

I. Location and type of prolapse:

Location	Type	
(1) Anterior compartment:	a] Bladder neck descent:	Grade:
	b] Bladder base descent:	Grade:
(2) Middle compartment:	a] Uterine descent:	Grade:
	b] Enterocele/Peritoneocele:	Grade:
(3) Posterior compartment:	a] Anorectal junction descent:	Grade:
	b] Rectocele:	Grade:

II. Defects in the pelvic organ support system:

Urethral supporting structures

a] Ligament/s:	Type of injury	Side:
b] Fascia level III:		
c] Puborectails:	Type of injury and/or weakness:	Side:

Vaginal supporting structures

a] Vaginal fascia level I and II:	Side:
b] Iliococcygeus: Type of injury and/or weakness	Side

III. Measurements of supporting structures:

H Line: M Line: Levator plate angle:

Width of levator hiatus:

Iliococcygeus angle:

<u>Opinion</u>

The predominant defect(s):

For SUI : Ligaments: Fascia: Muscles:

For POP: Fascia: Muscles:

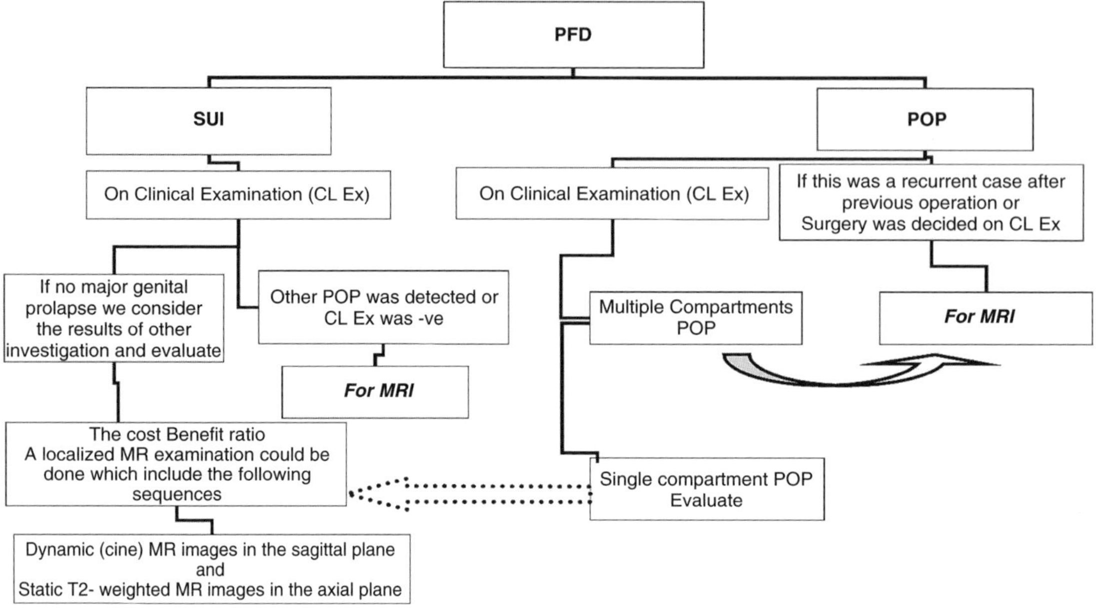

Figure 18.4   A diagnostic algorithm for MR imaging of patients with pelvic floor dysfunction.

Imaging protocol

- MR imaging is performed with the patient supine, using a pelvic phased-array coil and high magnetic filed strength.

  - Patient preparation

    - No oral or intravenous contrast agent is administered.

    - All patients should have a cleansing rectal enema (using warm water) the night before the MR examination.

    - The examination is performed while the urinary bladder is comfortably full. The patient is routinely asked to micturate 2 h before the examination.

    - The rectum is opacified with 90 to 120 cc of ultrasound gel.

  - Imaging parameters for static images

    - Static images of the pelvis are acquired in three planes using T2-weighted turbo spin-echo (TSE) sequences (TR/TE, 5000/132; field of view [FOV], 240–260 mm; slice thickness, 5 mm; gap, 0.7 mm; number of signals acquired [NSA], 2; flip angle, 90°; matrix, 512 × 512; acquisition time, 3.12 min for each sequence).

  - Imaging parameters for dynamic (cine) images

    - Dynamic sequences are performed in the sagittal, axial, and coronal planes, using BFFE sequence (TR/TE, 5.0/1.6 ms; FOV, 300 mm; slice thickness, 6–7 mm; gap, 0.7 mm).

    - In each plane five slices during six phases are acquired; each phase takes 10 s. These six phases are acquired (1) with the patient at rest, (2) during contraction of the pelvic floor (the patient was instructed to squeeze the buttocks as if trying to prevent the escape of urine), (3) during mild straining, (4) during moderate straining, (5) during maximum straining, and (6) during a repeated maximum straining sequence to ensure a maximal Valsalva maneuver (the patient was instructed to bear down as much as she could, as though she were constipated and trying to defecate).

Analysis of static MR images

- *The urethral supporting system* (Fig. 18.5)

  - In the axial plane, the urethral ligament abnormalities are classified into:

    - distortion, when internal architectural changes with waviness of the ligaments are seen

    - defect, defined by discontinuity of the ligament with visualization of the torn parts.

  - Level III fascial defect is recognized by the drooping moustache sign which is formed by the fat in the prevesical space against the bilateral sagging of the detached lower third of the anterior vaginal wall from the arcus tendineus fascia pelvis (ATFP).

  - Puborectalis muscle defect is recognized through disruption of the normal symmetrical appearance of the muscle slings or of its attachment to the symphysis pubis.

- *The vaginal supporting system* (Fig. 18.6)

  - Level I & II endopelvic fascial vaginal defect are visualized as sagging of the fluid-filled posterior urinary bladder wall into the bilaterally detached vaginal supporting fascia from the lateral pelvic wall (saddlebags sign).Central defect is also indicated by sagging of the central part of the urinary bladder posterior wall.

  - The iliococcygeus muscle is assessed for loss of the normal symmetrical appearance of its muscle slings or defect and/or disruption of its attachment to the obturator internus muscle.

Analysis of dynamic MR images

- *Sagittal plane*

  - In the sagittal plane the pubococcygeal line (PCL) is used as the reference line. This line extended from the inferior border of the symphysis pubis anteriorly to the tip of coccyx posteriorly.

  - The descent of the bladder neck, bladder base, uterus and anorectal junction below the PCL is recorded.

  - SUI is recorded when loss of urine through the urethra is visualized at maximum straining (however, absence of urine loss during MR imaging does not preclude the patient complaints).

  - Other measurements in the sagittal plane (Fig. 18.6) during maximum straining include:

    - the H-line (extends from the inferior aspect of pubic symphysis to the anorectal junction)

    - the M-line (dropped as perpendicular line from PCL to the posterior aspect of the H-Line)

    - the levator plate angle, enclosed between the levator pate and the PCL.

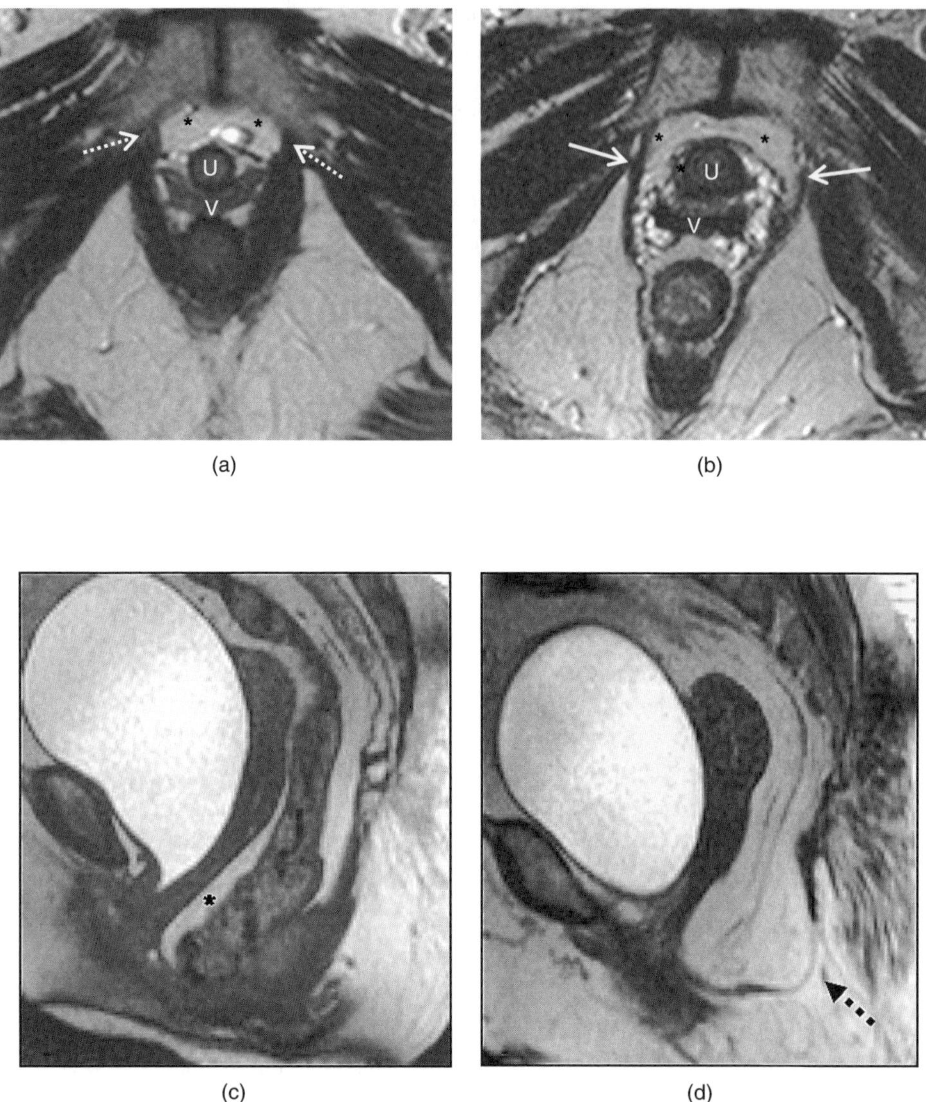

Figure 18.5 Normal and patterns of defect of urethral supporting structures at MR imaging [T2-weighted Turbo Spin Echo (TSE) MR images (TR/TE 5000/132) at the level of the proximal urethra (U), vagina (V)]. (a) Axial image obtained from a 27-year-old healthy continent volunteer shows normal level III endoplevic fascial support (**); dashed arrows, point to the attachment of the puborectalis slings to the pubic bone. (b) Axial image obtained from a 55-year-old patient with grade II SUI shows the typical MR imaging appearance of 'the drooping moustache sign', (**); thinning of the puborectalis muscle slings (arrows) more on the left side. (c,d) Dynamic balanced fast field echo (BFFE) MR images (TR/TE 9/4) (c) mid-sagittal, (d) parasagittal at maximum straining, peritoneocele (*), absence of small bowel content and the focal area of localized thinning and bulge of the iliococcygeus muscle (dashed arrow) are shown.

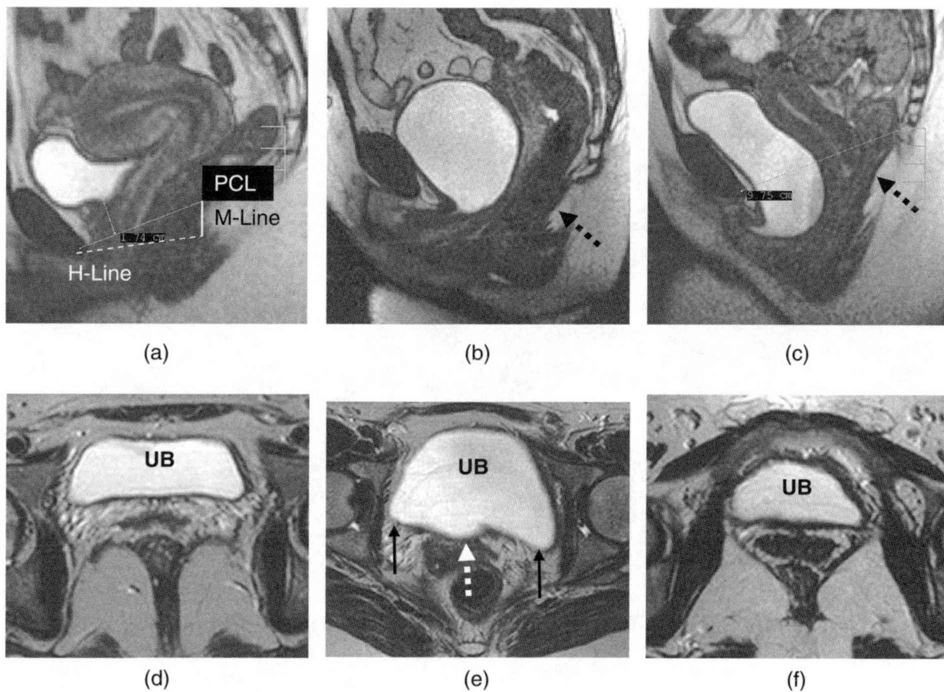

Figure 18.6 Normal plus patterns of defect of the vaginal supporting structures and how to correlate between static and dynamic MR images [Dynamic mid-sagittal balanced fast field echo BFFE (TR/T 9/4)] (a) Image obtained in a 30-year-old- healthy volunteer with no pelvic organ descent below the pubococcygeal line (PCL). (b,c) Images obtained in two patients with pelvic floor dysfunction, both images show cystocele with different grades and sagging of the levator plate (arrows) more advanced in C with uterine descent. It is not possible from these midline images to see the specific differentiating structural defects for each cystocele. (d,e,f) The corresponding axial T2-weighted turbo spin echo (TSE) MR images (5000/132) at level II endopelvic fascial support; (d) shows normal fascial support indicated by the straight posterior wall of the urine filled urinary bladder (UB); (e) shows fascial defects: bilateral paravaginal (saddlebags sign) more on the left side (solid arrows) and central defect (white arrow); (f) shows no gross evidence of fascial defect. Correlation between static and dynamic MR imaging findings reveals that in images B&E, POP is due to the more advanced fascial defect compared with the moderate sagging of the levator plate; while in C&F, the excessive sagging of levator plate relative to the fascial defect indicates that levator muscle weakness is the predominant defect responsible for POP. This analytic approach allows a defect- specific approach to disease management and surgical technique.

- *Axial and coronal planes*

  - In the axial and coronal planes (Fig. 18.7), the width of the levator hiatus (enclosed between the puborectalis muscle slings) and the iliococcygeus angle were measured, respectively, at rest and during maximum straining.

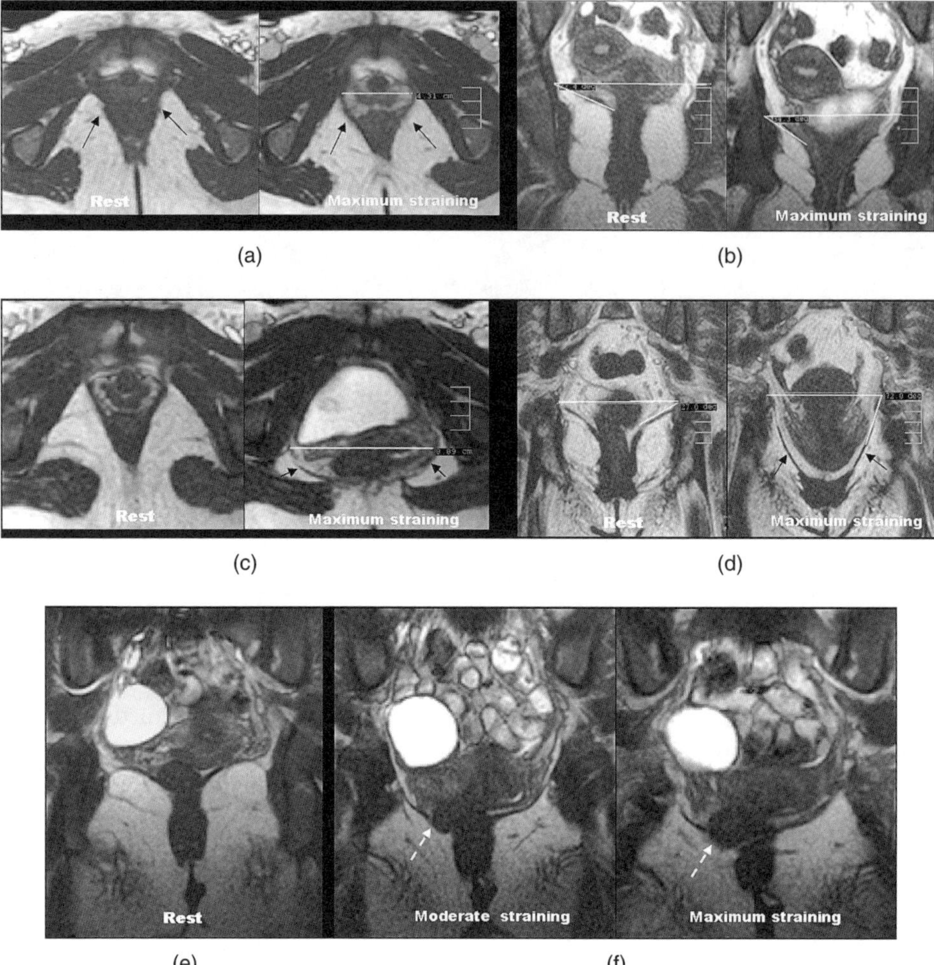

Figure 18.7 Patterns of pelvic floor muscle weakness and defect [Dynamic balanced fast field echo BFFE (TR/TE 9/4)] (a), axial (b) coronal images obtained in a 28-year-old healthy volunteer show normal width of the levator hiatus(WLH) (straight line) measuring 4.3 cm at maximum straining; arrows, point to the puborectalis (PR) slings in A, iliococcygeus angle(IL A) measured 34.3⁰ (enclosed between the joined lines in B). (c) axial (d) coronal images obtained in a 54-year-old female patient with SUI, and POP show weakness of the pelvic floor muscle indicated by ballooning of the PR muscle (arrows in C); WLH measuring 9 cm; excessive downward vertical descent of the iliococcygeus muscle (arrows in D) with the IL A reaching 72⁰. (e,f) Coronal images obtained in a 25-year-old patient with POP; with progressive straining a right levator defect is seen containing the rectum (dashed arrows).

○ The mean and SD of the H-line is 5.8 cm $\pm$ −0.5; the M-line 1.3 $\pm$ 0.5; the levator plate angle 11.7° $\pm$ 4.8°, the width of the levator hiatus 4.5 cm $\pm$ 0.7 and the iliococcygeus angle 33.4° $\pm$ 8.2° measured in healthy volunteers with no symptoms of lower genitourinary abnormalities at maximum straining. These measurements were proved to be of value in identification of pelvic floor laxity and quantification of the degree of the weakness. They are also useful for follow-up assessment.

Correlation between static and dynamic MR images

- Static and dynamic MR images in the same patient are analyzed simultaneously and findings obtained are correlated to determine the most marked type of pelvic supporting system defects This defect is reported as the predominant defect.

- Based on this approach it was possible to differentiate whether POP was due to defects in the endopelvic fascia, levator muscle weakness (Fig. 18.6), or due to abnormalities in both the endopelvic fascia and levator muscles.

- SUI was found to be associated with structural defects in the urethral supporting elements and not with bladder neck descent.

- This imaging correlation converts static and dynamic MR imaging from two types of images that record abnormalities separately, into an integrated system that can more precisely delineate the underlying anatomic defect responsible for symptoms in patients with pelvic floor dysfunction (even allowing differentiation of the underlying anatomic defect when any two patients have the same symptoms).

References

Bartram CI, DeLancey JO (eds), Halligan S, Kelvin FM, Stoker J (Assoc. eds) (2003) *Imaging Pelvic Floor Disorders*. Springer, Berlin, Heidelberg, New York.

El Sayed RF, Fielding JR, El Mashed SE, Morsy MM, Azim MS (2005) Preoperative and postoperative magnetic resonance imaging of female pelvic floor dysfunction: correlation with clinical findings. *J Women's Imaging* **7**: 163–180.

El Sayed RF, Morsy MM, El Mashed S, Abd El Azim MS (in press) Anatomy of the Urethral Supporting Ligaments Defined by Dissection, Histology, and MRI of Female Cadavers and MRI of Healthy Nulliparous Women (AJR 2007; 189:1145–1157).

Petros PP (2007) *The Female Pelvic Floor: Function Dysfunction and Management according to the Integral Theory*, Springer, Berlin, Heidelberg, New York.

Raz S and Rodriguez LV (2001) Diagnostic imaging of pelvic floor dysfunction. *Curr. Opin. Urol.* **11**: 423–428.

Assessing Pelvic Floor Dysfunction: Combined analysis of Static and Dynamic Magnetic Resonance Imaging Findings (Radiology August 2008: Volume 248: Number 2, 528–530).

19
Imaging of female infertility

Ahmed-Emad Mahfouz and Hanan Sherif

Radiology Departments, Hamad Medical Corporation, Qatar and Cairo University, Egypt

19.1 Introduction

Female infertility may be caused by several factors including functional causes related to hormonal disorders or organic causes related to the ovaries, uterus, fallopian tubes, and pelvic cavity. Among the imaging modalities currently used, ultrasonography and magnetic resonance imaging are the most widely used modalities for diagnosis of the cause of infertility. This chapter covers only imaging of abnormalities of the female pelvic organs that can cause infertility.

19.2 Polycystic ovary syndrome

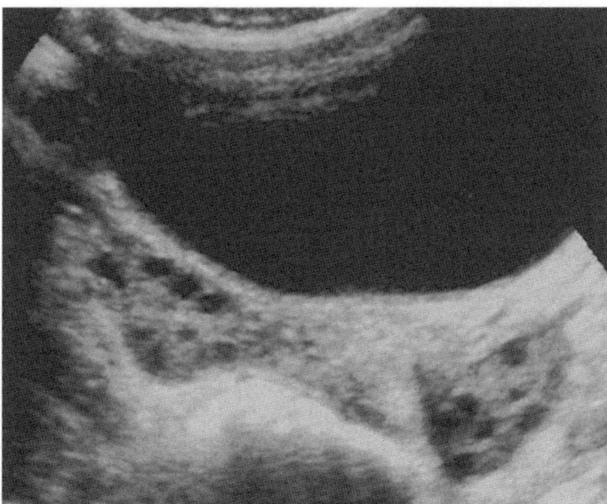

Figure 19.1 Transabdominal ultrasonography of a patient with polycystic ovary syndrome demonstrates enlarged ovaries and peripheral uniform small sized follicles.

Urogenital Imaging: A Problem-oriented Approach   Edited by Sameh K. Morcos and Henrik S. Thomsen
© 2009 John Wiley & Sons, Ltd

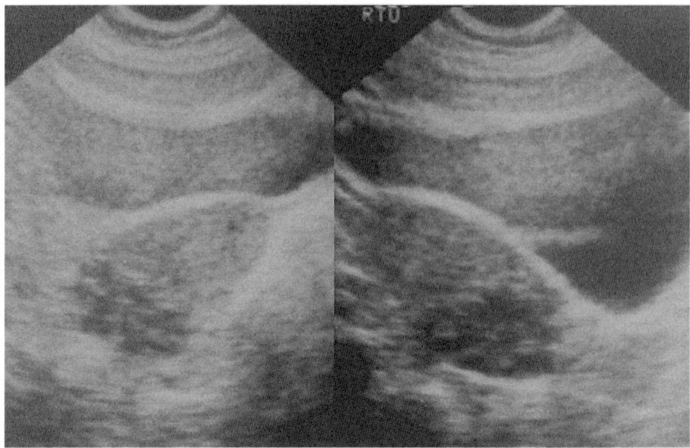

Figure 19.2 Transabdominal ultrasonography of another patient with polycystic ovary syndrome. The ovaries are mildly enlarged. The peripherally located follicles could not be adequately delineated.

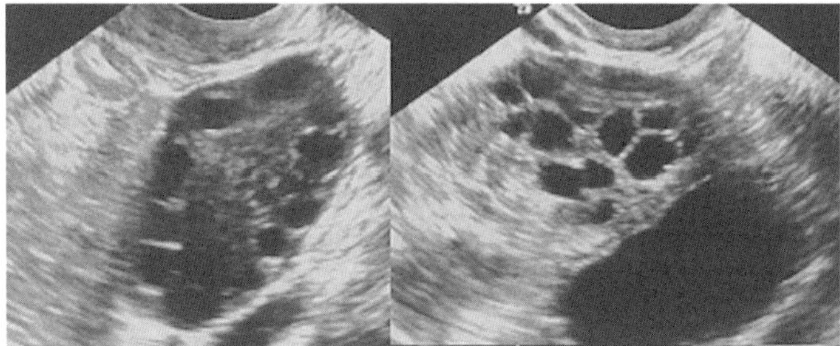

Figure 19.3 Transvaginal ultrasonography of a patient with polycystic ovary syndrome. The peripheral small follicles are demonstrated in high resolution.

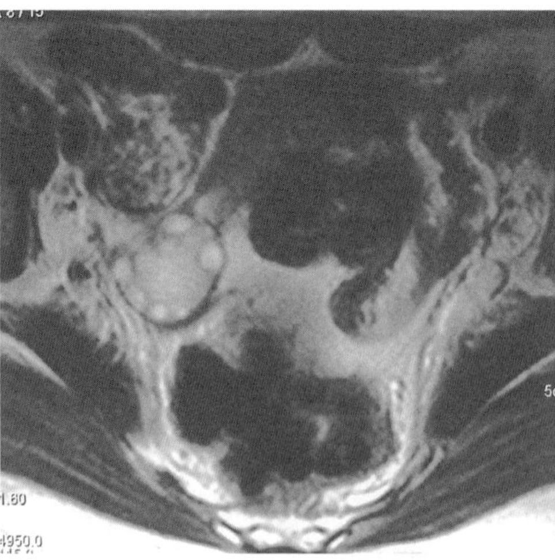

Figure 19.4 Transverse T2-weighted image demonstrates morphological features of polycystic ovary syndrome in an infertile patient: enlarged right ovary, spherical shape, thick capsule, peripheral follicles, and central solid component (transverse T2w image).

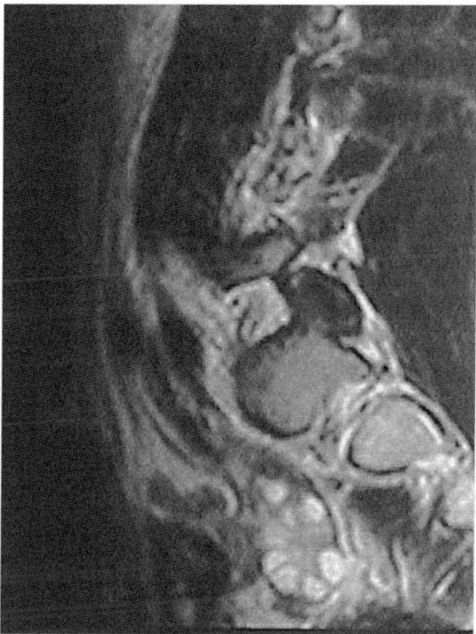

Figure 19.5 Polycystic ovary, incidentally discovered in a patient with normal fertility during MR imaging of the lumbosacral spine (parasagittal T2 w image).

Clinical features

- Polycystic ovary syndrome is the combination of chronic anovulation, clinical or biochemical signs of hyperandrogenism, and morphological features of polycystic ovary on imaging.

- It may present by infertility, menstrual disorders, obesity, acne, or hirsutism.

- It may be clinically silent, discovered only as incidental finding on ultrasonography or MR imaging.

Pathology

- Pathogenesis unknown. May be related to insulin resistance, abnormal ovarian steroidogenesis, excess extraovarian androgen, or adrenocortical dysfunction.

Imaging

- *Ultrasound*

  - Enlarged ovaries (more than 10 cc).
  - Multiple follicles (at least six per ovary) peripherally located and small (average 3 mm). Transabdominal ultrasonography may fail to detect the follicles. They are better seen by transvaginal ultrasonography.
  - Thick capsule.
  - Solid central component.
  - Spherical configuration of the ovary.

- *MRI*
  - The same morphological features can be demonstrated on MRI, best demonstrated on T2-weighted images (the follicles being seen as rounded markedly hyperintense peripheral small cysts).

19.3 Abnormalities of the fallopian tubes (Hydrosalpinx/Hematosalpinx, tubal block)

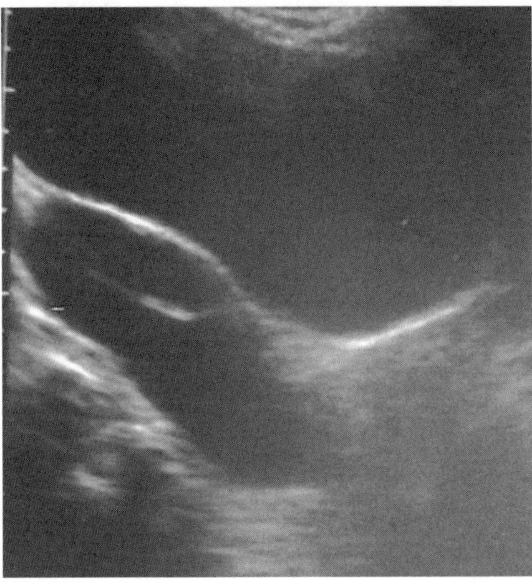

Figure 19.6 Longitudinal ultrasonography of an adnexal mass demonstrates oblong cystic lesion consistent with dilated fluid-filled fallopian tube.

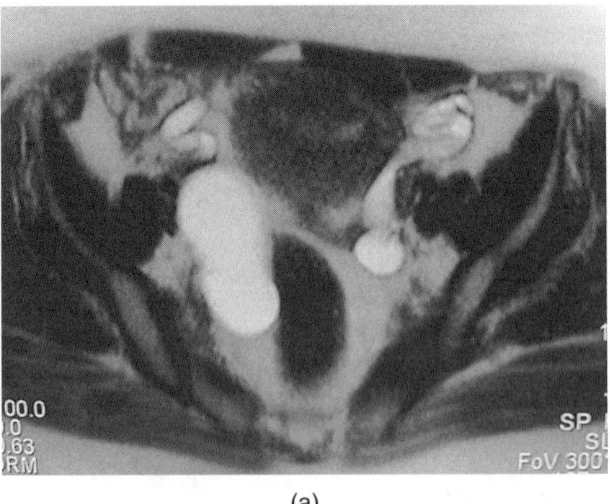

(a)

Figure 19.7 Transverse T2-weighted (a) and fat-saturated T1-weighted (b) images demonstrate bilateral dilated fluid-filled fallopian tubes. The fluid has low signal intensity on T1-weighted image and high signal intensity on T2-weighted image denoting hydrosalpinx.

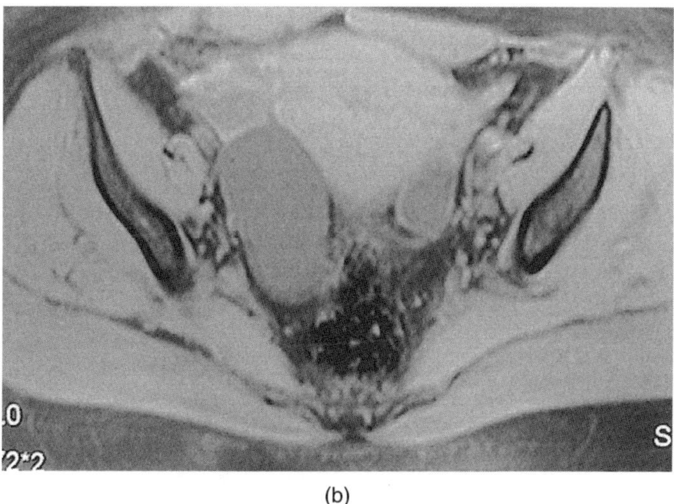

(b)

Figure 19.7 *(continued)*

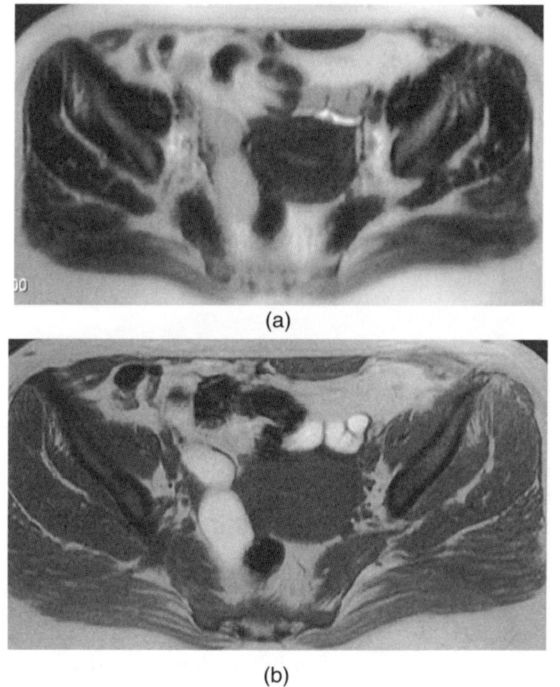

(a)

(b)

Figure 19.8 Transverse T2-weighted (a), T1-weighted (b), and fat-saturated T1-weighted (c) images demonstrate bilaterally dilated fluid-filled fallopian tubes. The fluid within the tubes has relatively low signal intensity on T2-weighted image and high signal intensity on T1-weighted images before and after fat saturation, denoting blood-degradation products within hematosalpinx.

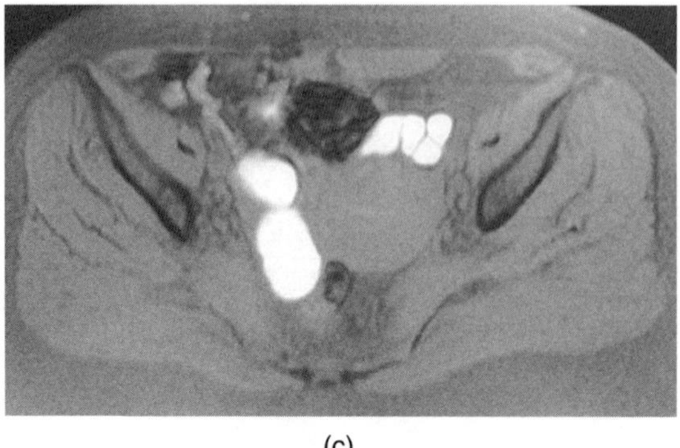

(c)

Figure 19.8   *(continued)*

Clinical features

- Pelvic pain, infertility

Pathology

- Obstruction of the fallopian tube due to adhesive inflammatory reactions in response to previous infection results in tubal obstruction and accumulation of fluid within the distended tube (hydrosalpinx), Hemorrhagic changes may occur and result in hematosalpinx.

- Hematosalpinx may be associated with pelvic endometriosis due to implantation of endometriotic foci in the tubes.

Imaging

- *Ultrasound*

  - Elongated fluid-filled adnexal structure, which may be folded over itself.

  - Clear anechoic fluid suggests hydrosalpinx. Echogenic fluid may suggest hematosalpinx or pyosalpinx.

- *Hysterosalpingography*

  - Failure to opacify the tubes or to achieve peritoneal spill by the contrast agent injected into the uterine cervix.

- *MRI*

  - Dilated fluid-filled fallopian tube. Non-hemorrhagic fluid has low signal intensity on T1-weighted images and extremely high signal intensity on T2-weighted images. Hemorrhagic fluid has high signal intensity on T1-weighted images before and after fat saturation and relatively low signal intensity on T2-weighted images.

  - Pyosalpinx and tuboovarian abscess show thickening of their wall and abnormal enhancement after injection of contrast agent.

19.4 Fibroids

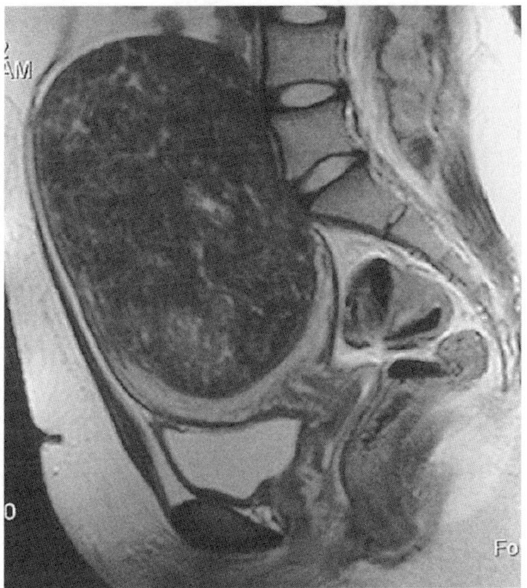

Figure 19.9 Sagittal T2-weighted MR image demonstrates large hypointense mass of the myometrium impressive of intramural fibroid. High signal intensity spots within the fibroid due degenerative changes.

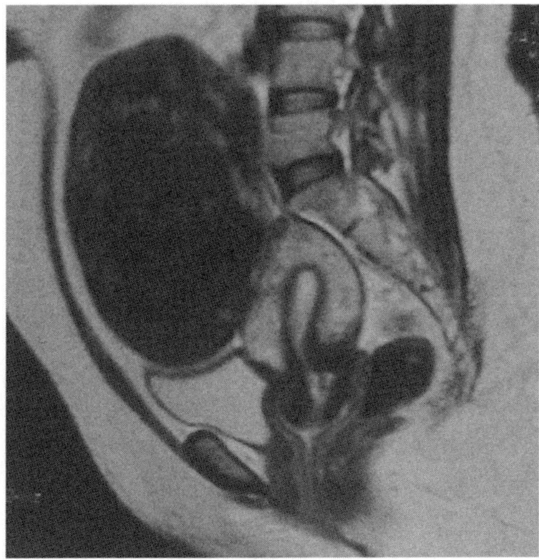

Figure 19.10 Sagittal T2-weighted image demonstrates large anterior subserous fibroid.

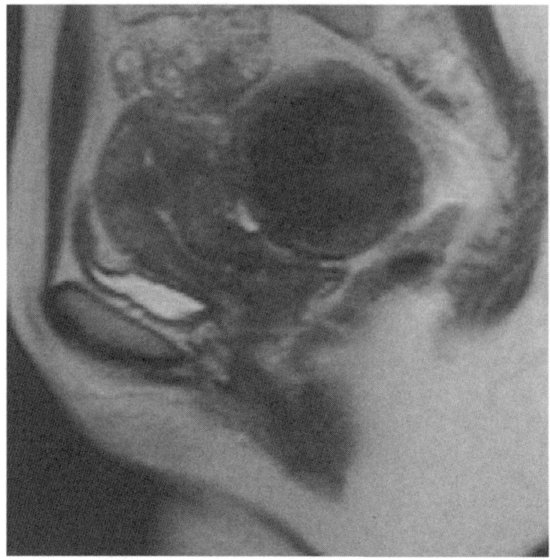

Figure 19.11 Sagittal T2-weighted MR image demonstrates posterior subserous fibroid and submucosal fibroid. In the clinical setting of infertility, submucosal fibroid is more significant than intramural and subserous fibroid.

Clinical features

- Menorrhagia, dysmenorrhea, pelvic pain, infertility

- May be clinically silent

- Pressure symptoms related to the urinary bladder, dyspareunia.

Pathology

- Benign neoplasm of the smooth muscles of the uterus

- Frequently multiple

- May undergo degeneration.

Imaging

- *Plain X-ray and intravenous urogram*

  - Calcified mass of the pelvic cavity

  - Indentation of the contrast filled urinary bladder.

- *Ultrasound*

  - Well defined hypoechoic or isoechoic uterine mass submucosal, intramural, or subserous in location.

  - Frequently there is posterior attenuation of ultrasound by the lesion.

  - May be calcified, causing acoustic shadow.

- o Linear artefact due to diffraction of ultrasound at the tissue interfaces at the boundaries of the lesion and within the lesion. When isoechoic to the myometrium, it may be recognized only by these diffraction artifacts.

- o Submucosal fibroids are better demonstrated by transvaginal ultrasonography especially if small.

- **CT**

  - o Bulky uterus with irregular outline. May show calcification within uterine mass.

- **MRI**

  - o Solid uterine mass, hypointense on T2-weighted images due to high fibrous tissue and muscle content, isointense to the uterus on T1-weighted images.

  - o Hyperintense foci within the mass on T2-weighted images may denote degenerative changes.

19.5 Adenomyosis

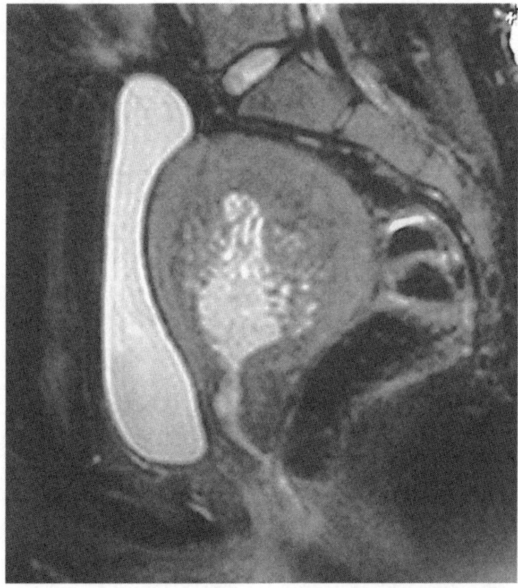

Figure 19.12 Sagittal T2-weighted MR image demonstrates multiple hyperintense foci within the junctional zone and myometrium of the uterus similar in signal intensity to that of the endometrium, consistent with adenomyosis. There is associated endometrial hyperplasia evidence by thickened endometrium.

Clinical features

- Menorrhagia, metrorrhagia, dysmenorrhea, dyspareunia, infertility

- It affects females late in their child-bearing period.

Pathology

- Adenomyosis is the ectopic presence of endometrium within the myometrium and the junctional zone between the myometrium and endometrium. The uterus becomes large and globular in shape.

- It may be associated with endometriosis.

Imaging

- *Ultrasound*

  o Enlarged globular uterus.

  o Heterogeneous echopattern of the involved myometrium. Focal forms of adenomyosis may be mistaken for fibroids.

- *MRI*

  o Enlarged globular uterus.

  o Thickened junctional zone between myometrium and endometrium (more than 12 mm). This may need to be differentiated from pseudothickening of the junctional zone caused by uterine contractions during ovulation or menstruation.

  o Multiple foci of endometrium within the myometrium and junctional zone, hyperintense on T2-weighted images and isointense or hyperintense on T1-weighted images.

  o It is easier to differentiate between adenomyosis and fibroids on MRI than on ultrasonography. On T2-weighted images, adenomyosis appears hyperintense while fibroids appear hypointense. On T1-weighted images, adenomyosis may appear hyperintense if associated with endometrial bleeding while fibroids appear isointense.

19.6 Developmental anomalies of the uterus

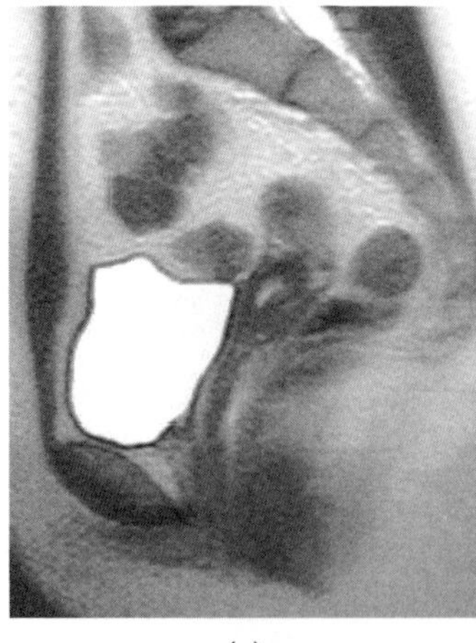 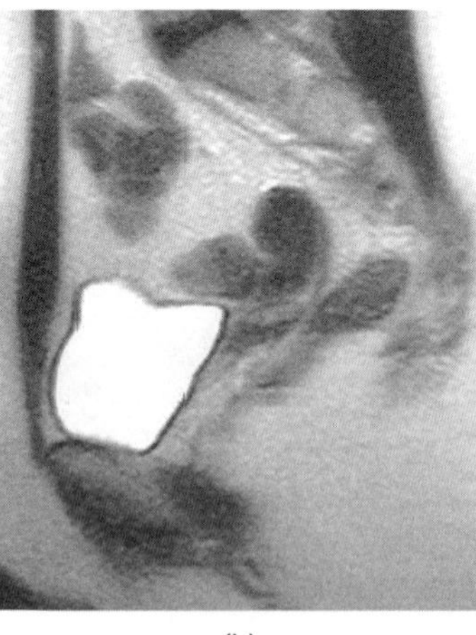

(a)   (b)

Figure 19.13 Sagittal (A, B) and transverse (C) T2-weighted MR images demonstrate small size of the uterine body and fundus in relation to the uterine cervix, a case of uterine hypoplasia.

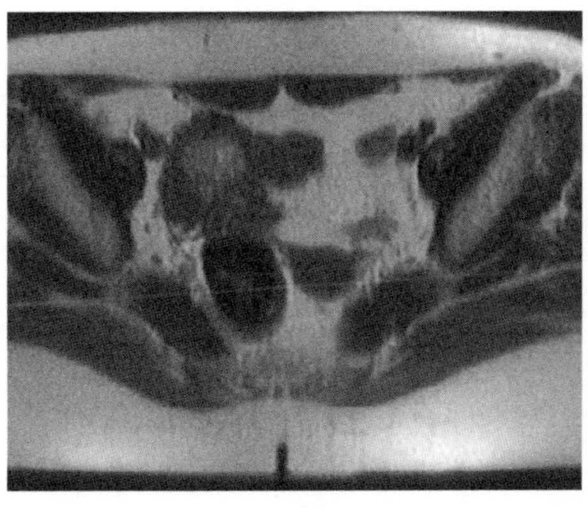

(c)

Figure 19.13 *(continued)*

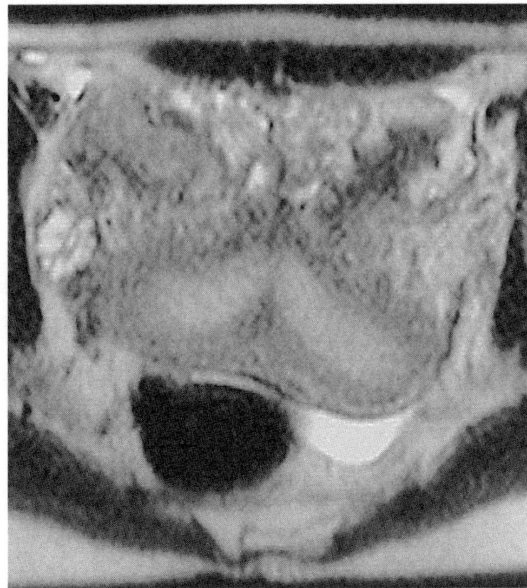

Figure 19.14 Transverse T2-weighted image demonstrates septate uterus. The two endometrial divisions are separated by a partially muscular septum. The outer surface of the uterus shows no corresponding separation of the two sides of the uterus.

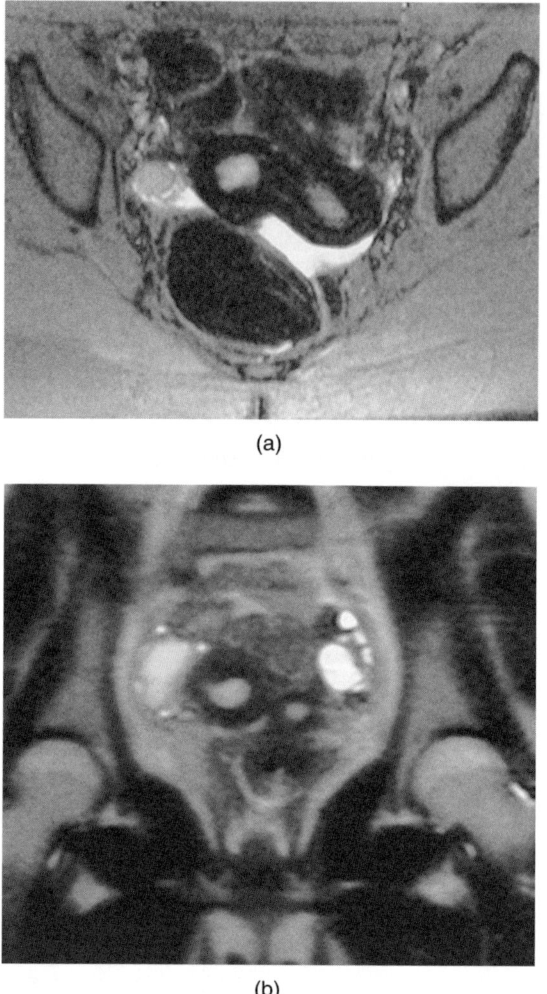

Figure 19.15 Transverse short TI inversion recovery (STIR) MR image (a) and coronal T2-weighted image (b) show bicornuate uterus. Unlike septate uterus, there is separation of the two horns on the outer uterine surface. Note the associated polycystic ovaries.

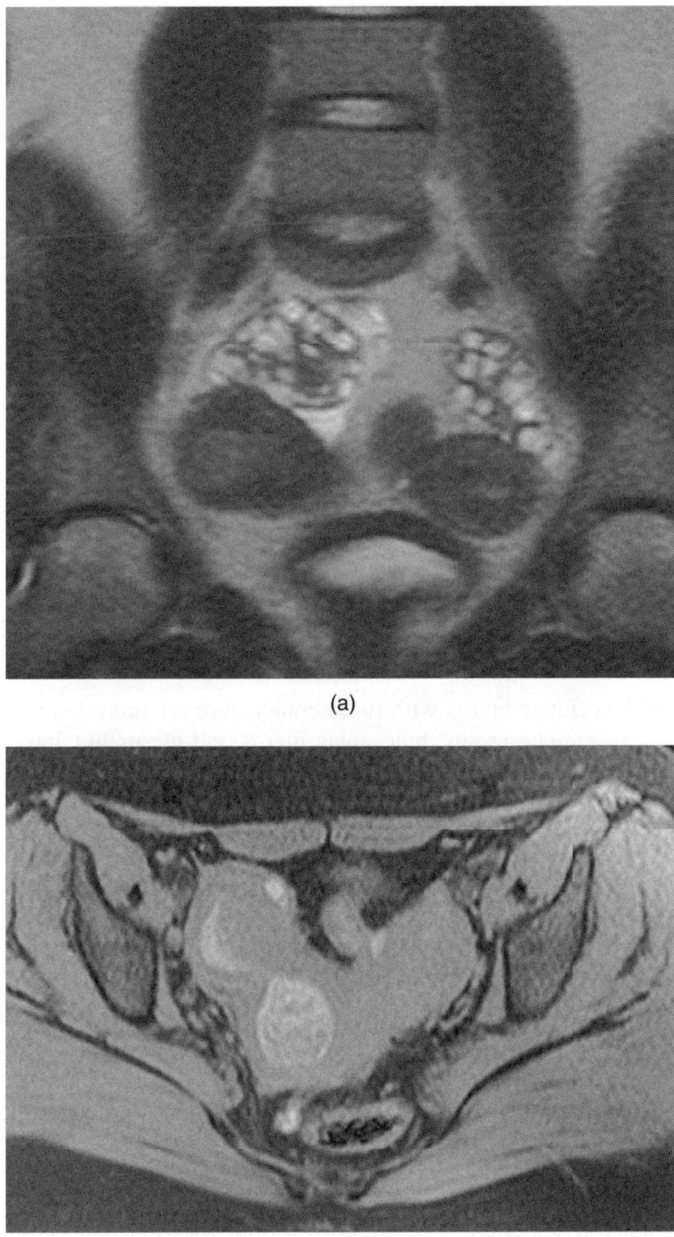

(a)

(b)

Figure 19.16 Coronal T2-weighted (a) and transverse fat-saturated T1-weighted (b) images demonstrate uterus didelphys bicornis bicolpos with right hemi-hematocolpos and hemi-hematometra due to imperforate right hymen. This 20-year-old female has been menstruating normally through the left side of the uterus, cervix, and vagina. Note also the associated polycystic ovaries.

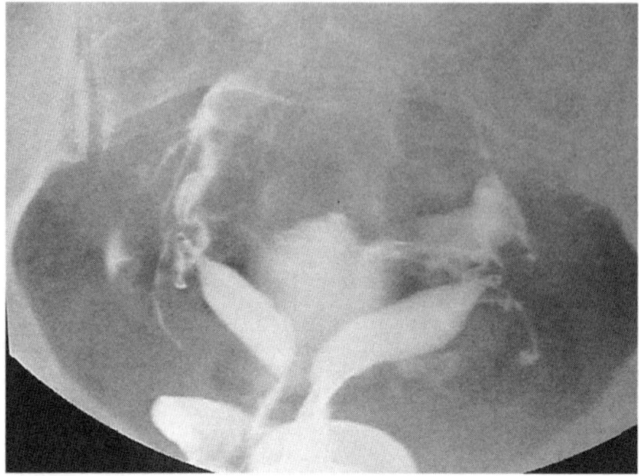

Figure 19.17   Hysterosalpingography demonstrates uterine duplication anomaly with a common external cervical os, through which the injection of contrast agent has been performed.

Clinical features

- Uterine hypoplasia is a recognized cause of primary infertility.

- Septate uterus may present by disfavorable outcome of pregnancy if implantation occurs at the septum.

- Unicornuate and bicornuate uterus with rudimentary horn are more likely to be associated with infertility than arcuate uterus, bicornuate uterus and uterus didelphys.

Pathology

- Developmental anomalies of the uterus result from anomalous development of the Mullerian ducts. According to the degree of fusion of the Mullerian duct anomalies are classified as: Class I: Uterine agenesis or hypoplasia, Class II: Unicornuate uterus, Class III: Uterus didelphys, Class IV: Bicornuate uterus, Class V: Septate uterus, Class VI: Arcuate uterus, Class VII: Diethylstilbestrol-exposed uterus (T-shaped endometrial cavity due to in utero exposure to diethylstilbestrol).

Imaging

- *Hysterosalpingography*

  - Demonstrates uterine hypoplasia as small size of the uterine cavity.
  - Demonstrates arcuate shape of the uterine fundus in cases of arcuate uterus.
  - When it demonstrates a single uterine horn, further imaging may be needed to differentiate between unicornuate uterus and other causes mimicking unicornuate uterus due to lack of filling of the other cavity with contrast agent.
  - When it demonstrates two cavities, further imaging may be needed to differentiate between septated, bicornuate, or didelphic uterus.

- *Ultrasound*

  - Assessment of external contour of the fundus differentiates septate uterus from bicornuate uterus.

- o The thickness and the myometrial content of the septum can be assessed by ultrasonography.
- o Transvaginal ultrasonography is superior to transabdominal ultrasonography in demonstration of the uterine septum.

- **MRI**

  - o MRI offers excellent anatomical details of the type of the anomaly. It demonstrates the outer contour of the uterus, the extent of the duplication in the uterus and cervix, and differentiates a fibrous from a muscular septum.
  - o The ability of MRI to recognize the signal intensity of blood degradation products makes it the best modality for demonstration of hemihematocolpos-hemihematometra.

19.7 Endometriosis

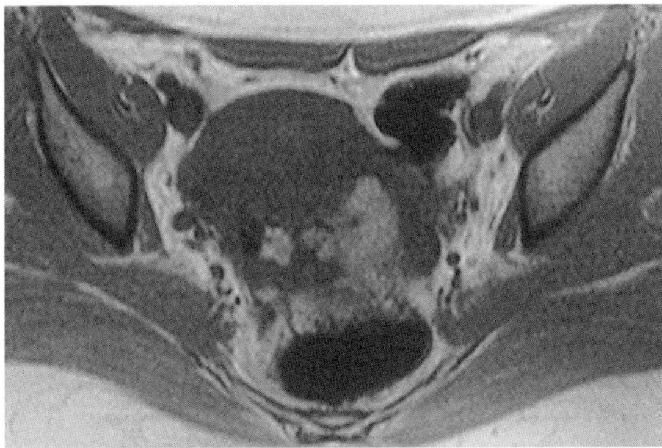

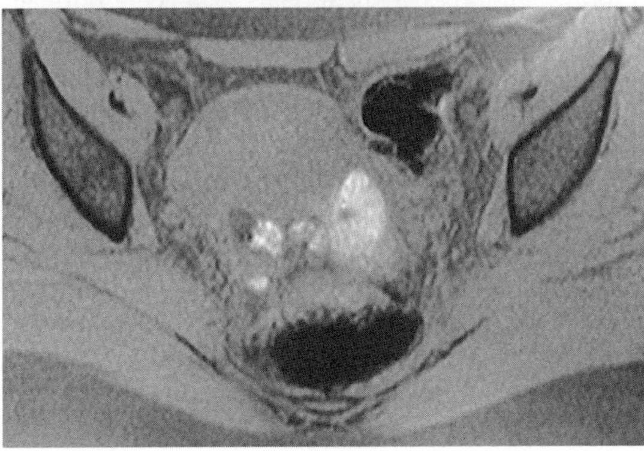

Figure 19.18 Transverse T1-weighted images of the pelvis before and after fat saturation in a female with infertility demonstrates hyperintense lesions posterior to the uterus, which show no loss of signal intensity after suppression of he bright signal intensity of fat. Findings are impressive of blood degradation products due to endometriosis.

Clinical features

- Pelvic pain and infertility.

- It affects females late in their child-bearing period.

Pathology

- Endometriosis is the extrauterine presence of endometrium, usually within the pelvic cavity, but distant location may also be involved.

- With the menstrual cycle, the extrauterine endometrial tissue undergoes the same cyclic changes of the normal endometrium. Shedding of the surface endometrium and bleeding may result in endometrial masses within the pelvic cavity composed of central hemorrhagic fluid surrounded by endometrial tissue and fibrous tissue.

19.8 Imaging

- *Ultrasound*

  - Cystic adnexal mass with echogenic fluid within the cyst. Occasionally sediment-fluid levels and thick walls.

- *MRI*

  - Abnormal adnexal and pelvic masses with high signal intensity on T1-weighted images before and after fat saturation.

  - Fat-saturated T1-weighted images are important to differentiate between dermoid cyst and endometrioma when a hyperintense lesion is identified on T1-weighted images. The high signal within dermoid cyst will disappear on the fat-saturated images. The high signal of endometriosis will not.

  - On T2-weighted images, endometriosis appears relatively dark. Particularly at the most dependent part of the hemorrhagic cystic masses.

  - MRI may demonstrate endometriosis at odd sites like the urinary bladder wall and the anterior abdominal wall. Hydroureter/hydronephrosis may be demonstrated in case of lower ureteric involvement by endometriosis.

Index

abdominal aorta 3, 21, 25, 33–4
abnormal uterine bleeding (AUB) 381–97
abscesses 39, 40–1, 159, 168, 170–3, 197, 319
   adnexal 354, 356, 366, 421
   children 151–2, 154, 158, 159, 160–1
   immunocompromised patients 177–8
   prostate 313–14, 319
   renal 68, 70, 76, 96, 107, 114, 128, 159
   TB 179–81
   urethritis 191–2
ACE (angiotensin converting enzymes)
      inhibitors 8, 44–5, 48–9
acquired cystic kidney disease (ACKD) 76, 87,
      94–5, 96
actinomycosis 379
acute renal failure (ARF) 197
adenocarcinomas 239, 241, 326, 392, 396
adenofribromas 354, 371
adenomas 3, 15, 16–17, 95, 131, 326, 340
   adrenal imaging 1–2, 4–6, 8, 15–17, 20
adenomyosis 370, 372, 381, 382–8, 390, 397,
      423–4
adnexal masses 183, 351–79, 393, 418, 420,
      430
adrenal cortical carcinomas 1, 8, 12–15, 20
adrenal glands 1–20, 21, 28, 45, 66, 130–1,
      417
adrenal hemorrhage 15, 17, 18–19
adrenal hyperplasia 4–5, 7–8, 348–9
adrenal incidentalomas 15–20
adrenal myelolipomas 1, 15, 17–19
adrenal rests 347–9
adrenocorticotropic hormone (ACTH) 2–4, 13,
      348
age 12, 15–16, 44, 276, 423, 430
   adnexal masses 352–3, 355–7, 360, 363

AUB 381–2, 388, 396
   bladder cancer 235, 242
   hematuria 221, 223, 226
   hemospermia 323–5, 330, 334, 336–7
   renal cystic lesions 76, 90, 92
   retroperitoneal tumours 30, 32
   scrotal masses 339–40
   urinary diversion 261, 264
   UTIs 166–7, 174, 183
   see also children
aldosterone 7, 13, 16, 45, 104
aldosteronoma 7–8, 16
allergy to contrast 40, 82, 226
amenorrhea 2
American Association for the Surgery of
      Trauma (AAST) 122–3
ampullae 274, 275, 278, 282, 308, 318
   hemospermia 325, 327, 328, 329–30
amputation of penis 143, 146
amyloidosis 32
anastomosis 104, 105, 106, 107, 142, 147
aneurysms 33, 68, 91, 92, 356
angio-computer tomography 24
angiography 24, 36–8, 46, 77, 92, 107, 128
   computed tomography 45, 48–51
angio-magnetic resonance imaging 24
angiomyolipoma (AML) 26, 55, 57,
      59–60, 72
angioplasty 43, 46, 100, 103–7
angiotensin 44, 45, 48, 104
angiotensin receptor blocker (ARB) 44
anorchia 329
anovulation 394, 417
antibiotics 41, 70, 146, 281, 314, 337
   UTIs 150, 153–6, 166, 168, 172–3, 178
anticoagulants 18, 37, 222, 229, 237, 324

432 INDEX

antigens 116
antiplatelet therapy 237, 324
aniline 235
anuria 33, 100, 107, 111, 117
appendicitis 198, 208, 378–9
appendix 258–9, 356, 377
aplasia 328
arcuate uterus 428
arcus tendineus fascia pelvis (ATFP) 400
arteriography 10, 45, 100–1, 105–6
ascending cystography 110, 112
ascites 351, 360, 374, 377
Aspergillus sp 177
atherosclerosis 46, 48–51, 104
attenuation 30–2, 39–41, 88, 114, 333–4, 389, 422
  adenomyosis 384, 386
  adrenal imaging 2, 8, 10, 14–15, 17, 19
  bladder cancer 248, 254
  renal masses 55, 57, 59–60, 63–5, 68, 70, 72
  urinary tract injury 124–8, 130, 131
  UTIs 159, 168, 170
avulsion 123, 127, 129, 132, 143–4
azoospermia 328, 329, 314, 320
azotemia 44

bacteria 77, 312–13, 316, 324
  UTIs 149–53, 162, 166–8, 172–4, 176–7, 178–9
bacteriuria 167, 174, 239, 337
balanced fast field echo (BFFE) MRI 408, 410, 411–12
barium 23, 89, 270
BCG 278, 284
benign prostate hypertrophy (BPH) 273–6, 278–81, 285, 287, 290–1, 294, 305
  hemospermia 326, 328, 332, 334–5
bicornate uterus 426, 427–9
bilharzial infection *see* schistosomiasis
biopsy 16, 179, 184, 281–3, 378
  adnexal masses 355, 366, 373, 376, 378
  AUB 382, 390, 395, 397
  bladder cancer 238, 242–3, 254
  hematuria 223, 226
  hemospermia 325, 326, 328–9, 332, 336
  prostate cancer 273, 276, 278–9, 281–7, 289–91, 293–302, 308
  renal masses 59, 62, 64, 66, 67, 73
  renal transplantation 116–20
  retroperitoneal tumors 25, 27, 40

bladder 8–9, 34, 133–6, 315–16, 318, 422, 430
  adnexal masses 351, 355, 356, 365
  hematuria 224–5, 228–30, 231–2
  hemospermia 325, 327–9, 333, 335–6
  PFD 401–2, 404–9, 411, 413
  renal transplantation 107–8, 114–15, 119–20
  stones 81, 170, 197, 199, 202, 208, 210, 214
  urethral trauma 137–42
  urinary diversion 257, 258–9, 261
  UTIs 166–7, 169–70, 172, 177–81, 183–4, 186–7, 192
  UTIs in children 149–50, 156, 162–5
bladder cancer 32, 184, 187, 235–54, 267, 326
  hematuria 222, 223–5, 228, 231, 233
  prostate cancer 278, 302, 308
  renal transplantation 100, 119–20
bleeding diathesis 18, 237, 324, 326
blood pressure *see* hypertension
bone extension of prostate cancer 273, 298, 304, 312
bone metastases 55, 241, 298, 304, 312, 327
Bosniak classification 57, 59, 65
bowel 23, 26, 37, 40, 184, 201
  adnexal masses 351, 356, 365–6, 374–5, 377, 379
  metastases 33, 377
  PFD 403, 405–6, 410
  trauma 128, 135
  urinary diversion 257, 258, 264, 269
brachytherapy 297, 326
breast cancer 16, 19, 32, 65, 243, 378
Brenner tumour 373
bronchogenic carcinoma 66–7
brucellosis 346
Buck's fascia 141, 143

calcification and calculi 128, 152, 175–6, 189, 195–218, 271
  adnexal masses 353, 357–8, 362, 365, 377–8
  adrenal imaging 10, 14–15, 17–18
  bladder cancer 235, 241–2, 248, 252
  fibroids 422–3
  hemospermia 325–8, 334–6
  immunocompromised patients 177–8
  leiomyomas 389
  prostate 278, 284, 313, 316, 320, 325–6, 334, 336

RAS 49, 51
renal cystic lesions 78, 80, 84–6, 88, 91–2, 94
renal masses 55, 57–9, 68, 70, 72
retroperitoneal tumors 23–3, 27–8, 30–1, 40
schistosomiasis 183–4, 186–7
scrotal masses 344, 347, 348–9
TB 179–82
see also stones
calcium oxalate stones 196
calcium phosphate stones 196–7
calical clubbing 158, 160
caliectasis 75
calyces 199–201, 203–5, 210, 218
Camey I and II 261–2
Candida albicans 177
carcinomas 33, 53–6, 57–8, 326, 336, 391–2, 395–7
adrenocortical 12–15, 16
adnexal masses 354
AUB 381, 391
bladder cancer 239–40, 242–3, 246, 253
endometrial 381–2, 391–2, 393, 395–7
hemospermia 323, 324–6, 328, 332, 336
prostate 283, 287, 291–2, 297–8, 304–7, 324–5, 328, 323, 332, 336
renal 53–63, 65, 68–70, 72–3
see also renal cell carcinoma; transitional cell carcinoma
carcinomatosis 378
cardiovascular disease 43–4
Caroli syndrome 88, 90
Castelman tumor 28
caudal junction 277, 299, 301, 306, 320
cavernosography 144
central gland (CG) 328, 332, 335–6
cervix 243, 387, 393, 420, 425, 427–9
chemical exposure 221, 235, 240
chemotherapy 66–7, 253–4, 325, 373
children 3, 9, 12, 101, 149–66, 213, 258
adnexal masses 352, 355
renal cystic lesions 76, 82, 86–90, 92–3
scrotal masses 342, 347
urinary tract injuries 132, 133
UTIs 149–66, 167–8, 172, 174, 182–4
chlamydia 190
cholangiography 89–90
choline 253, 290–1, 293
chondrogenic neoplasms 28
chordoma 26

choriocarcinams 340
chromotubation 316
chronic non-bacterial prostatitis–pelvic pain syndrome (CNBP/CPPS) 312, 316
chronic renal impairment (CRI) 198
cirrhosis 32
citrate 196, 290–1, 293
cloacal extrophy 257
coagulation 281, 381
anticoagulants 18, 37, 222, 229, 237, 324
coarctation of the aorta 44
coccygeus muscles 401
collagen 385
collecting system 38, 168, 170–5, 177–8, 188–9, 224
bladder cancer 248, 252, 253
children 153–4, 157
duplication 204, 310, 318
renal cystic lesions 75–7, 80–1, 82, 84, 88–9
renal masses 68, 71
renal trauma 123, 125, 126, 128
renal transplantation 108, 117
stones 203–7, 209–10, 212, 215–16
TB 179–80, 181
colon 21, 34, 37, 258–61, 266–7, 375, 406
colon cancer 3, 16, 33, 65, 243, 377
color Doppler ultrasound 48, 57, 60, 77, 124, 356
adnexal masses 359, 363
AUB 385, 386–7, 389, 393, 395, 396
hemospermia 327, 336
prostate 275, 278–9, 280
renal transplantation 101–2, 112, 117–18
scrotal masses 340–1, 344–5, 347–8
comedonecrosis 278, 283
computed tomography (CT) 121, 208–10, 227, 243–8, 317, 373–9
adnexal masses 354–5, 366–7, 373–9
adrenal imaging 1–2, 4–6, 8, 9, 11, 14–15
adrenal incidentalomas 15–20
bladder cancer 120, 236, 243–8, 252–4
children's UTIs 152, 154, 158–60, 161
fibroids 423
hemospermia 328, 333, 334
renal cystic lesions 75, 77–9, 81–2, 84–5, 88–9, 92, 94–6
renal masses 54–72
renal transplantation 100, 114–15, 120
renal trauma 122–5, 127–8
retroperitoneal tumors 21, 23–40

computed tomography (CT) (*continued*)
  stones 199–200, 204, 209–18
  trauma 122–5, 127–8, 130–5
  urinary diversion 269
  UTIs 167–76, 177, 180–1, 184–7, 189,
    191
computer tomography angiography (CTA) 45,
  48–51
computed tomography urography (CTU) 132,
  135, 180, 182, 248–50, 224–5
  bladder cancer 248–50, 254
  hematuria 223, 224–5, 226, 228–33
  renal cystic lesions 81–2, 84–5, 92
  renal transplantation 114–15
  stones 200, 210, 214, 218
  urinary diversion 268, 271
congenital bilateral absence of the vas deferens
  (CBAVD) 309, 316–17
congenital unilateral absence of the vas
  deference (CUAVD) 309, 318
Conn's syndrome 4–5, 8
continent catheterizing pouches 258–60
continent cutaneous urinary diversion 258–60
contraception 355, 365, 379
contrast 49–50, 224–6, 269–70, 342, 375, 408
  adnexal masses 359–60, 367–8, 372, 375,
    377
  adrenal imaging 1–2, 4–6, 11, 14–15,
    17–20
  allergy 40, 82, 226
  AUB 384, 386–8, 390–2, 394–5, 397
  bladder cancer 236, 243–6, 248, 251–4
  children's UTIs 154, 157–62, 164–5
  hemospermia 327, 329–31, 333–4
  infertility 420–1, 422, 428
  prostate 281, 284–6, 287–90, 292
  renal cystic lesions 77–8, 80–2, 84–6,
    88–9, 92, 94–5
  renal masses 54–61, 64–6, 68–71
  renal transplantation 103, 105, 114, 118–19
  retroperitoneal tumors 24–31, 33, 34–5,
    37–8, 39–40
  stones 199–200, 204–5, 215–17
  trauma 123–8, 131, 132, 134–5, 138–41,
    144
  UTUIs 169–71, 173, 175–6, 177, 180–2,
    184, 190–2
  see also iodinated contrast
corporea amylacea 274, 278–9, 316, 320
corpus luteum 352–3
cortisol 3–4, 7, 13, 16

Cowper's glands 327
C-reactive protein (CRP) 151, 167
creatinine 40, 82, 167, 216, 264, 290, 293
  children's UTIs 151, 153
  renal transplantation 107–8, 111, 113, 116
Crohn's disease 32, 264
cryotherapy 64, 73, 326
crystadenocarcinoma 377
Cushing's syndrome 2–5, 8, 13, 16, 44, 348
cyclosporine 101, 116, 119
cyst accident 354, 360
cystadenoma 30, 31, 354, 371
cystatine C 151
cystectomy 100, 120, 253, 257, 266–7
cystic fibrosis 309, 318
cystic glandular hyperplasia 390
cystic hygroma 97
cystic lymphangioma 30
cystic teratoma 30, 31
cystine stones 196–8
cystitis 149–51, 177, 178, 184, 239, 241
  hematuria 222, 229, 231
cystocele 401, 402, 403–6, 411
cystography 134–5, 138, 161–2, 163–5, 166
cystolitholapaxy 199
cystometry 402
cystoproctogram 405–6
cystoprostatectomy 241
cystoscopy 142, 223, 225, 231, 238–9, 244–7,
  254
cystourethrography (CUG) 93, 404, 405
cystourethroscopy 237, 329
cysts and cystic lesions 17–18, 30–2, 72–3,
  75–97, 212, 242, 305
  adnexal 352–4, 356–63, 365–7, 369–73,
    377–8
  adrenal 10–11, 15, 17–18
  AUB 387, 389, 392, 393–4, 395
  classification 75–6
  endometriosis 430
  fallopian tubes 418
  hematuria 222, 226, 227, 233
  hemospermia 325–8, 330–1, 333, 335
  hydatid disease 187–9
  ovarian 352–4, 356–63, 365–6, 372,
    415–18, 426–8
  pancreatic 72
  prostate 285, 305, 307–17, 319, 325–6,
    328
  renal 11, 55, 57–9, 61, 65, 72–3, 75–97
  retroperitoneal 22, 25, 28, 30–2

scrotal 342, 343, 346–8
    utricular 326–7, 330, 333
cytology 77, 374

debridement 146, 147
deep vein thrombosis (DVT) 100, 113
defecatory dysfunction 399, 401, 403
dehydroepiandrosterone (DHEA) 16
delayed graft function (DGF) 100, 116–19
dermoid cysts 430
dermoid mesh and plug 363–4
dermoid tumors 361–2, 363–4, 368–71
devascularization 123, 125, 128
dexamethasone suppression test 3, 13, 16
diabetes 101, 83, 166, 168, 172–4, 334, 396
diagnostic peritoneal lavage (DPL) 36
dialysis 72–3, 94–5, 100–1, 116, 178
diaphragm 21–2, 122, 131, 137–41, 180–1,
    401
diet 196, 199
diethylstilbestrol-exposed uterus 428
diffusion-weighted imaging 284, 292–6, 298,
    304, 309, 312
digital rectal examination (DRE) 137, 276,
    314, 324
digital subtraction arteriography (DSA) 45,
    100–1, 105–6
displacement of organs 23–4, 26, 31, 34, 141,
    212
diuretics 8, 82, 157, 252
diverticulitis 57, 198, 208, 378–9
diverticulosis 91
DMSA scintigraphy 152, 154–8, 161, 166, 172
Doppler ultrasound 45, 46–8, 55, 71, 145,
    171, 253
    renal transplantation 100–1, 103–5, 107,
        111, 116–18
    see also color Doppler; power Doppler
doxycycline 115, 337
drug abuse 33, 83, 221, 235
duodenum 21, 35–6, 188, 375
dysfunctional anovulatory bleeding 381
dysgenetic tumors 25, 26, 27
dysgerminoma 354
dysmenorrhea 382, 422, 423
dyspareunia 403, 422, 423
dysuria 80, 197, 237
    UTIs 150, 167, 184, 188, 190

echinococcosis 68, 70, 187–9
Echinococcosus sp 187

echocardiography 91
edema 25, 34, 44, 100, 254, 342, 354
    UTIs 151, 168, 169, 184
ejaculate 183, 307, 309, 314, 316, 319–20,
    323–37
ejaculatory ducts (ED) 307–8, 314–16, 318,
    325–31, 333–4
    obstruction 314, 316, 319–20, 325, 331
    prostate cancer 273–8, 280, 282, 290, 292,
        305
embryonal disorders 25, 28, 305, 309
emphysematous pyelitis 173
emphysematous pyelonephritis 170, 173–4
endometrial hyperplasia 423, 390, 393, 394–5,
    396–7
endometrial polyps 381–2, 389, 393–4,
    397
endmetriomas 358, 362, 367, 369, 372, 430
endometriosis 352, 358, 362, 370, 420, 424,
    429–30
endometrium 354, 381–2, 391–2, 393, 395–7,
    423–4
    AUB 381–97
    zona basalis 385
endopyelotomy 217
endorectal coil 276, 285, 300, 324–5, 327–8,
    331–2, 337
endoscopic retrograde
        cholangiopancreatography (ERCP)
        89–90
endoscopy 237–8, 247, 254, 308, 319
endoureterotomy 133
end-stage renal disease 83, 90, 95, 99, 152
enemas 23, 34, 281, 408
Enterobacter 151, 166
enterocele 402, 403, 404, 406, 407
enterococci 151, 166
epidermoid cyst 30, 31, 346–8
epididymides 325
epididymis 178, 180–1, 190, 340–1, 343,
    346–7, 349
epididymitis 177, 179, 345, 347
epididymo-orchitis 326, 339, 345
erythropoietin 91
Escherichia coli 151, 153, 166, 173–4, 177
estrogen 389, 394, 396
ethnicity 235, 340, 349
exercise 221, 229, 230
extracorporeal shock wave lithotripsy (ESWL)
    198–203, 211
extraparenchymal renal cysts 76, 96–7

fallopian tubes 179, 415, 418–21
fat 17–19, 79, 131, 409
  adnexal masses 361–2, 363, 367–8,
      370–1, 377–8
  AUB 384, 386–7, 390–2
  bladder cancer 239–40, 245
  infertility 419–21, 429–30
  prostate cancer 276–7, 280, 297, 299–301,
      305–6, 310–11
  renal masses 56, 57, 60
  retroperitoneal tumors 21, 25, 27, 30, 32,
      33, 35
  scrotal masses 341, 348, 350
  UTIs 151, 158, 161, 169, 175
fat suppression T1 weighted (FST1W) MRI
      367–9, 371–2, 384, 386–7, 390–2
  infertility 419–21, 427–8, 429–30
fat suppression T2 weighted (FSE-T2) 284,
      287, 289, 291, 293
fibroids 356, 365, 367, 373, 381, 421–3, 424
fibromas 26, 354, 360, 365, 367–8, 370, 373
fibromuscular dysplasia 48–51
fibromuscular stroma (FMS) 274–6, 279, 328
fibrosarcoma 24–5, 26
fibrosis 28–9, 33–5, 38, 111, 267, 313, 319
  bladder cancer 246, 254
  renal cystic lesions 83, 88, 89, 91
  UTIs 152, 171, 179, 184, 187, 190
fibrous histiocytoma 26, 340
fimbrial cyst 356
fistula 107–10, 128, 179
fluorodeoxyglucose (FDG) 1, 20, 29, 61, 253
fluoroscopy 162–3, 202, 217, 270, 328
focused abdominal sonography for trauma
    (FAST) 36
folded rectosigmoid bladder 260–1
Foley catheter 135–6, 140, 191, 214, 246, 270,
    405
follicular cysts 352–4, 356, 360
frequency 119, 197, 237, 401
  UTIs 151, 167, 177, 178, 183
fructose 307, 309, 330, 333
fungi and fungal infections 32 176–8, 346

gadolinium 14–15, 55–6, 105, 216, 251, 287,
    367, 372
  renal cystic lesions 79–80, 82
  UTIs 160–1, 172
gall stones 201, 209
gamma camera 156, 163–4
ganglioneuroma 26

gastro-intestinal tract tumors 3, 19, 22, 378
Gastrografin 375
gender 12, 44, 221, 235, 241, 242
  retroperitoneal tumors 25, 27, 28, 30, 31
  UTIs 149, 168, 173–4, 179–81, 184, 190,
    192
germ cell tumors 340, 344, 354
Gerota's fascia 21–2, 37, 169
Gleason grades 276, 283, 286, 288, 293,
    295–8, 301–7
glomerular filtration rate (GFR) 48, 83, 119
gonococci and gonococcal infection 190
granulomatous prostatitis 278, 284
granulosa cell tumors 354, 365, 375, 394
grayscale ultrasound 45–7, 104, 117, 333–5,
    359, 362

Hautmann urinary diversion 261–2
hemangiomas 26, 222, 235, 326
hemangiopericytomas 26, 28
hemangiosarcomas 26
hematoceles 145, 146
hematomas 35–8, 70, 101, 114, 299, 342
  renal cystic lesions 76, 87, 91, 96
  retroperitoneal 22, 30, 35–8, 39
  trauma 123–9, 130–1, 135, 137, 140–1,
    143–6
  urinary diversion 265, 269
hematosalpinx 358, 368, 418, 420–1
hematuria 13, 197, 219–33
  bladder cancer 120, 237–8, 243–5, 248,
    250, 253–4
  hemospermia 324, 329, 333, 337
  renal cystic lesions 76, 83, 90, 94
  renal masses 53–4, 56, 64–5, 67–9, 71
  renal transplant 100, 116, 120
  trauma 122–3, 132, 133, 136
  UTIs 167, 174, 178, 183, 187, 221
hemihematocolpos and hemihematometra
    427–9
hemodialysis *see* dialysis
hemorrhage 121, 247, 307, 381–97, 430
  adnexal masses 354, 360–3, 369–71, 378
  adrenal trauma 130–1
  hydatid disease 188, 189
  penile and scrotal trauma 144, 146
  post-coital 323, 327, 330, 331–2
  prostate cancer 281, 302
  renal cystic lesions 79–80, 91, 92, 94–5
  renal trauma 122, 126, 128, 129
  retroperitoneal 24–5, 30, 35–8, 94

scrotal masses 341, 342, 344–5, 350
hemosiderin 80, 370
hemospermia (HS) 183, 316, 323–37
hemothorax 131
heparinization 114
hepatitis 32
high intensity focused ultrasound therapy 326
histiocytoma 26, 27, 340
history 16, 82, 198, 230, 289, 345
    adnexal masses 355, 356, 359, 378
    bladder cancer 236, 237, 243, 254
    hemospermia 324–5, 328–9, 331–5
    RAS 43, 44, 69
    retroperitoneal tumors 30, 40
    TB 178, 182
HIV/AIDS 27, 32, 176, 177–8
Hodgkin's lymphoma 27
hormone replacement therapy (HRT) 355,
    381–2, 394
hormones 12–13, 15, 23, 415
horseshoe kidney 197, 204, 210–11, 218, 235
hydatid disease 76, 96, 187–9
hydatidotis 187–9
hydrocalicosis 179, 180
hydrocele 145, 342
hydronephrosis 33, 34, 39, 68, 128, 269, 430
    adnexal masses 377, 379
    renal cystic lesions 75, 94
    renal transplantation 100, 108, 111–15
    stones 200, 206–7, 209, 212, 215
    urinary diversion 265–6, 269
    UTIs 169, 171–2, 177, 179–80, 183–4,
        187, 189
hydropyosalpinx 354, 356
hydrosalpinx 418–21
hydroureter 169, 171, 179, 266, 430
hydroureteronephrosis 112
hyperaldosteronism 5–8, 44
hyperandrogenism 417
hypercalciuria 196, 222
hyperchlorenic acidosis 260, 267
hyperglycemia 3, 9–10
hyperparathyroidism 197
hyperoxaluria 196
hyperstradiolemia 394
hypertension 3, 5, 7–8, 9–10, 16, 222, 396
    bladder cancer 236, 237
    hemospermia 34, 325, 326
    RAS 43–5
    renal cystic lesions 76, 87, 89–90, 91, 93
    renal transplantation 100, 103–5, 113

renal trauma 128, 129
    UTIs 149, 166, 167
hyperuricosuria 196, 222
hypochloremic acidosis 267
hypocitraturia 196
hypofertility 307, 309, 310, 316
hypokalemia 7, 44, 261, 267
hyponatremic metabolic acidosis 267
hypospadias 330
hypotension 122, 167
hysterectomy 381, 382, 387, 388, 394, 404
hysterosalpingography 420, 428–9
hysteroscopy 386–7, 388–9, 395, 397

intra-arterial digital subtraction angiography
    (IA-DSA) 100–1, 105–6
ileo-urethrography 270
ileum 26, 38, 258–64, 267–8, 270
iliococcygeus muscle 401, 407, 409–12
iliopsoas abscess 40
image-guided percutaneous drainage (PCD)
    107, 114–15
impotence and sexual dysfunction 2, 142, 399
immunosuppression 168, 175–8, 314
    renal transplantation 99, 11, 103, 114, 120
Indiana pouch 259
indinavir 177–8, 197, 209
infarction 144, 146, 170, 222, 226–7, 265, 345
    renal transplantation 101–3
    renal trauma 124–7
infections 40, 68, 96, 144, 379, 388, 420
    bladder cancer 235, 237, 241
    hematuria 220, 222
    hemospermia 324–7
    ovarian cysts 356, 360
    prostate 281, 307, 310, 313, 314, 316
    renal cystic lesions 76–7, 80, 83, 85, 87,
        90–1, 93, 96
    renal transplantation 99–100, 111, 112, 120
    scrotal masses 346
    stones 197–8
    trauma 128, 131
    urinary diversion 261, 265
    see also urinary tract infections (UTIs)
inferior vena cava 15, 21, 25, 27, 34–5, 56,
    128
infertility 147, 316, 388, 415–30
inflammation 22, 32, 40, 116, 133, 264, 420
    adnexal masses 352, 354, 365–6, 379
    bladder cancer 235, 249, 254
    children's UTIs 151, 155, 161, 166

inflammation (*continued*)
   hemospermia 326, 327, 332, 335
   prostate 282, 287, 304–5, 308, 311–14,
      316, 319–20
   retroperitoneal fibrosis 33, 35
   scrotal masses 345, 346
   UTIs 167–9, 171–6, 177
interferon 116
intersex 330
intravenous urography (IVU) 123–4, 129, 135,
      253, 315–16, 355, 422
   hematuria 224, 225, 231
   renal cystic lesions 80–1, 84–6
   stones 199–200, 203–6, 210–11, 213, 218
   urinary diversion 267, 268, 271
intrinsic sphincter deficiency (ISD) 401, 402
iodinated contrast 1, 49–50, 55, 82, 246,
      269–70, 328
   allergy 226
irritable bowel syndrome 264
ischemia 124, 144, 147, 265, 379
   renal transplantation 104, 107, 111

jejunum 264, 267
Jewett–Strong–Marshall (ABCD)
      classification 239–40
juvenile nephronophthisis 82–3

Kaposi's sarcoma 32
kidneys 53–73, 75–97, 121–9, 132, 318, 375
   bladder cancer 237, 243
   children's UTIs 149–51, 154–66
   ectopic 157, 204–5, 209–10, 218
   hematuria 219–28, 233
   hemospermia 324, 327, 333
   horseshoe 197, 204, 210–11, 218, 235
   multicystic dysplastic (MCDK) 59, 61, 76,
      87, 92–4
   prostatic cysts 309, 316–17
   RAS 43–51
   retroperitoneal tumors 21, 25, 35–6, 38–40
   stones 170, 179, 197, 199–200, 205, 207,
      210–18
   transplantation 32, 39–40, 95, 99–120
   urinary diversion 261, 265, 266, 269
   urine leakage after transplantation 107–10
   UTIs 167–76, 177, 178–82, 183–4, 187,
      189
   see also polycystic kidney disease; renal
      cell carcinoma
Klebsiella 151, 166
Kock's pouch 259–60

lacerations 123–8, 132, 137, 140–2, 144, 146
laparoscopy 7, 13, 73, 113, 378
laparotomy 129
leiomyomas 25, 26, 59, 235, 388–9, 392–3
   AUB 382–5, 389, 392–3, 397
leiomyosarcoma 25–6, 242
lentigines 3
leukemia 170, 222, 229, 340
levator ani 280, 401
levator hiatus 401, 411–13
lipids 1–2, 4–6, 8, 17, 19–20, 59
lipomas 25, 26, 340–2, 350
liposarcomas 25, 26, 340, 350
lithium nephropathy 76, 87, 96
lithotripsy 85
Littré's glands 190, 191
liver 18, 87–91, 174, 184, 187–8
   adnexal masses 374, 376, 377–8
   metastases 55–6, 66, 241, 376–8
   trauma 123, 128, 131
loop diathermy 238
loopograms 216, 265, 268–71
loop ureterostomy 257, 265
lung cancer 3, 243
   metastases 16, 19, 32, 55, 66–7, 241, 375
luteal cysts 352–4, 360
lymph nodes 114, 178, 201, 209, 377
   bladder cancer 241, 246, 248
   metastases 32–3, 304, 309, 377
   prostate cancer 273, 298, 304, 309, 310
   retroperitoneal tumors 21, 24, 27, 29, 30,
      32–3, 40
lymphadenectomy 32
lymphadenopathy 67, 248, 267, 360, 375, 378
   hemospermia 327, 336
lymphangiography 29
lymphangioma 26, 28, 30–1
lymphangiomatosis 28
lymphangiosarcoma 26
lymphoceles 30, 32, 113–15, 265, 356
   renal transplantation 100–1, 108, 111,
      113–15
lymphoma 27, 29–30, 32, 62, 67, 326
   adnexal masses 354, 371
   bladder cancer 239, 242
   hematuria 222, 229
   scrotal masses 340, 342, 350
lymphoscintigraphy 304

magnetic resonance angiography (MRA) 45,
      49–51, 100–3, 105, 107

magnetic resonance imaging (MRI) 119, 200, 215–16, 276, 284, 287–99, 366–73
  adnexal masses 354–5, 357, 362, 365–74, 377–8
  adrenal masses 1–2, 3–6, 8, 11, 14–15, 17–18, 20
  AUB 382–4, 386–8, 390–7
  bladder cancer 120, 244, 249, 251–2, 254
  children's UTIs 152, 154, 160–1
  dynamic 285, 287–90, 293–6, 298, 408, 411–13
  ectopic ureter 318
  ejaculatory ducts 316, 320
  endorectal 314, 316, 320, 324–5, 327–8, 331–2, 337
  hematuria 224, 226, 227, 231–2
  hemospermia 324–5, 327–32, 334–7
  infertility 416–30
  PFD 399, 404–5, 407–13
  prostate cancer 273, 276, 280–5, 287–304, 309–12, 316
  prostate cysts 308, 314, 315–16
  renal cystic lesions 75, 77–80, 82–3, 85–6, 89, 92, 94–6
  renal masses 55–6, 59, 60, 68, 71
  renal transplantation 100–1, 108, 111, 113–15, 118–20
  retroperitoneal tumors 21, 23, 25, 28–30, 32, 35
  scrotal masses 341, 342–4, 346–50
  trauma 124, 144, 146
  urinary diversion 266, 269
  UTIs 171–2, 175, 181–2, 184, 189, 191
magnetic resonance spectroscopic imaging (MRSI) 290–5
magnetic resonance urography (MRU) 172, 215–16, 218, 226, 252–4
  renal transplantation 108–15
  urinary diversion 266, 269
malacoplakia 177–8
malignancy 119–20, 23–33, 261, 393, 395–6
  adnexal masses 352–5, 357–62, 365–6, 368, 370, 372–4, 377
  adrenal masses 1–2, 3, 8–10, 12, 15–17, 20
  bladder cancer 235, 239, 241–3
  hematuria 221–4, 227–9, 230–1
  hemospermia 323, 327, 336
  prostate cancer 278, 281
  renal cystic lesions 75, 77, 92
  renal masses 53, 55, 57, 59, 73

scrotal masses 339–40, 343, 344, 345
  UTIs 166, 174, 176, 189
marsupialisation 100, 113, 115
matrix stones 209
maximum intensity projection (MIP) 51, 102, 105, 160, 266
medullary necrosis 76, 82, 83–5
medullary sponge kidney 76, 80–2, 89, 171, 222, 227
  stones 197, 204, 211
megaseminal vesicles 309, 317
melanoma 3, 16, 20, 32, 326, 369, 378
  bladder cancer 243, 246
menopause 352–3, 355–7, 381–2, 388–9, 391, 393–4, 396–7
menorrhagia 382, 422, 423
menstruation 381–2, 388, 396, 417, 424, 427–8, 430
  adnexal masses 352, 355, 357, 360
mesenchymal tumors 25, 26, 27, 235, 239, 242
mesothelioma 31, 340
metabolic alkalosis 7
metachronous lesions 241, 253
metastases 19–20, 32–3, 222, 229, 242–3, 327, 336
  adnexal masses 354, 367, 369, 371, 373–8
  adrenal 1, 10, 12–13, 15–16, 19–20
  bladder cancer 239–41, 242–3, 248, 253
  bone 55, 241, 298, 304, 312, 327
  bowel 33, 377
  liver 55–6, 66, 241, 376, 377–8
  lung 16, 19, 32, 55, 66–7, 241, 375
  lymph nodes 32–3, 304, 309, 377
  prostate cancer 16, 32, 298, 304, 309, 311–12
  renal masses 55–6, 59, 61, 62, 66–7
  retroperitoneal 24, 27, 32–3
  scrotal masses 340
methemoglobin 79–80, 370
metrorrhagia 382, 423
Mitrofanoff technique 258–9
mitotane 13
mixed urinary incontinence 401–2
mucin and mucinous tumors 30, 31, 242, 357, 367, 369
Müllerian ducts 30–1, 307–8, 313–14, 354, 428
  hemospermia 326–7, 330, 331, 333
multicystic dysplastic kidney (MCDK) 59, 61, 76, 87, 92–4

multi-detector computed tomography (MDCT)
95, 195, 243–8, 375
bladder cancer 236, 243–8, 254
UTIs 158, 160, 167–8, 171, 173, 182
multilocular cystic nephroma 59
multiplanar reconstruction (MPR) 160, 309
multiple endocrine neoplasia (MEN) 9, 11, 23
mycobacteria 179, 237
myeloma 170
myomectomy 388
myometrium 381–2, 383–5, 387–93, 395–7,
421, 423–4, 429

necrosis 14–15, 59, 68, 266, 342, 344, 393
acute tubular (ATN) 116, 118–19
adnexal masses 356, 359, 365, 371, 373,
377
medullary 76, 82, 83–5
renal transplantation 107, 116, 118, 119
retroperitoneal tumors 24–5, 27, 28,
33, 41
UTIs 159, 171, 173–5, 179, 188–9
neobladders 258–60, 261–4, 265–70
neoplasms 22, 28, 30–1, 58, 71, 395, 422
adnexal masses 354, 371–2
bladder cancer 120, 235, 241, 243, 246,
248, 253
hemospermia 325–7
renal cystic lesions 75, 77–8
scrotal masses 339–40, 345, 350
UTIs 167, 170, 176, 179, 183
nephogram 125, 128, 157, 159, 169–70,
205
nephrectomy 100, 103, 129, 173, 176, 217
renal masses 54, 58, 61, 63, 68–9, 73
nephritic syndrome 25
nephritis 179, 222, 229
nephrolithiasis 222
nephrological pathology (nephropathy) 49–50,
83, 221–3, 229, 231, 261
nephrostogram 216
nephrostomy 132, 133, 168, 198
neurinoma 26
neuroblastoma 26, 28
neurofibroma 26, 235
neurofibromatosis 23, 27, 28
neurofibrosarcoma 26, 27
neurogenic bladder dysfunction 257, 258, 261
neurogenic tumors 25, 26, 27, 28
neurovascular bundles (NVB) 275, 280, 299,
301, 304–5, 336

nitrite 151, 167
nitrofurantoin 219
nocturia 82, 119
nomograms 297, 301, 303
non-continent cutaneous urinary diversion 258
non-contrast helical CT (NCHCT) 208–10,
211–13, 218
non-germ cell tumors 340, 344
non-Hodgkin's lymphoma 27, 29, 32
non-neoplastic cystic masses 30
non-orthotopic continent urinary diversion 258,
260–1
nuclear imaging 45, 48–9, 63, 217, 253, 269

obesity 2–3, 171, 394, 396, 417
obstruction 25, 83–5, 97, 188, 269, 403
bladder cancer 237, 248
bowel 375, 379, 403
children's UTIs 149, 152–4, 157, 161, 166
ejaculatory ducts 314, 316, 319, 320, 325,
331
fallopian tubes 418, 420
hemospermia 325, 327, 331–2, 335
renal transplantation 111, 113, 115
stones 197–200, 204–5, 208–9, 212, 215,
217
ureter 83–4, 111, 113, 166, 168, 237
UTIs 166–76, 177, 179, 182, 183–4, 186
oliguria 107, 111, 116
omentum 374–6, 378
oncocytoma 55, 59, 62–4
orchiectomy 144, 147, 326, 347
orchitis 177, 345
organ transplantation 27, 32, 39–40, 95,
99–120, 176, 178
Ormond's disease 33–5
orthotopic diversion to native, intact urethra
258, 261–4
orthotopic Kock's ileal reservoir 262–3, 265
ovarian cysts 31, 91, 352–4, 356–63, 365–6,
372, 377
ovaries 351–79, 404, 415–18, 421, 424,
426–8
cancer 3, 32, 243, 351–5, 360–1, 365–6,
369–70, 373–9
cysts 31, 91, 352–4, 356–63, 365–6, 372,
377
oxalate stones 196, 199

page kidney 128
pancreas 21–2, 30, 35–7, 39–40, 72, 91, 128
cancer 3, 19, 243, 377

papillae and papillarities 16, 81, 222, 326,
359–60, 396
lesions 238–9, 243–5, 247
papillomas 184, 228, 230, 231
paraganglioma 26, 31
paralytic ileus 39, 264
parasites 176–7, 182–7, 187–9, 346
parathyroid disorders 44
parietal peritoneum 22
pelvic floor dysfunction (PFD) 399–413
pelvic fracture 133–4, 136–7, 140
pelvic inflammatory disease(PID) 352, 365–6,
379
pelvic ligaments and muscles 399–400, 407,
409, 411–13
pelvic organ prolapsed (POP) 399, 401,
402–4, 405–6, 408, 411–13
penis 135, 141, 142–7, 191, 324
percutaneous nephrolithotomy (PCNL) 198,
201–2, 204, 208, 210, 217
percutaneous nephrostomy (PCN) 100,
107–11, 129, 133
percutaneous transluminal angioplasty (PTA)
100, 103, 105, 106–7
pericalyceal lymphangiectasia 96–7
perineum 135, 137, 141, 324, 402, 406
peritoneal inclusion cyst 356
peritonitis 379
peritonocele 407, 410
Phenacetin 221
pheochromocytomas 1, 3, 8–12, 15–16, 28,
44, 72
bladder cancer 235, 236
phleboliths 201, 209
pituitary gland 2–4
plain radiography 36, 38, 81, 84–5, 190, 355,
375, 422
stones 196, 199–204, 207, 211
trauma 121–2, 129, 135, 141, 144
urinary diversion 267–8, 270, 271
UTIs 162, 170–2, 178, 182, 184, 188–9,
190–1
pleural effusion 360, 374, 375, 377
polycystic kidney disease 75–6, 86–8, 90–2,
309, 317, 333
hematuria 222, 227
polycystic ovary syndrome 391, 415–18,
426–8
polycythemia 76
polydipsia 7, 82, 96
polyorchidism 350

polyuria 7, 96, 82, 83
positron emission tomography (PET) 20, 29,
59, 61–2, 65, 253
posterior vericourethral angle (PVUA) 404
post-menopausal bleeding (PMB) 381, 391,
396
potassium 8, 16, 267
Potter faces 87, 93
pouchography 262–3, 265, 268–71
povidine-iodine 115
power Doppler ultrasound 77, 124, 154, 275,
280
renal transplantation 101, 103–4, 117–18
pregnancy 9, 38, 226, 352–3, 381, 385, 428
ectopic 198, 360
UTIs 149, 166, 168, 171–2
preprostatic sphincter (PPS) 275, 276, 279–80
progesterone 389, 394
prolapses 91, 351, 399, 401–4, 406–8, 411–13
prostate 112, 137–41, 178, 226, 239,
273–320, 325–6
bladder cancer 238, 241
hermospermia 324–8, 330, 332, 334–6
hyperplasia 166, 222, 226
inflammatory disease 311–14, 316, 319–20
UTIs 181, 183, 184, 190
prostate cancer (PCa) 3, 16, 243, 273–5,
276–312, 316
extra capsular extension (ECE) 297–303,
305–6
hematuria 222, 226, 233
hemospermia 323–6, 328, 332, 336
metastases 16, 32, 298, 304, 309, 311–12
prostate cysts 285, 305, 307–9, 313–16
hemospermia 325–6, 328, 331, 333
prostate specific antigen (PSA) 226, 273,
278–9, 284–94, 297–304, 324, 335
prostatectomy 278, 283, 296
prostatitis 222, 237, 239, 311–12, 316, 319
hemospermia 325–6, 328, 334, 335–6
prostate cancer 274, 278, 287–91, 293–4,
311–12, 316, 319
UTIs 177, 179
Proteus sp 151, 166, 168, 174, 197
proteinuria 220–1, 223, 264
pseudoaneurysm 128
pseudocysts 17–18, 30, 31, 39, 97
Pseudomonas sp 151, 166
pseudotumors 349
psoas muscle 24, 26, 38, 40, 179–80
pubococcygeal line (PCL) 405–6, 409, 411

puborectalis muscle 401, 407, 409–12
pyelitis 154, 173
pyelogenic cyst 76, 85–6
pyelography 34, 100, 108–12, 132–3,
    216–17, 225, 230
pyelonephritis 68, 128, 150, 174–6, 222, 226,
    261
    children's UTIs 149–58, 162, 166
    UTIs 167–8, 170–2, 173–7, 186
pyeloplasty 217
pyelostomy 152, 168, 257
pyeloureterography 84
pyogenic infections 68, 70, 76, 96
pyonephrosis 154, 171, 197
pyosalpinx 420–1
pyuria 151, 167, 174, 178

quinolones 281, 337

radiation therapy 253–4, 325
radionuclide studies 12, 100, 101, 110, 118,
    119, 171
    crystography 163–5, 166
rectoceles 401–2, 403, 404, 406–7
rectum 34, 142, 166, 183–4, 299–302, 328
    PFD 403, 405, 406, 408, 412
reflux 149, 258, 260–5, 268–70, 319
    see also vesico-ureteral reflux
rejection of transplant 99, 101, 103–4, 111,
    114, 116–19
renal arteriovenous malformations (AVM) 68,
    71
renal artery 68, 123–4, 126–7, 129
    stenosis (RAS) 43–51, 100, 103–7
    transplantation 101–2, 105, 113, 116
renal cell carcinoma (RCC) 53–6, 57–8,
    59–63, 65, 68–70, 72–3, 326
    adrenal metastases 16, 20
    cystic lesions 92, 93, 95
    hematuria 222, 22–9, 231, 233
    UTIs 170, 175
renal colic 197, 209, 218
renal failure 33–4, 44, 166, 179, 183, 197,
    261
    cystic lesions 83, 87, 89, 94
renal trauma 121–9
renal tubular acidosis 197
renal vein 101, 113, 116–17, 123, 127–9
renin 7, 16, 45, 91, 104, 128
renography 45, 48–9, 152, 154, 156–7, 164,
    172

resection 4, 10, 13, 120, 238, 319, 354, 388
    renal masses 54, 56, 72–3
    transurethral (TUS) 238, 246, 254, 325
rete testis 343–4
retrograde pyelography 216–17, 225
retrograde urethrogaphy (RUG) 135, 138–40,
    329, 330
retroperitoneum 21–41, 94, 123, 131, 209,
    265, 267
    adnexal masses 374, 378
    renal masses 62, 67, 69
    TB 179, 180
rhabdomiomas 26
rhabdomyosarcomas 26, 242, 340
risk of malignancy index (RMI) 352

sarcoidosis 32, 349
sarcomas 23, 242, 326, 389
scarring 116, 167–8, 172, 179–82, 184, 190
    children 152, 154–5, 158
Schistosoma sp (bilharzias) 182–4, 187, 222,
    235
schistosomiasis (bilharzial infection) 179–80,
    182–7, 237, 241, 324
scintigraphy 12, 40, 105, 110, 119, 172, 304
    DMSA 152, 154–8, 161, 166, 172
sclerotherapy 100, 113, 115, 326
scrotum 135, 142–7, 177, 180, 324, 328,
    339–50
seminal vesicles (SV) 34, 241, 316, 317–18,
    320
    hemospermia 325–9, 330, 331–4, 336
    prostate cancer 274, 276–82, 285, 297,
        299, 301–3, 306–8
    prostate cysts 308–9, 313–17
    UTIs 183, 184, 190
seminomas 32, 340, 342, 344–5, 346
sepsis 18, 128, 173, 239, 281, 365
septate uterus 425–6, 428–9
septicemia 83, 107, 150, 152, 154, 167, 172
seroma 108
sessile lesions 243, 244–5, 248
sex cord stromal tumor 354
sexual history 166, 221, 237, 323–4, 365
short TI inversion recovery (STIR) MRI 304,
    426
sigmoid 260–1, 243
sigmoidcele 406
simple renal cysts 76–80
smoking 68, 221, 235, 240, 244
sonography 54–5, 57, 60, 71, 348, 394

spectroscopy 284, 290–3

spermatic cord 147, 324, 340, 350

spermogram 309

sphincters 191–2, 258, 260–1, 275, 276, 279–80, 401–2

spina bifida 212, 218

spongiitis 190

squamous cell carcinoma (SCC) 183, 235, 239, 241, 242, 396

squamous metaplasia 240

staphylococci 151

steinstrasse 203

stents 43, 46, 129, 132–3, 198, 202
    renal transplantation 100, 105, 108, 110–11

stoma 258, 259–60, 270

stomach cancer 23, 243, 377

stones 38, 61, 195–218, 266, 271, 253
    hematuria 224, 226, 231
    prostate 313, 316
    renal cystic lesions 80–2, 85–6
    staghorn 175–6, 198, 201, 207
    UTIs 166, 168, 170–7, 179, 190
    see also calcification and calculi

straddle injuries 136–7

stress urinary incontinence (SUI) 401, 402–5, 408–10, 412–13

stroma 340, 353, 363, 365, 373, 385, 393–5

struvite stones 196–7

Studer ileal bladder substitute 261, 263, 269

surgery 217, 242, 254, 325, 383, 389
    adnexal masses 354–6, 366, 373, 376, 378
    adrenal masses 4, 7–8, 13
    PFD 404, 407, 408, 411
    prostate 300, 304
    renal masses 62, 73
    renal transplantation 100, 102–3, 107, 110, 116
    retroperitoneal tumors 24, 25, 36–9, 41
    trauma 122–3, 128–9, 131, 133, 136, 144–7
    urinary diversion 264, 269
    UTIs 160, 162, 166–7
    see also resection

surgical capsule 275, 279, 280

sympathicoblastoma 26

symphysis pubis 134, 138, 181, 375, 404–5, 409

tamoxifen 355, 393, 396

tapeworms 187–9

teratoma 25–6, 30–1, 354, 358, 367–8, 378

testicles (testes) 32, 143–7, 325–6, 328–9, 339–50
    UTIs 180, 183, 184

thecomas 365, 373, 394

thermo-ablative technique 388

thermotherapy 326

thrombectomy 100

thrombosis 99–103, 126–8, 147, 170, 190
    adnexal masses 354, 377, 379
    renal transplantation 99–103, 107, 113, 116, 117

thyroid disorders 3, 44

tissue harmonic imaging 165

tomography 96, 124, 213

torsion 353–4, 360, 370, 378, 388

T-pouch ileal neobladder 263–4

transforming growth factor beta 116, 120

transitional cell carcinoma (TCC) 65, 68–9, 170, 222, 230, 240–1
    bladder cancer 239–42, 245, 248–9, 252–3

transrectal ultrasonography (TRUS) 308–9, 313–16, 320
    hemospermia 324, 327–8, 330, 333–7
    prostate cancer 273–4, 276–9, 281–7, 295, 297, 299, 302

transvaginal ultrasound (TVS) 180, 404–5, 416–17, 423, 429
    adnexal masses 353, 355, 357–60, 362–4, 366
    AUB 381–7, 389, 390, 391, 393–7

trauma 17–18, 35–7, 38, 96–7, 121–47, 169, 257
    bladder cancer 237, 239
    hematuria 221, 222, 227
    hemospermia 324, 326

trematodes 183

tuberculosis (TB) 32, 177, 178–82, 187, 190, 278, 346
    hematuria 222, 226
    renal cystic lesions 76, 96
    renal masses 68, 70
    salpingitis 179
    spondylitis 40

tuberous sclerosis 23, 28, 72, 76, 77

tubo-ovarian disorders 354, 366, 378, 379

tumor, nodes, metastases (TNM) staging classification 239–40

tunica albuginea 141, 143–7, 341, 343, 349–50

tunica vaginalis 145, 342, 349

turbo spin-echo (TSE) 408, 410, 411

ultrasound (ultrasonography) (US) 1, 15, 253,
355–66, 406
adnexal masses 352–67, 369, 372, 374,
376–8, 418, 420
children's UTIs 152, 153–5, 157, 164–5,
166
hematuria 223, 226, 229
infertility 415–18, 420, 422–4, 429–30
prostate 273, 279
RAS 45, 46–8
renal cystic lesions 75, 77–8, 81, 83–6,
88–9, 91–6
renal masses 59, 68
renal transplantation 100–1, 104–5, 108,
110–20
retroperitoneal 21, 24, 29, 30, 34, 38
scrotal masses 180, 340–1, 342–50
stones 199–200, 206–8, 217
trauma 124, 142, 144–7
urinary diversion 268, 269, 271
UTIs 168, 171, 175, 177, 180, 183–7, 189,
191–2
see also Doppler ultrasound
unicornate uterus 428
urachus 241–2
uremic medullary cystic disease 76, 82–3
ureteral stones 81, 197–203, 205–6, 208–10,
215–18
UTIs 166, 168, 170–1, 173, 179
ureters 21, 33–4, 38–9, 131–3, 110–13, 317
adnexal masses 351, 356, 377
bladder cancer 237, 243
children's UTIs 149, 151, 154, 162, 164–5
ectopic 206, 310, 318, 333
hematuria 222–3, 225, 228, 230
obstruction 83–4, 97, 403
renal cystic lesions 76, 83–4, 88, 93, 96–7
renal transplantation 100, 107, 109–16, 119
urinary diversion 258–63, 265–70
UTIs 166, 168–71, 173, 177–82, 183–4,
186–7, 189
ureteritis 111, 154
ureterocele 222, 226, 333, 356
ureteropelvic junction (UPJ) 129, 132, 212,
217
ureterorenoscopy (URS) 199, 201
ureteroscopy 217
ureterosigmoidostomy 260–1
urethras 38, 135, 136–42, 190–2, 238–9, 326
children 149, 154, 162–3, 165–6
hemospermia 325–30

penile and scrotum trauma 143, 145–6
PFD 401, 404, 409–10, 413
prostate 273–5, 301, 305, 314, 318, 325–6
urinary diversion 258, 261–4, 270
urethritis 177, 190–2, 222, 239, 326
urethrography 135, 138–41, 190–2, 329–30
urge urinary incontinence (UUI) 401–2
urgency 119, 177, 178, 184, 197, 237
uric acid stones 196
urinary diversion 100, 120, 133, 197, 239,
257–71
urinary incontinence (UI) 140, 142, 310, 399,
401–5, 408–10, 412–13
diversion 258–62, 264, 267, 269
urinary retention 133, 177, 403
urinary tract anomalies 149–53, 157–8, 10–2,
166, 204
urinary tract infections (UTIs) 68, 80, 90,
149–92, 170, 175, 402–3
children 149–66, 167
hematuria 167, 174, 178, 183, 187, 221
renal transplantation 100, 111, 112
stones 166, 170–7, 179, 190, 197–8
urinary tract trauma 121–47
urinomas 96, 97, 128, 132, 265, 269
renal transplantation 100, 107, 108
retroperitoneal 22, 30, 38–40
urodynamic studies 269
urography 23, 34, 121, 190, 224–5, 253, 269
children's UTIs 152, 157–8, 160, 161
renal cystic lesions 77, 80–2, 84–6, 92, 96
stones 199–200, 203–6, 210–11, 213–14
UTIs 168, 171, 173, 175, 177, 180, 184,
190
see also intravenous urography (IVU);
CTU; MRU
urolithiasis 64, 195–218, 248
see also calcification and calculi; stones
urological pathology 219–23, 231
uromucoid stones 196
urothelium 65, 69, 220, 324
bladder cancer 235, 239–41, 243, 248–9,
252–3
uterus 34, 171, 183, 330, 381–97, 424–9
adnexal masses 356, 362, 365, 366–7, 370,
372–4
didelphys 383, 427–9
hypoplasia 424–5, 428
infertility 415, 422–30
masses 16, 32, 381, 393
PFD 400, 401–4, 407, 409, 411

vagina 184, 206, 241, 351, 375, 427–8
    PFD 400–7, 409–11
    trauma 136, 137, 142
valsalva leak point pressure(VLPP) 402
valsalva maneuver 409
varicocele 342
vas deferens (VD) 25, 183, 309, 317–18, 320,
    329–30
    hemospermia 325, 327–8, 329–30, 333
    prostate cancer 274, 277–8, 281–2, 29,
        301, 306
    prostate cysts 308, 314, 315–17
vascular endothelial growth factor (VEGF) 120
vasectomy 326
vasograms 328
venography 128
veru montanum (VM) 274, 276–7, 280,
    318–19, 330
vesicostomy 257
vesico-ureteric junction (VUJ) 162, 186, 197,
    201, 206, 208, 210

vesico-ureteral reflux (VUR) 93, 167, 179,
    184, 186
    children 149–50, 12–4, 161–3, 165, 166
vesiculography 316, 328–9, 330, 331
viruses 176–7
voiding cystourethrography (VCUG) 152, 154,
    156, 162–6, 172, 329–30
voiding urosonography (VUS) 164
Von Hippel–Lindau (VHL) disease 9, 11, 23,
    28, 72, 76–7
Von Recklinghausen neurofibromatosis 9, 11

Wilm's tumor 76, 93, 222
Wolffian cysts 308, 315–16

xanthine stones 196
xanthogranuloma 26, 28
    pyelonephritis (XGP) 174–6

yolk-sac tumors 340, 342

Index compiled by Alison Waggitt